GI/LIVER SECRETS

GI/LIVER SECRETS

PETER R. McNALLY, DO, FACP, FACG

Gastroenterology Service
Fitzsimons Army Medical Center
Aurora, Colorado

HANLEY & BELFUS, INC./ Philadelphia

Publisher: **HANLEY & BELFUS, INC.**
                   Medical Publishers
                   210 South 13th Street
                   Philadelphia, PA 19107
                   (215) 546-7293; 800-962-1892
                   FAX (215) 790-9330

Library of Congress Cataloging-in-Publication Data

GI/Liver Secrets: questions you will be asked on rounds, in the clinic, and on oral exams /
    editor, Lt. Colonel Peter R. McNally
      p.   cm.
    Includes bibliographical references and index.
    ISBN 1-56053-150-9 (soft : alk. paper)
      1. Digestive organs-Diseases-Examinations, questions, etc.
    I. McNally, Peter R., 1954–
    RC802.G52 1995
    616.3' 3' 0076-dc20
    DNLM/DLC
    for Library of Congress
                                                                                95-47442
                                                                                CIP

Disclaimer: The opinions and assertions contained in this book are the private views of the authors and are not to be construed as reflecting the view of the Department of the Army or the Department of Defense.

GI/LIVER SECRETS   ISBN 1-56053-150-9

Last digit is the print number: 9 8 7 6 5 4 3 2

DEDICATION

The editor dedicates this book to his wife,
Cynthia; children, Alex, Meghan, Amanda,
Genevieve, and Bridgette; and parents,
Jeanette and Rusel.

CONTENTS

III. LIVER AND BILIARY TRACT DISORDERS

CONTRIBUTORS

Matthew S.Z. Bachinski, M.D.
Associate Professor of Medicine, Uniformed Services University of the Health Sciences, Bethesda, Maryland; Gastroenterology Service, Dwight D. Eisenhower Army Medical Center, Fort Gordon, Georgia

Bruce R. Bacon, M.D.
Professor of Internal Medicine, and Director, Division of Gastroenterology and Hepatology, Saint Louis University School of Medicine, St. Louis, Missouri

Vijayan Balan, M.B.B.S.
Assistant Professor of Medicine, Department of Transplant Medicine, Gastroenterology and Hepatology, University of Pittsburgh Medical Center, Pittsburgh, Pennsylvania

Jamie S. Barkin, M.D., FACP, MACG
Professor of Medicine, University of Miami School of Medicine, Miami; Chief, Division of Gastroenterology, Mt. Sinai Medical Center, Miami, Florida

David W. Bean, Jr., M.D.
Staff, Diagnostic Radiology, Department of Radiology, Fitzsimons Army Medical Center, Aurora, Colorado

Bahri Bilir, M.D.
Division of Gastroenterology, University of Colorado Health Sciences Center, Denver, Colorado

Nuray Bilir, M.D.
Division of Gastroenterology, University of Colorado Health Sciences Center, Denver, Colorado

John H. Bloor, M.D., Ph.D.
Instructor, Department of Medicine, Division of Gastroenterology, University of Colorado Health Sciences Center; Staff Physician, Denver General Hospital, Denver, Colorado

Bradley G. Bute, M.D., FACS, FASCRS
Colon and Rectal Surgical Associates of Long Island, Great Neck, New York

Steven D. Caras, M.D., Ph.D.
Fellow in Gastroenterology, University of Virginia School of Medicine, Charlottesville, Virginia

Donald O. Castell, M.D.
Kimbel Professor and Chairman, Department of Medicine, The Graduate Hospital, Philadelphia; Clinical Professor of Medicine, University of Pennsylvania School of Medicine, Philadelphia, Pennsylvania

Jeffrey Clark, M.D.
Director of Surgery Education, Saint Joseph Hospital, Denver, Colorado

James E. Cremins, M.D., FACP
Assistant Chief of Gastroenterology, Fitzsimons Army Medical Center, Aurora; Clinical Instructor of Medicine, University of Colorado Health Sciences Center, Denver, Colorado

Albert J. Czaja, M.D.
Professor of Medicine and Consultant in Gastroenterology, Division of Gastroenterology, Mayo Clinic and Mayo Medical School, Rochester, Minnesota

Dirk R. Davis, M.D., FACP
Director of Hepatology, Fitzsimons Army Medical Center, Aurora; Clinical Instructor, University of Colorado Health Sciences Center, Denver, Colorado

John C. Deutsch, M.D.
Associate Professor of Medicine, University of Colorado Health Sciences Center, Denver, Colorado

P. Dennis Dyer, M.D.
Chief, Allergy/Immunology Service, Department of Medicine, Fitzsimons Army Medical Center, Aurora, Colorado

Ben Eiseman, M.D.
Emeritus Professor of Surgery and Medicine, University of Colorado Health Science Centers, Denver, Colorado

Gulchin A. Ergun, M.D.
Assistant Professor of Medicine, Northwestern University Medical School, Chicago, Illinois

Gregory T. Everson, M.D.
Director, Section of Hepatology, and Associate Professor of Medicine, Division of Gastroenterology/Hepatology, University of Colorado Health Sciences Center, Denver, Colorado

Albert George Fedalei, M.D.
Staff Gastroenterologist, Brook Army Medical Center, Ft. Sam Houston, Texas

Anne M. Flynn, M.D.
Director, SICU, and Clinical Assistant Professor of Surgery, Uniformed Services University of the Health Sciences, Bethesda, Maryland

Stephen R. Freeman, M.D.
Assistant Clincical Professor of Medicine, University of Colorado Health Sciences Center, Denver, Colorado

Gregory G. Ginsberg, M.D.
Assistant Professor of Medicine and Director of Endoscopic Services, Division of Gastroenterology, University of Pennsylvania Health Systems, Philadelphia, Pennsylvania

John S. Goff, M.D.
Clinical Professor of Medicine, University of Colorado Health Sciences Center, Denver, Colorado

Ian M. Gralnek, M.D.
Fellow, Division of Digestive Diseases, Department of Medicine, UCLA School of Medicine, Los Angeles, California

Carlos Guarner, M.D.
Associate Professor of Medicine, Medico Adjunto Servicio de Patologia Digestiva, Hospital de Sant Pau, Autonomous University of Barcelona, Spain

Steven W. Hammond, M.D.
Staff Gastroenterologist, Gastroenterology Service, Department of Medicine, Tripler Army
Medical Center, Honolulu, Hawaii

Jorge L. Herrera, M.D.
Associate Professor of Medicine, Division of Gastroenterology, University of South Alabama
College of Medicine, Mobile, Alabama

Kent C. Holtzmuller, M.D.
Department of Gastroenterology, Walter Reed Army Medical Center, Washington, D.C.

Eugene Donald Jacobson, M.D.
Professor of Medicine and Physiology, University of Colorado Health Sciences Center, Denver,
Colorado

Dennis M. Jensen, M.D.
Professor of Medicine, UCLA School of Medicine, Los Angeles, California

Lawrence F. Johnson, M.D.
Professor of Medicine and Director, Digestive Disease Division, Department of Medicine,
Uniformed Services University of the Health Sciences, Bethesda, Maryland

Brian T. Johnston, M.D., MRCP
Senior Tutor, Department of Medicine, The Queen's University, and Senior Registrar, Royal
Victoria Hospital, Belfast, United Kingdom

Dan Michael Jones, M.D.
Chairman, Department of Gastroenterology, National Naval Medical Center, Bethesda, Maryland

Shailesh C. Kadakia, M.D.
Chief, Gastroenterology Service, Brooke Army Medical Center, Fort Sam Houston; Clinical
Associate Professor of Medicine, University of Texas Health Sciences Center at San Antonio, San
Antonio, Texas

Peter J. Kahrilas, M.D.
Professor of Medicine, Northwestern University Medical School, Chicago, Illinois

Thomas Kepczyk, M.D., FACP
Gastroenterology of San Marcos/New Braunfels, Central Texas Medical Center, San Marcos,
Texas

James Walter Kikendall, M.D.
Associate Professor of Medicine, Uniformed Services University of the Health Sciences,
Bethesda, Maryland; Director of Clinical Services, GI Service, Walter Reed Army Medical
Center, Washington, D.C.

Jonathan P. Kushner, M.D.
Assistant Professor of Medicine, Uniformed Services University of the Health Sciences,
Bethesda, Maryland; Staff Endocrinologist and Director of Nutrition Support, Walter Reed Army
Medical Center, Washington, D.C.

Anthony J. LaPorta, M.D.
Associate Professor of Surgery, Uniformed Services University of the Health Sciences, Bethesda,
Maryland; Chief, Department of Surgery, Fitzsimons Army Medical Center, Aurora, Colorado

Nicholas F. LaRusso, M.D.
Professor of Medicine, Department of Gastroenterology, Mayo Clinic and Mayo Foundation, Rochester, Minnesota

Steven P. Lawrence, M.D.
Chief, Gastroenterology Service, Department of Medicine, Tripler Army Medical Center, Honolulu, Hawaii

Donald J. Lazas, Jr., M.D.
Associate Professor of Medicine, Uniformed Services University of Health Sciences, Bethesda, Maryland; Gastroenterology Service, Dwight D. Eisenhower Army Medical Center, Fort Gordon, Georgia

Randall E. Lee, M.D.
Assistant Professor of Medicine, Division of Gastroenterology/Hepatology, University of Colorado Health Sciences Center; Medical Director, GI Endoscopy Unit, Denver Veterans Affairs Medical Center, Denver, Colorado

John Charles Lemon, M.D., FACR
Chief of Gastrointestinal Radiology, Fitzsimons Army Medical Center, Aurora, Colorado

Scot Michael Lewey, D.O.
Clinical Instructor, Department of Medicine, University of Colorado Health Sciences Center, Denver, Colorado; Fitzsimons Army Medical Center, Aurora, Colorado

Michael F. Lyons, II, M.D.
Clincial Assistant Professor of Medicine, University of Washington School of Medicine, Seattle, Washington

Phillip L. Mallory, II, M.D.
Chief, General Surgery Service, and Residency Program Director, Fitzsimons Army Medical Center, Aurora; Assistant Clinical Professor of Surgery, University of Colorado Health Sciences Center, Denver, Colorado

Michael R. Marohn, D.O.
Assistant Professor of Surgery, Uniformed Services University of the Health Sciences, Bethesda, Maryland; Chief of General Surgery, Malcolm Grove USAF Medical Center, Andrews Air Force Base, Maryland

Michael McBiles, M.D.
Assistant Chief, Nuclear Medical Service, Brooke Army Medical Center, San Antonio, Texas

Dale L. McCarter, M.D.
Interventional Radiologist, Department of Radiology, St. John Medical Center, Tulsa, Oklahoma

Robert C. McIntyre, Jr., M.D.
Assistant Professor of Surgery, University of Colorado Health Sciences Center and Veterans Affairs Medical Center, Denver, Colorado

Peter R. McNally, D.O., FACG, FACP
Gastroenterology Service, Fitzsimons Army Medical Center, Aurora, Colorado

John H. Meier, M.D.
Staff Physician, Department of Gastroenterology, Frye Regional Medical Center, Hickory, North Carolina

John A. Merenich, M.D.
Clinical Assistant Professor of Medicine, University of Colorado Health Sciences Center, Denver; Staff, St. Joseph Hospital, Denver, Colorado

Frank M. Moses, M.D.
Associate Professor of Medicine, Uniformed Services University of the Health Sciences, Bethesda, Maryland; Gastroenterology Service, Walter Reed Army Medical Center, Washington, D.C.

Bret R. Neustater, M.D.
Gastroenterology Fellow, Department of Medicine, Mt. Sinai Medical Center, Miami, Florida

Allan L. Parker, D.O.
Assistant Chief of Gastroenterology, Brooke Army Medical Center, San Antonio, Texas

Steven H. Peck, M.D.
Staff, Diagnostic Radiology, Department of Radiology, Fitzsimons Army Medical Center, Aurora, Colorado

David A. Peura, M.D.
Associate Professor of Medicine, Division of Gastroenterology, University of Virginia School of Medicine, Charlottesville, Virginia

Kevin Rak, M.D.
Department of Radiology, Fitzsimons Army Medical Center, Aurora, Colorado

Robert Matthew Reveille, M.D.
Clinical Assistant Professor of Medicine, University of Colorado Health Sciences Center, Denver, Colorado

Ingram M. Roberts, M.D.
Associate Clinical Professor of Medicine, Yale University School of Medicine, New Haven; Chief, Section of Gastroenterology, Bridgeport Hospital, Bridgeport, Connecticut

Spencer S. Root, M.D.
Staff Gastroenterologist, Brooke Army Medical Center; Clinical Instructor of Medicine, University of Texas at San Antonio Health Sciences Center, San Antonio, Texas

Bruce A. Runyon, M.D.
Professor of Medicine, Director of Liver Service, and Medical Director of Liver Transplantation, University of Louisville School of Medicine, University of Louisville Hospital and Jewish Hospital, Louisville, Kentucky

John W. Schaefer, M.D.
Professor of Medicine, University of Colorado Health Sciences Center, and Chief of Gastroenterology, Denver General Hospital, Denver, Colorado

Theodore R. Schrock, M.D.
Professor of Surgery, University of California, San Francisco, School of Medicine, San Francisco, California

Sal Senzatimore, M.D.
Gastroenterology Fellow, University of Miami School of Medicine, Miami, Florida

Steven S. Shay, M.D.
Department of Gastroenterology, The Cleveland Clinic Foundation, Cleveland, Ohio

Kenneth E. Sherman, M.D., Ph.D.
Associate Professor of Medicine, Liver Unit, Divison of Digestive Diseases, University of Cincinnati Medical Center, Cincinnati, Ohio

Keith M. Shonnard, M.D.
Director, Interventional Radiology Section, Department of Radiology, Fitzsimons Army Medical Center, Aurora, Colorado

Roshan Shrestha, M.D.
Assistant Professor of Medicine, Division of Gastroenterology/Hepatology, University of Colorado Health Sciences Center, Denver, Colorado

John Singleton, M.D.
Professor of Medicine, University of Colorado Health Sciences Center, Denver, Colorado

Maria Sjogren, M.D.
Chief, Department of Clinical Investigation, Walter Reed Army Medical Center, Washington, D.C.; Associate Professor of Preventive Medicine, Uniformed Services University of Health Sciences, Bethesda, Maryland

Donald R. Skillman, M.D.
Assistant Professor of Medicine, and Chief, Infectious Disease Service, Fitzsimons Army Medical Center, Aurora, Colorado

Milton T. Smith, M.D.
Staff Gastroenterologist, Department of Medicine, Walter Reed Army Medical Center, Washington, D.C.

Sandra E. Smith, M.S., R.D.
Nutrition Support Dietitian, Nutrition Care Directorate, Walter Reed Army Medical Center, Washington, D.C.

Stuart Jon Spechler, M.D.
Division of Gastroenterology, Beth Israel Hospital, Boston, Massachusetts

Philip E. Tanner, M.D.
Gastroenterology Fellow, Brooke Army Medical Center, Fort Sam Houston, Texas

Paul J. Thuluvath, M.B.B.S., M.D., MRCP
Medical Director, Liver Transplantation, The Johns Hopkins University School of Medicine, Baltimore, Maryland

Tuanh Tonnu, M.D.
Private practice, Woodbridge, Virginia

Amy M. Tsuchida, M.D.
Chief of Gastroenterology, Madigan Army Medical Center, Tacoma, Washington; Assistant Professor of Medicine, Uniformed Services University of Health Sciences, Bethesda, Maryland

Gregory Van Stiegmann, M.D.
Associate Professor of Surgery, and Chief, GI Tumor and Endocrine Surgery, University of Colorado Health Sciences Center and University Hospital, Denver, Colorado

Michael H. Walter, M.D.
Associate Professor of Medicine, Loma Linda University School of Medicine, Loma Linda, California

George H. Warren, II, M.D.
Department of Pathology, Rose Medical Center, Denver, Colorado

Sterling G. West, M.D.
Professor of Medicine, Division of Rheumatology, University of Colorado Health Sciences Center; Clinical Director, Autoimmune Disease Center, National Jewish Center for Immunology and Respiratory Medicine, Denver, Colorado

Wheaton John Williams, M.D.
Assistant Professor of Medicine, University of Colorado Health Sciences Center, Denver, Colorado

Roy K. H. Wong, M.D.
Professor of Medicine and Chief of Gastroenterology, Walter Reed Army Medical Center, Washington, D.C.; Uniformed Services University of the Health Sciences, Bethesda, Maryland

Arlene J. Zaloznik, M.D.
Deputy Commander for Clinical Services, Fitzsimons Army Medical Center, Aurora, Colorado

Gregory Zuccaro, Jr., M.D.
Head, Section of Gastrointestinal Endoscopy, Department of Gastroenterology, The Cleveland Clinic Foundation, Cleveland, Ohio

PREFACE

To practice the art of medicine, one must learn the secrets of physiology, disease, and therapy. In this text you will find the answers to many questions about the hepatic and digestive diseases. We hope that medical students, residents, fellows and, yes, even attending physicians will find this book instructive and insightful.

As editor, I am very appreciative of all of my contributors who have parted with their invaluable secrets and made this book an enjoyable and educational experience.

ACKNOWLEDGMENTS

The Editor extends thanks to Mr. Brian Long, Ms. Keri Mann, and Ms. Rayma Helton for administrative assistance in the preparation of this book.

The Editor thanks Ms. Judy A. Grubaugh for preparation of most of the illustrations that appear in this book.

LTC Peter R. McNally, DO, FACG, FACP

I. Esophageal Disorders

1. SWALLOWING DISORDERS AND DYSPHAGIA

Gulchin A. Ergun, M.D., and Peter J. Kahrilas, M.D.

1. How accurate is patient localization of the site of dysphagia?

Patients with oropharyngeal dysphagia accurately localize swallow dysfunction to the oropharynx; they may perceive uncontrollable accumulation of food in the mouth or an inability to initiate a pharyngeal swallow. Similarly, they generally recognize aspiration before, during, or after a swallow. Such is not the case, however, with esophageal dysphagia, wherein patients identify the location of obstruction with limited accuracy. Only 60–70% of patients correctly identify the location of esophageal dysfunction; the remainder mistakenly localize the dysfunction proximal to the actual site. Because the differentiation between proximal and distal lesions may be difficult on the basis of patient localization, associated oropharyngeal symptoms, such as difficulty with chewing, drooling, nasopharyngeal regurgitation, aspiration, or postswallow coughing or choking, are of great value in placing the problem in the oropharynx vs. the esophagus.

2. What are the symptoms of oropharyngeal dysphagia?

- Nasopharyngeal regurgitation
- Coughing or choking (aspiration) during swallowing
- Inability to initiate a swallow
- Sensation of food getting stuck in the throat
- Changes in speech or voice (nasality)
- Ptosis
- Photophobia or visual changes
- Weakness, especially progressive weakness toward the end of the day

3. Distinguish between globus sensation (globus hystericus) and dysphagia.

Globus sensation is the feeling of a lump in the throat. This sensation should not be confused with dysphagia, which is difficulty in swallowing. Globus sensation is not related to swallowing but is present continually and may even be temporarily alleviated during swallowing. Dysphagia, on the other hand, is noted by the patient only during swallowing.

4. List the causes of globus sensation in order of frequency (most common to least common).

- Gastroesophageal reflux disease
- Anxiety disorder (should not be diagnosed without a thorough exam to exclude organic disease)
- Early hypopharyngeal cancer
- Goiter

5. Categorize the causes of oropharyngeal dysphagia.

In the broadest sense oropharyngeal dysphagia results from propulsive failure or structural abnormalities of either the oropharynx or esophagus (see table on p. 2). Propulsive abnormalities may result from dysfunction of central nervous system control mechanisms, intrinsic musculature, or peripheral nerves. Structural abnormalities may result from neoplasm, surgery, trauma, caustic injury, or congenital anomalies. In some instances, dysphagia occurs in the absence of radiographic findings; motor abnormalities may be demonstrable by more sensitive methods such as electromyography (EMG) or nerve stimulation studies. However, if all studies are normal, impaired swallowing sensation may be the primary abnormality.

Causes of Oropharyngeal Dysphagia

PROPULSIVE	STRUCTURAL	IATROGENIC
Neurologic	Neoplasm	Oropharyngeal resections
Cerebrovascular accident	Cricopharyngeal bars	Mucositis due to chemotherapeutic regimens (drugs)
(medulla, large territory cortical)		
Parkinson's disease	Hypopharyngeal diverticula (Zenker's)	Radiation-induced xerostomia
Amyotrophic lateral sclerosis	Cervical vertebral body osteophytes	Radiation-induced myopathy
Multiple sclerosis	Bullous skin diseases (epidermolysis bullosa, pemphigoid, graft vs. host disease)	Neck stabilizations (hardware including halo or surgery
Degenerative diseases (e.g. Alzheimer's, Huntington's, Friedreich's ataxia)	Cervical esophageal webs	Steroid myopathy
Brain neoplasm (brainstem)	Lymphadenopathy	Tardive dyskinesia
Polio and postpolio syndrome	Goiter	Ill-fitting dental or intraoral prostheses
Cerebral palsy	Caustic injury	
Cranial nerve palsies	Lye	
Recurrent laryngeal nerve palsy	Pill-induced	
Muscular	Infections	
Muscular dystrophy	Abscess	
(Duchenne, oculopharyngeal)		
Myositis and dermatomyositis	Ulceration	
Myasthenia gravis	Pharyngitis	
Eaton-Lambert syndrome	Autoimmune—oral ulcerations with Crohn's, Behçet's disease	
Metabolic	Poor dentition/dental anomalies	
Hypothyroidism with myxedema		
Hyperthyroidism		
Inflammatory/Autoimmune		
Systemic lupus erythematosus		
Amyloid		
Sarcoid		
Infectious		
Acquired immunodeficiency syndrome with CNS involvement		
Syphilis (tabes dorsalis)		
Botulism		
Rabies		
Diphtheria		
Meningitis		
Viral (coxsackie, herpes simplex virus)		

6. Can development of dysphagia later in life be related to childhood illness such as polio?
Yes—even if the initial presentation did not include bulbar involvement. The postpolio syndrome is recognized as a disorder of the medullary motor neuron resulting from new or continuing instability of previously injured motor neurons. Typically the postpolio syndrome consists of new musculoskeletal symptoms such as weakness and atrophy in previously affected muscles. Patients become symptomatic 25–35 years after the original illness, and even muscular units (limb or bulbar) that appeared untouched by the original infection may develop signs of clinical weakness. Bulbar neuron involvement has been reported in only 15% of patients with acute infection, but recent studies have demonstrated that some bulbar muscle dysfunction can be demonstrated in all patients with the postpolio syndrome, although few report dysphagia. Swallowing problems are most severe in patients with bulbar involvement at onset of the original infection.

7. When a patient with stroke develops stroke-related dysphagia, what is the appropriate time frame for evaluation of swallowing function?

About 25–50% of strokes result in oropharyngeal dysphagia. Therefore, it is important to recognize that most stroke-related swallowing dysfunction improves spontaneously within the first 2 weeks; thus unnecessary diagnostic procedures can be avoided. If symptoms persist beyond this period, swallowing function should be evaluated.

8. Brainstem strokes are more likely to cause severe oropharyngeal dysphagia than hemispheral strokes. Why?

The swallowing center is situated bilaterally in the reticular substance below the nucleus of the solitary tract in the brainstem. Efferent fibers from the swallow centers travel either directly or via relay to the motor neurons controlling the swallow musculature located in the nucleus ambiguus. Therefore, brainstem strokes are likely to cause the most severe impairment of swallowing; the swallow response may be absent, or patients may have difficulty in initiating a swallow.

9. Describe the evaluation of patients with dysphagia that worsens with solids as well as later in the day, a nasal vocal tone, and ptosis.

Such symptoms are a classic presentation of myasthenia gravis. Myasthenia gravis is an autoimmune disorder characterized by progressive destruction of acetylcholine receptors at the neuromuscular junction. The most striking feature is fluctuating weakness of certain voluntary muscles, particularly those innervated by brainstem motor nuclei. Consequently, the cranial nerves are almost always involved, particularly the ocular muscles; this pattern accounts for the frequency of ptosis and diplopia as initial symptoms. The second most common presentation involves muscles of facial expression, mastication, and swallowing; dysphagia is a prominent symptom in more than one-third of cases. The disease is characterized by increasing muscle weakness with repetitive muscle contraction. A test for anticholinesterase antibody should be obtained, although it is only about 90% sensitive in diagnosing myasthenia gravis. If myasthenia gravis is strongly suspected, a trial of therapy with acetylcholinesterase inhibitors, such as edrophonium chloride (Tensilon) or pyridostigmine bromide (Mestinon), should be considered even in the absence of an anticholinesterase antibody.

10. Does a barium swallow exam adequately evaluate oropharyngeal dysphagia? Why or why not?

Oropharyngeal dysphagia is best evaluated with a cineradiographic or videofluoroscopic swallowing study. The patient should be in an upright position. Because the oropharyngeal swallow transpires in less than a second, it is essential that images be obtained and recorded at a rate of 15–30/sec to adequately detail the motor events. Moreover, when the swallow is recorded at this rate, the study can be played in slow motion for careful evaluation. This type of study is not synonymous with a barium swallow radiograph. The barium swallow focuses on the esophagus, is done in a supine position, and takes at best a few still images as the barium passes through the oropharynx.

11. Why is it extremely unusual for any disease process (other than infection) to involve the oropharynx and esophagus simultaneously?

The oropharynx and esophagus are fundamentally different with respect to musculature, innervation, and neural regulation.

Oropharynx	Esophagus
Striated muscle	Striated and smooth muscle (proximally)
	Smooth muscle (middle to distal portion)
Direct nicotinic innervation	Myenteric plexus within longitudinal and circular smooth muscles
Cholinergic regulation	Cholinergic regulation, nitric oxide, vasoinhibitory peptide

Because most disease processes are specific for a particular type of muscle or nervous system element, a single process is highly unlikely to involve such diverse systems.

12. What are the indications and risks of a cricopharyngeal myotomy?
Indications
  Cricopharyngeal bar with symptoms
  Zenker's diverticulum
  Parkinson's disease (?)
Risks
  Aspiration in a patient with gastroesophageal reflux disease
  Worsening swallow function

13. Which causes of dysphagia should be considered in a patient who has had surgery and other therapy (usually radiation and chemotherapy) for head and neck cancer?
  • Radiation myositis and/or fibrosis
  • Xerostomia (hyposalivation)
  • Anatomic defects due to surgery
  • Recurrence of malignancy disease

14. What is the most difficult substance to swallow? Why?
Water. Swallowing involves several phases. First is a preparatory phase that involves chewing, sizing, shaping, and positioning of the bolus on the tongue. During the oral phase, the bolus is propelled from the oral cavity into the pharynx while the airway is protected. From this location the bolus is transported from the oral cavity first into the pharynx and finally into the esophagus. Water is the most difficult substance to size, shape, and contain in the oral cavity. Similarly it is the hardest to control as it is passed from the oral cavity into the pharynx. For these reasons more viscous foods are used to feed patients with oropharyngeal dysphagia.

15. Which patients with which dysfunctions are the best candidates for swallow therapy?

Patients	Dysfunction
Intact mentation	Aspiration (during and after swallow)
Motivated	Unilateral pharyngeal paresis

16. What are the mechanisms by which gastroesophageal reflux disease is associated with dysphagia? List from most to least common.
  • Inflammation—30% of patients with esophagitis experience dysphagia
  • Stricture
  • Peristaltic dysfunction—related to severity of disease
  • Hiatal hernia (?)

17. Why is "cricopharyngeal achalasia" a misnomer? Contrast with achalasia of the cardia.
The upper esophageal sphincter (UES) is a striated muscle that depends on tonic excitation to maintain contractility. If innervation to the cricopharyngeus is lost, the sphincter becomes flaccid, not contracted. In direct contrast, achalasia in the lower esophageal sphincter (LES) is caused by loss of the inhibitory myenteric plexus neurons; thus there is no mechanism to inhibit myogenic contraction.

	LES	*UES*
Resting tone	Myogenic	None
Denervation results in	Contraction	Relaxation
Impaired opening results from	Failure of relaxation	Failure of traction (pulling open)
Opening force provided by	Bolus	Supra- and infrahyoid musculature

18. Describe the inheritance pattern and clinical presentation of oculopharyngeal dystrophy.
- Sex-linked, autosomal dominant
- Onset in fifth decade
- French Canadian ancestry
- Ptosis
- Less involvement of muscles other than oculopharyngeal muscles
- Slowly progressive

19. List the common symptoms and causes of xerostomia.

Symptoms	Causes
Dysphagia	Sjögren's syndrome
Dry mouth with viscous saliva	Rheumatoid arthritis
Bad taste in mouth	Drugs (e.g., anticholinergics)
Oral burning	Radiation therapy
Dental decay	
Bad breath	

20. What are the potential extraesophageal manifestations of gastroesophageal reflux disease?
- Asthma
- Laryngitis
- Pharyngitis
- Dental decay with loss of dental enamel
- Globus sensation
- Otitis (?)

21. Define Zenker's diverticulum.
Diverticula may occur throughout the hypopharynx. When hypopharyngeal diverticula are located posteriorly in an area of potential weakness at the intersection of the transverse fibers of the cricopharyngeus and oblique fibers of the inferior pharyngeal constrictors (Killian's dehiscence), they are called Zenker's diverticula.

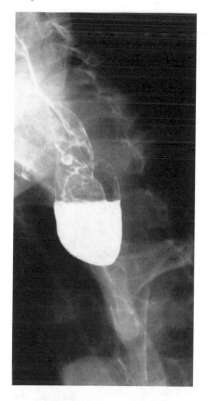

Radiograph of Zenker's diverticulum. (From Ergun GA, Kahrilas PJ: Oropharyngeal dysphagia in the elderly. Pract Gastroenterol 17:9–16, 1993, with permission.)

22. Is Zenker's diverticulum a result of obstructive or propulsive disease? Explain.

Previously it was believed that Zenker's diverticulum was caused by abnormally high hypopharyngeal pressures due to defective coordination of UES relaxation during pharyngeal bolus propulsion. It is now known that the cause is a constrictive myopathy of the cricopharyngeus (poor sphincter compliance) rather than pharyngeal-sphincter incoordination, impaired opening forces on the sphincter, or cricopharyngeal spasm. Increased resistance at the cricopharyngeus and increased intrabolus pressures above this relative obstruction cause muscular stress in the hypopharynx with herniation and diverticulum formation. Thus Zenker's diverticulum is an obstructive rather than propulsive disease.

23. Contrast esophageal and oropharyngeal dysphagia.

Esophageal dysphagia	Oropharyngeal dysphagia
Associated symptoms	Associated symptoms
Chest pain	Weakness
Water brash	Ptosis
Regurgitation	Nasal voice
	Pneumonia
	Cough
Organ-specific diseases	Systemic diseases
Esophageal cancer	Myasthenia gravis
Esophageal motor disorder	Parkinson's disease
Treatable (e.g., dilation)	Rarely treatable
Expendable organ (only 1 function)	Nonexpendable—functions include speech, respiration, and swallowing

BIBLIOGRAPHY

1. Alberts MJ, Horner J, Gray L, Brazer S: Aspiration after stroke: lesion analysis by brain MRI. Dysphagia 7:170–173, 1992.
2. Cook IJ, Blumbergs P, Cash K, et al: Structural abnormalities of the cricopharyngeus muscle in patients with pharyngeal (Zenker's) diverticulum. J Gastroenterol Hepatol 7:556–562, 1992.
3. Cook IJ, Gabb M, Panagopoulos V, et al: Pharyngeal (Zenker's) diverticulum is a disorder of upper esophageal sphincter opening. Gastroenterology 103:1229–1235, 1992.
4. Dodds WJ, Stewart ET, Logemann JA: Physiology and radiology of the normal oral and pharyngeal phases of swallowing. AJR 154:953–963, 1990.
5. Gordon C, Hewer R, Wade D: Dysphagia in acute stroke. BMJ 295:411–414, 1987.
6. Horner J, Massey E, Riski J, et al: Aspiration following stroke: Clinical correlates and outcome. Neurology 38:1359–1362, 1988.
7. Jacob P, Kahrilas PJ, Logemann JA, et al: Upper esophageal sphincter opening and modulation during swallowing. Gastroenterology 97:1469–1478, 1989.
8. Kahrilas PJ, Lin S, Logemann JA, et al: Deglutitive tongue action: Volume accommodation and bolus propulsion. Gastroenterology 104:152–162, 1993.
9. Kahrilas PJ, Logemann JA, Lin S, Ergun G: Pharyngeal clearance during swallowing: a combined manometric and videofluoroscopic study. Gastroenterology 103;128–136, 1992.
10. Logemann J: Evaluation and Treatment of Swallowing Disorders. San Diego, College-Hill Press, 1983.
11. Osserman KE: Myasthenia Gravis. New York, Grune & Stratton, 1958.
12. Robbins J, Hamilton JW, Lof GL, Kempster GB: Oropharyngeal swallowing in normal adults of different ages. Gastroenterology 103:823–829, 1992.
13. Siebens H, Trupe E, Siebens A, et al: Correlates and consequences of eating dependency in the institutionalized elderly. J Am Geriatr Soc 34:192–198, 1986.
14. Sonies BC, Dalakas MC: Dysphagia in patients with the post-polio syndrome. N Engl J Med 324:1162–1167, 1991.
15. Trupe EH, Siebens H, Siebens A: Prevalence of feeding and swallowing disorders in a nursing home. Arch Phys Med Rehabil 65:651–652, 1984.

2. GASTROESOPHAGEAL REFLUX DISEASE

Lawrence F. Johnson, M.D., and Peter R. McNally, D.O.

1. What is gastroesophageal reflux disease (GERD)? How common is it?

The term GERD is used to describe a pathologic condition of symptoms or histopathologic injury to the esophagus caused by percolation of gastric or gastroduodenal contents into the esophagus. GERD is extremely common. One survey of hospital employees showed that 7% experienced heartburn daily and 36% experienced symptoms at least monthly. Other studies have suggested a 3–4% prevalence of GERD among the general population, with a prevalence increase to ~5% in people older than 55 years. Pregnant women have the highest incidence of daily heartburn at 48–79%. The distribution of GERD between the sexes is equal, but men are more likely to suffer complications of GERD, esophagitis (2–3:1), and Barrett's esophagus (10:1).

2. What are the typical symptoms of GERD?

Heartburn is usually characterized as a midline retrosternal burning sensation that radiates to the throat and occasionally to the intrascapular region. Patients often place the open hand over the sternal area and flip the wrist in a up-and-down motion to simulate the nature and location of the heartburn symptoms. Mild symptoms of heartburn are often relieved within 3–5 minutes of ingesting milk or antacids. Other symptoms of GERD include the following:

Regurgitation consists of eructation of gastric juice or stomach contents into the pharynx and often is accompanied by a noxious bitter taste. Regurgitation is most common after a large meal and usually occurs with stooping or assuming a recumbent posture.

Dysphagia is defined as difficulty in swallowing. In patients with longstanding GERD, dysphagia is usually caused by a benign stricture of the esophagus. Solid foods, such as meat and bread, are often precipitants of dysphagia. Dysphagia implies significant narrowing of the esophageal lumen, usually to a luminal diameter < 13 mm. Prolonged dysphagia, associated with inability to swallow saliva, requires prompt evaluation and often endoscopic removal (see chapter on foreign body ingestion).

Gastrointestinal hemorrhage is an uncommon symptom of GERD. Endoscopic evaluation of patients with upper GI hemorrhage have identified erosive GERD as the cause in only 2–6% of cases.

Odynophagia is a painful substernal sensation associated with swallowing that should not be confused with dysphagia. Odynophagia rarely results from GERD. Instead, odynophagia is caused by infections (monilia, herpes simplex virus, cytomegalovirus), ingestion of corrosive agents or pills (tetracycline, vitamin C, iron, quinidine, estrogen, aspirin or NSAIDs), or cancer.

Waterbrash is an uncommon symptom, but highly suggestive of GERD. Patients literally foam at the mouth as the salivary glands produce up to 10 ml of saliva per minute as an esophago-salivary reflex response to acid reflux.

Atypical symptoms and signs of GERD include hoarseness, throat tightness, asthma, cough, hiccups, throat-clearing, recurrent otitis in children, and lingual dental erosions.

3. What clues about GERD can be gleaned from the physical exam?

- Severe kyphosis is often associated with hiatal hernia and GER, especially when a body brace is necessary.
- Tight-fitting corsets or clothing (in men or women) can increase intraabdominal pressure and may cause stress reflux.
- Abnormal phonation may suggest high GER and vocal cord injury. When hoarseness is due to high GER, the voice is often coarse or gravelly and often worse in the morning, whereas in other causes of hoarseness voice use or abuse leads to worsening later in the day.

- Wheezing or asthma and pulmonary fibrosis have been associated with GER. Patients often give a history of postprandial or nocturnal regurgitation with episodes of coughing or choking caused by near or partial aspiration.
- Loss of the enamel on the lingual surface of the teeth can be seen in severe GERD, although it is more common in patients with rumination syndrome or bulimia.
- Esophageal dysfunction may be the predominant component of scleroderma or mixed connective tissue disease. Inquiry about symptoms of Raynaud's syndrome and examination for sclerodactyly, taut skin, and calcinosis are important.
- Cerebral palsy, Down syndrome, and mental retardation are commonly associated with GERD.
- Children with peculiar head movements during swallowing may have Sandifer's syndrome.
- Some patients unknowingly swallow air (aerophagia) that triggers a burp, belch, and heartburn cycle. The observant clinician may detect this behavior during the interview and physical exam.

4. Do healthy persons have GER?

Yes. Healthy persons may regurgitate acid or food contents into the esophagus, especially after a large meal late at night. In normal persons, the natural defense mechanisms of the lower esophageal sphincter barrier and esophageal clearance are not overwhelmed and symptoms and injury do not occur. Ambulatory esophageal pH studies have shown that healthy persons have acid reflux into the esophagus < 2% of the daytime (upright position) and < 0.3% of the nighttime (supine position).

5. How can swallowing and salivary production be associated with GERD?

Reflux of gastric contents into the esophagus often stimulates salivary production and increased swallowing. Saliva has a neutral pH, which helps to neutralize the gastric refluxate. Furthermore, the swallowed saliva initiates a peristaltic wave that strips the esophagus of refluxed material (clearance). During the awake upright period, persons swallow $72 \times$/hr, and increase to $192 \times$/hr during meals. Swallowing is least common during sleep ($< 7 \times$/hr), and arousal from sleep to swallow during GER may be reduced by sedatives or alcohol ingestion. Patients with Sjögren's syndrome and smokers have reduced salivary production and prolonged esophageal acid clearance times.

6. What are the two defective anatomic mechanisms in patients with GERD?

1. Ineffective clearance and a defective gastroesophageal barrier
2. Clearance
   - **Esophageal:** Normally reflux of gastric contents into the esophagus stimulates a secondary peristaltic or clearance wave to remove the injurious refluxate from the esophagus. The worst case of ineffective esophageal clearance is seen in patients with "scleroderma" esophagus. In such patients the lower esophageal sphincter barrier is non-existent and there is no primary or secondary peristalsis of the esophagus — no clearance.
   - **Gastric:** Gastroparesis may lead to excessive quantities of retained gastroduodenal and food contents. Larger volumes of stagnate gastric contents predispose to esophageal reflux.
3. Gastroesophageal barrier: The normal lower esophageal sphincter (LES) is 3–4 cm long and maintains a resting tone of 10–30 mmHg pressure. The LES acts as a barrier against GER. When the LES pressure is less than 6 mmHg, GERD is common; however, the presence of "normal" LES pressure does not predict absence of GERD. Recent studies have shown that transient relaxations in the LES (tLESRs) are important in the pathogenesis of GERD. During a tLESR, the sphincter inappropriately relaxes and free gastric reflux occurs. The normal LES is susceptible to many factors that can influence resting pressure.

Factors Influencing LES Tone

	INCREASE LES PRESSURE	DECREASE LES PRESSURE
Neural agents	Alpha-adrenergic agonists	Alpha-adrenergic antagonists
	Beta-adrenergic antagonists	Beta-adrenergic agonists
	Cholinergic agonists	Cholinergic antagonists
Food	Protein	Fat
		Chocolate
		Ethanol
		Peppermint
Hormones/	Gastrin	Cholecystokinin
mediators	Motilin	Secretin
	Substance P	Glucagon
	Prostaglandin F_2alpha	Gastric inhibitory factor
		Progesterone
		Vasoactive intestinal peptide
Medications	Antacids	Calcium channel antagonists
	Metoclopromaide	Theophylline
	Cisapride	Diazepam
	Domperidone	Meperidine
		Morphine
		Dopamine
		Diazepam
		Barbiturates

7. What is the natural history of GERD?

Most patients with confirmed GERD have experienced symptoms for several years before seeking medical attention. Before the introduction of potent antireflux medications that inhibit the gastric proton pump, it was common for patients to experience recurrent symptoms even on therapy—antacids, histamine-2 antagonists, and prokinetic drugs. Most patients with GERD can now be successfully managed by the administration of a proton pump inhibitor (omeprazole or lansoprazole), but GERD is recurrent in > 80% of patients within 30 weeks of discontinuation of the drug.

Erosive GERD should be considered a chronic disease. The likelihood of recurrent symptoms after discontinuation of medical therapy is high. The goals of medical therapy should be relief of symptoms and avoidance of the major complications of esophagitis: stricture formation, Barrett's esophagus, and hemorrhage.

8. What other medical conditions may mimic symptoms of GERD?

The differential diagnosis of GERD includes coronary artery disease, gastritis, gastroparesis, infectious and pill-induced esophagitis, peptic ulcer disease, biliary tract disease, and esophageal motor diseases.

In the evaluation of patients with retrosternal chest pain, the clinician must always be mindful that patients with GERD do not die, but patients with new-onset angina or an acute myocardial infarction with symptoms mimicking GERD can. Clues that a patient's chest pain is cardiac in origin include radiation of the pain to the neck, jaw, or left shoulder/upper extremity; associated shortness of breath and/or diaphoresis; precipitation of pain by exertion; and relief of pain with sublingual nitroglycerin. Physical findings of new murmurs or gallops or abnormal rhythms are also suggestive of a cardiac origin. Although positive findings on a electrocardiogram are helpful in the evaluation of patients with chest pain, the absence of ischemic ECG changes should not discourage the clinician from excluding a cardiac etiology for the patient's symptoms.

9. How should patients with symptoms of GERD be evaluated?

Evaluation of patients with GER may be guided by the severity of symptoms. Patients without symptoms of high GER (aspiration or hoarseness) or dysphagia may be given careful instruction on lifestyle modification and a diagnostic trial of H-2 blocker therapy and followed clinically.

When the patient's symptoms persist or recur after a 2–3-month trial, further evaluation is warranted. Barium esophagram and upper GI series are safe and cost-effective first tests. These tests are helpful in evaluating for other diseases and in defining anatomic abnormalities such as hiatal hernia but rather insensitive in defining the degree of mucosal injury to the esophagus. The presence of a hiatal hernia does not accurately predict GERD; up to 33% of asymptomatic volunteers undergoing an upper GI study have been shown to have a hiatal hernia, and the presence of a hiatal hernia increases dramatically with age—up to 70% in some series. The finding of *spontaneous* reflux of heavy barium to the level of the thoracic inlet is helpful in predicting GERD. The upper GI study sometimes detects subtle esophageal strictures not seen on endoscopic examination.

A more expensive but more sensitive alternative test is esophagogastroduodenoscopy (EGD). Up to 50% of patients with GERD do not have macroscopic evidence of esophagitis at the time of endoscopy. In this group more sensitive GER testing may be necessary or alternative diagnoses considered. A commonly used endoscopic grading system for GERD appears below.

Endoscopic System of Scoring Esophagitis

Grade 0	Macroscopically normal esophagus; only histologic evidence of GERD
Grade 1	One or more nonconfluent lesions with erythema or exudate above the gastroesophageal junction
Grade 2	Confluent, noncircumferential, erosive, and exudative lesions
Grade 3	Circumferential erosive and exudative lesions
Grade 4	Chronic mucosal lesions (ulceration, stricture, or Barrett's esophagus)

10. What are some of the more sophisticated esophageal function tests? How can they be used appropriately in the evaluation of patients with GERD?

Clinical tests of GERD may be divided into three categories:

1. Acid sensitivity	Acid perfusion (Bernstein) test
	24-hour ambulatory esophageal pH monitoring
2. Esophageal barrier and motility	Esophageal manometry
	Gastroesophageal scintiscanning
	Standard acid reflux (modified Tuttle) test
	24-hr ambulatory esophageal pH monitoring
3. Esophageal acid clearance time	Standard acid reflux clearance test (SART)
	24-hr ambulatory esophageal pH monitoring

All patients with GERD do not need esophageal function testing. This testing should be reserved for patients who fail medical therapy or in whom the correlation of reflux symptoms is in doubt. The **Bernstein test** is helpful in confirming that symptoms are due to esophageal sensitivity to acid. The test is performed by alternatively infusing sterile water and dilute 0.1 N HCL in the distal esophagus. **Ambulatory 24-hr esophageal pH monitoring** is helpful in evaluating patients refractory to standard medical therapy. Acid hypersecretion is often seen in patients with GERD and esophageal pH monitoring may be helpful in titrating the dose of H-2 blocker of proton pump inhibitors (PPIs). Persistence of acid reflux on "adequate" doses of a PPI should raise the possibility of patient noncompliance or Zollinger-Ellison syndrome. **Esophageal manometry** is helpful in evaluating the competency of the LES barrier and the body of the esophagus for motor function. Severe esophagitis may be the sole manifestation of early scleroderma. Some have reported ambulatory 24-hr pH monitoring with distal and proximal esophageal pH electrodes to be helpful in the evaluation of patients with atypical reflux symptoms, such as hoarseness, throat tightness, asthma, and interstitial lung disease. When ambulatory pH testing is not available, **scintiscanning** has been shown to be helpful.

11. Are nonprescription therapies available to help patients with GERD?

Absolutely. Population studies have estimated that ~40% of adult Americans suffer from heartburn at least once a month and one-fourth of American adults take antacids more than twice a month. For patients with mild periodic heartburn, antacid tablets are an effective and convenient treatment. Instructions on lifestyle modifications are also helpful, including avoidance of tight-fiting garments; reduction or elimination of alcohol and tobacco; avoidance of common precipitation foods (chocolate, mints, tomato-based foods, and hyperosmolar liquids such as orange juice and pineapple juice); avoidance of chewing gum or sucking on lozenges, and refraining from eating 2–4 hours before sleep or recumbency. Some recommend elevation of the head of the bed with 4–6-inch blocks to promote gravity clearance of nocturnal reflux. Weight reduction is the most difficult but often the most useful lifestyle modification.

12. Define the various types of medical therapy for GERD and give a logical approach to prescription therapy for patients with long-standing GERD.

Medical Therapy for GERD

TOPICAL	DOSAGE	SIDE EFFECTS
Antacids	1–2 tablets after meals and at bedtime, as needed	Diarrhea (magnesium-containing) and constipation (aluminum-and calcium-containing)
Sucralfate	1 gm 4 times a day	Incomplete passage of pill, especially in patients with esophageal strictures, constipation, dysgeusia
H-2 blockers		
Cimetidine	400–800 mg 2–4 times/day	Gynecomastia, impotence, psychosis, hepatitis, drug, interactions with warfarin, theophylline
Ranitidine	150–300 mg 2–4 times/day	Same, less common
Famotidine	20–40 mg 1–2 times/day	Same, less common
Proton pump inhibitors (PPIs)		
Omeprazole	20–60 mg/day	Theoretical risk of carcinoid tumors; drug interaction due to cytochrome p-450 interaction (warfarin, phenytoin, diazepam)
Lansoprazole	30 mg/day	Probably the same—not yet released in U.S.
Prokinetic agents		
Bethanechol	10–25 mg 4 times/day or at bedtime	Urinary retention in patients with detrusor–external sphincter dyssynergia or prostatic hypertrophy, worsening asthma
Metoclopramide	10 mg 3 times/day or at bedtime	Extrapyramidal dysfunction, parkinsonianlike reaction; cases of irreversible tardive dyskinesia have been reported
Cisapride	10–20 mg 3 times/day and at bedtime	Abdominal cramping, intestinal gas, dry mouth

For the patient with mild uncomplicated symptoms of heartburn, empiric H-2 blocker therapy without costly and sophisticated diagnostic testing is reasonable. For patients recalcitrant to conventional therapy or with complications of high GERD (aspiration, asthma, hoarseness), Barrett's esophagus, or stricture, diagnostic and management decisions become more complicated. The medical or surgical therapy offered to such patients depends on patient preference, health care cost, risk of medical or surgical complications, and related factors.

13. Describe the commonly recommended approach to graded treatment.

Stage I	Lifestyle modifications
	Antacids, prokinetics, or sucralfate
Stage II	H-2 blocker therapy
	Reinforce need for lifestyle modifications
Stage III	Proton pump inhibitors (omeprazole or lansoperazole)
	Reinforce need for lifestyle modifications
Stage IV	Surgical antireflux procedure

The authors favor initiation of aggressive lifestyle modification (especially weight reduction and dietary changes) and pharmacologic therapy to achieve endoscopic healing of esophagitis (usually omeprazole, 20–40 mg twice daily). When esophagitis is healed, an effective dose of an intermediate potency H-2 blocker is substituted for the PPI. Then the patient is counseled about the risks, benefits, and alternatives to long-term medical therapy. Surgery is encouraged for the fit patient who requires chronic high doses of pharmacologic therapy to control GERD or dislikes taking medicines.

14. Do patients scheduled for surgical antireflux procedures need to undergo sophisticated esophageal function testing before surgery?
There is no absolute correct answer. However, it is prudent to do esophageal motility studies to ensure that esophageal motor disease is not present. Patients with scleroderma esophagus may have a paucity of systemic complaints, and the diagnosis may go undetected without esophageal manometry. Generally, surgical antireflux procedures are avoided or modified in such patients. In addition, esophageal motility studies and ambulatory 24-hr pH monitoring may confirm that the patient's symptoms are attributable to GERD, before performance of a surgical procedure.

15. The most serious long-term complications of GERD include esophageal stricture and Barrett's esophagus. How should these complications be managed?
Esophageal Stricture
- Prevention of peptic stricture with early institution of effective medical or surgical therapy appears to be particularly important for patients with scleroderma.
- For patients suffering symptoms of dysphagia due to peptic stricture, esophageal dilation is effective management. Dilation can be accomplished using mercury-filled, polyvinyl, Maloney bougies, wire-guided hollow Savary-Gulliard or American dilators, or through-the-scope (TTS) pneumatic balloons. Usually the esophagus is dilated to a diameter of 14 mm or 44 F. After successful dilation of a peptic stricture the patient should be placed on aggressive H-2 or PPI therapy to avoid recurrent stricture formation.
- Surgery, is an effective method of managing esophageal strictures. Usually pre-and intra-operative dilation is combined with a definitive antireflux procedure.

Barrett's Esophagus
- Barrett's esophagus is a metaplastic degeneration of the normal esophageal lining, which is replaced with a premalignant, specialized columnar epithelium. It is seen in roughly 5–7% of patients with uncomplicated reflux but in up to 30–40% of patients with scleroderma or dysphagia.
- Currently, there is no proven method to eliminate Barrett's esophagus. Preliminary studies of laser or bicap ablation of the metaplastic segment followed by alkalization of the gastroesophageal refluxate are encouraging. The need for cancer surveillance is discussed elsewhere in this book.

BIBLIOGRAPHY

1. Bainbridge ET, Temple JG, Nicholas SP, et al: Symptomatic gastroesophageal reflux in pregnancy: A comparative study of white Europeans and Asians in Birmingham. Br J Clin Pract 37:53, 1983.
2. Brunnen PL, Karmody AM, Needham CD: Severe peptic esophagitis. Gut 10:831, 1969.
3. Collen MJ, Lewis JH, Benjaman SB. Gastric acid hypersecretion in refractory gastroesophageal reflux disease. Gastroenterology 98:654, 1990.
4. Deemester TR, Wang CI, Wernly JA, et al: Technique, indications, and clinical use of 24 hour esophageal pH monitoring. J Thorac Cardiovasc Surg. 79:656, 1980.
5. Dodds WJ, Kahrilas PJ, Dent J, et al: Analysis of spontaneous gastroesophageal reflux and esophageal acid clearance in patients with reflux esophagitis. J Gastrointest Motil 2:79, 1989.
6. Graham DY, Smith JL, Patterson DJ: Why do apparently healthy people use antacid tablets? Am J Gastroenterol 78:257–260, 1983.
7. Johnson LF: Gastroesophageal reflux. In Spittell JA Jr (ed): Clinical Medicine. New York, Harper & Row, 1982, pp 1–39.

8. Kahrilas PJ, Gupta RR: The effect of cigarette smoking on salivation and esophageal acid clearance. J Lab Clin Med 114:431, 1989.

9. Kahrilas PJ, Hogan WJ: Gastroesophageal reflux. In Sleisenger MH, Fordtran JS (eds): Gastrointestinal Disease, 5th ed. Philadelphia, W. B. Saunders, 1993, pp 379–401.

10. Korsten MA, Rosman AS, Fishbein S, et al: Chronic xerostomia increases esophageal acid exposure and is associated with esophageal injury. Am J Med 90:701, 1991.

11. Marks RM, Richter JE, Rizzo J, et al: Omeprazole vs H2 receptor antagonists in treating patients with peptic stricture and esophagitis. 106:907–915, 1994.

12. McNally PR, Maydonovitch CL, Prosek RA, et al: Evaluation of gastroesophageal reflux as a cause of idiopathic hoarseness. Dig Dis Sci 34:1900–1904, 1989.

13. Meier JH, McNally PR, Freeman SR, et al: Does omeprazole (Prilosec) improve asthma in patients with gastroesophageal reflux: A double blind crossover study. Dig Dis Sci 39:1900–1904, 1994.

14. Nebel OT, Fornes MF, Castell DO: Symptomatic gastroesophageal reflux: Incidence and precipitating factors. Am J Dig Dis 21:953, 1976.

15. Ogrek CP: Gastroesophageal reflux. In Haubrich WS, Schaffner F (eds): Bockus Gastroenterology, 5th ed. Philadelphia, W. B. Saunders, 1995, pp 445–463.

16. Ott DJ: Barium esophagram. In Castell DO, Wu WC, Ott DJ (eds): Gastroesophageal Reflux Disease. Mt Kisco, NY, Futura, 1985, pp 109–128.

17. Richter JE, Castell DO: Gastroesophageal reflux. Pathogenesis, diagnosis, and therapy. Ann Intern Med 97:93, 1982.

18. Sontag SJ, O'Commell S, Khandelwal S, et al: Most asthmatics have gastroesophageal reflux with or without brochodilator therapy. Gastroenterology 99:613, 1990.

19. Winnan GR, Meyer CT, McCallum RW: Interpretation of Bernstein test: A reappraisal. Ann Intern Med 96:320–322, 1982.

3. ESOPHAGEAL INFECTIONS

Dirk R. Davis, M.D.

1. Is a positive culture for *Candida* sp. after endoscopic brushings diagnostic of monilial esophagitis?

Candida sp. is a commensal organism in the gastrointestinal tract of humans. To document infection, demonstration of mycelial forms on direct smear or cytologic brushings and evidence of mucosal invasion on tissue biopsy are required (see figure below).

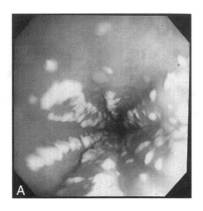 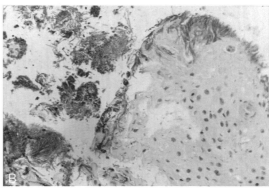

A, Endoscopic appearance of candida esophagitis. Pearly white exudate with erythema of adjacent mucosa.
B, Histologic example of hyphal elements suggesting candida infection.

2. Does acid suppression therapy predispose an immunocompetent patient to monilial esophagitis?

An increased incidence of culture-proven colonization of the esophagus with *Candida* sp., an obvious precursor of infection, has been shown in patients using H2 receptor antagonists.

3. Is systemic antifungal therapy required for the treatment of invasive candida esophagitis in patients with AIDS?

Although imidazole antifungal agents are recommended in immunocompromised patients with candida esophagitis (fluconazole, 100–200 mg/day orally, or ketoconazole, 400–800 mg/day orally), it is reasonable to use topical therapy. Administration of clotrimazole vaginal tablets (100 mg orally, 3 times/day for 1 week) was successful in healing esophagitis in all patients.

4. What would be considered first-line therapy in the granulocytopenic patient with documented monilial esophagitis?

Granulocytopenic patients should receive intravenous amphotericin B because of the high risk of fungal dissemination. The dose and duration of treatment are based on the patient's clinical status. Febrile patients with extensive fungal esophagitis or evidence of other visceral involvement should receive 0.5 mg/kg body weight/day. Patients without fever and milder mucosal disease may be treated with doses of 0.3 mg/kg/day.

5. In treating fungal esophagitis, is the eradication rate improved by using a combination of amphotericin B with an imidazole antibiotic (e.g., fluconazole)?
Despite a potentiation of some antibiotics (e.g., 5-fluorocytosine, tetracycline, rifampin) in combination with amphotericin B, this synergism does not exist with the imidazole drugs. The combined use of amphotericin B and imidazole agents may be antagonistic and should be avoided.

6. Are the sensitivities of musocal biopsies and cytologic brushings equivalent in diagnosing herpes simplex virus (HSV) and cytomegalovirus (CMV) infections in the esophagus?
Although mucosal biopsies and cytologic brushings are equally effective in the diagnosis of HSV esophagitis, brush cytology is seldom helpful in CMV infections. CMV, which is localized to submucosal fibroblasts and vascular epithelium, requires biopsies from the center of the ulcer. HSV infects squamous epithelium, and histologic evidence of HSV infection may be demonstrated in exfoliated squamous cells and mucosal biopsies from the edge of the ulcer. Brushings and biopsies also should be placed in viral transport media, because culture is more sensitive than histologic evaluation for both HSV and CMV.

7. Is it possible to differentiate HSV and CMV esophagitis based on endoscopic appearance?
Yes. In early stages of infection, the diagnosis of one or the other virus may be suggested by gross appearance. In the initial stages of infection with HSV, the small vesicles typical of nasolabial infections can be seen. These progress to form circumscribed ulcer craters that range in diameter from 0.5–2 cm and have raised granular yellowish edges — the so-called volcano ulcers. In CMV esophagitis, the early lesions are linear, serpiginous ulcers in the middle and/or distal esophagus. Concomitant infections with both HSV and CMV have been reported in immunocompromised hosts.

8. Cowdry type A inclusion bodies and ground glass nuclear staining pattern indicate infection with which of the three herpes viruses known to infect the esophagus?
The characteristic histologic features of HSV esophagitis are the presence of multinucleated giant cells, ballooning degeneration of squamous cells, margination of chromatin, and ground-glass nuclei. The Cowdry type A intranuclear inclusions are pathognomonic.

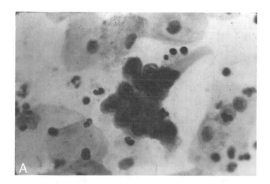 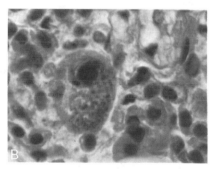

A, Cytologic specimen illustrating Cowdry type A intranuclear inclusions consistent with herpes simplex virus. *B,* Histologic specimen illustrating both intracytoplasmic and intranuclear inclusions consistent with cytomegalovirus infection.

The sensitivity of histologic staining for CMV is significantly less than that for HSV. Diagnostic yield by light microscopy ranges from 2–40%. If only squamous epithelium is present on biopsy specimens, CMV cannot be excluded, because such tissue cannot be evaluated adequately.

The typical histologic features of CMV infection are large cells containing intracytoplasmic inclusions and amphophilic intranuclear inclusions. The use of immunohistochemical stains and in situ hybridization for CMV DNA improves diagnostic sensitivity of tissue biopsies. Viral culture remains the standard for diagnosis of both HSV and CMV.

9. Is ulcerative distal esophagitis in a patient with AIDS more likely to be HSV or CMV?
If the nasolabial lesions of HSV are present, a presumptive diagnosis of HSV esophagitis is reasonable, but absence of the cutaneous lesions does not exclude HSV infection in the esophagus. Of interest in patients with AIDS, CMV is more likely to manifest ulcerative disease in the right colon than in the esophagus. In immunosuppressed recipients of bone marrow transplants and in leukemic patients, HSV and CMV occur in the esophagus with equal frequency. Although HSV may be disseminated, visceral involvement occurs less often than with CMV, for which widespread visceral infection tends to be the rule.

10. A large, flat, ovoid ulcer in the midesophagus occurring coincidentally with HIV seroconversion is most likely due to what organism?
In patients with AIDS, *Candida* sp., HSV, and CMV are potential causes of infectious esophageal ulcers. Early infection and seroconversion to HIV antibody-positive status are seldom associated with opportunistic infections. There have been multiple case reports of giant, HIV-associated ulcers that present with the same symptoms as other esophageal infections. Biopsies, brushings, and cultures fail to demonstrate the common organisms seen in immunocompromised patients. Electron microscopy has shown viral particles consistent with HIV in biopsies from the ulcer margin. There are reports of prompt resolution of such ulcers with corticosteroid therapy.

11. How often are esophageal infections due to bacterial agents?
In the series by Walsh and colleagues, 33 patients underwent esophageal biopsies, and 19 were diagnosed with infectious esophagitis. Of the 19, 2 (11%) met criteria for bacterial esophagitis. In an immunocompromised autopsy population, 20 of 123 (16%) were bacterial infections.

12. Can a diagnosis of bacterial esophagitis be made when fungal or viral organisms are present in tissue or culture?
Strict diagnostic criteria for bacterial esophagitis eliminate the possibility of concomitant viral, fungal, or neoplastic involvement in the esophagus. To make the diagnosis of bacterial esophagitis, bacterial invasion of esophageal mucosa must be demonstrated on tissue Gram stain. Periodic acid-Schiff (PAS) and Gomori-methanamine silver (GMS) stains are used to exclude the presence of fungi. Viral cultures for HSV and CMV, as well as the absence of viral inclusion bodies on histologic evaluation, exclude the common viral etiologies.

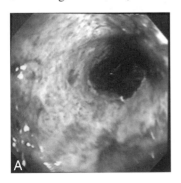 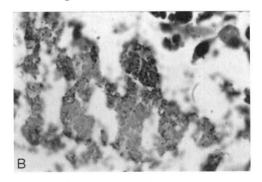

A, Endoscopic illustration of pyogenic esophagitis. Characteristic endoluminal features include diffuse mucoid exudate, mucosal edema with bullous formation, and cyanotic discoloration. *B*, Brown-Hopps stain of esophageal mucosa demonstrates numerous gram-positive organisms lining the surface of the mucosa.

13. What are the most common organisms isolated in bacterial esophagitis?
It makes sense that oropharyngeal flora are the most common bacteria to infect the esophagus. The Brown-Hopps stain demonstrates gram-positive cocci most frequently, followed by mixed infections with gram-positive cocci and gram-negative bacilli. Gram-negative bacilli alone are less common; rarely are gram-positive bacilli identified. Blood cultures should be obtained in patients in whom the diagnosis of bacterial esophagitis is considered. Bacteremia and sepsis are not uncommon in the setting of bacterial esophagitis, and isolation of an organism may help to direct therapy.

14. Does *Mycobacterium tuburculosis* need to be considered in the differential diagnosis of ulcerative esophagitis?
Tuberculosis (TB) of the esophagus is rare. In one review, 46 of 54 cases of TB involving the esophagus were secondary infections. Some authors suggest that in cases of primary TB of the esophagus, exclusion of TB involving other sites has not been well documented. The esophagus may be involved by direct extension from infected structures in the mediastinum, by inoculation with swallowed sputum, and by hematogenous or lymphatic spread. In general, esophageal TB responds to antituberculous antibiotics. Diffuse esophagitis due to TB and *Mycobacterium avium-intracellulare* has been reported in patients with AIDS and as a rule responds poorly to therapy.

15. Can the diagnosis of Chagas' disease be based on classic manometric findings and confirmed by histologic evaluation of deep mucosal biopsies from the distal esophagus?
Chagas' disease is caused by infection with *Trypanosoma cruzi*, which is endemic in South America. The organism destroys ganglion cells, and multiple organs are involved. The esophageal abnormalities resemble achalasia, but the lower esophageal sphincter pressure is not elevated and, in fact, may be low. Symptoms typically occur years to decades after the acute infection. Diagnosis requires typical manometric findings, positive serologic tests for the parasite, and evidence of other organ involvement. Mucosal biopsies are of no value in the diagnosis. The esophagus in Chagas' disease is more responsive to nitrates and calcium channel antagonists, which improve esophageal emptying. Unlike primary achalasia, Chagas' disease is often associated with cardiac, renal, intestinal, and biliary abnormalities.

16. Is it prudent to treat an immunocompromised patient presenting with odynophagia empirically for infectious esophagitis?
Odynophagia is the primary complaint in nearly all patients with infectious esophagitis, regardless of etiology. In patients with oral thrush or with perioral HSV infections, the decision to treat for fungal or HSV esophagitis is not difficult. In immunocompromised hosts, the leading cause of odynophagia is due to *Candida* sp. infection, and an empiric trial of topical therapy (clotrimazole, nystatin, or systemic antifungal imidazole antibiotics) for one week is reasonable. In patients failing to respond to a therapeutic trial of antifungal therapy, acyclovir treatment should be considered. If symptoms progress during treatment for *Candida* sp. or HSV or persist despite treatment, endoscopic assessment with biopsies, cytologic brushings, and cultures are indicated.

17. What are the recommendations for treatment of HSV esophagitis?
In immunocompetent patients with HSV esophagitis, the esophageal lesions parallel resolution of nasolabial and oral vesicles. Although resolution without treatment may be anticipated, most experts recommend acyclovir, 200 mg orally, 5 times daily, to shorten duration of symptoms. In immunocompromised patients, the dose of acyclovir is doubled to 400 mg orally, 5 times daily, or may be given intravenously in a dose of 250 mg/m^2 every 8 hours. Acyclovir may be used prophylactically to decrease the risk of HSV infection in immunosuppressed patients. Prophylactic doses are 200 mg orally, 4–5 times daily, or 800 mg orally, twice daily.

18. What are the treatment options for CMV esophagitis?
CMV infections occur in immunosuppressed individuals through reactivation of dormant virus or may be acquired by blood-product transfusions and organ transplantation. In CMV esophagitis,

two drugs have been shown to be effective. Ganciclovir may be administered IV in a dose of 5 mg/kg every 12 hours for 2 weeks, then daily for an additional week. In patients who become granulocytopenic during ganciclovir therapy or do not respond, foscarnet should be prescribed in a dose of 60 mg/kg every 8 hours for 2 weeks, followed by an additional 2 weeks at a dose of 90–120 mg/kg/day.

BIBLIOGRAPHY

1. Agha FP, Horching HL, Norstrant TT: Herpetic esophagitis: A diagnostic challenge in immunocompromised patients. Am J Gastroenterol 81:246, 1986.
2. Baehr PH, McDonald GB: Esophageal infections: Risk factors, presentation, diagnosis and treatment. Gastroenterology 106:509, 1994.
3. Buckner FS, Pomeroy C: Cytomegalovirus disease of the gastrointestinal tract in patients without AIDS. Clin Infect Dis 17:644, 1993.
4. Deshmukh M, Shah R, McCallum RW: Experience with herpes esophagitis in otherwise healthy patients. Am J Gastroenterol 79:173, 1984.
5. Eng J, Sabaratnam S: Tuberculosis of the esophagus. Dig Dis Sci 36:536, 1991.
6. Lalor E, Rabeneck L: Esophageal candidiasis in AIDS. Successful therapy with clotrimazole vaginal tablets taken by mouth. Dig Dis Sci 36:279, 1991.
7. Levine MS, Gudrun L, Katzka DA, et al: Giant, human immunodeficiency virus-related ulcers in the esophagus. Radiology 180:323, 1991.
8. Meyers JD: Prevention and treatment of cytomegalovirus infection. Annu Rev Med 42:179, 1991.
9. Porro GB, Parentie F, Cernuschi M: The diagnosis of esophageal candidiasis in patients with acquired immunodeficiency syndrome: Is endoscopy always necessary? Am J Gastroenterol 84:143, 1989.
10. Sutton FM, Graham DY, Goodgame RW: Infectious esophagitis. Gastrointest Endosc Clin North Am 4:713, 1994.
11. Vermeersch B, Rysselaere M, Dekeyser K, et al: Fungal colonization of the esophagus. Am J Gastroenterol 84:1079, 1989.
12. Walsh TJ, Belitsus NJ, Hamilton SR: Bacterial esophagitis in immunocompromised patients. Arch Intern Med 146:1345, 1986.

4. ESOPHAGEAL CAUSES OF CHEST PAIN

Brian T. Johnston, M.D., and Donald O. Castell, M.D.

1. When should the clinician consider an esophageal cause of chest pain?

Coronary artery disease is common in the developed world. In the United States 1.5 million patients/year suffer an acute myocardial infarction, and one-fourth of all deaths are attributed to myocardial infarction. Esophageal disease is also a common problem. However, esophageal causes of chest pain are rarely life-threatening and do not necessitate emergency diagnosis. Therefore, the initial approach must be to exclude coronary artery disease.

A normal electrocardiogram (EKG) during the episode of pain is reassuring. However, a pain episode sufficiently severe to warrant admission to hospital merits serial EKGs and assessment of cardiac enzyme levels. Further investigations after the acute episode include an exercise stress test (EST), thallium EST, or coronary angiography. Because a routine EST has a false-negative rate of 34%, only the last two investigations exclude coronary artery disease. At this stage, esophageal chest pain may be considered.

The concept of the esophagus as the origin of chest pain is not new. A century ago, Sir William Osler hypothesized that esophageal spasm represented one cause of chest pain in soldiers during wartime.

2. Does exclusion of coronary artery disease exclude all cardiac diagnoses?

No. Cardiac abnormalities other than coronary artery disease can be found in patients with chest pain, including mitral valve prolapse and microvascular angina. Exclusion of mitral valve prolapse requires echocardiography, whereas microvascular angina can be excluded only by the complicated procedure of measuring coronary artery resistance during stimulation with ergonovine and rapid atrial pacing.

However, studies suggesting that pain is no more common in patients with mitral valve prolapse or microvascular angina than in the general population question whether in fact these abnormalities produce pain. Even if they cause pain, the mechanism is unclear. Furthermore, the prognosis is excellent; the mortality rate is no different from that of the general population. Finally, a positive association between these abnormalities and esophageal motility disorders suggests a common or associated cause—either a generalized smooth muscle defect or heightened visceral nociception. It is therefore appropriate to search first for an esophageal cause that may be more common and more responsive to treatment.

3. Does history help to discriminate cardiac from esophageal chest pain?

Yes and no. A sharp pain localized by one finger at the fifth intercostal space in the midclavicular line with onset at rest in a 20-year-old woman is unlikely to be caused by coronary artery disease. Certain features in a patient's presenting history clearly help to differentiate between causes. However, many studies have shown sufficient overlap of all features to preclude certain diagnosis on the basis of symptoms alone. The description of pain by some patients with a known esophageal source and no cardiac disease mimics exactly the classical description of angina pectoris, including pain on exertion. One study from Belgium documented normal coronary angiograms in 25% of patients regarded by cardiologists as having myocardial ischemia on the basis of symptoms. In one-half of these patients, a probable esophageal cause could be identified.

4. What are the noncardiac causes of chest pain? How common are they?

Gastroesophageal reflux disease (GERD) is the most frequent esophageal cause for chest pain. In most studies it accounts for up to 50% of all cases of unexplained chest pain. Esophageal dysmotility can be diagnosed in a further 25–30%. Of the remaining 20–30%, one-third to one-half can be explained by a musculoskeletal source, such as costochondritis (Tietze's syndrome) and chest-wall pain syndromes. As discussed below, psychologic disorders, acting either independently or as cofactors, may account for a certain proportion of diagnoses. Panic disorder, in particular, must be considered.

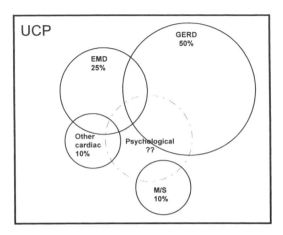

Venn diagram of the various causes of unexplained chest pain and their frequency of diagnosis. EMD=esophageal motility disorders, M/S=musculoskeletal.

5. Because GERD is the most likely diagnosis, is a therapeutic trial of acid suppression acceptable?
A therapeutic trial of acid suppression is relatively inexpensive and easy to perform and may avoid further investigation. However, adequate doses of appropriate medication must be used. Currently, we recommend omeprazole, 20 mg twice daily, or lansoprazole, 30 mg twice daily for a period of 4–8 weeks. This test produces both false-negative and false-positive results. Resistance to omeprazole has been described recently with persistent acid secretion in patients receiving the recommended dose. In such patients, the tendency is to conclude that GERD is not the cause of the pain. This conclusion cannot be made without ambulatory monitoring of intragastric and intraesophageal pH while the patient is taking omeprazole. False positives may occur because of the placebo response, especially in patients with unexplained chest pain (UCP). One study of patients with presumed esophageal chest pain noted a placebo response in 36%.

6. What is the most useful esophageal investigation?
Because GERD is the most common cause cause of UCP, it should be the first diagnosis considered. Ambulatory pH monitoring of the esophagus is the gold standard for diagnosing GERD and is the test most likely to yield a positive result in patients with UCP. For reasons outlined above, it remains the appropriate initial investigation even when a trial of acid suppression has appeared ineffective.

If ambulatory pH monitoring is abnormal (defined below), esophagogastroduodenoscopy (EGD) may be indicated to exclude the more serious consequences of GERD, such as esophagitis and Barrett's esophagus. EGDs should be considered when the total esophageal acid exposure for a 24-hour period exceeds 10% or when supine acid exposure is even slightly above normal limits. If ambulatory pH monitoring is negative, investigation for esophageal motility abnormalities is indicated.

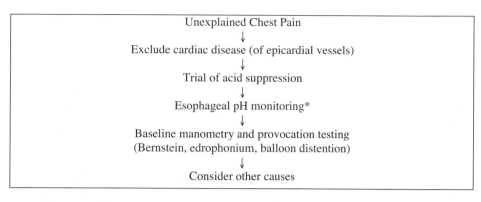

Unexplained Chest Pain
↓
Exclude cardiac disease (of epicardial vessels)
↓
Trial of acid suppression
↓
Esophageal pH monitoring*
↓
Baseline manometry and provocation testing
(Bernstein, edrophonium, balloon distention)
↓
Consider other causes

*EGD is indicated for severe reflux on pH monitoring (see text).

Other more unusual causes of UCP, such as biliary tract disease and gastric or duodenal ulceration, have been reported. Therefore, further gastrointestinal investigation, including abdominal ultrasound, occasionally is warranted, especially if anything in the history points to such diagnoses.

7. How is esophageal pH monitoring performed?

Esophageal pH monitoring is performed after an overnight fast. The level of acidity is measured by an intraesophageal electrode of either glass or antimony. The electrode is traditionally placed 5 cm above the upper border of the lower esophageal sphincter (LES), as previously determined by manometry.

An antimony electrode is thinner (2-mm diameter) but requires the use of a silver/silver chloride reference electrode attached to the patient's chest. The electrode is passed transnasally, and pH is recorded for a minimum of 16 hours. Patients are encouraged to follow their usual routine. Data are recorded on a portable recording device with marker buttons that allow the patient to indicate timing of meals, bedrest, and symptoms. A diary card is also completed to corroborate the timings. All information is transferred to a computer the next day and analysed both visually and by specialized software.

8. What abnormalities may be found with pH monitoring?

Analysis of the tracing includes both duration of esophageal acid exposure (i.e., time when esophageal pH is < 4) and its association with symptoms. Objective GERD is diagnosed when the duration of acid exposure for the total time or for either the upright or recumbent periods exceeds the 95th percentile of normal values. In our laboratory, these limits are defined as exposures to a pH <4 for 4.2% of the total time, 6.3% of the upright period, and 1.2% of the recumbent period.

Although an abnormal degree of acid reflux suggests the cause of the patient's symptoms, the case is not proved. For this reason, the occurrence of symptoms during the monitoring period is extremely valuable. If all symptoms coincide with episodes of acid reflux, the diagnosis can be made even when absolute levels of acid exposure do not exceed the 95th percentile of normal. Similarly, failure of all symptoms to correlate with acid reflux is strong evidence against reflux-related chest pain.

The situation is more difficult when some but not all symptoms are associated with episodes of acid reflux. Various "symptom indices" have been introduced in an attempt to quantify the symptom-reflux association. The simplest index uses the total number of symptoms as its denominator and symptoms that coincide with acid reflux as its numerator:

$$\text{Symptom Index} = \frac{\text{No. of symptoms occurring during acid reflux}}{\text{Total no. of symptoms during pH monitoring}}$$

A value of 50% or greater (e.g., two of four symptoms occur during episodes of acid reflux) is regarded as positive.

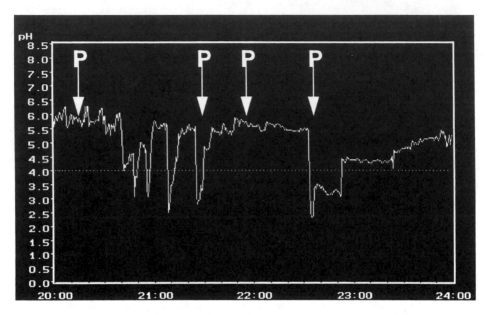

A 4-hour sample of esophageal pH monitoring. During this period 2 of 4 symptoms (P) were associated with episodes of acid reflux, yielding a symptom index of 2/4, 50%.

The approach to reflux-induced chest pain is no different from the normal management of GERD (see chapter 2).

9. If reflux has been excluded, which esophageal motility disorders may be found in patients with chest pain?

Abnormal esophageal motility disorders are found in 25–30% of patients with UCP. They may be categorized into the following types:

1. **Nutcracker esophagus** is the most common manometric abnormality. It has been so named because of the extremely high pressures generated during esophageal peristalsis. The diagnosis requires an average peristalic amplitude > 180 mmHg during 10 wet swallows over both distal channels.

2. **Nonspecific esophageal dysmotility** is a diagnostic category that includes patients with weak or poorly conducted waves; it is the second most common manometric finding.

3. **Diffuse esophageal spasm** is diagnosed when at least 2 of 10 water swallows produce simultaneous contractions instead of normal peristalsis. It also may be associated with other abnormalities, such as multipeaked or prolonged duration contractions. Although frequently suggested as a factor, this manometric pattern is found in only approximately 10% of patients with UCP and a diagnosis of esophageal manometric abnormality.

4. **An abnormally high basal LES pressure** is also on occasions associated with UCP.

5. **Achalasia** occasionally presents with chest pain and is further discussed in chapter 5. The relative frequencies with which these diagnoses are made in patients with UCP is illustrated on p. 24.

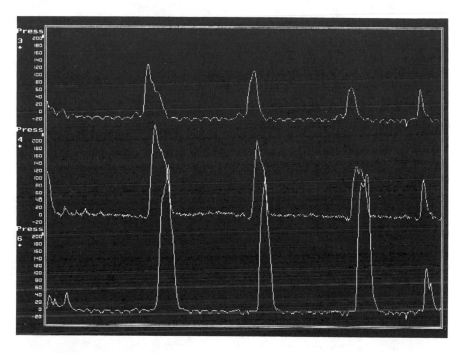

Nutcracker esophagus. The patient's average peristaltic amplitude was 250 mmHg. She experienced pain synchronous with most of her swallows.

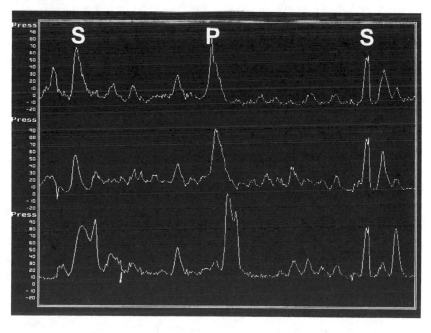

Diffuse esophageal spasm. Both simultaneous (S) and peristaltic (P) contractions occur in response to water swallows.

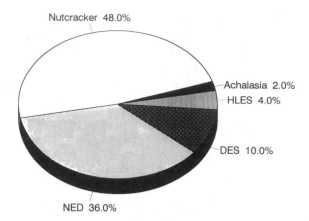

Relative frequencies of different diagnoses in patients with an esophageal dysmotility cause for chest pain. HLES=hypertensive lower esophageal sphincter, DES=diffuse esophageal spasm, NED = nonspecific esophageal dysmotility. (Adapted from Katz PO, Dalton CB, Richter JE, et al: Esophageal testing of patients with noncardiac chest pain or dysphagia. Results of three years' experience with 1161 patients. Ann Intern Med 106:593–597, 1987, with permission.)

10. What is the relationship of esophageal motility disorders to chest pain?

The mechanism or mechanisms by which motility disorders may cause chest pain are poorly understood. Specific mechanoreceptors have been identified in the esophageal mucosal and muscle layers. Abnormal contractions per se may be sufficient to stimulate these receptors and cause pain. Alternatively, the mechanoreceptors may be stimulated by esophageal distention, secondary to failed LES relaxation or retention of the bolus within the esophageal body. Yet another possibility is alteration of the threshold for esophageal sensation, which "tunes in" the patient to changes in esophageal pressure. A final theory is that high tension in the esophageal wall inhibits esophageal blood flow, causing myoischemia. However, the esophagus has an extensive blood supply, and contractions are unlikely to be sufficiently prolonged to induce ischemia. It is possible that dysmotility per se is not the cause of pain. Rather, it may represent an epiphenomenon that, like pain, is induced by another, unrecognized process.

11. What is esophageal provocation testing?

As with GERD, the demonstration of an esophageal motility disorder is not conclusive proof that dysmotility is the source of the pain. Occasionally, during routine manometry, a patient develops pain coincident with abnormal waveforms. More typically, the patient remains asymptomatic.

In an attempt to provoke symptoms, additional measures analogous to the exercise stress test used by cardiologists may be used to stimulate the esophagus. Options include acid infusion, pharmacologic stimulation, and intraesophageal balloon distention. For many years, it was believed that GERD caused chest pain by inducing dysmotility. Although this theory does not appear to be correct, acid perfusion (Bernstein test) is still used as a diagnostic test in UCP. Typically, 60–80 ml of 0.1 N hydrochloric acid are infused into the esophagus at a rate of 6–8 ml/min without the patient's knowledge, followed by a similar infusion of saline. The test is positive only if it (1) reproduces the patient's typical symptoms during acid infusion and (2) the symptoms disappear or do not recur during saline infusion. Chemoreceptors are present in the esophageal mucosa. Patients with a positive Bernstein test demonstrate acid sensitivity and should be treated for GERD-induced chest pain.

Various pharmacologic agents have been used to stimulate the esophageal smooth muscle. The current choice is the cholinesterase inhibitor, edrophonium (80 μg/kg intravenously). After injection, even in normal subjects, esophageal smooth muscle responds with increased peristaltic amplitude and duration during swallows. The test is regarded as positive only if it reproduces the patient's typical pain.

Intraesophageal balloon distention (IEBD) involves the graduated inflation of a latex balloon within the esophagus until pain or a predetermined maximal volume is reached. This test has the advantage of being specific to the esophagus and may reproduce the pain by a mechanism not dissimilar to that of dysmotility. It is positive only if it induces a patient's typical pain at an inflation volume that does not induce pain in normal subjects. Balloon distention has been shown to be reproducible and has the highest yield of all available provocation tests. Of the three forms of provocation, acid and edrophonium typically induce symptoms in 20% of cases; balloon distention has double this yield.

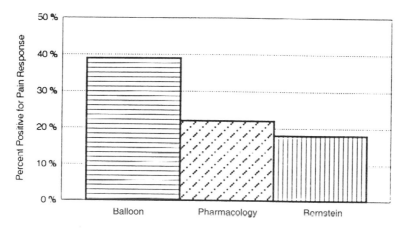

Mean values of seven reported studies of the percentage of positive pain response achieved by provocation with balloon distention, edrophonium and acid in patients with unexplained chest pain

12. How does provocation testing compare with combined ambulatory monitoring of both motility and pH?

All esophageal provocation tests have one major drawback—they are not physiologic. In an attempt to record the motility tracing during spontaneous chest pain, longer periods of manometry have been performed. Technology has now made it possible to record esophageal motility over a 24-hour period in an outpatient setting with minimal inconvenience to the patient.

Such a recording provides a large quantity of data. Currently, however, the best method of analysis is unclear. Whatever method is adopted, it must somehow compare the tracing during symptomatic and asymptomatic periods. Although ambulatory monitoring demonstrates the physiologic association between pain and dysmotility, it has not superseded the bank of esophageal provocation testing in most laboratories. Practitioners who have the most experience with ambulatory monitoring suggest that it should be reserved until after provocation testing has been performed and used only in patients with a positive result to delineate further the exact nature of the disorder.

13. What is visceral hypersensitivity? Define the "irritable esophagus."

Many patients with UCP have lower thresholds to pain in response to IEBD than normal individuals. This finding is believed to be due to visceral hypersensitivity or altered nociception. For some patients, the problem may not be due to abnormal contractions but rather to abnormal perception of normal events, including peristaltic muscle contractions, physiologic quantities of acid reflux, and luminal distention by air or food. Combined pH and manometric monitoring has identified patients who are sensitive to both acid and motility events. This condition is described as the irritable esophagus. Research analysing cerebral evoked potential responses to esophageal stimulation suggests that the abnormality is due to central interpretation rather than abnormal firing of the peripheral nociceptors.

14. Does UCP have a psychological component?

All disease has a psychological element; illness is interpreted according to personality and previous experiences. This appears to be particularly true for UCP. Psychological abnormalities have been documented in 34–59% of patients with UCP and are present in all of the causes described above. Psychiatric diagnoses are probably most prevalent in patients with esophageal motility disorders (84% in one study). Psychological factors therefore must be considered in the management of patients with UCP. Patients with high psychological scores are particularly susceptible to an initial placebo response to most medication, but in the long term treatment is ineffective; if such patients are identified, specific therapies can address the problem. Patients with high psychological scores have a worse prognosis and experience increased disability attributed to the illness.

15. What are the treatment options for nonreflux esophageal chest pain?

Medical treatment of diagnoses other than achalasia may target the motility abnormalities or the visceral hypersensitivity. Treatment for psychological factors also needs consideration. Finally, if medical therapy fails, more aggressive options may be considered for some patients.

Calcium antagonists, nitrates, and anticholinergic agents are the primary treatments aimed at motility dysfunction, i.e., the spastic component. If the pain is only occasional, short-acting nitrates or calcium antagonists may be taken sublingually as needed. More frequent episodes of chest pain are better managed by regular therapy with a long-acting preparation. Although such medications may have a dramatic effect on esophageal pressures, their symptomatic efficacy is often disappointing. Benzodiazepines both reduce skeletal muscular contractions and modify sensory pathways. They have had limited success in esophageal motility disorders. Of the other drugs used to modify sensory pathways, including anxiolytics and antidepressants, imipramine recently has been shown to be effective. It is used in low doses, suggesting that its effect is not due to antidepressant activity.

Various psychological and behavioral therapies have been tried in small-scale studies and are not readily available to most physicians. Relaxation therapy has met with some success and can easily be taught to patients who are willing to acknowledge the psychological element in their disease. Reassurance is available to all physicians. The ability to demonstrate a definite esophageal abnormality as an explanation for chest pain is of significant therapeutic benefit. The frequency of both pain and office visits for treatment of pain decreases after such reassurances.

Both empiric dilatation with a bougie and more specific targeting of a hypertensive LES with pneumatic dilatation have had limited success in some patients. Surgical myotomy may be of benefit to some patients with diffuse esophageal spasm or nutcracker esophagus. However, such interventions have documented complications and should be reserved for the rare severely disabled patient. The treatment of achalasia is discussed in chapter 5.

16. Can abnormal belching or aerophagia cause chest pain?

Esophageal distention, whether by reflux of gastric contents, impaction of a food bolus, or entrapment of air, can cause chest pain. In several well-documented cases gaseous esophageal distention was secondary to an abnormal belch reflex. Normally, the UES relaxes in response to distention with air. When this response fails, pain may occur.

17. What is the prognosis for patients with UCP?

Patients with UCP have a poor functional outcome. They consult a physician or visit the emergency department an average of twice per year, with an average of one hospitalization per year. If the patient does not have coronary artery disease, a positive esophageal diagnosis significantly reduces such behavior. Despite ongoing morbidity, the mortality rate of these patients (<1% per annum) is the same as for the general population.

BIBLIOGRAPHY

1. Cannon RO, Cattau EL, Yakshe PN, et al: Coronary flow reserve, esophageal motility, and chest pain in patients with angiographically normal coronary arteries. Am J Med 88:217–222, 1990.
2. Cannon RO III, Quyyumi AA, Mincemoyer R, et al: Imipramine in patients with chest pain despite normal coronary angiograms. N Engl J Med 330:1411–1417, 1994.
3. Castell DO: Chest pain of undetermined etiology. Proceedings of a symposium. Am J Med 92(Suppl 5A), 1992.
4. Castell DO, Castell JA (eds): Esophageal Motility Testing, 2nd ed. Norwalk, CT, Appleton & Lange, 1994.
5. Chambers J, Bass C: Chest pain and normal coronary anatomy: A review of natural history and possible etiologic factors. Progr Cardiovasc Dis 33:161–184, 1990.
6. Gignoux C, Bost R, Hostein J, et al: Role of upper esophageal reflex and belch reflex dysfunctions in noncardiac chest pain. Dig Dis Sci 38:1909–1914, 1993.
7. Katz PO, Dalton CB, Richter JE, et al: Esophageal testing of patients with noncardiac chest pain or dysphagia. Results of three years' experience with 1161 patients. Ann Intern Med 106:593–597, 1987.
8. Kemp HG, Kronmal RA, Vlietstra RE, Frye RL: Seven year survival of patients with normal or near normal coronary arteriograms: A CASS registry study. J Am Coll Cardiol 7:479–483, 1986.
9. Lam HG, Dekker W, Kan G, et al: Acute noncardiac chest pain in a coronary care unit. Evaluation by 24-hour pressure and pH recording of the esophagus. Gastroenterology 102:453–460, 1992.
10. Lantinga LJ, Sprafkin RP, McCroskery JH, et al: One-year psychosocial follow-up of patients with chest pain and angiographically normal coronary arteries. Am J Cardiol 62:209–213, 1985.
11. MacKenzie J, Belch J, Land D, et al: Oesophageal ischaemia in motility disorders associated with chest pain. Lancet ii:592–595, 1988.
12. Mayou R: Invited review: Atypical chest pain. J Psychosom Res 33:393–406, 1989.
13. Richter JE: The esophagus and noncardiac chest pain. In Castell DO (ed): The Esophagus. Boston, Little, Brown, 1992; pp. 715–746.
14. Richter JE, Barish CF, Castell DO: Abnormal sensory perception in patients with esophageal chest pain. Gastroenterology 91:845–852, 1986.
15. Semble E, Wise CM: Chest pain: A rheumatologist's perspective. South Med J 81:64–68, 1988.
16. Shapiro LM, Crake T, Poole-Wilson PA: Is altered cardiac sensation responsible for chest pain in patients with normal coronary arteries? Clinical observation during cardiac catheterisation. BMJ 296:170–171, 1988.
17. Smout AJPM, DeVore MS, Dalton CB, Castell DO: Cerebral potentials evoked by oesophageal distension in patients with non-cardiac chest pain. Gut 33:298–302, 1992.
18. Spears DF, Koch KL: Esophageal disorders in patients with chest pain and mitral valve prolapse. Am J Gastroenterol 81:951–954, 1986.
19. Vantrappen G, Janssens J, Ghillebert G: The irritable oesophagus—a frequent cause of angina-like pain. Lancet i:1232–1234, 1987.
20. Ward BW, Wu WC, Richter JE, et al: Long-term follow-up of symptomatic status of patients with noncardiac chest pain: Is diagnosis of esophageal etiology helpful? Am J Gastroenterol 82:215–218, 1987.

5. ACHALASIA

Donald J. Lazas, M.D., and Roy K.H. Wong, M.D.

1. Define achalasia.
Achalasia is a motor disorder of the esophagus characterized by loss of peristalsis and failure of the lower esophageal sphincter (LES) to relax completely with deglutition. The disease is an uncommon cause of dysphagia (incidence = 1:100,000); most patients present between the ages of 30 and 50 years.

2. What is the etiologic classification of achalasia?
Idiopathic achalasia comprises the largest etiologic category (95% of all documented cases). Familial achalasia represents 2–5% of all cases. Most cases of familial achalasia are transmitted horizontally and follow an autosomal recessive mode of inheritance in patients less than 4 years of age. Associated anomalies may include adrenocorticotrophic hormone insensitivity, alacrima, microcephaly, and nerve deafness. A small proportion of cases are associated with degenerative neurologic diseases such as Parkinson's disease and hereditary cerebellar ataxia.

3. What is the differential diagnosis of achalasia?
The differential diagnosis for achalasia usually begins with the broad differential diagnosis for dysphagia. Several diagnostic tests, including barium swallow, endoscopy, and esophageal manometry help to narrow the diagnostic possibilities. Once a diagnosis of achalasia is suggested, two major differential diagnosis must be revisited. Chagas' disease is a protozoal infection caused by the parasite *Trypanosoma cruzi*. This endemic disease should be suspected in patients who have travelled or lived in rural areas of South or Central America. Gastric adenocarcinoma involving the distal esophagus is the most common and worrisome disease that may mimic achalasia. Important clinical clues include age greater than 50 years, recent onset of dysphagia, and progressive weight loss. In highly suspicious cases, endoscopy with retroflex exam of the gastroesophageal junction should be performed and multiple biopsies obtained. Additional studies such as computed tomography (CT) and endoscopic ultrasound should be considered if the diagnosis of malignancy is still entertained.

4. What are the most common causes of secondary achalasia?
The table below lists several reported causes of secondary achalasia. These conditions may mimic the symptoms or manometric findings in patients with classic achalasia. A review of the list reveals the following broad diagnostic categories: malignancy, infection, infiltrative processes, inflammatory processes, and external compression.

Adenocarcinoma of stomach/distal esophagus	Chagas' disease
Adenocarcinoma of lung	Amyloidosis
Gastric or esophageal lymphoma	Anderson-Fabry's disease
Hepatocellular carcinoma	Esophageal leiomyomatosis
Hodgkin's disease	Eosinophilic esophagitis
Mesothelioma	Sarcoidosis
Prostate carcinoma	
Squamous cell carcinoma of esophagus	
Pancreatic pseudocyst	

5. How may the differential diagnosis influence the evaluation of patients with presumed achalasia?
Patients who are clearly at risk for adenocarcinoma involving the gastroesophageal junction should undergo endoscopic evaluation. Risk factors include (1) age greater than 50, (2) familial

history of carcinoma, (3) strong history of smoking and alcohol intake, (4) history of gastro-esophageal reflux, and (5) suspicious barium swallow.

6. Which six neuropathic lesions have been described in association with achalasia?

1. Loss of ganglion cell within the myenteric plexus of the distal esophagus
2. Degenerative changes of the vagus nerve
3. Quantitative and qualitative changes in the dorsal motor nucleus of the vagus
4. Marked decreases in small intramuscular nerve fibers
5. Paucity of vesicles in small nerve fibers
6. Occasional intracytoplasmic inclusions (Lewy bodies) in the dorsal motor nucleus of the vagus and myenteric plexus

7. What role does the LES play in the pathophysiology of achalasia?

The normal LES is in a relative state of constant contraction. Swallowing initiates esophageal peristalsis, which results in transient LES relaxation. The signals that initiate esophageal peristalis originate in the dorsal motor nuclei of the vagus and are transmitted through long preganglionic vagal neurons to shorter postganglionic inhibitory neurons located near the LES. Animal studies have shown that inhibitory neurons release vasoactive intestinal peptide (VIP) and/or nitric oxide on stimulation, which causes relaxation of LES smooth muscle through an intracellular pathway dependent on cyclic adenosine monophosphate (cAMP). In humans with achalasia, intravenous VIP infusion results in decreased LES pressure and improved LES relaxation, a finding that implicates a defective neurohumoral response of the inhibitory neuron. Furthermore, a paradoxical increase in LES pressure after intravenous infusion of cholecystokinin in patients with achalasia has been explained by a defect in the inhibitory neuron. In summary, it appears that the defect in LES relaxation results from dysfunction of the postganglionic inhibitory neurons.

8. What are the most common symptoms of achalasia?

Dysphagia is the most common symptom and is present in nearly all patients with achalasia. The interval from onset of symptoms to initial medical consultation is quite variable, ranging from 1–12 years. The second most commonly described symptom is regurgitation, which is due to accumulation of substances within the esophagus. Regurgitated food is described as undigested, nonbilious, and nonacidic. Patients frequently awaken at night with coughing or choking after an episode of regurgitation. Regurgitated fluid may have a characteristic white, foamy appearance and probably represents the nocturnal accumulation of saliva within the esophagus. Chest pain and heartburn occur with a similar frequency (in approximately 40% of patients). The pain is typically substernal and described as squeezing or pressurelike, with frequent radiation to the neck, jaw, or back. When the symptom of heartburn is present, achalasia may be misdiagnosed as gastroesophageal reflux. Achalasia-associated heartburn, however, does not occur postprandially and usually is not relieved by antacids.

9. Do patients with achalasia have dysphagia for solids, liquids, or both?

Most patients with achalasia have dysphagia for both solids and liquids. This finding agrees with the classic teaching that motility disturbances of the esophagus are manifested by symptoms of both solid and liquid dysphagia. In achalasia, however, the initial symptom is usually dysphagia for solids; liquid dysphagia occurs later in the clinical course.

10. Do patients with achalasia experience weight loss?

Weight loss is noted in as many as 85% of patients diagnosed with achalasia and is a good indicator of disease severity. The combination of progressive dysphagia and weight loss may mimic the clinical presentation of esophageal carcinoma. Weight gain after treatment correlates well with the degree of improvement in esophageal emptying.

11. What other historical clues are helpful in diagnosing achalasia?
Patients with achalasia report a progressive increase in the time that it takes to consume a meal. They characteristically drink a large volume of liquid during meals to assist in clearing food from the esophagus. Some patients report that consumption of carbonated beverages and warm liquids improves symptoms of dysphagia. Another technique that relieves symptoms is to perform the Valsalva maneuver while the patient maintains an upright posture in the head-back position.

12. List the complications of achalasia.

- Bezoar of the esophagus
- Distal esophagus diverticulum
- Esophageal foreign body
- Esophageal squamous cell carcinoma
- Esophageal varices
- Esophagocardiac fistula
- Neck mass (bullfrog neck)

- Pneumopericardium
- Pulmonary *Mycobacterium fortuitum*
- Postmyotomy Barrett's esophagus
- Stridor with upper airway obstruction
- Submucosal dissection of the esophagus
- Suppurative pericarditis

Some of the potential complications, such as pulmonary aspiration and bezoar formation, result from the accumulation of food and secretions within the aperistaltic esophagus. In longstanding achalasia, the esophagus may become massively dilated; a neck mass or stridor may result from local compression of the upper airway. As the esophagus dilates, thinning of the wall may predispose to microperforation, resulting in submucosal dissection, pneumopericardium, suppurative pericarditis, or fistula formation. Squamous cell carcinoma of the esophagus appears to occur with increased frequency in patients with achalasia. One prospective study found an overall incidence of 3.4 cancers per 1000 patient years (33-fold increase compared with controls).

13. What are the roles of the barium esophagram and upper endoscopy in the evaluation of patients with possible achalasia?
The barium esophagram is often performed early in the evaluation of achalasia; it is the preferred initial study in all patients presenting with dysphagia. The scout film of the chest may reveal an air fluid level in the mediastinum that represents retained food material in the esophagus. Plain radiographs also may reveal mediastinal widening without a gastric air bubble. Barium images may demonstrate a dilated, tortuous proximal esophagus with tapering and narrowing of the distal esophagus. This characteristic "bird-beak" appearance is found in patients with longstanding symptoms. Endoscopy is recommended in most patients with achalasia, especially in patients at risk for esophageal malignancy (age greater than 50, history of alcohol or tobacco use), patients with reflux symptoms, and patients in whom pneumatic dilation is considered. Most often the esophageal mucosa appear normal, but retained food may cause mucosal abnormalities such as erythema and superficial ulcerations in the distal esophagus. Resistance may be encountered at the gastroesophageal junction, but the endoscope usually passes with gentle forward pressure. A careful retroflexed examination of the gastric cardia and gastroesophageal junction should be performed, and biopsies of any suspicious mucosal lesions must be done to exclude malignancy. A hiatal hernia may have clinical significance; one study showed an added risk of perforation during pneumatic dilation.

14. How does esophageal manometry contribute to the diagnostic evaluation of possible achalasia?
Esophageal manometry confirms the diagnosis of achalasia and definitively distinguishes it from other esophageal motor disorders. Characteristic manometric findings include (1) hypertensive LES, (2) incomplete LES relaxation, and (3) aperistalsis of the esophageal body. Although the majority of patients exhibit a hypertensive resting LES pressure, occasionally the resting LES pressure is normal. In 70% of cases, the LES relaxes incompletely with deglutition. The remaining 30% demonstrate complete relaxation, but the duration of relaxation is shorter than normal. In normal subjects, swallowing induces orderly peristaltic contractions that propagate from the proximal esophagus to the LES. Peristalsis is absent in achalasia and is replaced by nonperistaltic,

simultaneous muscle contractions of the esophageal body. Of importance, distal esophageal obstruction from malignancy or previous antireflux surgery may produce manometric findings identical to those of achalasia. Individual manometric findings listed above may be seen in patients with isolated hypertensive LES, esophageal spasm, collagen vascular diseases, and scleroderma.

15. What are the available treatment options for patients with achalasia?

Treatment options include pharmacologic therapy, pneumatic balloon dilation of the LES, surgical myotomy, and intrasphincteric injection therapy.

16. How is pneumatic dilation performed?

Preparation for pneumatic dilation includes a 12–16 hour fast. Antibiotic prophylaxis is indicated in the appropriate clinical setting because of the >50% incidence of bacteremia after esophageal dilation. The procedure is initiated with an endoscopic exam, and the esophagus and stomach are cleared of all retained secretions, thus minimizing the risk of aspiration during the procedure. A guidewire is inserted through the endoscope and positioned in the antrum under fluoroscopic guidance. The guidewire is maintained in position while the endoscope is withdrawn. The dilator is then passed over the guidewire, and the bag is centered at the point at which the diaphragms converge. As the bag is slowly inflated, an indentation or waist is created by the LES. Repositioning of the dilator may be necessary to ensure that the waist is located in the center of the bag. Accurate positioning of the bag is extremely important to ensure that the 3-cm long LES is maximally ruptured by the dilation. Once centered, the bag is rapidly inflated and held in place for 60 seconds. Air is inflated until the bag is fully expanded and the waist deformity is obliterated (7–8 psi). Most experts now favor the use of the graduated technique, which uses serial dilations with bags ranging in diameter from 3.0–4.0 cm. Treatment is initiated with the smallest bag; increasing sizes are used in accordance with clinical response.

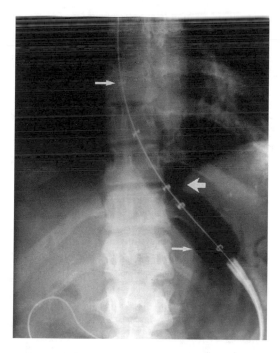

Pneumatic dilation of the LES in a patient with achalasia. The proximal and distal aspects of the bag are marked with radiodense bands (small arrows). The two central radiodense bands mark the center of the bag. The waist (large arrow) indicates the position of the LES on which the bag is centered before full inflation.

17. How effective is graded pneumatic dilation in treating achalasia?

The overall success rate in recent series has ranged from 86–100%. Initial success with the smallest bag (3.0 cm) is >60%. Patients are treated with increasing bag sizes if their symptoms are unresponsive or recur. Eventually >90% of patients have a good to excellent response, as measured by improvement in the dysphagia score. The need for redilation depends on the size of the last bag used; reported rates of redilation are 38%, 21%, and 7% for dilators of 3.0, 3.4, and 4.0 cm, respectively. The overall long-term response is >80%.

18. How is the efficacy of pneumatic dilation determined?

Improvement in dysphagia and weight gain are the two most important indicators of successful dilation. Dysphagia may not improve immediately because of the edema and inflammation due to the trauma of dilation. A postdilation decrement in LES pressure of >50% correlates with symptomatic improvement and also has been shown to predict long-term outcome.

19. Do certain subgroups of patients respond more favorably to pneumatic dilation?

Several authorities have noted that older patients (>50 years) respond significantly better than younger patients. A longer history of dysphagia may also be predictive of a better response to pneumatic dilation. From 2–5% of patients with achalasia have a hiatal hernia; such patients respond well to a single dilation.

20. What are the complications of pneumatic dilation? How are they diagnosed and managed?

The goal of pneumatic dilation is to generate a controlled tear of the LES musculature. An unfortunate but predictable complication is esophageal perforation. Although the incidence of esophageal perforation has ranged from 0–15%, most studies report rates of 0–4%. The decreasing incidence of esophageal perforation may relate to the use of fixed-size polyethylene dilators and the implementation of graded pneumatic dilation. Severe chest pain occurs frequently during dilation but usually resolves within 5 minutes after the procedure is completed. Persistent chest pain is an ominous sign and the first clinical clue to free esophageal perforation. Other clinical hallmarks include fever, diaphoresis, tachycardia, and shock. As a precaution, gastrografin swallow and a barium swallow are performed immediately after the procedure with the patient positioned at 45° on the fluoroscopy table. The radiologic findings associated with mucosal disruption are (1) linear mucosal tears, (2) contained perforations that penetrate beyond the muscular wall, (3) mucosal diverticular outpouchings, and (4) free perforation into the mediastinal, pleural, or peritoneal cavity. Mucosal tears and diverticula require only symptomatic monitoring. Contained perforations usually can be managed conservatively with nasogastric suction, no oral intake, and intravenous antibiotics. Free esophageal perforations, on the other hand, require immediate thoracic surgery.

21. What surgical treatment options are available?

The most commonly performed surgical procedure for the treatment of achalasia is the modified Heller myotomy in which a single, anteriolateral, longitudinal incision is made through the LES musculature. A critical aspect is the length of the myotomy. Enough muscle must be incised to relieve dysphagia, but some LES function must be preserved to prevent iatrogenic gastroesophageal reflux. The incidence of gastroesophageal reflux after myotomy ranges from 3–52%. Some surgeons perform longer myotomies together with an antireflux procedure to maximize relief of dysphagia and to avoid reflux. Significant improvement in dysphagia is reported in > 80% of patients undergoing myotomy. Of interest, dysphagia tends to worsen over time, thus paralleling the trend after pneumatic dilation. Recently, laparoscopic esophagomyotomy has been introduced as a less invasive surgical alternative. Initial series have reported good results in >80% of patients. The results, however, must be considered preliminary until larger series with extended follow-up are available.

22. Compare pneumatic dilation and surgery for treatment of achalasia.
No randomized control trials compare pneumatic dilation with myotomy in the initial treatment of achalasia. Although both procedures offer similar long-term efficacy in >80% of patients, pneumatic dilation offers several advantages as a first-line treatment:

1. Pneumatic dilation is far less invasive and does not entail the major operative risk of esophagomyotomy. Older patients with associated comorbid illness, who may have substantial surgical risk, respond most favorably to pneumatic dilation.

2. Treatment with pneumatic dilation is not complicated by gastroesophageal reflux, a problem that occurs in up to 50% of patients after esophagomyotomy. Some develop erosive esophagitis and stricture formation.

3. Cost comparison analysis has shown that pneumatic dilation is one-half as costly as esophagomyotomy, an important factor in the era of medical cost containment. Pneumatic dilation therapy is unsuccessful in 10–15% of patients; these patients should be referred for surgery.

23. What pharmacologic measures are effective in the treatment of achalasia?
Studies have shown that nifedipine and isosorbide dinitrate may improve symptoms in achalasia. Improvement in radionuclide esophageal emptying and a reduction in LES pressure have also been demonstrated. No study, however, has reported substantial weight gain in patients treated with pharmacologic agents. The aggregate clinical experience indicates that pharmacotherapy should be used as a temporizing measure before more definitive treatment.

24. Are any new treatment modalities available?
Intrasphincteric injection of botulinum toxin is currently under evaluation as a primary treatment of achalasia. An open-label, uncontrolled pilot trial in humans demonstrated significant improvement in symptoms and a substantial reduction in LES pressure. The response was sustained for 12 months in more than one-half of treated patients. Profound inhibition of acetylcholine release is the proposed mechanism for the smooth muscle relaxation. Placebo-controlled trials are needed to validate preliminary data.

BIBLIOGRAPHY

1. Eckardt VF, Aignherr C, Bernhard G: Predictors of outcome in patients with achalasia treated by pneumatic dilation. Gastroenterology 103:1732–1738, 1992.
2. Kadakia SC, Wong RKH: Graded pneumatic dilation using Rigiflex achalasia dilators in patients with primary esophageal achalasia. Am J Gastroenterol 88:34–38, 1993.
3. Pai GP, Ellison RG, Rubin JW: Two decades of experience with modified Heller's myotomy for achalasia. Ann Thorac Surg 38:201–204, 1984.
4. Pasricha PJ, Ravich WJ, Hendrix TR, Kalloo AN: Treatment of achalasia with intrasphincteric injection of botulinum toxin. Ann Intern Med 121:590–591, 1994.
5. Richter JE: Surgery or pneumatic dilatation for achalasia: A head-to-head comparison. Now are all the questions answered? Gastroenterology 97:1340–1341, 1989.
6. Traube M: On drugs and dilators for achalasia. Dig Dis Sci 36:257–259, 1991.
7. Wong RKH, Maydonovitch CL: Achalasia–new knowledge about an old disease. Semin Gastrointest Dis 3(3):156–165, 1992.
8. Wong RKH: Achalasia. In Bayless MD (ed): Current Therapy in Gastroenterology and Liver Disease, 4th ed. St. Louis, Mosby, 1994, pp. 64–68.
9. Wong RKH, Maydonovitch CL: Achalasia. In Castell DO (ed): The Esophagus, 2nd ed. Boston, Little, Brown, 1995.

6. ESOPHAGEAL CANCER

Albert G. Fedalei, M.D., and Shailesh C. Kadakia, M.D.

1. Are all esophageal cancers the same?

No. Esophageal cancer can be divided into squamous cell carcinoma and adenocarcinoma. The esophagus is normally lined in its entirety by a nonkeratinized stratified squamous epithelium. Squamous cell carcinoma used to represent 95% of all esophageal cancers, but over the past 10–15 years the incidence of adenocarcinoma of the esophagus has risen dramatically. Adenocarcinoma accounts for one-third or more of esophageal cancers. The vast majority arise in areas of heterotopic columnar mucosa, primarily Barrett's epithelium. A small number probably arise from the columnar mucosa of the esophageal mucous glands. Esophageal cancer is one of the most lethal malignancies with a grim long-term prognosis. The 5-year survival rate is only 3–6% and is not affected by tumor histology or degree of differentiation. There are several reasons for the poor prognosis: (1) by the time a patient becomes symptomatic, the tumor is advanced; (2) even small tumors spread early via the rich submucosal lymphatics; (3) and because the esophagus has no serosa, unlike most of the tubular GI tract, direct extension of tumor into the mediastinum and surrounding structures is common.

2. How common is esophageal cancer?

Esophageal cancer is one of the most common cancers worldwide but relatively uncommon in North America and Western Europe. Over 10,000 new cases are diagnosed in the United States each year, and esophageal cancer accounts for about 4% of all cancer deaths. There is a large variation in prevalence between sexes, races, and geographic regions. In the United States the male-to-female ratio for esophageal cancer is 3:1. Black men are four times more likely to develop squamous cell carcinoma than white men. However, white men are at greatest risk for developing adenocarcinoma. In France the male-to-female ratio is 20:1, whereas it is 1:1 in many other countries. The prevalence is between 5 and 7 new cases of esophageal cancer per 100,000 in U.S. men. The prevalence varies dramatically, with 100–200 new cases per 100,000 population in high-risk areas such as Iran, China, India, and Sri Lanka. In Sri Lanka esophageal cancer is the most common GI neoplasm, whereas colon cancer is by far the most common GI neoplasm in North America. The Asian esophageal cancer belt encompasses an area from Iran through Afghanistan to Mongolia and northwest China, where the incidence of esophageal cancer is extremely high.

3. What factors predispose to developing esophageal cancer?

Alcohol consumption and tobacco use are the best known risk factors. Either one alone increases the risk of developing esophageal cancer, but together there is a synergistic effect well beyond the additive risk. Dietary factors also have been implicated, such as vitamin A and riboflavin deficiency. Trace minerals such as zinc and molybdenum, a cofactor in nitrate reductase, may be protective. The role of other antioxidants, such as vitamins C and E, is not well known. Dietary carcinogens such as nitrosamines and aflatoxins may play a contributory role. The custom of consuming pickled vegetables infested with certain molds has been implicated in Linxian, China, where the incidence of esophageal cancer is high. It has been observed that chickens fed with pickled vegetables also develop esophageal cancer. Several other medical conditions are associated with an increased risk of esophageal cancer, including lye ingestion injury or stricture, tylosis (a rare autosomal-dominant disorder manifest by hyperkeratosis of palms and soles), Plummer-Vinson syndrome (triad of iron deficiency anemia, achlorhydria, and upper esophageal web), longstanding untreated achalasia, prior mediastinal irradiation, celiac sprue, and chronic nonreflux esophagitis (in Asia).

4. How do patients with esophageal cancer present clinically?

Dysphagia is by far the most common presenting symptom and is present in most cases. The onset of dysphagia is usually gradual and progressive, occurring initially with solids and then progressing to include liquids. Meats, bread, and apples are the most common foods causing dysphagia initially. Many patients alter their eating habits either consciously or subconsciously and adjust to the progressive dysphagia by changing to softer foods or liquids. There is often a significant component of weight loss. Odynophagia also may occur, perhaps due to superimposed infection or pill esophagitis secondary to the obstruction. Constant retrosternal, epigastric, or back pain is sometimes seen and implies invasion of mediastinal structures. Hiccups also may occur and signify diaphragmatic involvement. Excessive salivation may result from the progressive esophageal stenosis. Hoarseness is a less common symptom and is associated with tumor involvement of the recurrent laryngeal nerve. Neurologic and muscular symptoms also may be present as a result of hypercalcemia, which usually results from a paraneoplastic process rather than from bone metastases. Pulmonary symptoms, generally seen later in the course of the disease, include recurrent pulmonary infections due to aspiration or esophagorespiratory fistula. Hematemesis may result from a friable, oozing tumor (coffee grounds) or erosion into a vessel (frank blood).

5. Are any laboratory studies helpful in diagnosing esophageal cancer?

No particular lab tests are helpful. Anemia may be normochromic-normocytic (due to chronic disease), microcytic (due to iron deficiency), or macrocytic (reflecting underlying alcohol abuse). Hypoalbuminemia may occur with malnutrition. Liver-associated enzymes may be elevated because of metastatic disease or alcohol consumption. No tumor markers are helpful in diagnosis or management.

6. Do other diseases mimic the presentation of esophageal cancer?

This question may be rephrased as what is the differential diagnosis of dysphagia? Dysphagia is never psychosomatic. New-onset dysphagia in anyone over the age of 40 years should be treated as esophageal cancer until proved otherwise. The most common cause of dysphagia that mimics cancer is peptic stricture. Usually the dysphagia is slowly progressive and associated with a history of frequent pyrosis. Esophageal rings and webs usually cause dysphagia intermittently over a long period. Esophagitis also may cause dysphagia, but usually only with solids; a history of frequent pyrosis and regurgitation is typical. Achalasia and other motility disorders also may cause dysphagia, but they are generally not progressive and not accompanied by weight loss; usually they are distinguishable from cancer by a careful history.

7. How is esophageal cancer diagnosed?

A double-contrast barium esophagram allows a tentative diagnosis of cancer in most patients. Findings consistent with malignancy include nodularity, irregular or asymmetric narrowing, ulceration, abrupt luminal angulation, and rigid or aperistaltic areas on real time or cine (see figure A on next page). Peptic strictures generally have a symmetric, smooth, and tapered appearance. Dilation may occur proximal to the tumor but is generally less pronounced than with peptic strictures or achalasia. Endoscopy is more sensitive than barium esophagram and allows tissue to be obtained for histologic diagnosis (see figure B on next page). The extent of luminal involvement can be assessed, and if at least seven biopsy specimens of a lesion are taken, the diagnostic yield is 98%. Subtle abnormalities of the mucosa on endoscopy may indicate early or superficial carcinoma. This warrants brushings for cytology as well as biopsy to sample more mucosa and to increase diagnostic yield.

8. How is esophageal cancer staged?

The current primary tumor–regional nodes–metastasis (TNM) staging system was formulated by the American Joint Committee on Cancer in 1987. Under this system Tis stands for carcinoma in situ not extending below the basement membrane; T1 invades the lamina propria or submucosa; T2 invades the muscularis propria; T3 invades the adventitia; and T4 invades adjacent structures. N and M are designated 1 or positive, 0 or negative, and X is not accessible.

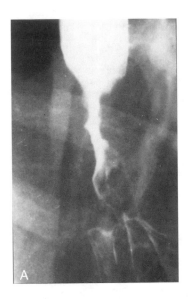
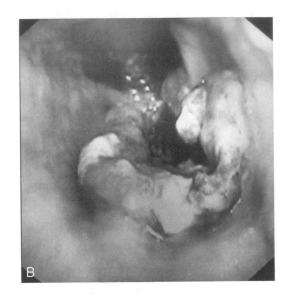

9. What should be done after the diagnosis of esophageal cancer has been made?

After a tissue diagnosis has been established, the next step is to determine whether the patient is a surgical candidate. If the patient is otherwise healthy enough to tolerate esophagectomy, the extent of malignant disease needs to be assessed. Although there is no established protocol, at the minimum a chest radiograph as well as a chest and abdominal CT scan probably should be performed. Such studies help to establish mediastinal and pulmonary involvement as well as to evaluate abdominal adenopathy or liver metastases. Endoscopic ultrasonography (EUS) is the most sensitive and accurate method for staging the primary esophageal tumor. It is technically difficult to master and not widely available but should be used in conjunction with studies such as CT whenever possible for optimal preoperative staging. Other procedures that may be useful in selected cases are bronchoscopy to rule out airway invasion, mediastinoscopy, and laparoscopy to rule out carcinomatosis of the liver or peritoneum. If the patient is deemed a surgical candidate based on staging, careful attention should be paid to nutrition. Significant malnutrition should be corrected; dilation to facilitate oral intake, nasogastric feeding, or total parenteral nutrition may be necessary. Pulmonary status should be assessed and optimized, because many patients have an extensive tobacco history. For this same reason a careful ear-nose-throat exam should be performed; 10–15% of patients with esophageal cancer have a synchronous cancer, usually of head, neck, or bronchial origin.

10. What features are helpful in predicting survival?

The primary determinants of survival are the size of the primary tumor at diagnosis and the presence of extraesophageal involvement. The mere fact that symptoms are present at presentation indicates a poor prognosis. In patients presenting symptomatically the 5-year survival rate is 2–8%. At the time of presentation 30–40% of patients already have evidence of advanced local disease or distant metastases and are therefore not operable for cure. Although 50–60% are believed to be operable for cure after staging, only 10% of these are resectable at the time of surgery. Tumors greater than 5 cm in size usually have metastasized to regional lymph nodes. Patients with tumors of less than 5 cm and no lymph node involvement have the best prognosis. The depth of invasion through the esophageal wall is the primary determinant of regional or local spread and therefore a major factor in predicting survival. Tumors limited to the submucosa have a 5-year survival rate of over 60%. If the muscularis propria is involved, the survival rate drops to 30%. Involvement of the adventitia by tumor reduces the 5-year survival rate to 10%. Early or superficially invasive cancers (limited to the mucosa and submucosa) carry an exceptionally good prognosis for surgical cure; a 5-year survival rate as high as 85% has been reported in China. In the United States early squamous cell cancers represent a small fraction of total cases. Vascular invasion indicates a poor prognosis and is associated with nodal metastases despite a small or superficial primary tumor. Because of the lack of a serosa, esophageal cancers directly invade adjacent structures with relative ease, including the trachea, bronchi, lungs, pleura, vascular structures, and diaphragm. Most squamous cell carcinomas occur in the middle third of the esophagus, followed by the lower third; a minority occur in the upper third. Histology (i.e., adenocarcinoma vs. squamous cell carcinoma) and degree of differentiation have no prognostic significance. Some evidence suggests that the degree of DNA aneuploidy may affect prognosis, at least in Asian populations.

11. How is esophageal cancer treated?

Surgery offers the best hope for cure but must be applied in a rational manner. The most common surgical procedure is esophagectomy with gastric pull-through and primary anastomosis. Occasionally colonic or small bowel interposition may be required for technical reasons to connect the esophageal and gastric remnants. In experienced hands the operative mortality ranges between 3 and 30% but may be higher in community hospitals. A significant amount of morbidity is associated with the procedure.

Surgical complications that cause death are primarily due to cardiac and pulmonary problems. Anastomotic leaks causing serious infection or death are not uncommon. A significant number of patients who would be surgical candidates based on staging are in too poor a state of health to tolerate the surgery. Close attention should be paid to optimizing nutrition, pulmonary status, and other active medical problems preoperatively. Radiation therapy, either palliative or curative, is another well accepted treatment.

Some studies have shown no difference in survival between surgery and radiation alone in patients who were considered operable by staging. There is no immediate mortality from radiation therapy, and treatment may be modified as side effects develop. Combined with the morbidity and mortality associated with surgery, this flexibility makes radiation therapy a frequent choice for treating squamous cell carcinoma of the esophagus. Radiation therapy may cause transient worsening of dysphagia early in treatment. Radiation esophagitis may develop with continued radiotherapy. Radiation therapy is much less effective for adenocarcinoma of the esophagus. Preoperative or postoperative radiation therapy does not seem to add any survival benefit over surgery alone. Over the past few years chemotherapy for squamous cell carcinomas has been shown to play a significant role.

12. What is the role of chemotherapy in treating esophageal cancer?

Cisplatin-based chemotherapy combined with radiation therapy has been shown to have a positive effect on survival when used preoperatively to reduce tumor burden. Patients with "sterilized" surgical specimens free of malignant cells after preoperative chemotherapy and radiation therapy have been shown to have enhanced disease-free survival after esophagectomy. In nonsurgical patients the combination of cisplatin chemotherapy and radiation therapy has been shown to be superior to radiation alone. In patients completing chemotherapy and radiation therapy without surgery, the 5-year survival rate has been reported to be 18% with squamous cell carcinoma; no patients with adenocarcinoma survived beyond 3 years.

13. What endoscopic modalities are available for palliation?

Severe dysphagia may be a major factor affecting quality of life. Bougie dilation with endoscopic or fluoroscopic assistance may be used for palliation, but the beneficial effects are often short-lived. Other modalities that reduce intraluminal tumor bulk, such as bipolar tumor probe application and endoscopic laser treatment, provide more prolonged results but at greater risk and expense. Photodynamic therapy uses an intravenously administered photosensitizing agent preferentially absorbed by tumor cells (e.g., hematoporphyrin). After administration the tumor is exposed intraluminally to low-energy laser light of a specific wavelength, which causes selective tumor cell death. Therapy is limited by cutaneous photosensitivity and is not generally available at present. Esophageal stenting with plastic or expandable metal stents is the treatment of choice for esophagorespiratory fistula. Dysphagia also may be treated with stenting, but this technique is more controversial and entails substantial risks. Complications are not uncommon and may be catastrophic (e.g., esophagoaortic fistula), especially in patients who have received prior radiation therapy. A percutaneous endoscopic gastrostomy (PEG) tube may be placed to facilitate nutrition in patients with severe dysphagia not amenable to other treatment modalities.

BIBLIOGRAPHY

1. Appleqvist P, Salmo M: Lye corrosion carcinoma of the esophagus: A review of 63 cases. Cancer 45:2655–2658, 1980.
2. Beahrs OH, Hensen DE, Hutter RV, Myers MH: Manual for Staging Cancer, 3rd ed. American Joint Committee of Cancer. Philadelphia, J. B. Lippincott, 1988.
3. Benrey J, Graham DY, Goyal RK: Hypercalcemia and carcinoma of the esophagus. Ann Intern Med 80:415, 1974.
4. Bogomoletz WV, Molas, G, Garet B, Potet F: Superficial squamous cell carcinoma of the esophagus. A report of 76 cases and review of the literature. Am J Surg Pathol 13:535–546, 1989.
5. Coordinating Group for Research of Esophageal Cancer in North China: The epidemiology and etiology of esophageal cancer in North China. Chin Med 1:167–183, 1975.
6. Day NE: The geographic pathology of cancer of the oesophagus. Br Med Bull 40:329, 1984.
7. Earlam R, Cunha-Melo JR: Oesophageal squamous cell carcinoma. II: A critical review of radiotherapy. Br J Surg 67:457, 1980.
8. Ellis FH: Current management of carcinoma of the esophagus. Compr Ther 19:219–19, 1993.
9. Galandiuk S, Hermann RE, Gassman JJ, Cosgrove DM: Cancer of the esophagus. The Cleveland Clinic experience. Ann Surg 203:101, 1986.
10. Geenen JE, Fleischer DE, Waye JD, et al (eds): Techniques in Therapeutic Endoscopy, 2nd ed. New York, Gower, 1992.
11. Graham DY, Schwartz JT, Cain CD, Gyorkey F: Prospective evaluation of biopsy number in the diagnosis of esophageal and gastric carcinoma. Gastroenterology 82:228, 1982.
12. Guojun H, Lingfang S, Dawei Z, et al: Diagnosis and surgical treatment of early esophageal carcinoma. Chin Med J (Engl) 94:229, 1981.
13. Harper PS, Harper RM, Howel-Evans AW: Carcinoma of the oesophagus with tylosis. Q J Med 39:317–333, 1970.
14. Herskovic A, Martz K, al-Sarraf M, et al: Combined chemotherpy and radiotherapy compared with radiotherapy alone in patients with cancer of the esophagus. N Engl J Med 326:1593–1598, 1992.
15. Iizuke T, Hirata K, Watanae H, Semba T: Factors controlling five-year survival in patients with esophageal carcinoma. Jpn J Clin Oncol 9:41–48, 1979.
15a. Kallimanis GE, Pradeep GK, Firas AH, et al: Endoscopic ultrasound for staging esophageal cancer, with or without dilation, is clinically important and safe. Gastrointest Endosc 41:540–546, 1995.
16. Lewis KJ, Riddell RH, Weinstein WM (eds): Gastrointestinal Pathology and Its Clinical Implications. New York, Igaku-Shoin, 1992.
17. Lightdale C, Botet J, Zauber A, Brennan M: Endoscopic ultrasonography (EUS) in the staging of esophageal cancer: Comparison with dynamic CT and surgical pathology. Gastrointest Endosc 36:191, 1990.
18. Mandard AM, Dalibard F, Mandard JC, et al: Pathologic assessment of tumor regression after preoperative chemoradiotherapy of esophageal carcinoma. Clinicopathologic correlations. Cancer 73: 2608–2616, 1994.
19. Maram ES, Kurland LT, Ludwig J, Brian DD: Esophageal carcinoma in Olmsted County, Minnesota, 1935–1970. Mayo Clin Proc 52:24, 1977.
20. Silverberg E, Boring CC, Squires TS: Cancer statistics 1990. Cancer 40:9, 1990.
21. Sleisenger MH, Fordtran JS (eds): Gastrointestinal Disease. Philadelphia, W. B. Saunders, 1993.
22. Sugimachi K, Koga Y, Mori M, et al: Comparative data on cytophotometric DNA in malignant lesions of the esophagus in the Chinese and Japanese. Cancer 59:1947–1950, 1987.
23. Wang HH, Antonioli DA, Goldman H: Comparative features of esophageal and gastric adenocarcinomas: Recent changes in type and frequency. Hum Pathol 17:482, 1986.
24. Wienbeck M, Berges W: Oesophageal lesions in the alcoholic. Clin Gastroenterol 10:375, 1981.
25. Wilke H, Siewert JR, Fink U, Stahl M: Current status and future directions in the treatment of localized esophageal cancer (review). Ann Oncol 5 (Suppl):26–32, 1994.
26. Wolfe WG, Vaughn AL, Seigler HG, et al: Survival of patients with carcinoma of the esophagus treated with combined-modality therapy. J Thorac Cardiovasc Surg 105:749–55, 1993.

7. PILL-INDUCED AND CORROSIVE INJURY OF THE ESOPHAGUS

Matthew Bachinski, M.D., and James Walter Kikendall, M.D., F.A.C.P.

1. Who is affected by pill-induced esophageal injury?

Anyone of any age who ingests caustic pills is susceptible to pill-induced injury. Reported cases range from 5–89 years old. Women outnumber men by a ratio of 1.5:1. It is not uncommon for pills to stick in a normal esophagus during transit. One study showed that 36 of 49 normal subjects who assumed a supine position after swallowing a round, nonsticky barium tablet with 15 ml of water retained the tablet in the esophagus for 5–45 minutes. A more sticky gelatin tablet remained in the esophagus for more than 10 minutes in over one-half of normal subjects who ingested the pill in a supine position. Esophageal dysmotility or prior esophageal lesions such as rings or strictures are clearly not required for pill-induced injury.

2. What factors contribute to esophageal retention of pills?

Esophageal clearance is determined by several factors, some of which can be modified to decrease the risk of pill-induced injury. Upright posture improves esophageal clearance of pills. The volume of water ingested with pills also affects clearance, although no study has identified the volume required to ensure passage through the esophagus. One study showed that 11 of 18 patients retained a barium pill swallowed with 15 ml of water compared with 3 of 18 who swallowed the pill with 120 ml of water. Other partially modifiable factors include structural abnormalities such as rings or strictures, which can be dilated as needed. Abnormal esophageal motility sometimes is improved with pharmacologic agents, but motility usually is normal in patients with pill-induced injury who are evaluated with formal esophageal manometry. Taking the pill with inadequate fluid and lying down immediately afterward are the only identifiable risk factors in most patients suffering pill-induced injury.

3. What are the risk factors for pill-induced injury?

Anyone who takes a caustic pill is at risk, but some patients are at particular risk for severe pill-induced esophageal injury, including those with structural abnormalities of the esophagus, both pathologic (stricture, tumor, ring) and physiologic (hiatal hernia, narrowing of the esophagus secondary to compression from the left atrium, aortic arch, left mainstem bronchus). Cardiac disease is a risk because of esophageal compression by a dilated left atrium and frequent use of inherently caustic medications (aspirin, potassium chloride, quinidine). Patients who have undergone thoracotomy are at increased risk because they are bedridden and may develop adhesions and fibrosis that trap the esophagus between the aorta and the vertebral column, making it more susceptible to compression by an enlarged left atrium and thus decreasing esophageal clearance. Supine positioning during pill ingestion impairs esophageal clearance and places patients at risk. The stickiness of the pill surface, the inherent caustic nature of certain drugs, and the volume of liquid consumed with pills affect risk. Elderly patients and patients with underlying gastroesophageal reflux disease (GERD) are at increased risk. GERD may cause a more acid environment; because many drugs, including nonsteroidal antiinflammatory drugs (NSAIDs), are weak acids, their absorption into tissues is increased in an acidic environment.

4. Describe the typical presentation of patients with pill-induced injury.

The typical patient has no prior history of esophageal disease and presents with the sudden onset of retrosternal pain, which may have awakened the patient from sleep (particularly if pills were ingested with little liquid just before or while lying down) and may be exacerbated by swallowing. The pain may be mild or so severe that swallowing is impossible. The pain typically increases over the first 3–4 days before gradually subsiding. Painless dysphagia is uncommon (20%) and may suggest an alternative diagnosis. Less common symptoms and signs include dehydration, weight loss, fever, and hematemesis. Patients with preexisting esophageal problems such as GERD frequently present with worsening symptoms of heartburn, regurgitation, and dysphagia.

5. How is the diagnosis of pill-induced esophageal injury made?
The diagnosis of pill-induced esophageal injury may be suspected on the basis of history alone when typical symptoms suddenly appear soon after the ingestion of a pill known to cause esophageal injury. In a typical and uncomplicated case, an invasive diagnostic test may not be required, and the diagnosis can be made on the basis of history and physical exam. A diagnostic study is indicated when symptoms are severe, persist longer than 3–4 days, have atypical features, or suggest a complication (stricture, hemorrhage) or when the history suggests an alternative diagnosis (foreign body obstruction, infectious esophagitis in an immunocompromised host). Upper endoscopy is the most sensitive test; results are abnormal in almost all cases of pill-induced esophageal injury. In addition, it allows the most accurate assessment of alternate diagnoses such as severe GERD, infectious esophagitis, or malignancy.

6. What does the typical pill-induced lesion look like at time of endoscopy?
The typical lesion of pill-induced esophageal injury is one or more discrete ulcers with normal surrounding mucosa. Ulcers range in size from pinpoint to circumferential lesions involving the entire esophagus and may be several centimeters long. Ulcers may have local surrounding inflammation. Pill fragments have been seen in ulcer craters.

7. What are the potential complications of pill-induced esophageal ulcers?
Typical ulcers involve only the mucosa, but deeper lesions may occur. Torrential hemorrhage has resulted from erosions into vascular structures, including the left atrium. Cases with penetration to the mediastinum have been reported. Deep circumferential ulceration may result in formation of a circumferential fibrotic stricture, but this occurs in less than 10% of reported cases. Probably the true incidence of stricture formation is much less, because severe or atypical cases are more likely to be reported.

8. What pills are frequently implicated or are particularly injurious?
Antibiotic pills are frequent offenders, accounting for more than one-half of all reported cases of pill-induced esophageal injury, because of the large number of prescriptions written and the caustic nature of the pills themselves. Doxycycline and tetracycline accounted for 293 of 454 reported cases of pill-induced esophageal injury in one recent review. Although frequent offenders, antibiotics rarely cause complicated injury to the esophagus. Patients with antibiotic-associated injury almost always present with acute, severe pain and local, circumscribed tissue injury due to mucosal ulceration. The ulceration is believed to be secondary to a single trapped pill.

Cardiac and vascular medications, including antihypertensive and antiarrhythmic, compose a large group of caustic drugs. Quinidine alone has been reported in 13 cases of pill-induced injury; 7 of the 13 patients later developed strictures, making quinidine a particularly injurious substance. An unusual feature of quinidine-induced injury is its tendency to form profuse, irregular exudate that is sufficiently thick and adherent, appearing as a filling defect suggestive of carcinoma on barium swallow. On endoscopy the exudate can be washed away and has not been shown to be predictive of late fibrotic stricture formation.

Antiinflammatory medications are relatively uncommon agents in pill-induced esophageal injury. A recent review reported only 71 cases of injury attributable to this class of drugs. In part because they are so widely prescribed, 22 different antiinflammatory agents have been reported to cause injury, but approximately 45% of these reports are secondary to aspirin, doleron, and indomethacin. No hallmark lesion is associated with NSAIDs.

Emepronium bromide, an anticholinergic pill not available in the United States, deserves separate mention because of the frequency with which it produces esophageal injury and because of the interesting mechanism of injury. A recent review reported that it was second only to doxycycline in the number of reported cases of esophageal injury. Emepronium, an anticholinergic often administered to relieve urinary frequency in patients with bladder irritability, is particularly likely to be taken at bedtime with little fluid. The standard-release preparation is formulated with a hydrophilic agent intended to cause rapid tablet break-up when exposed to water. If the pill is swallowed with insufficient water, the hydrophilic agent is attracted to and adheres to the moist esophageal mucosa, leading to mucosal desiccation and injury. In addition, the systemic anticholinergic effects of reduced amplitude to esophageal contractions and decreased salivation may decrease esophageal clearance and predispose patients to esophageal retention of subsequent doses.

9. What other mechanisms have been proposed to explain pill-induced injury?

Animal studies have demonstrated that certain pills placed in direct contact with esophageal tissue can cause ulceration. This finding has been verified in humans by esophagogastroduodenoscopy (EGD), which revealed an esophageal ulcer containing a retained pill and circumscribed to the location of the pill. It is believed that pills must be inherently caustic to cause injury. Local acid burn is proposed for pills (e.g., doxycycline, tetracycline, ascorbic acid, ferrous sulfate) that produce an acidic solution with a pH <3 when dissolved in 10 ml of water. Phenytoin dissolved in 10 ml of saliva raises the pH to 10.4, suggesting that it may cause an alkaline burn. Other proposed mechanisms of injury include induction of gastroesophageal reflux (theophylline and anticholenergics) and production of localized hyperosmolarity capable of tissue desiccation and vascular injury (potassium chloride). Finally, some medications appear to be absorbed locally into the esophageal mucosa, causing toxic intramucosal concentrations (doxycycline, NSAIDs, alprenolol).

10. What are the postulated mechanisms of NSAID-induced injury?

NSAIDs are used by 30 million people each day, and approximately 16% of patients report gastrointestinal side effects. Gastric injury is most common, although cases of esophageal injury are well-documented. In one study all patients with NSAID-induced esophageal injury who were tested with 24-hour pH monitoring had gastroesophageal reflux disease (GERD). In the presence of GERD associated with a pH < 4, NSAIDs may enter the mucosa and cause direct toxicity. NSAIDs may cause injury by inhibiting synthesis of mucosal prostaglandins. Prostaglandins are known to have a cytoprotective role in gastric mucosa, but it is unclear whether the same effect applies to esophageal mucosa. The role of the mucus and bicarbonate layer in protecting the esophagus is also unclear, but the deleterious effect of NSAIDs on the mucosal barrier of the stomach secondary to prostaglandin inhibition may also occur in the esophagus. Finally, NSAIDs may negatively affect lower esophageal sphincter pressure and function, thereby increasing GERD and potentiating their own absorption.

11. Where are the areas of physiologic narrowing of the esophagus?

The normal esophagus has areas, generally minor, of external compression and narrowing at the sphincters. Pills may be more likely to hang up and cause injury in these areas. External compression may be caused by bony prominence from the spinal column, which often worsens with age and degenerative spine disease. The aortic arch and the left mainstem bronchus may cause compression of the esophagus. The left atrium varies in size, depending on underlying heart disease, and may cause significant compression of the esophagus. Such compression is particularly troublesome because the medications often used to treat diseases associated with left atrial enlargement, such as potassium chloride in conjunction with diuretics and quinidine for atrial fibrillation, are particularly caustic agents.

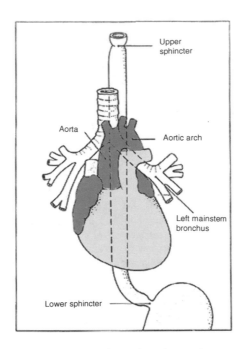

Areas of physiologic esophageal narrowing.

12. Does alcohol consumption play a role in pill-induced esophageal injury?

Alcohol appears to act synergistically with caustic agents to induce esophageal injury. In one study, healthy volunteers took 8 aspirins/day for 2 weeks. EGD showed no esophageal mucosal damage. After the same volunteers consumed a single dose of aspirin combined with alcohol, 33% had erythema and/or esophageal hemorrhage. Alcohol may affect the esophagus by interfering with esophageal clearance and thus prolonging aspirin contact with the mucosa. Alcohol is believed to decrease primary and secondary contractions of the esophagus.

13. What are the options for treating pill-induced esophageal injury?

Most cases of pill-induced injury heal without active intervention in 3 days to several weeks. Therapy starts with avoidance of the initial drug responsible for the injury and all other caustic drugs, when possible. When avoidance is not possible, every effort must be made to decrease the potential for reinjury by using elixir or other liquid preparations, administering medications in the upright position with at least 4 ounces of liquid, and maintaining an upright posture for at least 10 minutes after ingestion.

Medications that buffer acid, decrease production of acid, or create a barrier coat for the esophagus are frequently prescribed (antacids, H_2 blockers, sucralfate) but are of questionable value unless GERD contributes to symptoms. The use of topical anesthetics in various combinations (Bemylid—Benadryl, Mylanta, and Lidocaine in equal parts) may decrease symptoms, but their use is limited by potential systemic toxicity.

Patients with such severe symptoms that they cannot eat or drink require hydration. If symptoms persist, they may require parenteral nutrition and analgesia. Other supportive measures may also be required for treatment of complications (e.g., blood products for hemorrhage and antibiotics for bacterial superinfection).

Acute inflammatory stenosis may resolve spontaneously, but chronic stricture formation may require repeated esophageal dilation. Strictures that prove to be recalcitrant to repeated dilation may require surgical correction, but this is rare.

14. What is the epidemiology of caustic ingestion in the United States?

Chemical ingestion remains an important problem despite improvements in packaging (e.g., child-proof containers), product labelling and warnings. Approximately 26,000 caustic ingestions occur per year. Adolescents and adults who willfully ingest caustic agents as a suicidal gesture in general consume a larger volume and therefore have more serious injury than children, who ingest the agent accidentally and often expectorate most of it before swallowing. Children often have minimal esophageal damage, but their oral, pharyngeal, and laryngeal injury may be more severe. Approximately 80% of caustic ingestions occur accidentally in children less than 5 years of age, who most often consume household cleaners.

15. What are the common caustic agents? Where are they found?

Caustic agents are present in many common household products. The severity of the damage depends largely on the corrosive properties and concentration of the ingested agents. The caustic agents most often responsible for serious injury are the strong alkaline cleaning products, such as drain cleaners and lye soaps. Severe alkaline burns also result from the ingestion of disc batteries that contain concentrated sodium or potassium hydroxide. Concentrated acid compounds also cause severe injury but are not common household items; thus they are encountered less often. The severity of esophageal and gastric injury secondary to caustic ingestion depends not only on the concentration and corrosive properties of the agent but also on the quantity consumed.

Caustic Agents Found in Common Household Products

CLASS	CAUSTIC AGENT	PRODUCT CONTAINING AGENT
Strong alkalis	Ammonia	Cleaning products
	Lye (sodium hydroxide)	Clinitest tablets
	(potassium hydroxide)	Disc batteries
		Drain cleaners
		Nonphosphate detergents
		Paint removers
		Washing powders
Strong acids	Hydrochloric acid	Muriatic acid
		Soldering fluxes
		Swimming pool cleaners
		Toilet bowel cleaners
	Nitric acid	Gun barrel cleaners
	Oxalic acid	Antirust compounds
	Phosphoric acid	Toilet bowel cleaners
	Sulfuric acid	Battery acid
		Toilet bowel cleaners
Miscellaneous	Sodium hypochlorite	Liquid bleach

16. Lye (sodium hydroxide) is a common caustic ingestion. How has its formulation changed over the past 30 years? How has this change affected the pattern of injury?

Before the 1960s caustic ingestion frequently involved solid or crystalline lye products with concentrations > 50%. Such products were extremely corrosive and caused extensive damage on contact with the mucosa, but the immediate burning pain on contact with the oral mucosa often caused the victim to spit out the solid material. Injury was usually limited to the mouth, pharynx, and esophagus and rarely affected the stomach. Reports vary, but free esophageal perforation and mediastinitis were common complications. Such experiences led to the belief that lye injured the esophagus with relative sparing of the stomach compared with acids. This dictum did not hold true with concentrated liquid lye preparations, which can be swallowed more easily and quickly than solid lye. In the late 1960s such products were introduced as drain cleaners in concentrations of 25–36%, and they caused devastating injury. Complications included respiratory compromise, esophageal and gastric perforations, septicemia, and death. Patients who survived often developed esophageal stricture as a later complication of ingestion. By the mid 1970s highly concentrated liquid products had been replaced in the U.S. by moderately concentrated (<10%) liquid drain cleaners. If ingested in sufficient quantity, such products are strong enough to cause severe esophageal and gastric injury, including visceral perforation. More often a smaller volume is ingested, and the patient recovers from the acute injury; later, however, strictures may develop. Caustic materials currently available for industrial usage are often much more concentrated than household products. Children occasionally encounter cleaning products containing highly concentrated lyes or acids, particularly around farms, construction sites, and swimming pools.

17. Describe the pathophysiology of acute alkali esophagitis.
      When tissue is exposed to strong alkali, the immediate result is liquefactive necrosis, the complete destruction of entire cells and their membranes. Cell membranes are destroyed as their lipids are saponified and cellular proteins are denatured. Thrombosis of the local blood vessels also contributes to tissue damage. Tissue destruction and organ penetration progress rapidly until the alkali is diluted and neutralized by dilution with tissue fluids. Transmural necrosis of organs exposed to strong alkali occurs rapidly. Experimental exposure of cat esophagus to 5 ml of a 30.2% sodium hydroxide solution for only 3 seconds causes perforation and impending death.
      The severity of caustic injury to the esophagus can be graded as first-, second-, or third-degree, using a system similar to that for classifying burns of the skin. The table below correlates the degree of burn with the endoscopic and pathologic findings. Endoscopy within the first 24 hours may underestimate the severity of esophageal injury.

Degree of Esophageal Injury and Associated Findings

DEGREE	ENDOSCOPIC FINDINGS	PATHOLOGY
First	Erythema and edema of the mucosa only	Sloughing of the superficial layers of the mucosa
Second	Ulceration with membranous exudate	Ulcer extends through the mucosa and submucosa to muscularis tissue
Third	Deep ulceration with penetration, black discoloration	Transmural injury, erosions into mediastinum or peritoneal structures

18. What are the three phases of injury and healing associated with lye?
Experimental lye injury may be divided into three phases: the acute or liquefaction phase (approximately days 1–4), the subacute or reparative phase (days 5–14), and the scar retraction or cicatrization phase. The acute phase is characterized by liquefactive necrosis, vascular thrombosis, and progressive inflammation. Mucosal erythema and edema are intense, but even severely injured tissue may not exhibit sloughing or ulceration during the first 24 hours. The hallmark of the subacute or reparative phase is sloughing of the necrotic areas with obvious ulceration and development of granulation tissue. Fibroblasts appear, and collagen deposition peaks during the second week but may continue for months. Mucosal reepithelialization begins, and the wall of the esophagus is thinnest and most vulnerable during this period. The cicatrization phase, which begins about the end of the second week, is marked by continued proliferation of fibroblasts and further deposition of collagen. The recently formed collagen contracts both circumferentially and longitudinally, resulting in esophageal shortening and stricture formation. Reepithelialization is generally complete by 1–3 months after lye ingestion. The table below demonstrates the phases of lye injury. The evolution and outcome of a given lye ingestion involve a spectrum of events that may not follow the exact time course outlined above.

Phases of Lye Injury

PHASE	TIMING	PATHOLOGY	COMMENTS
Acute	Days 1–4	Liquefactive necrosis	Sloughing or ulcer not apparent <24 hr
		Vascular thrombosis	
		Increase inflammation	
Subacute	Days 5–14	Sloughing of casts	Esophageal wall is thinnest
		Granulation tissue	
		Fibroblast begin	
		Collagen deposition	
Cicatrization	Day 15–3 months	Fibroblasts proliferate	Reepithelialization in 1–3 months
		Further collagen deposition	Stricture formation

19. Contrast the effects of acid ingestion with the effects of lye ingestion.

Concentrated acid solutions cause more severe pain on contact with the oropharyngeal mucosa than liquid alkalis, which often are swallowed before protective mechanisms can take effect. This property tends to limit the amount of acid that is ingested by accident. In past decades it was often noted that acid caused the greatest damage in the stomach, whereas alkali preferentially injured the esophagus. This observation was largely due to the fact that granular or solid lye usually was swallowed in small quantities and failed to reach the stomach in sufficient volume to cause serious gastric injury. The highly concentrated liquid alkalis that were introduced in the 1970s were likely to cause penetrating injury to both esophagus and stomach. The moderately concentrated liquid acids and alkalis available today are less likely to cause acute perforation of either organ but often lead to late stricture formation.

Histologic examination of tissue exposed to acid reveals coagulation necrosis with clumping and opacification of the cellular cytoplasm. The cell boundaries are usually recognizable in contrast to the complete cellular destruction of the liquefactive necrosis induced by strong alkali. The coagulum formed during coagulative necrosis consists in part of consolidated connective tissue, thrombosis of vessels, and clumping of blood proteins. This coagulum may limit the depth of penetration of the acid. However, esophageal perforations due to acid ingestion have been reported.

20. Do acute signs and symptoms predict the severity and extent of caustic injury?

Clinicians should be aware when evaluating patients with caustic ingestion that early signs and symptoms are not reliable indicators of the severity of caustic injury. Caustic agents (acids and crystalline lye) frequently cause immediate pain on contact with the mucosa of the oropharynx and may be expectorated before they are swallowed. Therefore, patients who ingest such agents may exhibit signs and symptoms of damage to the oropharynx with no injury to the esophagus. In contrast, lethal esophageal burns may occur with minimal evidence of oropharyngeal damage. Therefore, signs and symptoms of injury to the oropharynx do not reliably indicate the severity of damage to the esophagus or stomach. The distribution and severity of injury with acid or alkali depend as much on the physical characteristics of the product (solid versus liquid, volatility, titratable acid or base) as the volume ingested and the duration of exposure.

21. Describe the presentation of a typical case of caustic ingestion.

The typical clinical course of uncomplicated caustic ingestion has three phases that closely parallel the phases of experimental caustic injury: acute, latent, and retractive. In the acute phase, immediate oral burning pain often limits the volume of ingestion. Caustic burns to the epiglottis and the larynx may lead to immediate or delayed wheezing, cough, stridor, hoarseness, dyspnea, or aphonia. Dyspnea also may result from aspiration with damage to the bronchial tree and lung parenchyma. If a significant volume of the agent is swallowed, chest pain, dysphagia, or odynophagia may develop within minutes. Secretions may not be handled because of injury to and swelling of the posterior pharynx; drooling may occur. Retching and emesis may follow, and vomitus may contain blood or tissue. Pain and dysphagia in the uncomplicated course are largely due to dysmotility and edema and may subside over 3–4 days.

The patient with a more complex course may have additional symptoms and a worsening course. Persistent substernal pain or back pain may indicate a third-degree burn of the esophagus with mediastinitis. Perforation of the esophagus or stomach may cause peritonitis with abdominal rigidity and rebound tenderness. Perforation may evolve over the first few days and manifest as increasing pain, fever, and shock.

22. Describe the common features of the patient's course after acute ingestion.
Initial pain and dysphagia may remit after a few days, ushering in the latent phase. Both physician and patient may be lulled into a false sense of security. The third phase, scar retraction, may begin as early as the end of the second week and last for several months. Clinically apparent esophageal strictures develop in 10–30% of patients with documented esophageal injury. Eighty percent of strictures become apparent during weeks 2–8, but occasionally patients may become symptomatic from stricture many months after the initial ingestion. Early strictures often progress rapidly, advancing from mild dysphagia to the inability to handle secretions in only a few days. The rapid progression of early strictures necessitates rapid evaluation and therapy to avoid the formation of dense, tight, constricting lesions. Therapy for such strictures is careful bougienage, as needed to maintain esophageal patency.

23. What is the mortality rate associated with caustic ingestion?
The mortality rate has decreased markedly over the last three decades from approximately 20% to 1–3%. The decreased mortality is probably due to improvements in supportive care (antibiotics and nutritional support), advances in surgery, anesthesia, and intensive care management as well as substitution of less concentrated alkali and acids for the highly concentrated products available in the 1950s and before.

24. What is the cancer risk to a patient with stricture after lye ingestion?
The association between esophageal cancer and caustic ingestion is strong. The expected incidence of esophageal carcinoma is higher in patients with caustic ingestion than in the general population. Approximately 1–7% of patients with carcinoma of the esophagus have a history of caustic ingestion. The latent period is long and in one study was on average 41 years. Currently no screening is recommended after lye ingestion.

25. Describe the emergency department management of a patient with caustic ingestion.
The initial steps in the management of a suspected caustic injury are similar to those used on an emergency basis to manage any toxic ingestion. First, airway, breathing, and circulation (ABCs) must be controlled. Patients with caustic ingestion may present with respiratory compromise and require endothracheal intubation to protect the airway and to provide adequate oxygenation. Intubation should be performed only under direct visualization and should not be attempted in a blind manner. Next, hypotension must be addressed with adequate fluid support and resuscitation, as needed. If obvious signs of mediastinitis or peritonitis suggest perforation of a viscus, the patient should be prepared for surgery.

When respiratory and hemodynamic status have been addressed and the patient is stable, an attempt should be made to determine the quantity and type of caustic agent and time of ingestion as well as any coingestions (more often with suicidal attempts than accidental ingestion). It is helpful to obtain the container of the caustic agent, which lists all active substances as well as concentrations of caustics. If the clinician is not familiar with management of poison ingestion or if the content of the caustic is in question, a poison control center should be contacted. Emesis should not be induced, because it will reexpose the esophagus and perhaps larynx to caustic materials. If a solid caustic has been ingested, a few sips of water may help to dislodge the solid particles from the esophageal mucosa and dissolve them in a larger volume of water in the thicker-walled stomach. This, of course, should not be done in patients at risk of aspiration or with clinical evidence of perforation.

By the time victims of ingestion present to the physician, it is usually too late to intervene effectively to reduce internal burns. Because of the rapid action of alkali agents, efforts to neutralize caustic substances are not likely to be effective in limiting injury. In addition, an attempt to neutralize the alkali agent may be dangerous. Neutralization may release significant amounts of heat and add thermal injury to chemical injury. Oral administration of any substance also may increase the risk of vomiting and aspiration. With acid injury, large volumes of water or milk within minutes of ingestion may dilute and neutralize the acid.

26. Should gastric lavage be performed on patients with caustic ingestion?

The answer is controversial. Patients most likely to benefit from gastric lavage present shortly after ingestion when a significant amount of caustic material may still be present in the stomach. In addition, patients with suspected coingestion of pills may benefit from lavage to decrease absorption. Such benefits must be weighed against the risks. Nasogastric intubation may induce retching and vomiting with recurrent exposure of the esophagus and oropharynx to caustics. Because the nasogastric tube may perforate the esophagus or stomach, strong consideration should be given to placement under fluoroscopic guidance. If the tube is placed, gastric contents should be aspirated before lavage. The stomach should be lavaged with cold water to dissipate any heat that is produced.

27. What is the role of endoscopic evaluation in patients with caustic ingestion?

Flexible upper endoscopy has a role in the early, emergent, and later, subacute management of caustic ingestion. Patients in whom perforation (diagnosed either radiographically or clinically) requires surgical exploration should undergo complete upper endoscopy to identify the extent of disease. For example, in patients with a normal esophagus but injured stomach, surgery may be limited to the abdomen. The risk of upper endoscopy is acceptable once the decision to operate has been made.

If surgery is not indicated, endoscopy still should be performed to identify uninjured patients who do not require prolonged hospital observation and to define the severity of burns in injured patients. Timing of endoscopy is based on clinical suspicion of severe injury. If significant esophageal injury is unlikely, EGD should be performed promptly to provide rapid reassurance and to avoid hospital observation. More than 50% of patients with a history of caustic injury are found on endoscopy to have no injury. If internal injury is likely but signs of perforation are absent, a delay of 48–72 hours permits development of the inflammatory reaction (little inflammation may be present in the first 24 hours) and easier assessment of the true extent of injury. Although endoscopic evaluation identifies the location of the mucosal injury, it may not accurately predict the depth of invasion.

Endoscopy classifies injuries into four categories, as outlined in the table below. The findings influence hospital stay and likelihood of stricture formation.

Classification of Injury by Endoscopic Findings

ENDOSCOPIC FINDINGS	HOSPITAL STAY	RISK OF STRICTURE
No injury	No observation in hospital	None
Gastric only	Observe 24–48 hours	None
Linear esophageal injury, oriented longitudinally	Observe 24–48 hours	Low
Circumferential esophageal injury	Observe at least 48 hours	High

28. What is the role of corticosteroids or antibiotics in the treatment of caustic ingestion?

Patients in whom endoscopy demonstrates near-circumferential or circumferential esophageal burns are at risk for strictures. Since the 1950s, corticosteroids have been the mainstay of prophylaxis against stricture formation. The rationale for their use was based on animal studies showing that steroid therapy begun within 24 hours after lye injury and continued for 6–8 weeks reduced the incidence of strictures by inhibiting formation of granulation tissue. Follow-up was short, however, and early death from septicemia was much more common in steriod-treated animals. A prospective, randomized, controlled trial in children with caustic ingestion, performed by Anderson in 1990, showed that corticosteroids did not decrease stricture formation. Clearly there is no consensus. If steroids are to be used, they should be reserved for patients with circumferential esophageal burns, who are at greatest risk of stricture formation. The dosage and length of therapy for corticosteroids have not been defined. Prednisone, 1.5–2.0 mg/kg/day, with a tapering period of 2 months, has been recommended.

In patients with significant caustic ingestion and clinical evidence of impending airway compromise, corticosteroids may help to decrease inflammation of the bronchopulmonary tree. Dexamethasone (pediatric dosage, 0.5–1.0 mg/kg; adult dosage, 2.0–3.0 mg/kg) is given intravenously to patients who have a high probability of impending airway compromise and may need intubation, cricothyrotomy, or tracheostomy for treatment of airway obstruction.

Empirical antibiotic therapy is even less established. It was originally advocated because antibiotics reduced the early mortality in animals treated with steroids for esophageal burns. The patients most likely to benefit are those who are treated with corticosteroids and appear to be at increased risk of systemic infection. Gram-positive organisms are most commonly implicated, but broad-spectrum coverage is generally prescribed.

29. Discuss the prophylactic role of bougienage and esophageal stents.

Once the acute injury has resolved, the next complication is likely to be stricture of the esophagus in patients who had circumferential burns. If such patients are left untreated, a long narrow stricture may develop. Such strictures may not be amenable to dilation and may require surgery. To avoid stricture formation, patients may undergo prophylactic dilation with a Maloney dilator or esophageal stenting. Dilation should be avoided during the acute phase of injury because of the increased risk of perforation. Dilation should be initiated in patients with circumferential burns at about the third week, before the stricture becomes symptomatic. Dilation is accomplished with a single pass of a moderately large (42 Fr) dilator several times a week. If resistance is encountered, the dilator is not forced through. Instead, progressive therapeutic dilations are initiated, starting with the largest dilator that passes without resistance. This method generally maintains patency of the esophageal lumen. Although some risk is associated with dilation, the procedure may prevent formation of the long narrow stricture commonly associated with caustic ingestion. An alternative to prophylactic dilation is close personal observation and questioning so that therapeutic dilation can be instituted at the onset of symptomatic dysphagia. Unfortunately, many injured patients are too young or too unreliable to be managed with this wait-and-see approach.

The use of prophylactic esophageal stents to maintain lumenal patency during the healing process is controversial and should be limited to centers with experience in placing stents and ongoing research interests. Stents are placed endoscopically or surgically and left in place for approximately 3 weeks. The theory is that stenting allows esophageal healing without cicatrization and stenosis. After 3 weeks the stent is removed. The stents are uncomfortable, and appreciable risk is associated with placement and removal. No randomized data evaluate the efficacy of stents, but anecdotal data have shown that most patients require subsequent esophageal dilation.

30. Review the controversies associated with the options for treatment of caustic ingestions.

Currently many sources promote different invasive and noninvasive therapies for caustic ingestions. Fortunately, the number of severe caustic ingestions seems to be decreasing. Because of decreasing experience and ethical concerns about testing experimental therapies on humans, few well-controlled data are available to guide the clinician. Withholding therapy, however, is also an ethical concern.

Nasogastric intubation and maintenance of a nasogastric tube (NGT) have several benefits. NGTs provide a mechanism to deliver adequate nutritional support and needed medications. They also allow the esophagus to rest and prevent wound trauma that may be associated with bolus food ingestion. Finally, NGTs maintain a lumen that can be used to assist dilation. Negative aspects include the possibility that the tube may cause continuous irritation and inflammation of the healing esophagus and lead to increased fibrosis and stricturing. Overall, a fluoroscopically placed, flexible NGT seems to be beneficial for the first 2 weeks in patients who are seriously ill and unlikely to maintain adequate nutrition.

Total parenteral nutrition (TPN) has been advocated to allow complete esophageal rest and maintain maximal nutrition for healing. No prospective data support TPN in all patients. Clear candidates are patients at high risk of aspiration and patients in whom passage of an NGT is contraindicated because of the severity of esophageal injuries.

Antibiotics were originally advocated to decrease long-term stricture formation, but this effect has not been reproducible in animal or human studies. Antibiotics may have a role in decreasing septicemia in steroid-treated patients at high risk of infection. Empirical therapy has not been shown to be more efficacious than monitoring for clinical signs of infection and using broad-spectrum antibiotics at their first appearance. If empirical therapy is chosen, antibiotics may be stopped after 5–7 days of infection-free observation.

Empirical corticosteroid therapy, although still controversial, is supported by experimental evidence. Animal studies have repeatedly shown a reduction in early stricture formation when corticosteroids are administered within 48 hours; this effect may be observed when they are used as late as 4–7 days after caustic ingestion. Based on animal data and uncontrolled human studies, corticosteroids are recommended for patients with circumferential esophageal burn who are at highest risk of stricture formation. The negative aspects of corticosteroids, including increased risk of infection and systemic side effects, also must be considered. In addition, controlled data indicate that corticosteroids do not reduce stricture formation secondary to caustic ingestion in children. The study, however, had a small number of patients, and although formation of esophageal stricture did not seem to be affected by corticosteroids, the need for total esophagectomy was decreased in the steroid-treated group (4 vs. 7 untreated patients).

The final area of controversy is the use and timing of prophylactic dilation. Most agree that oral esophageal dilation is the cornerstone of stricture prophylaxis. Others argue that repeated trauma to esophageal mucosa from dilation causes increased fibrosis and encourages stricture formation. Prophylactic dilation of all patients with caustic ingestion clearly subjects some patients to unneeded, potentially hazardous procedures. No data are available to resolve this issue. Because strictures rarely manifest before the second week after ingestion, it seems wise to wait 10–14 days before beginning bougienage.

BIBLIOGRAPHY

1. Anderson KD, Rouse TM, Randolph JG: A controlled trial of corticosteroids in children with corrosive injury of the esophagus: N Engl J Med 323:10, 1990.
2. Bozymski EM, London JF: Miscellaneous diseases of the esophagus. In Sleisinger MH, Fordtran JS (eds): Gastrointestinal Diseases, 5th ed. Philadelphia, W.B. Saunders, 1993.
3. Browne JD, Thompson JN: Caustic injuries of the esophagus. In Castell DO (ed): The Esophagus. Boston, Little, Brown, 1992.
4. Byrne WJ: Foreign bodies, bezoars, and caustic ingestions. Gastrointest Endosc Clin North Am 4:99–119, 1994.
5. Gumaste VV, Pradyuman BD: Ingestion of corrosive substances by adults. Am J Gastroenterol 87:1–5, 1991.
6. Kikendall JW: Caustic injury of the esophagus and stomach. In Current Therapy in Gastroenterology and Liver Disease, 3rd ed. Philadelphia, B.C. Decker, 1990.
7. Kikendall JW: Caustic ingestion injuries. Gastroenterol Clin North Am 20:847–857, 1991.
8. Kikendall JW, Johnson LF: Pill-induced esophageal injury. In Castell DO (ed): The Esophagus. Boston, Little, Brown, 1995.
9. Loeb PM, Eisenstein AM: Caustic injury to the upper gastrointestinal tract. In Scharschmidt BF (ed): Gastrointestinal Diseases, 5th ed. Philadelphia, W.B. Saunders, 1993, pp 293–301.
10. Minocha A, Greenbaum DS: Pill-esophagitis caused by nonsteroidal antiinflammatory drugs. Am J Gastroenterol 86:1086–1089, 1991.
11. Semble EL, Wu WC, Castell DO: Nonsteroidal antiinflammatory drugs and esophageal injury. Semin Arthritis Rheum 19:99–109, 1989.
12. Spechler SJ: Caustic ingestions. In Taylor MB (ed): Gastrointestinal Emergencies. Baltimore, Williams & Wilkins, 1990, pp 13–21.

8. BARRETT'S ESOPHAGUS

Stuart Jon Spechler, M.D.

1. What is Barrett's esophagus?

Barrett's esophagus is the condition in which a metaplastic columnar epithelium replaces the squamous epithelium that normally lines the distal esophagus. Ironically, the condition is named after a British surgeon, Norman Barrett, who wrote a treatise in 1950 contending that the esophagus could not be lined by columnar epithelium. Barrett's esophagus has clinical importance because of its strong association with two disorders: (1) gastroesophageal reflux disease (GERD) and (2) adenocarcinoma of the esophagus and gastroesophageal junction.

2. How does Barrett's esophagus develop?

The precise sequence of events that leads to the development of Barrett's esophagus is not known, but the condition appears to be acquired through the process of metaplasia wherein one kind of fully differentiated cell (columnar) replaces another kind of fully differentiated cell (squamous). Metaplasia results when tissue is exposed chronically to noxious factors that injure mature cells while simultaneously promoting the aberrant differentiation of immature, proliferating cells. For most patients with Barrett's esophagus, chronic gastroesophageal reflux appears to be the factor that both injures the mature esophageal squamous cells and promotes mucosal repair through columnar metaplasia. Some reports allege that Barrett's esophagus also may develop as a result of chronic chemotherapy with agents that injure squamous cells (e.g., cyclophosphamide, methotrexate, and 5-fluorouracil). However, the frequency and importance of chemotherapy-induced Barrett's esophagus is unclear and disputed. Metaplasia may be viewed as a protective process, because columnar epithelium is more resistant to injury induced by gastroesophageal reflux and chemotherapeutic agents than the native squamous epithelium. Unfortunately, columnar metaplasia in the esophagus also is a risk factor for cancer development.

3. What are the histologic features of Barrett's esophagus?

Any or all of three types of columnar epithelia may be found in Barrett's esophagus: (1) a gastric fundic-type epithelium, (2) a junctional-type epithelium, and (3) specialized intestinal metaplasia.

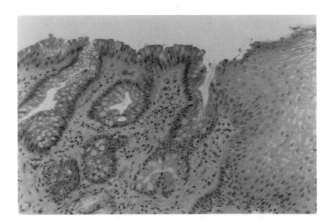

Biopsy specimen obtained at the squamocolumnar junction in the distal esophagus shows an abrupt transition from stratified squamous epithelium to specialized intestinal metaplasia. Both the surface and the intestinal-type glands of the specialized columnar epithelium are lined by mucus-secreting cells and goblet cells (H&E; original magnification × 200). (From Spechler SJ, Zeroogian JM, Antonioli DA, et al: Prevalence of metaplasia at the gastro-oesophageal junction. Lancet 344:1533–1536, 1994, with permission.)

The first two types resemble epithelia that normally are found in the gastric fundus and cardia, respectively. Specialized intestinal metaplasia, in contrast, has intestinal features, such as goblet cells, that readily distinguish it from normal gastric and esophageal mucosae. Specialized intestinal metaplasia also is the most common and important of the three epithelial types. Dysplasia and carcinoma in Barrett's esophagus invariably are associated with intestinal metaplasia.

4. What are the diagnostic criteria for Barrett's esophagus?

On endoscopic examination, columnar epithelium in the esophagus has a characteristic red color and velvetlike texture that contrast sharply with the pale, glossy appearance of the adjacent squamous epithelium. Endoscopists can recognize Barrett's esophagus easily when they see long segments of columnar epithelium extending up the esophagus, well above the junction with the stomach. This condition is recognized in 10–15% of patients who have endoscopic examinations for the evaluation of GERD symptoms. Diagnostic difficulties arise when patients are found to have short segments of columnar lining in the distal esophagus. Because gastric mucosa normally may extend a short distance into the distal esophagus, the finding of gastric type epithelia in the distal segment does not establish a diagnosis of Barrett's esophagus. Some authorities have proposed that Barrett's esophagus should be diagnosed only if there is a specific extent of columnar lining (e.g., columnar epithelium involving >3 cm of the distal esophagus). Diagnostic criteria based on extent alone are clearly arbitrary, however. For example, if one chooses 3 cm as the diagnostic criterion for Barrett's esophagus, patients with 2.5 cm of metaplastic columnar lining (with potential for neoplastic change) will be ignored. Furthermore, there can be considerable imprecision both in obtaining endoscopic measurements and in localizing the anatomic esophagogastric junction precisely. For patients with short segments of columnar lining in the distal esophagus, biopsy specimens may be obtained to look for specialized intestinal metaplasia. The finding of intestinal metaplasia in the distal esophagus clearly is abnormal, even if the aberrant mucosa extends only a short distance above the esophagogastric junction.

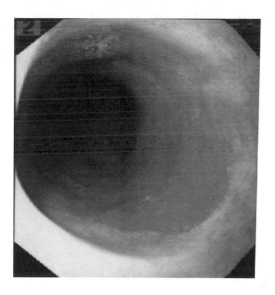

Characteristic appearance of Barrett's esophagus, with a long sheet of red, columnar epithelium extending well above the esophagogastric junction.

5. Is it common to find short segments of specialized intestinal metaplasia in the distal esophagus? What is the importance of this finding?

In one recent report, short segments of intestinal metaplasia (i.e., extending <3 cm above the esophagogastric junction) were found in 18% of unselected patients in a general endoscopy unit.

The distal esophagus did not appear to be abnormal in most of these cases, and the intestinal metaplasia would have gone unrecognized if the study protocol had not mandated the acquisition of biopsy specimens from a normal-appearing squamocolumnar junction. The importance of this condition has not been established. The vast majority of studies of Barrett's esophagus included only patients with endoscopically apparent disease in whom long segments of columnar epithelium extended well up the esophagus. The results of these studies may not be applicable to patients with short segments of intestinal metaplasia at the esophagogastric junction. Although intestinal metaplasia is thought to predispose to malignancy in the esophagus, it is not clear that the risk of carcinogenesis for patients with short segments of intestinal metaplasia is the same as for patients with endoscopically apparent Barrett's esophagus. Unlike endoscopically apparent Barrett's esophagus, furthermore, short segments of intestinal metaplasia may not be associated strongly with complicated GERD.

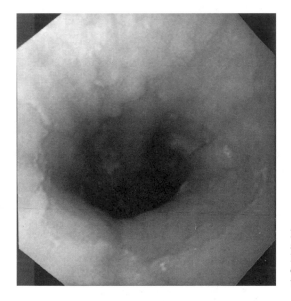

Normal-appearing distal esophagus lined by a short segment of columnar epithelium. Biopsy specimens obtained at the squamocolumnar junction showed specialized intestinal metaplasia.

6. Why is GERD so severe in patients who have endoscopically apparent Barrett's esophagus?

Patients with endoscopically apparent Barrett's esophagus often have GERD that is complicated by esophageal ulceration, stricture, and bleeding. A number of physiologic abnormalities have been described that may contribute to the severity of GERD. Some patients with Barrett's esophagus exhibit hypersecretion of gastric acid and duodenogastric reflux. Consequently, the gastric material available for reflux may be exceptionally caustic, containing high concentrations of acid, bile, and pancreatic digestive enzymes. Manometric studies of patients with Barrett's esophagus often reveal extreme hypotension of the lower esophageal sphincter that predisposes to gastroesophageal reflux and disordered esophageal motility that may delay esophageal acid clearance. Diminished esophageal sensitivity to pain has been described in some cases; consequently, the reflux of noxious material into the Barrett esophagus may not cause heartburn. Without heartburn, patients have no warning that they are experiencing gastroesophageal reflux and have little incentive to comply with antireflux therapy. Finally, decreased salivary secretion of epidermal growth factor, a peptide that enhances the healing of peptic ulcerations, has been found in some patients with Barrett's esophagus. Decreased secretion of this growth factor may delay the healing of reflux-induced esophageal injury.

7. With so many abnormalities predisposing to severe GERD, does Barrett's esophagus progress with time as columnar cells replace more and more reflux-damaged squamous cells?

Logically, one may assume that Barrett's esophagus should progress in extent over the years. Recent data suggest, however, that when Barrett's esophagus develops it does so quickly and does not progress substantially with time. Investigators at the Mayo Clinic reviewed the records of 377 patients with Barrett's esophagus. When the patients were grouped according to age, the length of esophagus lined by columnar epithelium was not found to differ significantly among the various age groups (i.e., 20-year-old patients had a segment of columnar-lined esophagus similar in length to that of 80-year-old patients). Furthermore, no significant change in the extent of columnar lining was found among 101 patients who had follow-up endoscopic examinations after a mean interval of 3.2 years. Although there are verified cases of progression, most studies have not found substantial change in the extent of Barrett's esophagus with time. For reasons that remain unclear, it appears that Barrett's esophagus usually does not progress in extent despite ongoing, severe GERD.

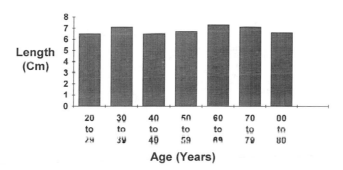

Relationship of the length of esophagus lined by columnar epithelium with age in 377 patients with Barrett's esophagus followed at the Mayo Clinic. (Data adapted from Cameron AJ, Lomboy CT: Barrett's esophagus: Age, prevalence, and extent of columnar epithelium. Gastroenterology 103:1241–1245, 1992.)

8. Since Barrett's esophagus develops as a consequence of GERD, can the columnar epithelium regress with effective GERD therapy?

Some patients treated with potent GERD therapies such as proton pump inhibitors or antireflux surgery have developed patchy areas where squamous epithelium has grown over columnar epithelium in the esophagus. The clinical importance of this phenomenon is not clear, because adenocarcinoma has developed in patients with Barrett's esophagus even after highly effective control of acid reflux by medical and surgical means. Anecdotal reports of complete regression of Barrett's esophagus with GERD therapy are unconvincing. It is not clear that the observed regression of columnar epithelium was real or only apparent, i.e., a result of biopsy sampling error. In the vast majority of cases, GERD therapy does not appear to effect substantial change in the extent of esophageal columnar epithelium.

9. Is there any specific treatment for Barrett's esophagus?

Treatment for patients with Barrett's esophagus usually is aimed at controlling the underlying GERD, a practice that appears to have little effect on the metaplastic epithelium. Recently, several reports have documented that it is possible to photoablate metaplastic epithelium with laser light. One report described the results of argon laser irradiation of Barrett's esophagus in 10 patients. All patients were treated with omeprazole for the duration of the study. Squamous mucosa was found to replace photoablated columnar epithelium in 38 of 40 treatment locations in the 10 patients. Most patients required multiple endoscopic laser treatments to achieve ablation of the irradiated segment. Although this and other reports document the feasibility of laser ablation of Barrett's epithelium, they do not establish the benefit of the technique. The procedure is expensive and entails some risk. Furthermore, it is not clear whether photoablation reduces the incidence of esophageal cancer or whether life-long, intensive acid suppression will be necessary to prevent return of the columnar epithelium. Further studies addressing such issues are necessary before laser ablation of Barrett's epithelium can be recommended for clinical application.

10. What is the risk of developing cancer in Barrett's esophagus?

Barrett's esophagus with intestinal metaplasia is the most important recognized risk factor for adenocarcinoma of the esophagus and gastroesophageal junction, tumors whose incidence has been increasing dramatically for the past 20 years. In patients who have endoscopically apparent Barrett's esophagus, cancers develop at the rate of approximately one case per 125 patient-years. Expressed as a percentage, the annual rate of cancer development in patients with Barrett's esophagus is approximately 0.8%, a rate more than 40-fold higher than that for the general population of the United States. As previously mentioned, it is not clear that the cancer risk for patients who have short segments of intestinal metaplasia in the distal esophagus is similar to that for patients with endoscopically apparent Barrett's esophagus.

11. How do cancers develop in Barrett's esophagus?

As in other tissues, cancers in Barrett's esophagus are thought to evolve through a sequence of genetic alterations. Carcinogenesis appears to begin with the activation of protooncogenes (e.g., c-erb-B) and the disablement of tumor suppressor genes (e.g., p53), changes that endow the cells with certain growth advantages. The advantaged cells hyperproliferate and in so doing acquire more genetic alterations that result in neoplasia with autonomous cell growth. Eventually, when enough DNA abnormalities accumulate, a clone of malignant cells emerges—malignant because they have the ability to invade adjacent tissues and to proliferate in unnatural locations. Molecular biologic techniques may be used to detect specific genetic alterations in the columnar cells of Barrett's esophagus. However, before the cells acquire enough DNA damage to become frankly malignant, the earlier genetic alterations often cause morphologic changes that can be recognized as dysplasia on routine histologic examination of biopsy specimens.

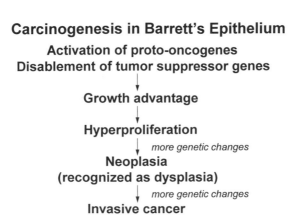

Proposed sequence of genetic alterations that result in cancer in Barrett's esophagus.

12. What is dysplasia in Barrett's esophagus?

Dysplasia in Barrett's esophagus is defined as a neoplastic alteration of columnar cells that remain confined within the basement membranes of the glands from which they arose. Histologically, dysplasia can be classified as low-grade or high-grade, depending on the degree of alteration in glandular architecture, nuclear pleomorphism, nuclear hyperchromatism, and nuclear polarity. Dysplasia is widely regarded as the precursor of invasive malignancy, and this is what makes the condition so interesting for the clinician. The finding of dysplasia in Barrett's esophagus may represent an opportunity to initiate therapy to interrupt the progression to invasive cancer.

13. What are the shortcomings of dysplasia as a biomarker for malignancy in Barrett's esophagus?

Although dysplasia is a clinically useful biomarker for malignancy in Barrett's esophagus, it is far from ideal. The grading of dysplasia is largely a subjective skill, and interobserver variation in grading may be considerable, even among skilled pathologists. Disagreement is especially likely when pathologists attempt to distinguish low-grade dysplastic changes from nonneoplastic regenerative changes in an epithelium recovering from inflammatory damage. Another problem with dysplasia as a biomarker is the fact that its natural history is not well defined. A number of reports have suggested that high-grade dysplasia often progresses quickly to invasive adenocarcinoma. The precise frequency and speed of that progression remain unclear, however, and there are verified cases of patients who have had high-grade dysplasia in Barrett's esophagus for years with no apparent malignant transformation. Finally, the use of dysplasia as a biomarker for malignancy is subject to biopsy sampling error. Patients found to have only high-grade dysplasia with no obvious tumor mass may already have an inapparent invasive carcinoma of the esophagus. Indeed, a number of studies found that esophageal resection revealed invasive carcinoma in approximately one-third of patients who were thought to have only high-grade dysplasia in Barrett's esophagus on preoperative endoscopic examinations.

14. Can the use of a rigorous biopsy protocol differentiate high-grade dysplasia from early adenocarcinoma in Barrett's esophagus?

As mentioned above, it may be difficult to differentiate high-grade dysplasia from early adenocarcinoma in Barrett's esophagus because of biopsy sampling error. Recently, investigators from Seattle reported that they could make this differentiation by adherence to a rigorous endoscopic biopsy protocol. They obtained four-quadrant "jumbo" biopsy specimens at 2-cm intervals throughout the columnar-lined esophagus and took many additional samples from sites of known dysplasia. After preoperative evaluation by this protocol, none of 7 patients who had an esophageal resection for high-grade dysplasia in Barrett's epithelium was found to have invasive cancer in the resected specimens. For each of the 7 patients, 29–185 preoperative biopsy specimens were available for review. One patient had 185 biopsy specimens obtained during 5 preoperative endoscopies from a segment of columnar epithelium that spanned only 3 cm, i.e., more than 60 biopsies per centimeter of metaplastic mucosa. Undoubtedly, this extensive sampling minimized the problem of biopsy sampling error. The authors also described 29 patients with high-grade dysplasia who had no esophageal resection and were followed for 2–46 months. Seven of the 29 patients (24%) were found to have invasive cancer during the follow-up period, whereas the other 22 had no apparent progression to malignancy. This study suggests that adherence to a very rigorous biopsy protocol for patients with high-grade dysplasia may exclude a synchronous malignancy with reasonable certainty, but the risk for developing invasive cancer remains high.

15. Are there other biomarkers that may be more useful than dysplasia for patients with Barrett's esophagus?

Much attention has focused on flow-cytometric abnormalities that may be earlier and more specific markers for cancer development than dysplasia in Barrett's esophagus. However, flow cytometry does not appear to provide sufficient additional information to justify its routine application in clinical practice. Indeed, none of the biomarkers listed in the table below provides such information. Despite the shortcomings, the finding of dysplasia remains the most appropriate biomarker for the clinical evaluation of patients with Barrett's esophagus.

Proposed Biomarkers for Malignancy in Barrett's Epithelium

Ornithine decarboxylase
Carcinoembryonic antigen (CEA)
Mucus abnormalities
Flow cytometry—aneuploidy
Flow cytometry—abnormal cellular proliferation
Chromosomal abnormalities (trisomy 7, 17p deletions)
Oncogenes (c-Ha-ras, c-erb-B)
Tumor suppressor genes (p53)
Growth regulatory factors (EGF, TGF-α, EGF-R)
Proliferating cell nuclear antigen and Ki67

Adapted from Spechler SJ: Barrett's esophagus. Semin Oncol 21:431–437, 1994.

16. Does brush cytology have a role in the evaluation of Barrett's esophagus?

Data suggest that examination of esophageal brush cytology specimens sometimes detects dysplastic changes and cancers missed by perendoscopic biopsy. In one study of 65 endoscopic examinations in which both biopsy specimens and brushings were obtained from Barrett's esophagus, the cytologic and histologic findings agreed in 47 cases (72%). In 13 cases, however, cytologic examination revealed a higher-grade lesion than histologic examination, whereas the histologic changes were more severe than the cytologic changes in 5 cases. This and other reports suggest that brush cytology and biopsy of Barrett's epithelium may be complementary tests for detecting dysplasia and adenocarcinoma.

17. What is the role of endoscopic ultrasonography?

With no interference caused by skin, bone, or air, endoscopic ultrasonography can use high-frequency ultrasonic waves that provide exquisitely detailed images of the esophageal mucosa. In theory, endosonography should be useful for detecting foci of occult carcinoma in patients with high-grade dysplasia in Barrett's esophagus. Unfortunately, the published experience to date has been disappointing. In one study from the Cleveland Clinic, for example, preoperative endosonography correctly staged the level of tumor invasion in only 4 of 9 patients who had esophageal resection for high-grade dysplasia in Barrett's esophagus. With further refinements in the technique, endosonography eventually may become a useful means for determining the need for esophageal resection in patients with dysplasia. Presently, however, the routine use of endosonography to decide when to operate on patients with Barrett's esophagus is not recommended.

18. What are the treatment options for patients with high-grade dysplasia in Barrett's esophagus?

Esophageal resection is the only therapy that clearly interrupts the progression from dysplasia to invasive cancer in Barrett's esophagus. Esophageal resection, unfortunately, is associated with substantial morbidity and mortality, and its role in patient management is disputed. Recently, photodynamic therapy has been proposed as a safer and easier alternative to esophageal resection. In photodynamic therapy, patients are given a systemic dose of a light-activated drug (porphyrin) that is concentrated in the neoplastic tissues. These tissues then are irradiated with laser light, stimulating the porphyrin to produce singlet oxygen that destroys the neoplastic cells. Presently, little is published about the use of photodynamic therapy for patients with high-grade dysplasia in Barrett's esophagus, but preliminary reports are encouraging. Nevertheless, use of this experimental therapy should be limited to patients enrolled in research protocols.

19. What are the arguments against esophageal resection for high-grade dysplasia in Barrett's esophagus?

There are verified cases of patients whose high-grade dysplasia in Barrett's esophagus persisted for years without progression to esophageal cancer. There also are documented cases of patients with high-grade dysplasia in whom rigorous endoscopic surveillance detected adenocarcinoma in an early, curable stage. The mortality rate for esophageal resection is in the range of 4–10%, and substantial, long-term morbidity is associated with the procedure. Such features suggest that some patients with high-grade dysplasia may not progress to adenocarcinoma and therefore can avoid the hazards of esophageal resection.

20. What are the arguments for esophageal resection for high-grade dysplasia in Barrett's esophagus?

As discussed above, patients found to have high-grade dysplasia in Barrett's esophagus already may have an invasive cancer. Frequent and extensive biopsy sampling is required to exclude the presence of adenocarcinoma with reasonable certainty. The progression to invasive cancer may be rapid and appears to occur quite frequently. The efficacy of endoscopic surveillance in detecting early, curable cancers is not clear. Established esophageal cancers have a tendency to metastasize frequently and often are not curable. Such features suggest that expectant management of high-grade dysplasia in Barrett's esophagus can be hazardous.

21. What are the recommendations for management of patients with Barrett's esophagus who do not have dysplasia?

Patients who have Barrett's esophagus without dysplasia are advised to have regular endoscopic surveillance, unless such surveillance is contraindicated by comorbidity. During the endoscopic examination, four-quadrant biopsy specimens are taken at intervals of at least every other centimeter throughout the columnar-lined esophagus. Brush cytology specimens are also obtained. The optimal interval between surveillance examinations has yet to be determined; the author recommends surveillance endoscopy every other year.

22. Describe the management of patients with high-grade dysplasia in Barrett's esophagus.

The finding of dysplasia should be confirmed by at least one other expert pathologist. As discussed above, there can be substantial disagreement, even among experienced pathologists, in the grading of dysplastic changes. If doubt remains after the biopsy material has been reviewed, the endoscopic examination is repeated to obtain more biopsy and cytology specimens for analysis. For otherwise healthy patients confirmed to have multiple foci of high-grade dysplasia, surgery is advised to resect all of the esophagus lined by columnar epithelium. If advanced age or comorbidity precludes such surgery, experimental treatments such as photodynamic therapy may be considered.

23. Describe the management of patients with low-grade dysplasia.

The finding of low-grade dysplasia also requires confirmation by another expert pathologists. For patients confirmed to have low-grade dysplasia, intensive medical antireflux therapy (including a proton pump inhibitor) should be instituted. The antireflux therapy is given to minimize the esophageal inflammation that may confound the interpretation of dysplastic changes. After 8–12 weeks of intensive medical therapy, the endoscopic examination is repeated to obtain multiple esophageal biopsy and cytology specimens. If histologic examination again reveals low-grade dysplasia, endoscopic surveillance should be intensified. In this context, the author usually repeats the endoscopic examination at intervals of 6 months. Presently, the risks of esophageal resection do not appear to be warranted for patients with only low-grade dysplasia in Barrett's esophagus.

24. What should be done when no dysplasia is found on follow-up examination of a patient previously found to have dysplasia in Barrett's esophagus?

There are several potential explanations for the apparent disappearance of dysplasia on follow-up examinations:

1. It is conceivable that dysplasia may regress as a result of antireflux therapy or other, unknown factors.

2. The histologic changes initially interpreted as dysplasia in fact may have been reactive changes caused by inflammation. Reactive changes clearly may regress with antireflux therapy.

3. Dysplasia may be missed because of biopsy sampling error. For patients whose dysplasia is not detected on follow-up examination, the author recommends intensive surveillance (e.g., endoscopic examinations every 6 months) until at least two consecutive examinations reveal no dysplastic epithelium.

BIBLIOGRAPHY

1. Berenson MM, Johnson TD, Markowitz NR, et al: Restoration of squamous mucosa after ablation of Barrett's esophageal epithelium. Gastroenterology 104:1686–1691, 1993.
2. Blot WJ, Devesa SS, Kneller RW, Fraumeni JF Jr: Rising incidence of adenocarcinoma of the esophagus and gastric cardia. JAMA 265:1287–1289, 1991.
3. Cameron AJ, Zinsmeister AR, Ballard DJ, Carney JA: Prevalence of columnar-lined (Barrett's) esophagus. Comparison of population-based clinical and autopsy findings. Gastroenterology 99:918–922, 1990.
4. Cameron AJ, Lomboy CT: Barrett's esophagus: Age, prevalence, and extent of columnar epithelium. Gastroenterology 103:1241–1245, 1992.
5. Dent J, Bremner CG, Collen MJ, et al: Working Party Report to the World Congresses of Gastroenterology, Sydney 1990: Barrett's oesophagus. J Gastroenterol Hepatol 6:1–22, 1991.
6. Geisinger KR, Teot LA, Richter JE: A comparative cytopathologic and histologic study of atypia, dysplasia, and adenocarcinoma in Barrett's esophagus. Cancer 69:8–16, 1992.
7. Hameeteman W, Tytgat GNJ, Houthoff HJ, van den Tweel JG: Barrett's esophagus: Development of dysplasia and adenocarcinoma. Gastroenterology 96:1249–1256, 1989.
8. Hassall E: Barrett's esophagus: New definitions and approaches in children. J Pediatr Gastroenterol Nutr 16:345–364, 1993.
9. Levine DS, Haggitt RC, Blount PL, et al: An endoscopic biopsy protocol can differentiate high-grade dysplasia from early adenocarcinoma in Barrett's esophagus. Gastroenterology 105:40–50, 1993.
10. Overholt B, Panjehpour M, Tefftellar E, Rose M: Photodynamic therapy for treatment of early adenocarinoma in Barrett's esophagus. Gastrointest Endosc 39:73–76, 1993.
11. Reid BJ, Blount PL, Rubin CE, et al: Flow-cytometric and histological progression to malignancy in Barrett's esophagus: Prospective endoscopic surveillance of a cohort. Gastroenterology 102:1212–1219, 1992.
12. Spechler SJ, Goyal RK: Barrett's esophagus. N Engl J Med 315:362–371, 1986.
13. Spechler SJ: Barrett's esophagus. Semin Oncol 21:431–437, 1994.
14. Spechler SJ: Laser photoablation of Barrett's epithelium: Burning issues about burning tissues. Gastroenterology 104:1855–1858, 1993.
15. Spechler SJ, Zeroogian JM, Antonioli DA, et al: Prevalence of metaplasia at the gastro-oesophageal junction. Lancet 344:1533–1536, 1994.

9. ESOPHAGEAL ANOMALIES

John H. Meier, M.D.

1. What is the best imaging method for demonstration of a web?
Barium esophagram with lateral views is best.

2. A patient with dysphagia is found to have a web by barium studies. What blood disorder must be sought and what is the best therapy for the dysphagia?
Esophageal webs are often, but not universally, associated with iron-deficiency anemia; this combination is known as Plummer-Vinson or Paterson-Brown Kelly syndrome. Esophageal bougienage is the preferred therapy, although many webs are probably ruptured at endoscopy.

3. For what cancer are patients with esophageal webs reportedly at increased risk?
Esophageal webs reportedly increase the risk of squamous cell carcinoma of the hypopharynx and upper esophagus, although the risk is not well-defined.

4. What types of esophageal rings are described? What is the difference between them?
Two types of esophageal rings have been described: the cleverly named A and B rings. A rings are muscular, whereas B rings (also known as Schatzki's rings) are mucosal and occur at the gastroesophageal junction. The pathogenesis of both is unknown, although A rings are associated with esophageal dysmotility and B rings are possibly related to reflux.

5. Are all Schatzki's rings symptomatic? What is the typical history of the symptomatic patient?
Such rings are usually symptomatic only when the luminal diameter is less than 13 mm. Even so, symptomatic patients usually describe only intermittent solid-food dysphagia induced by hurrying or anxiety.

6. What are the three types of esophageal diverticula?
  1. Upper esophageal, also called Zenker's diverticulum.
  2. Midesophageal, also called a traction diverticulum.
  3. Distal esophageal, also called an epiphrenic diverticulum.

7. What is the typical history of Zenker's diverticulum?
Patients may complain of regurgitation of undigested food, bad breath, a visible lump on the side of the neck, and dysphagia in the neck.

8. How is Zenker's diverticulum treated?
Symptomatic Zenker's diverticula should be surgically removed. Diverticulectomy is recommended because of possible persistence of symptoms and the small risk of carcinoma in the diverticulum. Cricopharyngeal myotomy is also recommended but not always performed.

9. Why are midesophageal diverticula called traction diverticula?
It was previously thought that midesophageal diverticula were formed by adhesion of the esophagus to tuberculous mediastinal lymph nodes; most are now thought to result from esophageal motility disorders. Few need specific therapy.

10. Should all epiphrenic diverticula be surgically treated?
No. Unusually large diverticula or those producing symptoms such as regurgitation or aspiration should be resected. Because of the high association with esophageal motility disorders, manometric evaluation and lower esophageal sphincter myotomy should be considered.

11. Define dysphagia lusoria.

Lusoria means "a trick of nature," and dysphagia lusoria refers to impingement of aberrant vasculature on the proximal esophagus. Most patients with aberrant vasculature are asymptomatic, but some have dysphagia. The most common anomaly is aberrant right subclavian artery, but double aortic arch, right aortic arch, and several other anomalies have been reported. Most are surgically manageable.

12. What are the most and least common types of esophageal atresia with tracheoesophageal fistula? Describe their presentations.

The most common type of tracheoesophageal fistula with atresia is the lower-pouch fistula. It typically presents in infancy with regurgitation and weight loss; pneumonias may occur because of communication of the gastric pouch with the trachea. The least common form is congenital esophageal stenosis, a forme fruste of atresia that may present as late as adulthood. Patients complain of dysphagia, and endoscopy may show multiple cartilaginous rings (presumably embryonic remnants) along the esophageal lumen. Bougienage or resection is advocated.

13. What is intramural pseudodiverticulosis?

Formed by dilatation of submucosal esophageal glands, small pseudodiverticula are commonly associated with *Candida* esophagitis (50%). Many patients have esophageal motor disorders, and many have esophageal strictures. The inciting event is unknown. Treatment with stricture dilation, antireflux medications, and possibly calcium blockers is said to be effective.

BIBLIOGRAPHY

1. Boyce GA, Boyce HW: Esophagus: Anatomy and structural anomalies. In Yamada T (ed): Textbook of Gastroenterology, Philadelphia, J.B. Lippincott, 1991.
2. Richter JE: The esophagus. In Rogers A (ed): Medical Knowledge Self-Assessment Program in the Subspecialty of Gastroenterology. Philadelphia, The American College of Physicians, 1993.

II. Stomach Disorders

10. GASTRITIS

R. Matthew Reveille, M.D.

1. What are the cardinal symptoms of gastritis?

Symptoms associated with gastritis include dyspepsia (epigastric discomfort or burning), nausea, vomiting, postprandial fullness or bloating, and occasionally GI bleeding. Many individuals with histologic evidence for gastritis are asymptomatic. Chronic gastritis increases in frequency with age, and some 60% of adults have histologic evidence of a nonspecific chronic gastritis.

2. What are the causes of acute gastritis?

Acute gastritis is usually seen endoscopically as scattered mucosal erosions and foci of intramucosal hemorrhage, termed "erosive" and "hemorrhagic" gastritis, respectively. Histologically, there is a minimal inflammatory component confined to the mucosa. Most cases of acute gastritis involve chemical or ischemic injury. Viruses that produce a gastroenteritis syndrome (e.g., enteroviruses, rotavirus, Norwalk agent) typically do not cause a true gastritis. Rarely, invasive bacterial infections cause an acute phlegmonous or emphysematous gastritis, which can be lethal

Causes of Acute Gastritis

Alcohol
NSAIDs, aspirin
"Stress" gastritis
Corrosive (alkali) ingestions
Viruses
    Cytomegalovirus
    Herpes viruses
Bacteria
    α-Hemolytic streptococci
    Clostridium septicum
Uremia
Radiation exposure

NSAIDs = nonsteroidal anti-inflammatory drugs.

3. In what clinical circumstances should one be concerned about stress gastritis?

The risk factors for stress gastritis include respiratory failure requiring mechanical ventilation, underlying liver or renal disease with coagulopathy, sepsis, extensive surgery or trauma, burns, and CNS injury. The erosions of stress gastritis often develop within 24 hours of a physiologic insult and can produce overt GI bleeding in up to 30% of patients, with potentially life-threatening hemorrhage occurring in about 3% of cases. With burns, unique lesions called Curling's ulcers are seen, and they appear to have a higher risk of bleeding and perforation, especially of the duodenum. In the setting of major head trauma, Cushing's ulcers often develop. These are particularly aggressive, owing to acid hypersecretion from hypergastrinemia, and are often deep. Cushing's ulcers bleed and perforate more often than any other form of stress gastropathy. The importance of identifying true high-risk patients and initiating prophylaxis against stress gastritis to prevent bleeding and perforation cannot be overstated.

4. What are the options for prophylaxis of stress gastritis in the intensive care setting?
A principal goal of stress prophylaxis has been to raise gastric luminal pH above 4.0. At pH >4, the proteolytic enzyme pepsin is inactivated and blood coagulation is enhanced.

A variety of methods are now acceptable in the prophylactic setting. Antacids instilled into the stomach via a nasogastric (NG) tube every 2–4 hours, with periodic monitoring of the gastric pH, is still an effective means of prophylaxis. Administration of intravenous H_2 blockers via bolus or continuous infusion is employed most commonly. The controversy as to whether the use of H_2 blockers increases the risk of nosocomial pneumonia in patients on ventilators remains to be settled. An alternative to H_2 blockers is gastric instillation of sucralfate suspension, 1 g every 4 hours via an NG tube. Misoprostol, a prostaglandin analogue, has also been used at 200 μg per NG every 4 hours. Periodic monitoring of gastric pH is probably prudent, with the addition of antacids to titrate the pH level back above 4.0.

5. Describe a classification scheme for the causes of chronic gastritis.
There continues to be considerable controversy as to the best method of classifying the various causes of chronic gastritis. The Sydney classification scheme of 1990 was an attempt to bring together endoscopic, anatomic, and histologic findings, but this scheme is not widely accepted. From a pathophysiologic perspective, chronic gastristis can be classified as follows:

Classification of Chronic Gastritides

Chemical gastritis	Hypertrophic gastropathies
Alkaline/bile reflux	Ménétrier's disease
NSAIDs (?)	Gastric pseudolymphoma
"Specific" gastritis	Zollinger-Ellison syndrome
Eosinophilic gastritis	Normal variant
Eosinophilic granuloma	Portal hypertensive/congestive gastropathy
Eosinophilic gastroenteritis	(not a true gastritis)
Granulomatous gastritis	"Nonspecific" gastritis
Crohn's disease	Nonerosive types
Tuberculosis	Type A autoimmune gastritis
Histoplasmosis	Type B environmental gastritis
Syphilis	*Helicobacter pylori*-related chronic gastritis
Sarcoidosis	Erosive types
Foreign body	Lymphocytic gastritis
Parasitic	Varioliform gastritis
Idiopathic	

6. What is the significance of chronic gastritis?
Chronic gastritis of the nonspecific, nonerosive type is associated with a risk of developing ulcer disease during one's lifetime. Some forms of specific chronic gastritis result in hypo/achlorhydria and vitamin B_{12} deficiency. Still other forms of gastritis are signs of more widespread GI disorders, such as Crohn's disease and eosinophilic gastroenteritis. The major clinical significance of chronic gastritis is that it is considered by many to be a very early premalignant lesion which progresses in time through atrophy, intestinal metaplasia, and on to carcinoma. Fortunately, most patients with chronic gastritis in the United States never go on to develop gastric carcinoma. Chronic gastritis also appears to be a risk factor for primary gastric lymphoma.

7. How are types A and B chronic nonspecific gastritis distinguished on anatomic and etiologic grounds?
Early in the course of these two disorders, there is an anatomic predilection for specific sites of inflammation. In **type A gastritis,** inflammation is associated with antiparietal cell antibodies and thus is autoimmune in nature. It involves the fundus and corpus of the stomach. With time, atrophy and loss of intrinsic factor production occur with B_{12} deficiency as a consequence. Patients develop achlorhydria and typically have hypergastrinemia. In **type B gastritis,** or antral gastritis, the inflammatory process and subsequent atrophy and metaplasia that can develop are largely con-

fined to the antrum. Infection of the antrum with the ulcer-causing bacterium *Helicobacter pylori* accounts for approximately 80% of all cases of type B gastritis. In other parts of the world, environmental exposures, such as diets high in nitrates and deficient in green vegetables, have been implicated in chronic type B gastritis. Interestingly, the anatomic distinctions of these two gastritic conditions tend to blur with time, such that advanced cases of either type can involve virtually the entire stomach and lead to diffuse atrophy and metaplasia. Both forms are associated with the formation of gastric hyperplastic polyps and adenomas. Type B gastritis is associated with gastric carcinoma and lymphoma.

8. In what clinical setting does one encounter portal hypertensive or congestive gastropathy?

Portal hypertensive gastropathy, as the name implies, refers to mucosal and submucosal changes in the stomach that develop as a result of cirrhosis and portal hypertension. After successful eradication of esophagogastric varices by endoscopic means, it is common to see subsequent development of this gastropathy. Endoscopically, gastric folds appear prominent and erythematous, with punctate intramucosal hemorrhages and a reticulated or "mosaic" mucosal pattern. Histologically, superficial capillary congestion, vascular ectasia, and perivascular fibrosis are seen, with no significant inflammatory component.

9. How is GI bleeding from congestive gastropathy managed?

Gastrointestinal blood loss can be either acute or chronic. Acute bleeding is often managed as for variceal bleeding—with an intravenous infusion of either vasopressin or the somatostatin analogue octreotide. H_2 blockers or proton-pump inhibitors are often given as well, although the benefits of antisecretory therapy in this setting have not been proved. For chronic blood loss, if no other cause is identified and there are no contraindications, often an effective approach is the administration of a β-blocker (e.g., propranolol) in divided doses, titrated to produce a resting pulse of 60 bpm. Rarely do patients with blood loss from portal hypertensive gastropathy require portosystemic shunt surgery, unless they have refractory or rebleeding varices that need surgical decompression.

10. What is meant by "alkaline reflux" gastritis?

Alkaline or bile reflux gastritis refers to a mucosal injury caused by reflux of duodenal or jejunal contents into the stomach. This condition is most commonly encountered after vagotomy and antrectomy for ulcer disease with either a Billroth I or II type anastomosis. The gastritis is nonerosive. Histologically, there is hyperplasia of gastric foveolar glands, islands of lipid-containing histiocytes, and, occasionally, cystic dilatations of the glands, along with edema in the lamina propria and minimal to mild chronic inflammation. The term *bile reflux gastritis* is probably more accurate in describing the etiology of this type of gastritis, because chronic exposure of gastric mucosa to bile can produce these changes.

11. What are the treatment options for patients with symptomatic alkaline reflux gastritis?

Most patients are asymptomatic from the gastritis per se, but some may complain of burning epigastric pain unrelieved by random use of antacids, worsened by meals, and associated with bilious vomiting. Various medical treatments have been tried, none with universal success. Rational treatments are based on attempts to neutralize the effects of refluxed bile, alter bile components, promote prompt gastric emptying, or divert bile from entering the stomach. Aluminum-containing antacids and sucralfate taken after meals and at bedtime bind bile acids and may offer protection for the mucosa, although they are seldom effective. Ursodiol, a component of bear bile, has been used to alter bile composition to more water-soluble forms, which are less injurious to the mucosa. Bile acid binders, such as cholestyramine and cholestid, are useful, but caution must be used in patients with prior vagotomy with gastric stasis so that bezoars do not form. Prokinetic drugs such as metoclopramide, bethanechol, and cisapride enhance gastric emptying and may be worth trying. If medical therapy fails to relieve symptoms, surgical diversion by Roux-en-Y gastrojejunostomy may be necessary.

12. Outline the approach to the patient with chronic dyspepsia and gastritis.

Evaluation and Management of Chronic Gastritis

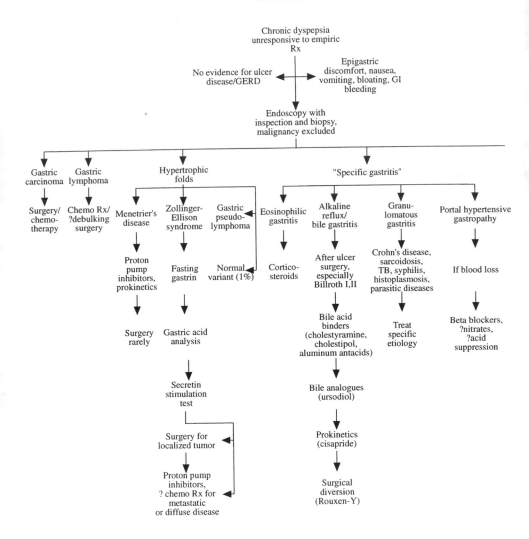

Evaluation and Management of Chronic Gastritis *(Continued)*

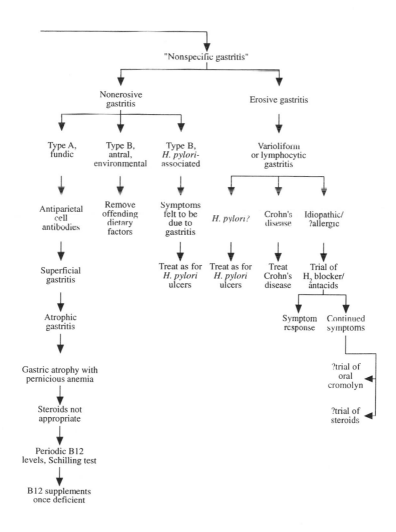

BIBLIOGRAPHY

1. Antonioli DA: Chronic gastritis: Classification. In Bayless TM (ed): Current Therapy in Gastroenterology and Liver Disease, 4th ed. St. Louis, Mosby, 1994.
2. Correa P: Chronic gastritis: A clinico-pathological classification. Am J Gastroenterol 83:504, 1988.
3. DeCross AJ, McCallum RW: Chronic gastritis: Management. In Bayless TM (ed): Current Therapy in Gastroenterology and Liver Disease, 4th ed. St. Louis, Mosby, 1994.
4. Dixon MF, et al: Reflux gastritis: Distinct histopathological entity. J Clin Pathol 39:524, 1986.
5. Dixon MF, et al: Lymphocytic gastritis—relationship to *Campylobacter pylori* infection. J Pathol 153: 125, 1989.
6. Dooley CP, et al: Prevalence of *Helicobacter pylori* infection and histologic gastritis in asymptomatic persons. N Engl J Med 321:1562, 1989.
7. Ectors NL, Dixon MF, Geboes KJ, et al: Granulomatous gastritis: A morphological and diagnostic approach. Histopathology 23:55, 1993.
8. Elta FG, Appelman HD, Behler EM, et al: A study of the correlation between endoscopic and histologic diagnoses in gastroduodenitis. Am J Gastroenterol 82:749, 1987.
9. Gostout CJ, Viggiano TR, Balm RK: Acute gastrointestinal bleeding from portal hypertensive gastropathy: Prevalence and clinical features. Am J Gastroenterol 88:2030, 1993.
10. Graham DY, Go MF: *Helicobacter pylori:* Current status. Gastroenterology 105:279, 1993.
11. Haot J, et al: Lymphocytic gastritis: Prospective study of its relationship with varioliform gastritis. Gut 31: 282, 1990.
12. Laine L, Weinstein WM: Histology of alcoholic hemorrhagic "gastritis": A prospective evaluation. Gastroenterology 94:1254, 1988.
13. McCormack TT, et al: Gastric lesions in portal hypertension: Inflammatory gastritis or congestive gastropathy? Gut 26:1226, 1985.
14. Reveille RM: Chronic gastritis. In Levine JS (ed): Decision Making in Gastroenterology, 2nd ed. St. Louis, Mosby, 1992.
15. Rubin CE: Histological classification of chronic gastritis: An iconoclastic view. Gastroenterology 102:360, 1992.
16. The Sydney System: A new classification of gastritis: The Working Party Report of the World Congresses of Gastroenterology. J Gastroenterol Hepatol 6:207, 1991.

11. GASTRIC CANCER

John Deutsch, M.D.

1. What are the usual cell types in primary gastric malignancies?
Approximately 90–95% of gastric malignancies are adenocarcinomas. Another 5% are due to lymphoma, whereas 1–2 % are squamous cell cancers, carcinoid tumors, and leiomyosarcomas.

2. Describe the geographic distribution of gastric cancer.
Gastric cancer is one of the most common malignancies in parts of Asia and South America. The incidence in Japan is approximately 8-fold greater than the incidence in the U.S.

3. What causes gastric cancer?
The cause is unknown. However, food preservation may play a role, since the incidence of gastric cancer is highest in regions of the world where salted and smoked fish and meat are common. Recent epidemiologic evidence has also linked *Helicobacter pylori* infection with the development of gastric cancer. In addition, the risk of gastric cancer appears to be increased in patients with pernicious anemia or atrophic gastritis with achlorhydria.

4. Does omeprazole cause gastric cancer?
Omeprazole is the most potent acid-suppressant used to treat peptic ulcer disease. One predictable side effect of acid suppression is an elevation in serum levels of gastrin. Elevated gastrin levels, particularly in rats, lead to the development of carcinoid tumors of the stomach. However, in humans, it does not appear to cause problems even after 5 years of continual use.

5. What is gastric stump cancer?
Gastric stump cancer is an adenocarcinoma at a gastrointestinal anastomosis. The risk of developing gastric cancer appears to be increased 15 or more years after partial gastrectomy.

6. Should high-risk patients be screened for gastric cancer?
Although screening programs appear to be successful in high-incidence areas of the world such as Japan, screening in the U.S., even of patients at a relative increased risk (pernicious anemia, previous gastric surgery), does not appear to be efficacious, possibly because of the low background incidence.

7. Should asymptomatic *Helicobacter pylori* infections be treated to decrease the risk of gastric cancer?
Not at this time, although the issue is somewhat controversial. Although *H. pylori* infection is associated with the development of gastric cancer, the risk appears to be low. *H. pylori* is commonly found in adult Americans; over 50% of men older than 60 years have serologic evidence of infection. Gastric cancer is uncommon compared with the number of adults with *Helicobacter* infection.

8. What genetic alterations commonly occur in gastric malignancies?
Abnormalities in the tumor suppressor genes p53 (chromosome 17) and DCC (chromosome 18) have been found in over 50% of gastric cancers. These mutations are also common in colonic tumors. However, mutations in the *ras*-oncogene family appear to be rare in gastric cancers, although they are common in colonic tumors.

9. Are aneuploid gastric cancers biologically more aggressive than diploid gastric cancers?
Aneuploid tissue contains an abnormal amount of DNA per nucleus, which is usually associated with more anaplastic lesions. Several studies have suggested that aneuploidy is a poor prognostic sign in gastric cancer, whereas several others have failed to confirm the association.

10. How is the incidence of gastric cancer changing in the U.S.?
The incidence of cancer of the body of the stomach has decreased over the last 50 years. However, the incidence of adenocarcinoma of the gastroesophageal junction has recently increased.

11. What is a gastric polyp?
Gastric polyps are growths in the stomach. There are three major types: adenomas, hamartomas, and hyperplastic polyps. Only adenomas are associated with gastric cancer.

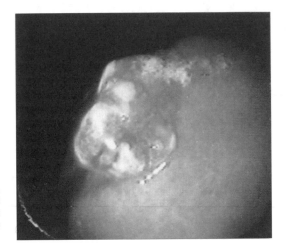

An endoscopic view of a large gastric polyp. It is impossible to tell whether it is malignant or benign without histology. This polyp was removed by snare cautery and found to be hyperplastic.

12. What is the malignant potential of the gastric polyps found in Peutz-Jeghers syndrome?
Gastric polyps in Peutz-Jeghers syndrome are usually hamartomas; their malignant potential is no greater than that of surrounding tissue.

13. What is a Krukenberg tumor?
Krukenberg tumors are metastases of gastric cancer to the ovaries. Women with gastric cancer sometimes present with tumorous infiltration of the ovaries before discovery of the gastric primary tumor.

14. What are the usual presenting symptoms of gastric cancer?
Gastric cancer often has no symptoms until late in the disease when patients have weight loss, abdominal pain, or symptoms from metastatic disease. Massive gastrointestinal bleeding is an abnormal presentation except for leiomyosarcomas.

15. Why is follow-up endoscopy recommended for benign gastric ulcers?
About 1–3% of gastric ulcers that are thought to be benign in fact are due to gastric cancer. Follow-up is performed to assess healing and to obtain biopsies of nonhealing lesions. This practice is somewhat controversial, because it rarely diagnoses a gastric cancer that is cured with resection.

16. How is gastric cancer usually diagnosed?

Patients with gastric cancer are usually evaluated late in the course of disease course for weight loss or abdominal pain. Often they have had either a barium radiograph or esophagogastroduo-denoscopy (EGD). Sometimes patients are found to have metastatic disease during an evaluation of abnormal blood levels of liver-associated enzymes. The diagnosis of gastric cancer requires a biopsy, which is almost always obtained during EGD.

17. Why are eight biopsies recommended for suspicious gastric lesions?

Gastric tumors are usually surrounded by inflammation, and the center of the tumor may be necrotic. It is easy to biopsy an abnormal area in the stomach that contains cancer without obtaining identifiable cancer cells. Studies have shown that multiple biopsies of suspicious gastric lesions increase the likelihood of correct diagnosis. For example, there is a 70% of diagnosing gastric cancer from a single biopsy of a malignant ulcer, but a 95–99% chance if eight biopsies are obtained. The yield does not appear to increase if more than eight biopsies are taken.

18. What is linitis plastica?

Linitis plastica is an infiltrating growth pattern seen in aggressive gastric adenocarcinomas. The stomach is poorly distendable and appears to be thickened with scar tissue. This pattern of growth is poorly contained; metastatic disease is invariably present at diagnosis.

19. Do any serum markers help to diagnose and manage patients with gastric cancer?

Although various serum markers have been evaluated in patients with gastric cancer, no marker appears to be elevated in more than approximately one-half of patients. Carcinoembryonic antigen (CEA) is elevated in about one-fourth of patients with gastric cancer.

20. How often can gastric adenocarcinoma be cured?

In general, gastric cancer cannot be cured, by the time of diagnosis patients have an advanced malignancy. Large series have shown an overall 5-year survival rate of 8%. Gastric cancer can be cured only by complete surgical resection, which is possible only if the cancer is found at an early stage.

21. Can gastric lymphoma be cured without surgery?

Some patients with gastric lymphoma can be cured without surgery, if they receive aggressive radiation therapy and chemotherapy. In patients with early-stage disease, the cure rate with chemotherapy and radiation therapy appears to be similar to the cure rate with surgical resections.

22. How should patients with a suspected gastric malignancy be evaluated?

First, the diagnosis must be established by biopsy; tissue usually can be obtained during EGD. Next, the patient should be evaluated for metastatic disease, which precludes complete surgical resection. A physical exam, with particular attention to the supraclavicular and axillary lymph nodes, is important. A chest radiograph should be obtained, along with a computed tomography scan of the abdomen. Laparoscopy decreases the number of laparotomies, but most patients require some type of resection to manage the primary tumor.

23. Does adjuvant therapy increase survival rates after attempts at curative resection of gastric adenocarcinoma?

This topic is controversial. Some studies have reported improved survival rates with adjuvant chemotherapy, whereas others have shown no benefit.

24. What role does chemotherapy play in treating gastric cancer?

Several chemotherapeutic regimens have significant activity in patients with adenocarcinoma, but chemotherapy should be considered palliative. Response rates of 50% and higher have been reported for protocols such as ELF (etoposide, leucovorin and 5-fluorouracil) and FAMTX (5-flu-orouracil, adriamycin and methotrexate). EAP (etoposide, adriamycin, cis-platinum) appears to be too toxic for routine use.

BIBLIOGRAPHY

1. Bruckner HW, Chesser MR, Wong H, et al: Folate biochemical modulation regimen for the treatment of gastric cancer. J Clin Gastroenterol 13:384–389, 1991.
2. Bruckner HW, Kondo T: Neoplasms of the stomach. In Holland JF, Frei E III, Bast RC Jr, et al (eds): Cancer Medicine. Philadelphia, Lea & Febiger, 1993.
3. Bytzer P: Endoscopic follow-up study of gastric ulcer to detect malignancy: Is it worthwhile? Scand J Gastroenterol 26:1193–1199, 1991.
4. Chyou PH, Nomura AM, Hankin JH, et al: A case-cohort study of diet and stomach cancer. Cancer Res 50:7501–7504, 1990.
5. Correa P, Fox J, Fontham E, et al: *Helicobacter pylori* and gastric carcinoma. Serum antibody prevalence in populations with contrasting cancer risks. Cancer 66:2569–2574, 1990.
6. Crucitti F, Doglietto GB, Bellantone R, et al: Stomach cancer: a study of 117 consecutive resected cases and results of R2–R3 gastrectomy. Int Surg 76:23–26, 1991.
7. Eckardt VF, Giessler W, Kanzler G, et al: Does endoscopic follow-up improve the outcome of patients with benign gastric ulcers and gastric cancers? Cancer 69:301–305, 1992.
8. Forman D, Mewell DG, Fullerton F, et al: Association between infection with *Helicobacter pylori* and risk of gastric cancer: Evidence from a prospective investigation. BMJ 302:1302–1305, 1991.
9. Haraguchi M, Korenaga D, Kakeji Y, et al: DNA ploidy is associated with growth potential in gastric carcinoma. Cancer 68:2608–2611, 1991.
10. Horii A, Nakatsura S, Miyoshi Y, et al: The APC gene, responsible for familial adenomatous polyposis, is mutated in human gastric cancer. Cancer Res 52:3231–3233, 1992.
11. Katz A, Gansl RC, Simon SD, et al: Phase II trial of etoposide (V), adriamycin (A), and cisplatinum (P) in patients with metastatic gastric cancer. Am J Clin Oncol 14:357–358, 1991.
12. Kelsen D, Atiq OT, Saltz L, et al: FAMTX versus etoposide, doxorubicin, and cisplatinum: A random assignment trial in gastric carcinoma. J Clin Oncol 10:541–548, 1992.
13. Kneller RW, McLaughlin JK, Bjelke E, et al: A cohort study of stomach cancer in a high-risk American population. Cancer 68:672–678, 1991.
14. Kriplani AK, Kapur BM: Laparoscopy for pre-operative staging and assessment of operability in gastric carcinoma. Gastrointest Endosc 37:441–443, 1991.
15. Lerner A, Gonin R, Steele GD Jr, et al: Etoposide, doxorubicin, and cisplatinum chemotherapy for advanced gastric adenocarcinoma: results of a phase II trial. J Clin Oncol 10:536–540, 1992.
16. Nomura A, Stemmermann GN, Chyou PH, et al: *Helicobacter pylori* infection and gastric carcinoma among Japanese Americans in Hawaii. N Engl J Med 325:1132–1136, 1991.
17. Parsonnet J, Friedman GD, Vandersteen DP, et al: *Helicobacter pylori* infection and the risk of gastric carcinoma. N Engl J Med 325:1127–1131, 1991.
18. Sano T, Tsujino T, Yoshida K, et al: Frequent loss of heterozygosity on chromosomes 1q, 5q, and 17p in human gastric cancers. Cancer Res 51:2926–2931, 1991.
19. Serucha R, David L, Holm R, et al: p53 mutations in gastric carcinoma. Br J Cancer 65:708–710, 1992.
20. Stael von Holstein C, Eriksson S, Huldt B, et al: Endoscopic screening during 17 years for gastric stump carcinoma. A prospective clinical trial. Scand J Gastroenterol 26:1020–1026, 1991.
21. Tamura G, Kihana T, Nomura K, et al: Detection of frequent p53 gene mutations in primary gastric cancer by cell sorting and polymerase chain reaction. Cancer Res 51:3056–3058, 1991.
22. Uchino S, Tsuda H, Noguchi M, et al: Frequent loss of heterozygosity at the DCC locus in gastric cancer. Cancer Res 52:3099–3102, 1992.
23. Wobbes T, Thomas CM, Segers MF, et al: Evaluation of seven tumor markers (CA 50, CA 19-9, CA 19-9 TruQuant, CA 72-4, CA 195, carcinoembryonic antigen, and tissue polypeptide antigen) in the pretreatment sera of patients with gastric carcinoma. Cancer 69:2036–2041, 1992.

12. PEPTIC ULCER DISEASE AND HELICOBACTER PYLORI

Steven D. Caras, M.D.,Ph.D., and David A. Peura, M.D.

1. What is *Helicobacter pylori?*

H. pylori (previously classified as *Campylobacter pylori*) is a spiral-shaped, gram-negative bacterium, 0.5 microns in width and ranging from 2–6.5 microns in length. Its main distinguishing features are multiple sheathed, unipolar flagella and potent urease activity. The organism's shape and flagella allow penetration of and movement through the gastric mucus layer. Its urease activity appears essential for colonization and survival. Urease also forms the basis for diagnostic testing for infection. Although gastric bacteria were first described in the human stomach at the turn of the century, their importance in peptic ulcer disease and chronic gastritis was not appreciated until the early 1980s.[12] *H. pylori* was first successfully cultured in 1982 by Marshall and Warren.[6]

2. Do any other Helicobacter-like organisms cause disease?

Four other spiral-shaped organisms have been identified in human gastrointestinal mucosa: *H. cinadei, H. fennelliae, Flexispira rappni,* and *Gastrospirillum hominis. G. hominis,* thought to be transmitted by close contact with dogs and cats, has been shown to cause chronic gastritis in humans. Whether the other organisms cause clinical gastrointestinal disease is presently unclear.

3. What is the worldwide prevalence of *H. pylori?*

The geographic distribution of *H. pylori* is closely correlated with socioeconomic development. In developing countries, the prevalence of infection may reach levels of 80–90% by 20 years of age.[7] This prevalence remains constant for the rest of adult life. In contrast, in developed countries the prevalence of *H. pylori* infection is less than 20% in people below the age of 25 years and increases about 1% per year to about 50–60% by age 70. Incidence data from developing countries appear to be subject to generational bias; primary infection is acquired during childhood, but each successive birth cohort is less likely to develop infection. Within a given geographic area, incidence appears to be affected by racial and ethnic factors. For example, in the United States, African-Americans and Hispanics acquire infection earlier in life and more frequently than Caucasians.

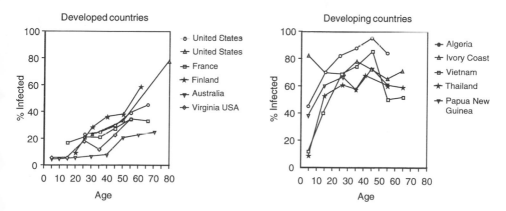

Seroprevalence of *H. pylori* infection in developed and developing countries. (From Marshall et al (eds): *H. pylori* in Peptic Ulceration and Gastritis. Boston, Blackwell, 1991, pp 46–58. Reprinted with permission of the American Digestive Health Foundation.)

4. Are children ever infected by *H. pylori*?

As noted above, most infection is probably acquired during childhood. *H. pylori* has been found to cause clinical symptoms of nausea, vomiting, abdominal pain, hematemesis, and melena in children between 8–16 years of age. The organism also has been isolated from the stool of children with diarrheal illnesses. Although antihelicobacter antibodies have been demonstrated in neonates, this most likely represents placental transfer of maternal antibodies. Primary infection before the age of 2 years is rare. Siblings and parents of infected children are more likely to be infected.[1]

5. What are the risk factors for *H. pylori* infection?

Low socioeconomic status, crowded living conditions, and suboptimal sanitary conditions appear to be major risk factors for acquiring *H. pylori*. Gastroenterologists have a higher than expected prevalence of infection, possibly from contact with infected gastric secretions and endoscopic equipment. Such transmission, however, is less likely now that most physicians adhere to universal precautions during endoscopic procedures. No evidence links *H. pylori* infection to gender, smoking, alcohol, or particular diet.

6. How is infection transmitted?

The exact mode of transmission is not known at present. However, most data support fecal-oral or oral-oral routes. The higher than anticipated prevalence in institutionalized individuals, familial clustering of infection, association with crowded living conditions, and documented transmission from contaminated devices such as endoscopes suggest person-to-person spread. In Peru, infection has been linked epidemiologically to the municipal water supply in low-income communities. The organism has been cultured from dental plaque of dyspeptic patients and from the feces of young children with diarrheal illnesses.

7. Where in the gastrointestinal tract does *H. pylori* live?

H. pylori infection is restricted to humans and primates. It colonizes primarily the stomach and is well adapted to survive in this otherwise hostile environment. The organism lives within or beneath the gastric mucus layer, somewhat protected from stomach acid, and its potent urease activity, which hydrolyzes urea to ammonia and bicarbonate, increases resistance to the stomach's low pH environment. *H. pylori* recognizes and binds to specific receptors expressed by gastric-type epithelial cells and, therefore, is able to adhere tightly to the epithelial cell surface.[10] The organism has been found adherent to ectopic gastric epithelium throughout the gastrointestinal tract, i.e., esophagus (Barrett's esophagus), duodenum (gastric metaplasia), small intestine (Meckel's diverticulum), and rectum (ectopic patches of gastric mucosa).

8. Can *H. pylori* be detected endoscopically? If so, how?

The organism was first cultured from endoscopically obtained gastric tissue. Culture of the organism, however, is difficult and requires appropriately enriched culture medium and prolonged incubation for 3–5 days in a controlled microaerophilic environment. For these reasons, direct culture of *H. pylori* is generally not useful for clinical diagnosis and should be reserved for special circumstances, such as determining antibiotic sensitivity profiles for treatment of resistant organisms.

An alternative method to detect organisms is histologic staining of gastric biopsy material. Organisms can be detected with standard hematoxylin and eosin stains but sensitivity may vary with staining technique, number of organisms present, and the experience of the histopathologist. Special stains that make organisms easier to identify include Giemsa, Warthin-Starry, and Genta. Sensitivity and specificity of histology are > 95%.

A third method to detect organisms in endoscopically obtained biopsy material uses the bacteria's potent urease activity. A biopsy specimen is placed on a template containing urea and a pH indicator. If *H. pylori* are present, the urease hydrolyzes urea to bicarbonate and ammonia, raising the pH and changing the color of the pH indicator. The sensitivity and specificity of biopsy urease testing are > 95%.[2]

Diagnostic Tests for H. pylori

TEST	SENSITIVITY (%)	SPECIFICITY (%)	RELATIVE COST
Noninvasive			
Serology	88–99	86–95	$
Urea breath test	90–97	90–100	$$
Invasive			
Rapid urease assay	89–98	93–98	$$$$*
Histology	93–99	95–99	$$$$$*
Culture	77–92	100	$$$$$*

*Includes cost of endoscopy
Reprinted with permission of the American Digestive Health Foundation. (Adapted from Brown and Peura, Gastroenterol Clin North Am 22:105, 1993.[2])

9. Is endoscopy necessary to diagnose infection?

Nonendoscopic methods to detect *H. pylori* infection include serology and urea breath testing. IgG or IgA antibodies directed at various bacterial antigens can be detected by enzyme-linked immunosorbant assay (ELISA). In addition, several office-based serologic methods are commercially available. Serologic methods detect evidence of primary *H. pylori* infection in untreated individuals with a sensitivity and specificity > 90%. Although antibody levels may fall after successful bacterial eradication, they remain elevated for up to 3 years. This "serologic scar" limits the usefulness of serology in assessing treatment and determining reinfection.

A urea breath test is another noninvasive method to detect *H. pylori* infection.[12] It is ideally suited to monitor treatment response and to assess reinfection, because it is positive only in a setting of active infection. The patient ingests a small amount of radiolabelled urea. *H. pylori*'s urease hydrolyzes the urea and liberates labelled carbon dioxide, which is absorbed and exhaled in the breath. Labelled carbon dioxide can be collected and quantified in breath samples. Sensitivity and specificity of urea breath testing are > 95%. At present, urea breath tests are not generally available; they have yet to be approved by the Food and Drug Administration for commercial use and distribution.

10. What is the best method to detect H. pylori in clinical practice?

To be cost-effective, the various diagnostic tests should be used appropriately to answer specific questions. If diagnostic endoscopy is indicated to establish a clinical diagnosis, the preferred method to detect *H. pylori* infection is the biopsy urease test, which adds little additional cost to that of the endoscopic procedure. Histologic examination also may be used, but tissue processing and histopathologic interpretation add additional costs. A biopsy urease test turns positive within 24 hours, but results often are available within 1 hour. Histologic interpretation usually takes several days. As noted previously, direct bacterial culture is rarely indicated.

If the clinical diagnosis has been established by prior endoscopy or upper gastrointestinal barium radiographs, serology is the test of choice to determine *H. pylori* status. It is noninvasive, simple to perform, and relatively inexpensive.

When breath testing becomes generally available, it will be the method of choice to confirm bacterial eradication in selected patients, such as patients with complicated ulcer disease or patients in whom symptoms return after antihelicobacter therapy. Alternatively, endoscopic techniques may be used to assess treatment success.

Recent use of antibiotics, bismuth-containing compounds, or acid pump inhibitors such as omeprazole suppress bacteria, leading to false-negative results with rapid urease analysis, histologic exam, culture, and breath test. Therefore, testing with these methods should be delayed until 4 weeks after treatment has been discontinued.

11. How does _H. pylori_ cause damage?
A number of potential mechanisms may play a role in the pathogenicity of _H. pylori_. Direct adherence of the organism to epithelial cells, ammonia produced by the urease enzyme, and bacterial cytotoxins may damage epithelial cell membranes. Other bacterial enzymes disrupt the protective mucus barrier, rendering the underlying mucosal surface more susceptible to acid injury. Further damage may occur as a result of the local and systemic inflammatory response to infection.[3]

12. Does infection cause physiologic abnormalities?
H. pylori has been found to increase serum gastrin levels, which in turn increase gastric acid production.[8] Although the mechanisms for such effects are unclear at present, most evidence suggests that they are due to interference with the inhibitory effects of somatostatin produced by the antral D-cell on the gastrin-producing G-cell.[11] After successful eradication of infection, physiologic abnormalities tend to normalize.

13. What is the association of _H. pylori_ with histologic gastritis?
Infection with _H. pylori_ is known to produce an active chronic gastritis with intraepithelial and interstitial neutrophils in addition to lymphocytes and plasma cells. In most individuals, gastritis remains confined to the antrum. In others, however, it may progress to involve the entire stomach. Patients with antral gastritis alone are more likely to develop subsequent duodenal ulcers, whereas patients with pangastritis, especially in association with atrophy and intestinal metaplasia, are at risk for gastric ulcers and adenocarcinoma.

14. What is the association of _H. pylori_ with duodenal ulcer disease?
The association between duodenal ulcer and _H. pylori_ gastritis is very strong. As many as 95% of patients with duodenal ulcer are infected with _H. pylori_.

15. What is the mechanism by which stomach infection causes duodenal ulcers?
As noted above, infection may result in excessive acid production. Over years, excessive acid, along with other unknown factors, may damage the duodenal mucosa, resulting in duodenal gastric metaplasia. The metaplastic epithelium becomes infected by _H. pylori,_ leading to duodenitis and eventual duodenal ulcer. Thus, one can prevent duodenal ulcers by eliminating acid (the traditional approach) or by eliminating _H. pylori_.

16. Does _H. pylori_ play a role in gastric ulcer?
Most gastric ulcers (60–90%) occur in the setting of _H. pylori_ gastritis. As noted above, _H. pylori_ makes the gastric mucosal layer more susceptible to acid injury through various mechanisms.

17. Are there other causes of ulcers besides _H. pylori?_
H. pylori-negative duodenal ulcer disease is rare and usually due to nonsteroidal antiinflammatory drugs (NSAIDs), hypersecretory conditions such as Zollinger-Ellison syndrome, or unusual manifestations of conditions such as Crohn's disease. True idiopathic duodenal ulcers may be genetically determined and are characterized by hypersecretion of acid, rapid gastric emptying, poor response to traditional treatment, and clinical complications. Most _H. pylori_-negative gastric ulcers are associated with NSAIDs. Nevertheless, gastric adenocarcinoma or lymphoma should be excluded in all patients with gastric ulcer.

18. Can infected individuals develop symptoms even without a detectable ulcer?
Nonulcer dyspepsia (NUD) is a poorly defined clinical entity, probably with multiple causes. Evidence that _H. pylori_ gastritis causes dyspepsia in the absence of an ulcer has been difficult to obtain, because no specific symptoms separate _H. pylori_-related dyspepsia from other forms of nonulcer dyspepsia. In addition, the effect of treatment for _H. pylori_ infection on NUD symptoms has been unreliable. Nevertheless, a subset of patients with NUD certainly has symptoms related to infection and responds to treatment. Unfortunately, at present we cannot reliably identify such patients.

19. Why do only a few infected individuals develop clinical disease?

All infected individuals develop histologic evidence of active chronic gastritis. However, only a minority develop clinically obvious symptoms. At present, it is unknown whether host factors, such as immune response or genetic susceptibility, or infection with more virulent bacterial strains is the major determinant of clinical illness.

20. In what situation is it appropriate to eradicate *H. pylori* infection?

The February 1994 Consensus Conference of the National Institutes of Health[19] recommended treatment of infected patients with ulcer disease with antimicrobial and antiulcer medication on initial presentation or recurrence. In addition, infected patients with ulcer disease who are on maintenance therapy with antisecretory agents should be treated for infection and maintenance therapy discontinued. Antimicrobial treatment is also recommended for infected patients in whom NSAIDs are a contributing factor. Current data are insufficient to recommend treatment of all infected patients with nonulcer dyspepsia or of asymptomatic infected individuals to prevent subsequent ulcer disease or gastric neoplasia.

21. What role does treatment of *H. pylori* infection play in complicated ulcer disease?

Complications such as bleeding from peptic ulcers are associated with significant morbidity and mortality. Data suggest that once complicated ulcers have healed, maintenance antisecretory therapy reduces the likelihood of recurrent complication; preliminary studies show that eradicating *H. pylori* also may be effective in preventing ulcer complications. However, until such studies have been confirmed, it may be prudent to continue maintenance antisecretory therapy in patients with complicated ulcer disease even after *H. pylori* has been eradicated.

22. What treatment regimens have been used to eradicate *H. pylori*?

A 2-week course of triple therapy, which combines bismuth, metronidazole, and either tetracycline or amoxicillin, eliminates infection in 75–90% of patients.[3] It is less effective in patients

Therapeutic Options

REGIMEN	DRUGS	DOSAGE	DURATION
Standard triple therapy	Pepto-Bismol Metronidazole Tetracycline *or* amoxicillin	2 tablets qid 250 mg qid 500 mg qid 500 mg qid	2 weeks
Triple therapy plus ranitidine (**acute ulcer**)	To standard triple therapy, add H₂RA	Full dose at bedtime	2 weeks, then 4–6 weeks treatment with H₂RA alone
Dual therapy with acid pump inhibitor	Omeprazole Amoxicillin (dosed concurrently) *or*	20 mg bid 500–750 mg qid	2 weeks
	Omeprazole Clarithromycin (dosed concurrently)	20 mg bid 500 mg tid	2 weeks
Dual therapy with acid pump inhibitor (**acute ulcer**)	Omeprazole Amoxicillin (dosed concurrently) *or*	20 mg bid 500–750 mg qid	2 weeks
	Omeprazole Clarithromycin (dosed concurrently)	20 mg bid 500 mg tid	2 weeks, then 2 weeks treatment with omeprazole alone (20 mg qd) *or* 4–6 weeks treatment with full dose H₂RA

Reproduced from *Helicobacter pylori:* The New Factor in Management of Ulcer Disease, 1994, The Digestive Health Initiative.

with metronidazole-resistant organisms. In addition, the regimen is complicated and associated with poor compliance as well as side effects.

Alternative regimens include a 2-week course of an acid pump inhibitor such as omeprazole and either amoxicillin or clarithromycin. Although simpler to take and associated with fewer side effects than triple therapy, such regimens are slightly less effective; eradication rates range from 70–80%. To achieve maximal efficacy, treatment with omeprazole and an antibiotic should be started at the same time.

23. What happens to peptic ulcer disease when *H. pylori* infection is eradicated?
The annual recurrence rate of duodenal ulcers after healing is approximately 75%. The rate can be reduced to 25% with chronic maintenance antiulcer treatment. If *H. pylori* is eradicated, recurrence of duodenal ulcers is less than 5% per year.[4] Gastric ulcers not associated with NSAIDs also recur infrequently after *H. pylori* eradication.

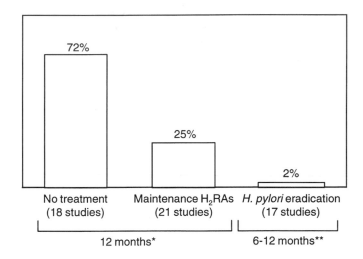

Duodenal ulcer recurrence: results of three strategies.
*Freston: Am J Gastroenterol 82(12):1242, 1987.
**Data from Tytgat and Rauws: Gastroenterol Clin North Am 19:183, 1993. Reprinted with permission of the American Digestive Health Foundation.

24. Is reinfection a common problem?
Rates of reinfection after eradication vary geographically. In developing countries, the annual recurrence rate may be as high as 15%. However, in developed countries such as the U.S., once infection has been eliminated, the annual rate of reinfection is low (0.5%–3%).

25. What economic benefits are associated with eradication of *H. pylori* infection?
To date, no studies have compared actual costs of treating ulcers with and without *H. pylori* eradication. However, computer modeling comparing the direct and indirect costs of various treatments clearly shows that antibiotic therapy is the least expensive option. This cost advantage holds true over a wide range of assumptions relative to the rate of *H. pylori* eradication, reinfection, and cost of treatment.

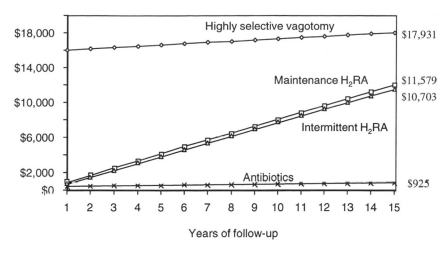

Projected total cost of duodenal ulcer therapy. (From Sonnenberg: NIH Consensus Conference on *H. pylori*, 1993. Reprinted with permission of the American Digestive Health Foundation.)

BIBLIOGRAPHY

1. Blecker U, Lanciers S, Mahta D, et al: Familial clusters of *Helicobacter pylori* infections. Clin Pediatr 33:307–308, 1994.
2. Brown K, Peura D: Diagnosis of *Helicobacter pylori* infection. Gastroenterol Clin North Am 22:105–116, 1993.
3. Dixon MF: Pathophysiology of *Helicobacter pylori* infection. Scand J Gastroenterol 29(Suppl 201).7–10, 1994.
4. Forbes GM, Gluner ME, Cullen DJ, et al: Duodenal ulcer treated with *H. pylori* eradication: Seven-year follow up. Lancet 343:258–260, 1994.
5. Marshall BJ: Treatment strategies for *H. pylori* infection. Gastrointest Clin North Am 22:183–198, 1993.
6. Marshall BJ, Warren JR: Unidentified curved bacilli in the stomach of patients with gastritis and peptic ulceration. Lancet 1(8390):1311–1315, 1984.
7. Marshall BJ, et al (eds): *Helicobacter pylori* in Peptic Ulceration and Gastritis. Boston, Blackwell Scientific, 1991.
8. Moss SF, Calam J: Acid secretion and sensitivity to gastrin in patients with duodenal ulcer: Effect of eradication of *H. pylori*. Gut 34:888–892, 1993.
9. NIH Consensus Development Panel on *Helicobacter pylori* in Peptic Ulcer Disease: *Helicobacter pylori* in peptic ulcer disease. JAMA 272:65–69, 1994.
10. Northfield TC, Mendall M, Goggin PM (eds): Helicobacter Infection: Pathophysiology, Epidemiology and Management. Boston, Kluwer Academic Publishers, 1993.
11. Odurn L, Petersen HD, Andersen IB, et al: Gastrin and somatostatin—*Helicobacter pylori*-infected antral mucosa. Gut 35:615–618, 1994.
12. Rathbone BJ, Heathley RV (eds): *Helicobacter pylori* and Gastrointestinal Disease. Boston, Blackwell Scientific, 1992.
13. Walsh JH, Peterson WI: The treatment of *Helicobacter pylori* infection in the management of peptic ulcer disease. N Engl J Med 333:984–991, 1995.

13. GASTRIC POLYPS AND THICKENED GASTRIC FOLDS

Gregory G. Ginsberg, M.D.

1. What are gastric polyps?

Gastric polyps are any abnormal growth of epithelial tissue arising from the otherwise smooth surface of the stomach. They may be sessile or pedunculated. Hyperplastic polyps account for 70–90% of gastric polyps. Adenomatous, fundic gland polyps, and hamartomas make up the rest.

2. Describe the histologic features of each type of gastric polyp.

Hyperplastic polyps consist of hyperplastic, elongated gastric glands with abundant edematous stroma. There is often cystic dilation of glandular portions but no alteration of the original cellular configuration. Adenomatous polyps are defined as true neoplastic growths composed of dysplastic epithelium not normally present in the stomach. They are composed of cells with hyperchromatic, elongated nuclei arranged in picket-fence patterns with increased mitotic figures. Fundic gland polyps are composed of hypertrophied fundic gland mucosa and are considered a normal variant. Hamartomatous polyps have branching bands of smooth muscle surrounded by glandular epithelium; the lamina propria is normal.

3. What is the risk of malignancy associated with gastric polyps?

The risk of malignant transformation in hyperplastic polyps is low (0.6–4.5%). Adenomas are true neoplasms. The risk of malignant transformation is as high as 75% and is size-dependent; size >2.0 cm is critically significant, although carcinomas have developed from adenomatous polyps <2.0 cm. Fundic gland polyps and gastric hamartomas have no malignant potential.

4. How should gastric polyps be managed?

Because polyp histology cannot be reliably distinguished by endoscopic appearance or forceps biopsy sampling, gastric epithelial polyps should be entirely excised endoscopically if feasible. Gastric epithelial polyps with a diameter of 3–5 mm may be removed entirely by multiple forceps biopsies. Sessile and pedunculated polyps >5.0 mm in diameter should be excised by snare resection and tissue retrieved for histologic evaluation. Larger, broad-based polyps that cannot be safely removed endoscopically should undergo surgical excision. Hyperplastic and adenomatous gastric polyps occur against a background of chronic gastritis and, in some instances, intestinal metaplasia. Thus the risk of cancer in the gastric mucosa apart from the polyp is increased. This association is greater with adenomatous rather than hyperplastic gastric polyps and increases with age. Therefore, in addition to removing all polyps, a careful exam should be performed to evaluate the remaining gastric mucosa, and biopsies should be obtained from any areas displaying surface abnormalities.

5. Is surveillance necessary in patients with gastric polyps?

Routine surveillance with endoscopy is not required for patients with gastric hyperplastic or fundic gland polyps. The recurrence rate of adenomatous polyps is 16%, and although the long-term benefits of surveillance have not been determined, patients may well benefit from interval surveillance with endoscopy.

6. What is the relationship between gastric polyps and chronic gastritis?

Gastric adenomatous and hyperplastic polyps commonly appear against a background of chronic gastritis and are late manifestations of *Helicobacter pylori* infection, or type A chronic gastritis (pernicious anemia). Multiple mucosal biopsies should be obtained to determine the presence and severity of underlying gastritis with the emphasis on identifying the presence and type of intestinal metaplasia. *H. pylori* eradication should be attempted for patients with *H. pylori* gastritis and gastric polyps, although it is uncertain whether eradication positively affects polyp recurrence or metaplasia.

7. What is the definition of large gastric folds?
Large gastric folds are defined as those that do not flatten with insufflation of air at the time of endoscopy. Radiographically, large gastric folds are >10 mm in width on standard barium upper GI series.

8. List the differential diagnosis for intrinsic causes of thickened gastric folds.
   Lymphoma
   Mucosa-associated lymphoid tissue (MALT) syndrome
   Linitis plastica
   Gastric adenocarcinoma
   Menetrier's disease
   H. pylori gastritis (acute)
   Zollinger-Ellison syndrome
   Lymphocytic gastritis
   Eosinophilic gastritis
   Gastric antral vascular ectasia
   Gastritis cystica profunda
   Kaposi's sarcoma
   Gastric varices

9. What systemic diseases may be associated with thickened gastric folds or granulomatous gastritis?
Crohn's disease and sarcoidosis may be associated with granulomatous inflammation of the stomach. Other potential causes of granulomatous gastritis include **histoplasmosis, candidiasis, actinomycoses,** and **blastomycoses. Secondary syphylis** may present with *Treponema pallidum* infiltration, producing perivascular plasmacytic response. Disseminated mycobacteria in **tuberculosis** may also cause gastric infiltration. Systemic **mastocytosis,** in addition to facial flushing, may be associated with hyperemic thickened gastric folds. Rarely, **amyloidosis** may cause gastric wall infiltration with thickened gastric folds.

10. Endoscopic ultrasonography (EUS) displays the gastric wall in five alternating hyperechoic and hypoechoic bands. Histologically, to what wall layers do they correlate?

Correlation of EUS Bands and Wall Layers

WALL LAYER	EUS BANDS	HISTOLOGIC CORRELATION
1st	Hyperechoic	Superficial mucosal
2nd	Hypoechoic	Deep mucosa, including the muscularis mucosa
3rd	Hyperechoic	Submucosa
4th	Hypoechoic	Muscularis propria
5th	Hyperechoic	Serosa

11. What is the role of EUS in the evaluation of thickened gastric folds?
Although EUS cannot differentiate between histologically benign and malignant processes, it is of value in the differential diagnosis of large gastric folds and identifies patients in whom further investigation is warranted either with repeated large-particle endoscopic biopsy or full-thickness

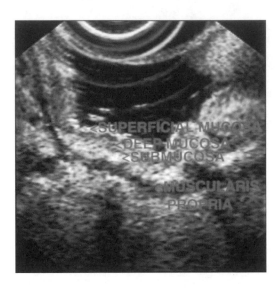

biopsy at laparotomy. EUS is a sensitive means of identifying gastric varices, thereby avoiding the potential dangers of endoscopic biopsy sampling. When EUS demonstrates enlargement limited to the superficial layers, multiple biopsies should confirm the presence of underlying malignancy. Conversely, when EUS documents enlargement involving primarily the deeper layers (i.e., the submucosa or muscularis propria), results of endoscopic biopsies for malignancy may prove negative. This EUS pattern, however, is highly sensitive for malignant invasion; therefore, surgery is recommended to obtain a full-thickness biopsy. Data about the utility of EUS-guided needle aspiration remain forthcoming.

12. What are the clinical features of gastric lymphoma?
Lymphomas account for <5% of all gastric malignancies but make up the largest group second to adenocarcinoma. Of primary gastrointestinal lymphomas, 40–60% arise in the stomach; 20–30% arise from the small bowel, with ilial disease being most common. Multiple sites are reported in 8–15% of cases. B-cell lymphomas make up the largest pathologic group of gastric lymphomas, followed by T-cell phenotype and other varieties. Endoscopically they may present as a discrete polypoid lesion, an ulcerated mass, or a diffuse submucosal infiltration with enlarged rugal folds. The most common presenting symptoms are abdominal pain, weight loss, nausea, anorexia, and hemorrhage. When standard biopsy techniques do not yield a diagnosis but gastric lymphoma is suspected, large-particle biopsies, snare biopsies, and needle aspirates should be attempted. EUS is useful in identifying abnormalities of the deeper wall layers, which raise further suspicion. EUS is also useful in establishing nodal involvement. When endoscopic biopsy techniques are unrevealing, surgical full-thickness biopsy should be obtained.

13. Describe the Ann Arbor Classification of non-Hodgkin's lymphoma as applied to gastric lymphoma.

Stage	Extent of Disease
I	Disease limited to the stomach
II	Extension to abdominal lymph nodes by biopsy or lymphangiography
III	Involvement of the stomach, abdominal lymph nodes, and nodular involvement above the diaphragm
IV	Disseminated lymphoma

14. Define Menetrier's disease.

Menetrier's disease is a rare condition characterized by giant gastric rugal folds that often spare the antrum. The histologic features are marked foveolar hyperplasia with cystic dilations that may penetrate into the submucosa. Symptoms may include abdominal pain, weight loss, gastrointestinal blood loss, and hyperalbuminemia. The cause is unclear. The diagnosis can be confirmed by EUS findings of thickening of the deep mucosal layer and large-particle biopsy specimens demonstrating the characteristic histology. Treatment with H_2 receptor antagonists is successful in some patients.

15. How is Menetrier's disease in children different from Menetrier's disease in adults?

Unlike Menetrier's disease in adults, which is characterized by chronicity of symptoms, Menetrier's disease of children is generally self-limited. Recurrence and sequelae are rare. Clinically, pediatric patients present with abrupt onset of vomiting associated with abdominal pain, anorexia, and hypoproteinemia. Gradual onset of edema and ascites results from this protein-losing enteropathy. Hypoalbuminemia, peripheral eosinophilia, and mild normochromic, normocytic anemia are often seen. Radiographic findings include thickened gastric folds in the fundus and body of the stomach, often with antral sparing. Such findings are confirmed in an upper GI barium meal, ultrasonography, and endoscopy. Histologically the gastric mucosa are hypertrophic with elongation of gastric pits and glandular atrophy. However, in pediatric patients, intranuclear inclusion bodies consistent with cytomegalovirus (CMV) infection are common; culture of gastric tissue is often positive for CMV. Pediatric patients generally respond to supportive, symptomatic treatment with complete resolution.

16. What is lymphocytic gastritis?

Lymphocytic gastritis is characterized by foveolar hyperplasia and abundant infiltration of lymphocytes. It is also termed variolaform gastritis. Gross inspection reveals thickened folds, mucosal nodularity, and multiple erosion, often volcanolike. The cause is unknown. Symptoms are vague, and no therapy has been proved effective. The most important aspect of management is to exclude lymphoma or other specific forms of gastritis.

17. What is the differential diagnosis for a submucosal mass seen on endoscopy?

Common	Less Common	Rare
Leiomyoma	Carcinoid	Leiomyoblastoma
Lipoma	Leiomyosarcoma	Liposarcoma
Aberrant pancreas	Granular cell tumor	Schwannoma
Gastric varix	Lymphoma	
	Splenic remnant	
	Submucosal cyst	
	Extraluminal compression	
	Splenic artery aneurysm	

18. What is the role of EUS in evaluating submucosal lesions?

Although EUS does not provide a histopathologic diagnosis, it allows reliable assumptions about the nature of certain lesions based on their location relative to the sonographic pattern of the gut wall and EUS appearance. EUS may determine whether a lesion is vascular and be used for aspiration cytology and biopsy with jumbo forceps. EUS is accurate in differentiating true submucosal tumors from extraluminal compression by adjacent organs or from varices. Leiomyomas and leiomyosarcomas are seen as hypoechoic structures arising from the fourth (hypoechoic) sonographic layers, which corresponds to the muscularis propria. No unique sonographic differences in size, shape, or appearance distinguish leiomyoma from leiomyosarcoma. Gastric lymphomas appear as diffuse hyperechoic lesions within the submucosal layer. Gastric wall cysts are seen as echo-free structures within the submucosa. Other less common submucosal lesions, such as pancreatic rests, carcinoids, fibromas, and granular cell tumors, have not been described in sufficient numbers to allow description of distinctive EUS findings. EUS findings in submucosal gastric lesions serve as a guide to therapeutic decisions based on lesion size. One management scheme is to follow lesions <2–4 cm in diameter that are without evidence of bleeding, obstruction, or malignancy, by serial endosonography. A significant change in size of the lesion by EUS should be considered an indication for surgery. Larger lesions should be considered for de novo resection.

19. A submucosal mass was identified during upper endoscopy. EUS was performed. A hypoechoic lesion was found to arise from the fourth wall layer or muscularis propria. What is the most likely diagnosis?

The most common lesion with such EUS findings is a leiomyoma. However, a leiomyosarcoma, although less common, may have similar characteristics. In addition, other rare lesions, such as schwannoma, liposarcoma and myxosarcoma, may arise from the muscularis propria and have a similar EUS appearances. EUS is not a substitute for histologic confirmation. When the lesion is well circumscribed, small (<3 cm), and without evidence of surrounding tissue invasion or adenopathy, the size of the lesion may be followed for interval stability, which confers benignity. Lesions that are greater than 3–4 cm, increase in size, or invade surrounding tissue should be considered for resection.

20. A 65-year-old woman presented with self-limited, coffee-ground emesis. Endoscopy reveals a single, pedunculated, 1-cm polyp in the gastric body. What is the best option for management?

The majority of gastric polyps are epithelial in origin; of these, 70–90% are hyperplastic and 10–20% are adenomatous. Although gastric polyps may cause abdominal pain or bleeding, up to 50% are asymptomatic. Complete removal of the lesion by snare polypectomy for histologic evaluation is both diagnostic and curative. Although the risk of complications is greater than for colonoscopic polypectomy, snare polypectomy is generally safe and well tolerated. An epinephrine solution diluted to 1:10,000 can be injected into the stalk of large polyps to lessen the risk of postpolypectomy bleeding. Glucagon may be used to prevent peristalsis from inhibiting retrieval. An overtube should be considered to avoid accidental dislodgement of the polyp into the airway during retrieval. Although not of proven benefit, a brief course of H_2 blocker or sucralfate therapy is generally recommended to promote healing.

21. The accompanying photograph demonstrates findings with upper endoscopy of a patient with familial adenomatous polyposis. What is the most likely histology of such polyps? What is their malignant potential? What other significant upper GI lesions may be detected at the time of upper endoscopy? What are the manifestations of gastric polyps in the other hereditary GI polyposis syndromes?

Nearly all patients with familial adenomatous polyposis have polyps in the upper GI tract. The majority of polyps are found in the proximal stomach or fundus; they are small, multiple, and hyperplastic. Although they carry no risk for carcinomatous conversion, they may cause bleeding. Forty to ninety percent of these patients, however, have adenomatous polyps in the distal stomach, antrum, or duodenum, particularly in the periampullary region. Risk of adenocarcinoma of the gastric antrum is not increased in U.S. families with adenomatous polyposis but appears to be increased in Japanese families. The relative risk of duodenal, particularly periampullary, cancer is markedly increased in patients with familial adenomatous polyposis and duodenal or ampulary adenomas. Patients with Gardner's syndrome have a preponderance of hyperplastic polyps in the proximal stomach. Patients with Peutz-Jeghers syndrome and juvenile polyposis syndromes may have hamartomatous polyps in the stomach. Although they may cause bleeding, an increased cancer risk is not apparent.

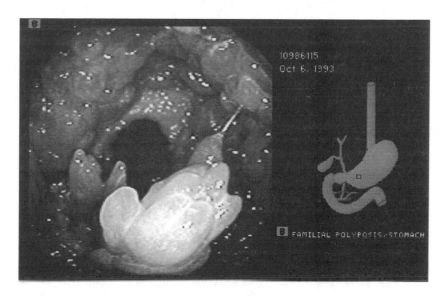

22. What is the relationship between carcinoid tumors of the stomach and atrophic gastritis?

Carcinoid tumors of the stomach occur primarily in the fundus and body. They are generally submucosal but often present as a polypoid structure. Although they can be observed in otherwise normal stomachs, they are found with much higher frequency in patients with achlorhydria secondary to atrophic gastritis. It is believed that carcinoids develop as a result of high concentrations of circulating gastrin, which is trophic for the enterochromaffin cells of the proximal stomach. Although carcinoids have been detected in rats given high doses of omeprazole for long periods, no such lesions have been observed in humans treated with long-term acid suppressive therapy. Gastric carcinoids in the setting of achlorhydria and hypergastrinemia may be treated with antrectomy to remove the source of gastrin. Carcinoids that are not the result of hypergastrinemia should undergo appropriate gastric resection for removal of large tumors. The stomach is the location of approximately 2–3% of all carcinoids, but carcinoids represent only 0.3% of all gastric tumors. Gastric carcinoids do not produce symptoms related to vasoactive peptides, and their discovery is frequently incidental. Complete excision is the treatment of choice, and many, if not most, can be removed endoscopically either with multiple forceps biopsies or snare resection. EUS is useful to assess the gastric wall layer of origin and depth of invasion when endoscopic excision is considered.

23. Endoscopy performed on a homosexual man with acquired immunodeficiency syndrome (AIDS) to evaluate abdominal pain reveals a serpiginous, reddish-purple, thickened fold in the body of the stomach. The patient has similar-appearing lesions on the roof of the mouth and lower extremities. What does this lesion represent? What is the risk of bleeding at biopsy? What histologic characteristics are the biopsies likely to reveal?

The lesion is most likely Kaposi's sarcoma (KS). Upper endoscopy or flexible sigmoidoscopy reveals GI lesions in 40% of patients with AIDS who have KS of the skin and lymph nodes. Endoscopic appearance is characteristic. There is no increased risk of bleeding from biopsies. Histologic confirmation is possible in only 23% of visibly inspected luminal KS because of the submucosal location. Because the vascular lesion is deep to the submucosa and not reached by biopsy forceps, the technique is safe but the results are nonspecific. Symptoms include pain, dysphasia, and occasionally bleeding and obstruction.

24. A 60-year-old woman is referred with nocturnal epigastric pain and secretory diarrhea. A fasting serum gastrin is >1,000 pg/ml. Endoscopy demonstrated diffusely thickened hyperemic antral folds with antral erosions. Forceps biopsies were nondiagnostic. Thiazin stain for _Helicobacter pylori_ was negative. What is the differential diagnosis? What series of tests should be ordered next?

Hypergastrinemia has several possible causes. The absence of a history of prior gastric surgery excludes the consideration of retained antrum syndrome. Spurious use of H_2 blockers or proton pump inhibitors may cause elevation of the serum gastrin level. Type A atrophic gastritis associated with pernicious anemia results in hypergastrinemia due to disinhibition of gastrin production. Finally, the patient may have antral gastrin cell hyperplasia or grastrinoma as part of Zollinger-Ellison syndrome. The endoscopic appearance is consistent only with the last two diagnoses. Gastric acid analysis will identify the presence of gastric acid hypersecretion, distinguishing between hypergastrinemia from Zollinger-Ellison syndrome and appropriate hypergastrinemia in response to achlorhydria. Patients with Zollinger-Ellison syndrome fail to respond to exogenous secretin, and show no decrease in serum gastrin level. However, a secretin stimulation test need not be done when gastric acid hypersecretion >1000 pg/ml accompanies hypergastrinemia.

25. A 40-year-old man has a history of chronic pancreatitis. He presents with a self-limited upper GI bleed. Endoscopy demonstrated a normal esophagus and duodenum.The accompanying photograph represents the gastric findings. What is the most likely diagnosis? What therapeutic options should be considered?

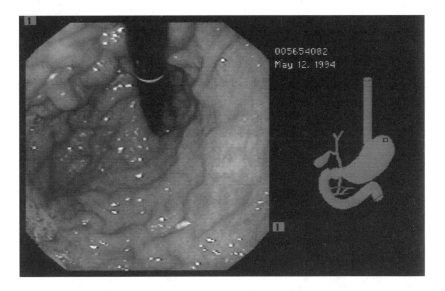

The patient has isolated gastric varices secondary to splenic vein thrombosis. Splenic vein thrombosis is a potential complication of acute and chronic pancreatitis, pancreatic carcinoma, lymphoma, trauma, and hypercoagulable states. The left gastric veins empty via the splenic vein. Esophageal venous flow is unaffected. Because endoscopic therapy is generally not effective for the prevention of gastric variceal bleeding, surgery with splenectomy is required. Gastric varices are submucosal or deep to the submucosa, whereas the esophageal varices lie superficial in the lamina propria. Gastric variceal bleeding accounts for 10–20% of acute variceal hemorrhage. The incidence of gastric variceal bleeding is 10–20% among patients with bleeding from esophagogastric varices. Acute bleeding may be treated endoscopically; however, rebleeding is the rule, and the mortality rate is as high as 55%. When bleeding is due to portal hypertension, transjugular intrahepatic or surgical shunting is effective. European and Canadian experience with intravascular injection of cyanoacrylate has been encouraging, but the drug is not currently available in the U.S. When not actively bleeding, gastric varices may be difficult to distinguish from benign prominent folds. EUS identifies hypoechoic, tortuous dilated blood vessels in the submucosa that are characteristic for gastric varices.

26. A 65-year-old woman is referred for evaluation of chronic iron deficiency anemia and Hemoccult-positive stool. Colonoscopy and upper GI series were negative. Findings of an upper endoscopy are noted in the accompanying photograph. Identify the immediately apparent diagnosis and appropriate treatment.

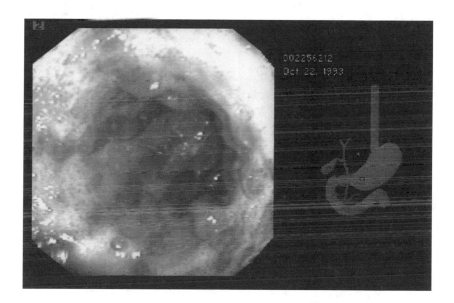

The striking endoscopic appearance of raised, convoluted thickened folds that radiate spoke-like from a pylorus covered by friable vascular malformations is characteristic of "watermelon stomach." The endoscopic appearance is diagnostic. Also referred to as gastric antral vascular ectasia (GAVE), this is a rare source of chronic occult GI bleeding; its incidence in the general population is unknown. It occurs more frequently in women and is often associated with autoimmune or connective tissue disorders. Underlying atrophic gastritis with hypergasteremia and pernicious anemia may be present. The pathogenesis is unclear. Histologic features include dilated mucosal capillaries with focal thrombosis; dilated, tortuous submucosal venous channels; and fibrous fibromuscular hyperplasia. Chronic GI blood loss responds to endoscopic coagulation therapy. The best experience has been with Nd:YAG laser. Lesions may recur but usually respond to repeat endoscopic therapy.

27. What is the most likely diagnosis for the lesion in the accompanying photograph?
The lesion is a pancreatic rest, also called aberrant or heterotopic pancreas. Such lesions occur typically in the prepyloric antrum and often have a central umbilication. Endoscopic appearance is usually diagnostic. EUS findings are variable but may demonstrate a relatively hyperechoic lesion arising from the mucosa or submucosa, with a central ductal structure in some cases. Pancreatic rests rarely produce symptoms.

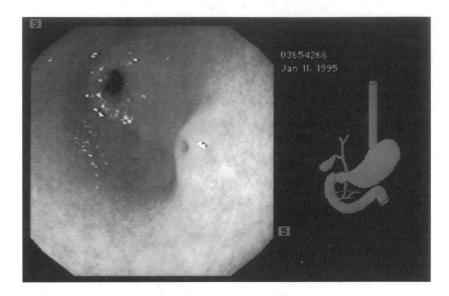

BIBLIOGRAPHY

1. Amer MH, el-Akkad S: Gastrointestinal lymphoma in adults: Clinical features and management of three hundred cases. Gastroenterology 106:846, 1994.
2. Caletti GC, Brocchie E, Baraldini M, et al: Assessment of portal hypertension by endosonography. Gastrointest Endosc 34:154–155, 1988.
3. Cristallini E, Ascani S, Bolis G: Association between histologic type of polyp and carcinoma of the stomach. Gastrointest Endosc 38:481–484, 1992.
4. d'Amore F, Brincker H, Gronback K: Non-Hodgkin's lymphoma of the gastrointestinal tract: a population-based analysis of incidence, geographic distribution, clinical pathologic presentation features, and prognosis. J Clin Oncol 12:1673, 1994.
5. Deppish LM, Rona VT: Gastric epithelial polyps: A ten year study. J Clin Gastroenterol 11:110–115, 1989.
6. Friedman SL, Wright, TL, Altman DF: Gastrointestinal Kaposi's sarcoma in patients with AIDS: Endoscopic and autopsy findings. Gastroenterology 89:102, 1985.
7. Frucht H, Howard JM, Slaff JL, et al: Secretin and calcium provocative tests in Zollinger-Ellison syndrome. Ann Intern Med 111:697–699, 1989.
8. Gilliam JH, Geisinger KR, Wu WC, et al: Endoscopic biopsies diagnostic of gastric antral vascular ectasia: The watermelon stomach. Dig Dis Sci 34:885–888, 1989.
9. Gostout CJ, Ahlquist DA, Radford CM, et al: Endoscopy laser therapy for watermelon stomach. Gastroenterology 96:1462–1465, 1989.
10. Hughes R: Diagnosis and treatment of gastric polyps. Gastrointest Endosc Clin North Am 2:457–467, 1993.
11. Kimmey ND, Martin RW, Haggit RC, et al: Histologic correlates of gastrointestinal ultrasound imaging. Gastroenterology 94:433, 1989.
12. Mendis RE, Gerdes H, Lightdale CJ, Botete JF: Large gastric folds: A diagnostic approach using endoscopic ultrasonography. Gastrointest Endosc 40:437–41, 1994.
13. Rustgi AK: Hereditary gastrointestinal polyposis in non-polyposis syndromes. N Engl J Med 331: 1694–1702, 1994.
14. Tio TL, Tytgat GNJ, der Hartog Jager FZA: Endoscopic ultrasonography for the evaluation of smooth muscle tumors in the upper gastrointestinal tract: An experience with 42 cases. Gastrointest Endosc 36:343–350, 1990.

14. GASTROPARESIS

Michael Walter, M.D.

1. Define gastroparesis.
Gastroparesis is a motility disorder of the stomach often associated with other intestinal motility disorders. It results from impairment of the normal gastric emptying mechanism.

2. What factors determine gastric motility and emptying?
The factors that determine gastric motility are (1) the composition of the meal, (2) neuroregulators, and (3) hormonal regulators. Liquid and solid meals empty at different rates from the stomach, and the content further influences emptying (e.g., fat slows emptying). Neural innervation is complex but largely involves the vagus nerve. The CNS pathways are only partly known, and the enteric nervous system through gastrointestinal reflexes is also important. Several hormones affect gastric smooth muscle. Motilin and neurotensin accelerate and secretin and cholecystokinin delay gastric emptying.

Gastrointestinal Reflexes

REFLEX	DESCRIPTION	EFFECT
Reflex relaxation	Stroking throat, distending esophagus	Relaxes gastric tone
Accommodation reflex	Distention of stomach	Relaxes gastric tone to maintain low pressures
Enterofundic reflex	Fat, protein in jejunum; sugar, protein in ileum	Relaxes fundic tone
Enterofundic reflex	Duodenojejunal distention	Relaxes fundic tone
Antral reflex	Distention of stomach	Stimulates antral peristalsis
Enterogastric reflex	Nutrients or acid in contact with proximal gut mucosa*	Inhibits antral peristalsis
Enterogastric reflex	Duodenojejunal distention	Inhibits antral peristalsis
Pyloric reflex	Acid and fat in contact with duodenojejunal mucosa*	Tonically narrows pylorus; increases frequency of pyloric phasic contractions
Gastroenteric reflex	Gastric distention, especially when food present in upper GI tract	Increases gut resistance to inflow

From Yamada T, Alpers DH, Owyang C, et al (eds): Textbook of Gastroenterology, 2nd ed. Philadelphia, J.B. Lippincott, 1995, with permission.

3. Describe the electric pacesetter in the stomach.
The rate of contraction of the stomach is controlled by the pacesetter, which oscillates at 3 cycles per minute. The cells with the highest frequency, which are located on the greater curve of the stomach, determine the 3-per-minute frequency (similar to the atrioventricular node in the heart). Stomach potentials differ from those in the heart in that, because of neurohormonal influences, not every potential results in a contraction.

4. What is the interdigestive myoelectric cycle (IDMEC)?
In the fasting state, the GI tract undergoes cycles of contractions with cycle lengths of 90–120 minutes. Most of this time is spent in the quiet phase (phase I). Muscle contractions begin to appear in phase II and build to a crescendo of maximal contractility in phase III, which lasts about 5 minutes. Phase III is a forceful burst of contractions that sweeps the antrum and continues along the entire GI tract. This is the migrating motor complex (MMC). Phase III is sometimes followed by a brief period of decreasing activity (phase IV).

5. What happens to the IDMEC during the fed state?

The fed pattern is continuous as long as food is in the stomach. During this time, the pattern is similar to phase II of the IDMEC in that the pacemaker stimuli are followed by submaximal contractions of the antrum.

6. Describe gastric motility and emptying.

The stomach serves as a reservoir for food and allows it to pass into the duodenum at a controlled rate. The proximal half of the stomach serves as the reservoir, and the volume is governed by the muscular tone of the stomach. Distention of the esophagus or stomach relaxes the muscular tone of the stomach; this reflex, called receptive relaxation, means simply that the volume of the stomach can be increased without a rise in pressure.

The contractions in the distal half of the stomach from the circumferential bands of muscle are forceful; they culminate in terminal antral contracts (TACs). TACs result in a to-and-fro movement that grinds food into smaller pieces. These hydrodynamic forces cause a sieving process whereby smaller 1-mm particles are selectively propelled more rapidly and thus pass the pylorus before it and the antrum close at the end of the TAC.

Liquid emptying is volume-dependent and follows first-order kinetics. During the first 30 minutes, emptying is rapid. From 30–120 minutes, emptying is constant but slower than the first 30 minutes. Solid emptying is volume-independent. Initially, while solids are reduced in size, there is no emptying. This is followed by a prolonged linear phase. Overall, gastric emptying is controlled by the activity in the proximal and distal halves of the stomach as well as the pyloric outlet, all of which act in sequence with one another. Exactly how they interact with each other is not completely understood.

7. What are the causes of gastroparesis?

As gastric motility becomes better understood, associated disorders increase. Some of these disorders are well established, whereas others are of uncertain significance. Idiopathic gastroparesis remains the most common cause of delayed gastric emptying.

8. What are the established associations with delayed gastric emptying?

1. GI symptoms are common in **diabetes mellitus** but are not always associated with gastroparesis. Although most believe that gastroparesis is a neuropathy, it is difficult to be certain about its relationship to the duration of disease, associated nausea, vomiting, neuropathy, retinopathy, and type of diabetes.

2. Delayed gastric emptying is common in **anorexia nervosa.** Nausea, vomiting, gastric dilation, and even perforation on feeding have been reported.

3. Gastric atony may occur after **gastric surgery.** This uncommon complication affects about 5% of patients, ranging from 1.25% of patients who undergo vagotomy and pyloroplasty to 9% of patients who undergo vagotomy and subtotal gastrectomy. Surgery should not be done acutely on a dilated, obstructed stomach, because atony is more likely to occur.

9. What associations are likely to be important in gastroparesis?

1. **Gastric dysrhythmias,** usually of an idiopathic nature, may delay gastric emptying. Various dysrhythmias have been described and may be measured with electrogastrography (see figure on next page). Tachygastria is associated with delayed gastric emptying. Secondary gastric dysrhythmias are associated with anorexia nervosa and motion sickness. They also have been reported in gastric ulcers and gastric cancers.

2. There is an inverse relationship between body size and gastric emptying. Slowing of gastric emptying occurs with **obesity.**

3. Various kinds of **stress** through the CNS modulate gastric emptying, including stress from pain or anxiety.

4. **Neurologic disorders,** including strokes, brain tumors, headaches, and high intracranial pressures, alter gastric emptying.

5. Diseases that involve the gastric wall may slow gastric emptying, including **scleroderma, amyloidosis, systemic lupus erythematosus** and **dermatomyositis.**

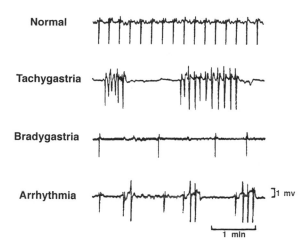

Gastric dysrhythmias. (From Yamada T, Alpers DH, Owyang C, et al (eds): Textbook of Gastroenterology, 2nd ed. Philadelphia, J.B. Lippincott, 1995, with permission.)

6. **Abdominal cancer** may delay gastric emptying by direct involvement of the stomach wall or by invading the surrounding nerves. Gastroparesis also may be a paraneoplastic effect.

10. What is the differential diagnosis of chronic nausea and vomiting?

Differential Diagnosis of Chronic Nausea and Vomiting

1. Gastric
    Causes of mechanical gastric outlet obstruction
        Chronic peptic ulcer disease
        Acute pyloric channel ulcer
        Gastric carcinoma
        Gatric lymphoma
        Duodenal carcinoma
        Pancreatic disease
        Crohn's disease
    Functional gastric outlet obstruction
        Gastroparesis: diabetes, scleroderma,
            metabolic, idiopathic
        Drug-induced
        Postviral
        Postgastric surgery
        Anorexia nervosa
2. Small intestine
    Mechanical obstruction: usually presents acutely
        or with intermittent acute symptoms
    Motilty disorder: intestinal pseudoobstruction
        Scleroderma
        Diabetes
        Jejunal diverticulosis
        Amyloidosis
        Peritoneal studding with metastases
        Oat cell tumor of the lung with paraneoplastic
            neuropathy involving intestine
        Familial visceral myopathy
        Familial visceral neuropathy
        Hypothyroidism

3. Psychogenic
        Bulimia
        Psychogenic, not bulimic
4. Central nervous system
        Increased intracranial pressure
            secondary to tumor
        Pseudotumor
5. Drugs
        Narcotic
        Cardiac glycosides
        Theophylline derivatives
6. Pregnancy
        Nausea and vomiting of pregnancy
        Hyperemesis gravidarum
7. Metabolic/endocrine
        Hyperthyroidism
        Addison's disease
8. Other
        Idiopathic cyclic vomiting
            (motility disorder)

From Yamada T, Alpers DH, Owyang C, et al (eds): Textbook of Gastroenterology, 2nd ed. Philadelphia, J.B. Lippincott, 1995, with permission.

11. What are the symptoms of gastroparesis?

Gastroparesis is part of the differential diagnosis of chronic nausea and vomiting. Symptoms, therefore, are nonspecific and include nausea, vomiting, early satiety, abdominal bloating, and weight loss.

12. What parts of the history and physical exam are important in establishing a diagnosis of gastroparesis?

The nonspecific symptoms listed in question 11 suggest gastroparesis. Nausea may be insidious and without vomiting. The timing of vomiting also may be important. Patients with gastroparesis may vomit undigested food several hours after eating. Patients with regurgitation do not have true nausea; therefore, other diagnoses should be considered. Associated symptoms, such as pain, fever, and diarrhea, are indicative of other causes. Gastric outlet obstruction and its causes should always be considered before making a diagnosis of gastroparesis. A drug history is always important, because many drugs slow gastric emptying, including pain medications and any drug with anticholinergic properties. A psychological history is also important, because patients with bulimia and anorexia nervosa may be quite difficult to identify and differentiate from patients with primary gastroparesis.

13. What tests should be done in patients suspected of having gastroparesis?

Gastroparesis is often a diagnosis of exclusion. A pregnancy test, along with tests to rule out Addison's disease and hyperthyroidism, should be done. An upper endoscopy is necessary to exclude gastric outlet obstruction. The presence of more than 100 ml of fluid in a fasting stomach is abnormal and also indicates gastroparesis. Partial small bowel obstruction also needs to be considered.

A quantitative gastric emptying study should be done next. Several tests are available. Gamma scintigraphy is the standard because of its precision, simplicity, and reproducibility. Be-

Tests for Gastric Emptying

TEST	DESCRIPTION	COMMENTS
Radiographic		
Upper GI series	$BaSO_4$ suspension	Insensitive; not quantitative
Barium burger	Barium-impregnated food	More sensitive; not quantitative
Radiopaque tubes	Barium-filled plastic	Sensitive; quantitative
Intubation		
Saline load	Saline	Semiquantitative; insensitive
Serial test meal	Liquid nutrients	Quantitative; somewhat sensitive impractical
Double sampling dye dilution	Liquid nutrients	Quantitative; somewhat sensitive
Intestinal dye dilution	Liquid or mixed meals	Quantitative; sensitive; cumbersome
Scintigraphic		
Scanner or single crystal	Liquid or mixed meals	Semiquantitative; sensitive
Gamma camera	Liquid or mixed meals; nondigestibles	Quantitative; sensitive; most versatile; now standard technique
Real-time ultrasound		
To measure gastric volume	Liquid meals	Quantitative; erect posture only; nonobese only
To measure gastric emptying time (antral cross-section)	Liquid or mixed meals	Semiquantitative; erect posture only; nonobese only
Gastric impedance		
Nontomographic; limited electrodes	Nonionic liquid or homogenized mixed meals	Quantitative; needs H_2 blockers
Tomographic	Nonionic liquid of homogenized mixed meals	Quantitative; needs H_2 blockers
Ferromagnetic	Iron suspension	Little experience

From Yamada T, Alpers DH, Owyang C, et al (eds): Textbook of Gastroenterology, 2nd ed. Philadelphia, J.B. Lippincott, 1995, with permission.

cause gastric emptying of solids is a better indicator of disease, a solid-meal study should be done. A convenient measure is the T50%, or the time it takes for one-half of the test meal to leave the stomach. The nature of the early emptying phase may also be important.

Antroduodenal manometry also may be used to measure gastric contractions as they progress along the antrum and into the duodenum. This test is more difficult to perform, is not as widely available, and gives different information from the nuclear medicine study of gastric emptying.

Electrogastrography (EGG) is becoming more readily available and measures the pacesetter potential at a frequency of 3 contractions per minute. Tachygastria correlates with gastroparesis, but more needs to be learned about this test before it can be used as a clinical tool.

Regardless of the method of measurement, many variables influence gastric emptying, including the type of marker, size and kind of meal composition, meal temperature, time of day at which the test is done, position of patient, age, sex, drug intake, and history of smoking.

14. Once gastroparesis is diagnosed, how should it be treated?

Electrolytes should be corrected, and any drug that potentially slows gastric emptying should be stopped. Several prokinetic drugs that facilitate gastric motility are available.

Bethanechol is a cholinergic drug that stimulates muscarinic receptors. Antral contractions increase but not phase III activity. Its usefulness in gastroparesis is limited.

Metoclopramide is a dopamine antagonist with potent cholinergic effects. It acts mainly on the proximal GI tract. In the stomach it increases antral contractions and relaxes the pylorus. It also has antiemetic properties. The usual dosage is 10 mg 4 times/day and it may be given orally or intravenously. Side effects are common, including drowsiness, dystonic reactions, and nervousness. It is significantly less expensive than cisapride.

Cisapride is a benzamide derivative that facilitates acetylcholine release at the myenteric plexus. It affects the entire GI tract and does not have the CNS side effects of metoclopramide. Starting dose is 10 mg 3–4 times daily. The IV form is not yet available.

Domperidone is a benzimidazole derivative with clinical effects similar to metoclopramide. It acts primarily on the proximal GI tract and has fewer side effects than metoclopramide. It is not yet available in the U.S.

Erythromycin in doses of 50 mg IV induces phase III contractions in the antrum and upper small bowel. It acts as a motilin agonist, and the effect on the stomach has been described as "pharmacologic antrectomy." Its effect becomes less dramatic after 4 weeks. More information is needed before its therapeutic role is established.

BIBLIOGRAPHY

1. Haubrich WS, Schaffner F, Berk JE (eds): Bockus Gastroenterology, 5th ed. Philadelphia, W.B. Saunders, 1995.
2. Sleisenger MH, Fordtran JS, (eds): Gastrointestinal Disease: Pathophysiology Diagnosis Management, 4th ed. Philadelphia, W.B. Saunders, 1993.
3. Yamada T, Alpers DH, Owyang C, et al (eds): Textbook of Gastroenterology, Philadelphia, J.B. Lippincott, 1995.

III. Liver and Biliary Tract Disorders

15. EVALUATION OF ABNORMAL LIVER TESTS

Kenneth E. Sherman, M.D., Ph.D

1. What are "liver tests?"

Many laboratory evaluations can be characterized as "liver tests." Most commonly, the term refers to the routine chemistry panel that includes alanine aminotransferase (ALT), aspartate aminotransferase (AST), gamma glutamyl transpeptidase (GGT), alkaline phosphatase (AP), bilirubin, albumin, and protein. Other terms for the same tests are liver function tests (LFTs) and liver-associated enzymes (LAEs), but neither descriptor is totally accurate. Only the first four are properly called enzymes, and only the last two provide a measure of liver function. These tests help to characterize injury patterns and provide a crude measure of the synthetic function of the liver. Various combinations can be helpful in diagnosing specific disease processes, but generally these tests are not diagnostic. Other liver function tests are described below. Finally, certain tests help to define specific causes of liver disease. They may be serologic (e.g., hepatitis C antibody) or biochemical (e.g., alpha-1 antitrypsin level) but generally are not used as screening assays or as part of general health profiles.

2. What are the true liver function tests?

True liver function tests evaluate the liver's synthetic capacity or measure the ability of the liver either to uptake and clear substances from the circulation or to metabolize and alter test reagents. Albumin is the most commonly used indicator of synthetic function, although it is not highly sensitive and may be affected by poor nutrition, renal disease, and other factors. In general, low albumin levels indicate poor synthetic function. The prothrombin time (PT) is another simple measure of the liver's capacity to synthesize clotting factors. The PT may be related to decreased synthetic ability or vitamin K deficiency. A high PT that does not correct with oral administration of vitamin K (5–10 mg for 3 days) may indicate liver disease, unless ductal obstruction or intrahepatic cholestasis prevents bile excretion into the duodenum and thus absorption of vitamin K. Administration of a subcutaneous or intravenous injection of vitamin K may help to sort through the possibilities.

Various uptake and excretion tests described in the literature profess to define liver function, including bromosulphothalein (BSP), indocyanine green, aminopyrine, caffeine, and monoethylglycinexylidide (MEGX). Research laboratories frequently use such tests to determine severity of liver disease and to predict survival outcomes, but currently they are not part of routine clinical practice.

3. What is the difference between cholestatic and hepatocellular injury?

The two main mechanisms of liver injury are damage or destruction of liver cells, which is classified as hepatocellular, and impaired transport of bile, which is classified as cholestatic. Hepatocellular injury is most often due to viral hepatitis, autoimmune hepatitis, and various toxins and drugs. Transport of bile may be impaired by extrahepatic duct obstruction (e.g., gallstone, postsurgical stricture), intrahepatic duct narrowing (e.g., primary sclerosing cholangitis), bile duct damage (e.g., primary biliary cirrhosis), or failed transport at the canalicular level (e.g., chlorpromazine effect). In some cases, elements of both types of damage are involved.

The most specific test for hepatocellular damage is the ALT level. The AST level also may be elevated but is not as specific. In contrast, cholestatic injury is best diagnosed by an elevated AP level. Bile acids stimulate AP production, but duct obstruction or damage prevents its excretion into the duodenum. Therefore, the level in serum rises dramatically. Serum AP levels may be slightly increased in early hepatocellular disease, but this increase is due to release of cellular enzyme without excessive stimulation of new enzyme. Because AP can be derived from other body tissue (e.g., bone, intestine), a concurrent elevation of GGT or 5'-nucleosidase helps to support a cholestatic mechanism.

4. What are serum transaminases? How are they used?

The two serum transaminases commonly assayed in clinical practice are ALT and AST. Many laboratories still use older terminology that refers to ALT as serum glutamic pyruvate transaminase (SGPT) and to AST as SGOT (serum glutamic oxaloacetic transaminase). The newer terms reflect more accurately their enzymatic action, which involves the transfer of amino groups from one structure to another.

As noted above, elevation of ALT and/or AST reflects the presence of hepatocellular injury. It is important to understand how the assays are performed and what confounding factors may alter interpretation of test results. The most commonly used test reaction for ALT is as follows:

$$\text{Alanine} + \text{alpha-ketoglutarate} \Longleftrightarrow \text{pyruvate} + \text{L=glutamate}$$

This reaction requires ALT and pyridoxal phosphate (vitamin B_6). A crucial point is that enzyme assays *do not measure how much enzyme is present*; instead, they *indirectly measure the catalytic activity* of the enzyme in performing a particular function. Therefore, the assay does not indicate how much ALT is present but how quickly it causes the above reaction to take place. The assumption is that the faster the reaction, the greater the amount of ALT. To complicate matters further, the assay does not measure the amount of reaction product that is created. Instead, a linked enzyme reaction is employed:

$$\text{Pyruvate} \Longleftrightarrow \text{lactic acid}$$

This reaction occurs in the presence of another enzyme, lactate dehydrogenase. The reaction requires the oxidation of reduced nicotinamide adenine dinucleotide (NADH) and creates the unreduced form (NAD+) as an additional reaction product. NAD+ absorbs light at 340-nm wavelength. This absorption, as measured by a spectrophotometer, is used to determine ALT activity. Therefore, the end-point measurement is several steps removed from the quantitative measurement of interest. The speed of a reaction, however, may be affected by several components of the process, including temperature, substrate concentration, amount of enzymes or cofactors, interfering substances in the reaction mix, and sensitivity of the spectrophotometer, to name a few. For example, if a patient is deficient in pyridoxal phosphate and this cofactor is not added in excess of the amount needed for the test reaction, the reaction rate will be slowed, and the final result will reveal a falsely low ALT activity. This confounding effect is probably common in malnourished alcoholics, in whom deficiency of vitamin B_6 rather than ALT level is the limiting step in the reaction.

The second major issue is the determination of normal vs. abnormal levels. This determination is generally made by the local laboratory in an arbitrary manner. A small set of "healthy" patients is selected, often from a blood bank. The ALT is determined in all members, and a mean and standard deviation are calculated. Arbitrary cut-offs are assigned, usually at values representing the top and bottom 2.5% of the sample population. This technique is unfortunate, because many demographic factors play a role in ALT level. Men have higher ALT levels than women, obese women have higher ALT levels than people close to ideal body weight, and certain racial groups have higher ALT activity than others. Therefore, if the test population consists mainly of thin, Caucasian women who happen to donate blood at an office drive, the cut-off values may be very low. Thus many overweight men may have ALT levels in the "high" range, even in the absence of disease. This problem applies to all of the enzyme tests described in this chapter. Therefore, the further a test result is from normal, the more likely that disease in fact exists. Conversely, patients with significant silent liver disease may have normal ALT levels.

The ALT level, therefore, is an imperfect marker of the liver process. In diseases that involve massive liver damage, such as in acute viral hepatitis, acetaminophen or solvent toxicity, or amanita mushroom poisoning, ALT may be increased to very high levels. For example, an ALT of 2000 IU/L (~50 times the upper limit of normal) is frequently seen in significant acetaminophen overdoses. This value reflects significant loss of ALT from damaged hepatocytes. In patients with chronic viral hepatitis, levels tend to be lower and frequently are 2–10 times normal.

5. What makes the AP level rise?

AP is a group of enzymes that catalyze the transfer of phosphate groups. Different isoenzymes can be identified from multiple sites in the body, including liver, bone, and intestine. Most hospital labs do not have the facilities to separate AP and identify the source. This inability may pose a problem for clinicians. In one large study of hospitalized patients, only about 65% of elevated AP was from the liver. When the source is the liver, the mechanism appears to be related to a stimulation of enzyme synthesis associated with local increases in bile acids. This finding results from drug-associated cholestasis and intrahepatic and extrahepatic obstruction. The test reaction for AP is:

$$\text{p-Nitrophenyl phosphate} <======> \text{phosphate} + \text{nitrophenyl}$$

The appearance of nitrophenyl indicates that AP is present. Although this assay is not a linked reaction, the problems associated with determining enzyme activity and establishing a normal range are analogous to those described for serum transaminases. The association of elevated AP with either GGT or 5'-nucleosidase helps to establish a liver source and suggests the presence of a cholestatic process.

6. What does an elevated bilirubin mean?

Bilirubin, a breakdown product of red blood cells, exists in two forms: **conjugated** and **unconjugated.** Unconjugated bilirubin appears in the serum when blood is broken down at a rate that overwhelms the processing ability of the liver. This finding is most common in patients with hemolysis. Several genetically acquired enzyme deficiency states result in improper or incomplete bilirubin conjugation in the liver. The most common is Gilbert's syndrome, which is characterized by a relative deficiency of glucuronyl transferase. Patients often have high-normal to borderline-elevated bilirubin levels. When they fast or decrease caloric intake (e.g., patients with viral gastroenteritis), the bilirubin rises, primarily because of increases in the unconjugated form. If a bilirubin fractionation is not done, a patient with abdominal pain, nausea and vomiting, and an elevated bilirubin may be misdiagnosed as having cholecystitis. The resulting cholecystectomy could easily have been avoided by obtaining the fractionation.

The most common test for bilirubin involves a biochemical reaction over time. Most labs report only total bilirubin. By stopping the reaction at a particular time and subtracting the result from the total bilirubin, the lab arrives at the **indirect** bilirubin, which is an approximation of unconjugated bilirubin. Exact measurement requires the use of chromatography, which is not routinely performed in clinical labs. Conjugated bilirubin is elevated in many diseases, including viral, chemical, and drug and alcohol-induced hepatitis; cirrhosis; metabolic disorders; and intrahepatic and extrahepatic biliary obstruction.

7. What tests are used to evaluate common metabolic disorders of the liver?

In patients with liver disease, specific lab tests are routinely used to evaluate whether certain metabolic disorders are likely. **Hemochromatosis** is a disease of iron overload in the liver and other organs. The defect is probably in a regulatory mechanism for iron absorption in the small intestine. Over many years, patients build up stored iron in the liver, heart, pancreas, and other organs. The most common screening test for hemochromatosis is serum ferritin; an elevated level suggests the possibility of iron overload. Unfortunately, ferritin is also an acute-phase reactant and may be falsely elevated in various inflammatory processes. If ferritin is elevated (usually ≥400 µg/L), serum iron and total iron binding capacity (TIBC) should be assessed. If the serum iron divided by TIBC is >50–55%, hemochromatosis should be strongly suspected instead of secondary iron overload (hemosiderosis). The definitive test is a quantitative assessment of iron. This requires a liver biopsy specimen to determine the amount of iron present in the liver tissue. An age-adjusted correction called the iron age index is then calculated:

$$\text{Iron age index} = \frac{(\text{Fe } (\mu g/gm) \ (\tfrac{1}{56})}{\text{patient's age}}$$

Studies suggest that magnetic resonance imaging of the liver also may be helpful and in the future may reduce the need for liver biopsy.

Alpha-1 antitrypsin is an enzyme made by the liver that helps to break down trypsin and other tissue proteases. Multiple variants are described in the literature. The variant is expressed as an allele from both parents. Therefore, a person may have one or two forms of alpha-1 antitrypsin in the blood. One particular variant, called Z because of its unique electrophoretic mobility on gel, is the product of a single amino acid gene mutation from the wild-type protein (M). The Z protein is difficult to excrete from the liver cell and causes local damage that may result in hepatitis and cirrhosis. Three tests help to make the diagnosis. The first is a serum protein electrophoresis (SPEP). When blood proteins are separated on the basis on electrical migration in gel, several bands are formed. One of these, the alpha-1 band, consists mostly of alpha-1 antitrypsin. Therefore, an alpha-1 antitrypsin deficiency results in a flattening of the alpha-1 band on SPEP. The second option is a direct assay that uses a monoclonal antibody against alpha-1 antitrypsin. The degree of binding can be measured in a spectrophotometer by rate nephelometry. The third option is to order an alpha-1 antitrypsin phenotype. Only a few labs in the U.S. run this test, which designates the allelic protein types in the serum (e.g., MM, ZZ, MZ, FZ). Patients with protein of the ZZ type are said to be homozygotic for Z-type alpha-1 antitrypsin deficiency. This is the form most frequently associated with significant liver disease. If Z protein is trapped in hepatocytes, it can be seen in liver tissue as small globules that stain with the periodic acid-Schiff (PAS) reaction and resist subsequent digestion with an enzyme called diastase. An immunostain is also available in some institutions.

Wilson's disease, a disorder of copper storage, is associated with deficiency of an enzyme derived from liver cells. Like iron, copper may accumulate in many tissues in the body. Its storage sites are somewhat different, however. Deposition may be seen in the eye (Kayser-Fleischer rings) and in parts of the brain. Many cholestatic diseases of the liver (e.g., primary biliary cirrhosis) also result in aberrant copper storage but not to the degree seen in true Wilson's disease. The main screening test is the serum ceruloplasmin level, which is low in over 95% of patients with Wilson's disease. Ceruloplasmin is also an acute-phase reactant and may be falsely elevated into a low-normal range in patients with an inflammatory process. Follow-up tests include assessments of urine and serum copper levels. A quantitative assessment of copper in liver tissue from liver biopsy provides definitive diagnosis. Copper is stained in the tissue with special stain processes (e.g., Rhodanine stain).

Tests for Common Metabolic Disorders of the Liver

DISEASE	PRIMARY TEST	SUPPORTIVE TEST	DEFINITIVE TEST
Hemochromatosis	Serum ferritin >400 µg/L	Iron saturation >55%	Iron age index ≥2
Alpha-1 antitrypsin deficiency	SPEP or Al-AT level	Phenotype (Pi type)	Liver biopsy with PAS-positive diastase-resistant granules
Wilson's disease	Ceruloplasmin <10 mg/dL	Urine/serum copper >80 µg/24 hr	Liver biopsy with quantitative copper >50 µg/g wet weight

There are numerous other hereditary diseases of the liver, including Gaucher's disease, Niemann-Pick disease, and hereditary tyrosinemia. These rare diseases are usually diagnosed in children. Specific tests are beyond the scope of this chapter.

8. What are autoimmune markers? How do they relate to diagnosis of liver disease?
Autoimmune markers are tests used to determine the presence of antibodies to specific cellular components that have been epidemiologically associated with the development of specific liver diseases. Autoimmune markers include antinuclear antibody (ANA), antismooth muscle antibody (ASMA; also called antiactin antibody), liver-kidney microsomal antibody, type 1 (LKM-1), antimitochondrial antibody (AMA), soluble liver antigen (SLA), and antiasialoglycoprotein re-

ceptor antibody. ANA, ASMA, and AMA are the most readily available tests and help to define the probability of the more common classes of autoimmune liver disease. Currently SLA is not easily obtained in the U.S.

The common antibody tests are performed by exposure of the patient's serum to cultured cells and labeling with a fluorescein-tagged antibody against human antibodies. The cells are examined by fluorescent microscopy and graded according to intensity of the signal and which part of the cell binds the antibody. Therefore, reading of antibody levels and determination of positive or negative results are highly subjective, and most hepatologists require positive results in dilution titers >1:80 or 1:160 before considering the tests as part of a diagnostic algorithm. ANA and ASMA are particularly common in older people, women, and patients with a wide spectrum of liver diseases. Therefore, the diagnosis of autoimmune liver disease depends on a broad clinical picture that takes into account age, sex, presence of other autoimmune processes, gammaglobulin levels, and liver biopsy findings. In addition, the overlap in antibodies present in different autoimmune liver diseases is considerable. The table below provides a crude representation of one classification scheme. A newer scoring system that tries to take into account the variables noted above also has been proposed.

Classification of Autoimmune Liver Disease

DISEASE	ANTIBODY
Type I classic lupoid hepatitis	ANA and/or ASMA
Type II autoimmune hepatitis	LKM-1
Type III autoimmune hepatitis	SLA
Primary biliary cirrhosis	AMA

9. When should screening or diagnostic tests be ordered for patients with suspected liver disease?

The transaminases, bilirubin, and alkaline phosphatase serve as screening tests when liver disease is suspected. The history, physical exam, and estimation of risk factors help to determine which specific diagnostic tests should be ordered. Some patients have occult liver disease with normal or near-normal enzymes, and occasionally patients with isolated enzyme elevations have no identifiable disease. In general, patients should have at least two sets of liver enzyme tests to eliminate lab error before a full work-up for liver disease is begun. Many diseases (hepatitis B and hepatitis C) generally require proof of chronicity (abnormality >6 months) before therapy is initiated or confirmatory and staging liver biopsies are obtained. The severity of enzyme abnormality and the likelihood of finding a treatable process may modify the typical waiting period. For example, a female patient with transaminase levels 10 times normal, a history of autoimmune thyroid disease, and an elevated globulin fraction probably has a flare of previously unrecognized chronic autoimmune hepatitis. An autoimmune profile and early liver biopsy may help to support this hypothesis and lead to prompt treatment with steroids and other immunosuppressants.

BIBLIOGRAPHY

1. Bassett ML, Halliday JW, Powell LW: Value of hepatic iron measurements in early hemochromatosis and determination of the critical iron level associated with fibrosis. Hepatology 6:24–29, 1986.
2. Brensilver HL, Kaplan MM: Significance of elevated liver alkaline phosphatase in serum. Gastroenterology 68:1556–1562, 1975.
3. Buffone GS, Beck JR: Cost-effectiveness analysis for evaluation of screening programs: Hereditary hemochromatosis. Clin Chem 40:1631–1636, 1994.
4. Eriksson S, Carlson J, Velez R: Risk of cirrhosis and primary liver cancer in alpha-1 antitrypsin deficiency. N Engl J Med 314:736–739, 1983.
5. Kaplan MM: Laboratory Tests in Diseases of the Liver, 6th ed. Philadelphia, J.B. Lippincott, 1987, pp 219–260.
6. Scharschmidt BF, Goldberg HI, Schmid R: Approach to the patient with cholestatic jaundice. N Engl J Med 308:1515–1519, 1983.
7. Sherman KE: Alanine aminotransferase in clinical practice: A review. Arch Intern Med 151:260–265, 1991.
8. Wroblewski F: The clinical significance of transaminase activities of serum. Am J Med 27:911–923, 1959.

16. VIRAL HEPATITIS

Kenneth E. Sherman, M.D., Ph.D.

1. What are the types of hepatitis viruses?
There are currently five identifiable forms of viral hepatitis: A, B, C, D, and E. All of these viruses are hepatotrophic; that is, the liver is the primary site of infection. Other viruses also infect the liver, but it is not their primary site of replication and cellular damage. Examples include cytomegalovirus (CMV), herpes simplex virus (HSV), Epstein-Barr virus (EBV), and many of the arthropod-borne flaviviruses (e.g., dengue virus and yellow fever virus).

Key Characteristics of the Hepatitis Viruses

TYPE	NUCLEIC ACID	GENE SHAPE	ENVELOPE	SIZE (NM)
A	RNA	Linear	No	28
B	DNA	Circular	Yes	42
C	RNA	Linear	Yes	?40–50
D	RNA	Circular	Yes	43
E	RNA	Linear	No	32

2. What is the difference between acute and chronic hepatitis?
All hepatitis viruses can cause acute infection, which is defined as clinical, biochemical, and serologic abnormalities present for up to 6 months. Hepatitis A and E are cleared from the body within 6 months and do not cause persistent infection for a longer period. In contrast, infection hepatitis B, C, and D can lead to chronic infection, which is more likely to be associated with development of cirrhosis and increased risk of primary hepatocellular carcinoma than acute viral infection in the liver.

The risk of chronicity for hepatitis B is highly dependent on the person's age at infection and immunologic status. Neonates infected with hepatitis B have a chronicity rate approaching 100%. The rate decreases to about 70% for young children. Healthy young adults probably have chronicity rates less than 1%, but patients taking steroids or with chronic illness (e.g., renal disease) are less likely to clear the viral infection.

Hepatitis D chronicity occurs only in the presence of simultaneous hepatitis B infection. In patients with chronic hepatitis B who become superinfected with hepatitis D, the risk of chronicity approaches 100%.

Hepatitis C chronicity may occur in up to 85% of patients. It is frequently but not always associated with the development of histologically identifiable hepatitis.

3. How are hepatitis viruses transmitted?
Hepatitis A and E are transmitted via a fecal-oral route. Both agents are prevalent in areas where sanitation standards are low. Large epidemics of both diseases frequently occur after floods and other natural disasters that disrupt already marginal sanitation systems. Hepatitis A is endemic in the United States and much of the world, whereas hepatitis E is not endemic in the United States. Large outbreaks of hepatitis E have been seen in Central and South America, Bangladesh, and India. The fecal-oral transmission route includes not only direct contamination of drinking water and food, but viral concentration and enteric acquisition by eating raw shellfish from sewage-contaminated waters.

4. What are the symptoms of hepatitis?
The classic symptoms of acute hepatitis include anorexia, nausea, vomiting, severe fatigue, abdominal pain, mild fever, jaundice, dark urine, and light stools. Some patients may have a serum

sickness–like presentation that includes arthralgias, arthritis, and skin lesions; this presentation is more common in hepatitis B than in other forms of acute viral hepatitis and may be seen in up to 20% of infected patients. Many patients with acute viral hepatitis do not have disease-specific symptoms. For many patients with all forms of viral hepatitis, the presentation is a mild-to-moderate flulike illness. In a recent national survey of the U.S. population, approximately 30% of participants had serologic evidence of past hepatitis A infection, but few were diagnosed with hepatitis A or reported an illness with classic hepatitis features.

Patients with chronic hepatitis B or C report fatigue as the leading symptom. Other common manifestations include arthralgias, anorexia, and vague, persistent right upper quadrant pain. Jaundice, easy bruisability, or prolonged bleeding after shaving or other small skin breaks usually mark the development of end-stage liver disease and often signify the presence of scarring and irreversible liver dysfunction.

5. What biochemical abnormalities are associated with viral hepatitis?

Elevation of serum transaminases (alanine aminotransferase [ALT], aspartate aminotransferase [AST]) is the hallmark of acute liver damage and identifies the presence of various processes caused by viral hepatitis. In patients with acute hepatitis A, B, D, and E, elevations of transaminases to several thousand are not uncommon; they usually are accompanied by more modest increases in alkaline phosphatase and gamma-glutamyl-transferase (GGT). As the disease progresses, the transaminases decrease. As the levels decrease slowly over a period of weeks, bilirubin often rises and may peak weeks after the transaminases peak. Bilirubin levels usually subside by 6 months after infection. Hepatitis C is not as frequently associated with a notable acute hepatitis, and transaminases rarely exceed 1000 IU/L.

Abnormalities that persist for longer than 6 months define the chronic process. In this stage of disease, transaminases range from mildly elevated to 10–15 times the upper limit of normal. Bilirubin is often normal or mildly elevated, as is alkaline phosphatase and GGT. Sudden elevations of transaminases in the chronic period often signify a virus flare rather than development of a new process superimposed on the preexisting chronic viral state.

6. How is hepatitis A diagnosed?

The diagnosis of hepatitis A depends on identifying a specific IgM antibody directed against the viral capsid protein. This is often identified as a HAVAB-M test (hepatitis A viral antibody—IgM class) on lab slips. The IgM antibody appears early in infection and persists for 3–6 months. The other available lab test is for the IgG form of the antibody, which diagnoses past infection and does not have a role in routine clinical practice.

7. How is hepatitis B diagnosed?

The incorrect interpretation of hepatitis B serologic markers is frequent and leads to many inappropriate laboratory tests and specialty consultations. It is important to understand the sequence of marker appearance and disappearance and the information that each marker provides. Tests of hepatitis B include both serologic and molecular markers:

1. **HBsAg** (hepatitis B surface antigen). This protein, which forms the outer coat of the hepatitis B virus, is produced in great excess during viral replication and aggregates to form noninfectious round and filamentous particles in the serum. It is detected by a radioimmunoassay (RIA) or enzyme-linked immunosorbent assay (ELISA) assay and indicates the presence of either acute or chronic infection. Its disappearance from the serum indicates viral clearance.

2. **HBcAb** (hepatitis B anticore antibody). This test detects antibody formation against the core protein of the hepatitis B virus. The core protein surrounds the viral DNA and is surrounded by HBsAg in the complete virion, which is called the Dane particle. An ELISA assay is used to detect HBcAb. The specific test comes in three forms, which must be differentiated to understand the meaning of the results: an IgG form, an IgM form, and a total form that measures both IgG and IgM. Most laboratories include the total test in hepatitis screening profiles, but it is important

to find out which test is routinely run. A positive total HBcAb indicates either current or past hepatitis B infection. A positive HB anti-HBc IgM usually indicates an acute hepatitis B infection, although it also may indicate viral reactivation associated with immunosuppression or chronic illness. In contrast, a positive HB anticore IgG is consistent with either resolved past infection or, if present in conjunction with HBsAg, a chronic carrier state.

3. **HBeAg** and **HBeAb** (hepatitis B "e" antigen and hepatitis B "e" antibody). The "e" antigen is a structural part of the core that can be detected by an ELISA assay. Its presence indicates active replication. Therefore, HBeAg is seen in both acute infection and actively replicating chronic hepatitis B. In patients with acute infection, this test is not necessary. In patients with chronic infection, a positive result indicates a replicative form of the disease. Only when HBsAg is present, and chronic liver disease is suspected, does this test help in decision making related to treatment and treatment outcomes. In a patient with a resolved acute infection or a relatively inactive (nonreplicative) chronic hepatitis B infection, HBeAg disappears and anti-HBe appears. Some patients with a point mutation in the precore coding region of the hepatitis B genome cannot make HBe and therefore do not develop an antibody response after resolution. The clinical significance of this mutation remains unclear.

4. **HBsAb** (hepatitis B surface antibody). This test detects an antibody directed against the surface antigen. This neutralizing antibody binds with and helps to clear the virus from the circulation. Its presence, therefore, indicates past infection with hepatitis B, which has been successfully cleared. The surface antibody also may appear in patients who are successfully vaccinated with the currently available recombinant hepatitis B vaccines. Its presence at a titer greater than 10 mIU/ml of serum confers protection against active infection.

5. **DNA polymerase assay.** The polymerase assay was one of the earliest molecular assays used to detect hepatitis B DNA in serum. It was based on the finding that the hepatitis B virus carries its own DNA polymerase enzyme within the core. The assay measures the enzyme activity as it directs the incorporation of radioactive-tagged nucleotides into new viral DNA. The test is not highly sensitive and is not in routine clinical use. However, it is frequently referenced in research about hepatitis B from the 1970s and 1980s as a marker of viral activity.

6. **Hybridization assays.** This class of assays includes various specific techniques that use a probe complementary to specific portions of the hepatitis B DNA genome. The actual hybridization may be performed on a filter paper matrix (dot blot) or in a column filled with beads that are impregnated with the probe material. The assay detects a marker substance on the probe, which sticks to the viral DNA. The marker is often a radioactive tracer (e.g., radioactive phosphorus [^{32}P]) but also may be a chemical reactant (e.g., horseradish peroxidase). The sensitivity of these assays is not as great as amplification techniques, but most detect HBV DNA in a range of 1.5–20 pg/ml of serum. This range seems to provide a good marker for distinguishing replicative from nonreplicative disease.

7. **bDNA assays.** In this hybridization assay the viral nucleic acid hybridizes with complementary bDNA ("branched-chain" DNA) attached to a microtiter well. The hybridized viral DNA is then further hybridized to specific complementary DNAs in a reaction mixture, which are arrayed in a manner analogous to a multibranched tree. On the tree are pods of a marker molecule that emit light in a chemiluminescent reaction that can be detected by a luminometer. Because the light emission is proportionate to the amount of bound DNA the test provides a highly reliable quantitative assay that is more sensitive than standard hybridization assays.

8. **Polymerase chain reaction (PCR) assays.** Whereas the bDNA assay amplifies the signal generated by hybridization, PCR amplifies a portion of the DNA itself and makes it more detectable. PCR is the most sensitive technique available for detection of hepatitis DNA. Unfortunately, this sensitivity has little clinical relevance. Regardless of whether the carrier state is replicative or nonreplicative, DNA is always detected by PCR amplification. There is a high correlation between PCR positivity and the presence of HBsAg in serum. The latter assay is cheaper and more reliable and should be the key test to determine whether active hepatitis B infection is present.

8. How is hepatitis C diagnosed?

The screening assay for hepatitis C is an ELISA assay that detects the presence of antibody to two regions of the hepatitis C genome. The currently available assay is in its second generation, and future modifications are likely. The test is highly sensitive but not specific; therefore, it gives many false-positive reactions. In populations with a low pretest probability of carrying hepatitis C, more than 40% of repeatedly reactive specimens are false positives. The antibody that is detected is nonneutralizing; that is, its presence does not confer immunity. If antibody is detected and the reaction is not a false positive, the patient almost always has active viral infection. Clearly, it is important to separate false positives from true positives. The cause of most false-positive reactions is binding of nonspecific immunoglobulin on the ELISA well surface. To avoid the use of serum, which requires obtaining drawn blood, oral fluid collection may have a role in screening populations for HCV antibodies in the future.

To support a true-positive reaction, the most commonly used test is a recombinant immunoblot assay (RIBA), which involves exposing the patient's serum to a nitrocellulose strip impregnated with bands of antigen. The currently available version has four antigens on the test strip as well as controls for nonspecific immunoglobulin binding and superoxide dismutase antibodies, which may confound the test results. The RIBA is not as sensitive as the ELISA, however, and therefore should not be used as a screening test for hepatitis C infection.

Other assays in specialized laboratories include a bDNA quantitative assay for hepatitis C RNA and a PCR assay (see hepatitis B tests). The PCR is more sensitive but not readily adaptable to quantitation. The presence of hepatitis C RNA in serum or liver tissue is the gold standard for diagnosis of hepatitis C infection. Recent data suggest that quantitative evaluation of hepatitis C RNA levels in serum may have prognostic value in determining who is likely to respond to therapeutic intervention and in following the course of a treatment cycle.

9. How is hepatitis D diagnosed?

Hepatitis D is diagnosed by an ELISA assay that detects the presence of antibody to hepatitis D in serum or plasma. The presence of the antibody in serum correlates with ongoing hepatitis D replication in the liver. Detection of hepatitis D antigen in liver tissue generally adds little to the diagnostic process. Early in the course of infection, acute hepatitis D may be detectable only by performing a test for the IgM form of the antibody. A PCR-based assay also may be performed to detect the presence of RNA from hepatitis D in serum or tissue. This assay is not commercially available, and its use seems to add little to the antibody testing. Because hepatitis D occurs only with concurrent acute hepatitis B infection or as a superinfection of chronic hepatitis B, there is little utility in testing for its presence at the initial work-up for viral causes of liver enzyme abnormalities.

10. How is hepatitis E diagnosed?

At this point, only experimental assays are available for the detection of hepatitis E virus. The original assays relied on a technique called an antibody-blocking assay, in which freshly infected primate tissue was exposed to serum from the patient, and then to serum from a known positive patient. If antibody is present in the unknown serum, it binds to the tissue and blocks the attachment of the second known antibody. This technique was difficult and will be supplanted by a commercial ELISA assay that should be available soon. Hepatitis E does not seem to occur naturally in the United States. However, there should be a high index of suspicion in patients who have an acute hepatitis A-like illness, test negative for hepatitis A antibody IgM, and have traveled to an endemic area.

11. Are there other hepatitis viruses not yet discovered?

Probably. Several lines of evidence suggest that there are more hepatotrophic viruses than are currently recognized. Epidemiologic studies suggest that a small percentage of posttransfusion cases and a higher percentage of community-acquired cases of hepatitis have no identifiable viral infection, even when molecular detection techniques are used. Forms of liver disease (e.g., giant cell hepatitis) have been associated with paramyxovirus infection, although its role remains speculative at best. The cause of fulminant hepatic failure, hepatitis-associated aplastic anemia, and cryptogenic cirrhosis cannot be defined in a significant proportion of cases. Such findings point to the presence of one or more as yet unidentified agents.

12. What is the treatment of acute viral hepatitis?

The primary treatment of acute hepatitis of any type is mainly supportive. Patients generally do not require hospitalization unless their disease is complicated by significant hepatic failure manifest by encephalopathy, coagulopathy with bleeding, renal failure, or an inability to maintain adequate nutrition and fluid intake. Efforts must be made to identify the form of hepatitis and, if necessary, to ensure that the patient is removed from situations in which he or she is a high risk to others. For example, a food-handler should be removed from the workplace when hepatitis A is diagnosed, and health authorities must be notified.

Specific antiviral treatment has been attempted in acute hepatitis cases. Recent literature about use of alpha and beta interferon in acute hepatitis C infection is conflicting. By general agreement, early drug intervention leads to a response in terms of both ALT level and viral load. Whether the rate of viral persistence associated with chronic HCV infection is lowered remains unclear. Because most patients with acute HCV infection are not identified, large-scale trials may be impossible. Alpha interferon also has been studied in patients with acute hepatitis D infection and fulminant hepatitis due to either coinfection or superinfection with hepatitis B. It appeared to have little value in this setting.

13. Is chronic viral hepatitis treatable?

Yes. The chronic forms of hepatitis B, C, and D have been studied with regard to a number of treatment modalities. Alpha interferon has been tested in multiple randomized, controlled trials and is currently the only treatment for hepatitis B and C approved by the Food and Drug Administration.

Patients with chronic hepatitis B, well-compensated liver disease, and evidence of viral replication (HBV DNA or HBeAg) are candidates for therapy. The goal of therapy is to reduce the level of replication and to change the infection to a relatively inactive disease. The clearance of HBsAg is not the immediate goal of therapy, although some evidence suggests that this may occur more frequently in successfully treated patients than in those that do not respond over subsequent years. The standard treatment is alpha interferon 2b at a dose of 30–35 MU/week for 16 weeks. Patients seem to tolerate a dosing of 5 MU 6 days/week better than other regimens. Side effects include a flulike syndrome, which is occasionally quite severe at this dose. Often a platelet count and absolute neutrophil count decrease significantly; thus the patient must be monitored closely and dose adjustments made. Response rates range up to 60%, although in some groups it may be as low as 5%. Poor response is seen in patients with chronic, longstanding infection since childhood and in patients with HIV infection or other immunosuppression. The ideal patients, in terms of response outcomes, are women with recent chronic infection, an ALT >200 IU/L, and a viral load <100 pg/ml by hybridization assay.

Treatment of chronic hepatitis C is also interferon-based, although a lower dose is generally used. The standard therapy for chronic hepatitis C infection in patients with well-compensated liver disease is 3 MU 3 times/week for 24 weeks. Although the side-effect profile is the same as for hepatitis B treatment, this regimen is usually better tolerated because of the lower interferon dosing. Response rates range from 30–50% for primary therapy when ALT normalization is used as a response criteria. Unfortunately, 50–70% of patients relapse after completion of therapy. Longer treatment times may decrease the relapse rates.

Alternative therapies for hepatitis C under investigation in many clinical research centers include ribavirin, ribavirin with interferon, thymosin alpha-1 with interferon, ursodeoxycholic acid, and phlebotomy in patients with borderline iron overload and HCV infection. Although results in some trials are promising, none of these alternatives can be recommended as standard therapies at present. For responders that relapse, several studies are evaluating long-term maintenance with interferon. At present this approach also should be reserved for patients in well-designed trials.

Hepatitis D also may be treated with interferon. Doses of 9 MU 3 times/week for 48 weeks was associated with a 50% response rate in one randomized, controlled trial. Relapse at the end of therapy was common, however.

14. Is viral hepatitis preventable?

Hepatitis A infection can be prevented by the use of pooled gamma globulin after acute exposure or a vaccine for long-term protection. A vaccine previously used in Europe, Canada, and elsewhere became available in the United States in 1995. The vaccine is prepared from an attenuated strain of the virus grown on tissue culture cells. It is chemically inactivated and seems to confer immunity in 80–90% of treated subjects. The vaccine has not been tested in young (<2 year old) children but is recommended for individuals who travel to hyperendemic areas with poor sanitation, child-care workers, deployable military personnel, and other high-risk individuals. Universal vaccination has not been studied adequately to determine its cost-benefit ratio. For individuals exposed in local outbreaks (shellfish, food-handler), gamma globulin should be adequate for short-term protection.

A vaccine for hepatitis B has been available since the early 1980s. It was originally prepared by isolation of the surface antigen protein. The current forms most widely used in the United States are surface antigen proteins made by recombinant techniques. The vaccine is more than 90% effective in providing long-term immunity after 3 doses. In 20–30% of vaccinees antibody titers drop to less than 10 mIU/ml within 5 years. This titer is believed to be the critical protective level. Current Public Health Service recommendations do not mandate either follow-up testing or boosters. These recommendations may change as future data become available. Acute hepatitis B exposure in nonvaccinated individuals requires treatment with hepatitis B immunoglobulin (HBIG). This hyperimmune gamma globulin has very high-titer antibodies against hepatitis B surface antigen. It may be administered simultaneously with the first dose of vaccine; this regimen is often followed in infants of HBsAg-positive mothers.

No vaccine is available for hepatitis C. Because of rapid mutation in the envelope region of the genome, a multivalent vaccine probably will be required and may take several years to develop and test before it is available for routine use.

CONTROVERSY

15. Should patients be treated for chronic hepatitis C infection, in light of the high cost, low response rates, and many sideeffects of interferon therapy?

Pro: Hepatitis C is a progressive disease that frequently leads to the development of cirrhosis. We are unable to predict adequately which patients will progress to symptomtic liver disease and which will not. Although the ultimate goal of therapy should be virus eradication, this goal has not been frequently achieved with interferon therapy. However, the majority of patients treated have some histologic improvement over the course of therapy or fail to show short-term progression of disease. Therefore, even "unsuccessful" therapy may be beneficial if it delays the disease process by reducing the inflamatory component that is thought to result in fibrosis. Hepatitis C has become the leading cause of liver transplantation in many centers.

Con: Long-term studies of hepatitis C infection are limited. One study in a Veterans' Administration population failed to show increased mortality among hepatitis C-infected patients vs. two control cohorts in long-term follow-up. The infected group had an excess of liver-related mortality, however. Current treatments for hepatitis C are inadequate. A sustained response to interferon therapy is seldom seen in patients with hepatitis C. Given the cost of this therapy and proclivity for side effects, enthusiasm for the use of this drug in the treatment of hepatitis C should be tempered.

BIBLIOGRAPHY

1. Alter MJ, Margolis HS, Krawczynski K, et al: The natural history of community-acquired hepatitis C in the United States. N Engl J Med 327:1899–1905, 1992.

2. Centers for Disease Control: Hepatitis B virus: A comprehensive strategy for eliminating transmission in the United States through universal childhood vaccination: Recommendations of the Immunization Practices Advisory Committee (ACIP). MMWR:40(no. RR-13), 1991.

3. Choo QL, Richman KH, Han JH, et al: Genetic organization and diversity of the hepatitis C virus. Proc Natl Acad Sci USA, 88:2451–2455, 1991.

4. Davis GL, Balart LA, Schiff E, et al: Treatment of chronic hepatitis C with recombinant interferon alfa. N Engl J Med 321:1501–1506, 1989.

5. Dawson GJ, Chau KH, Cabal CM, et al: Solid phase enzyme linked immunosorbent assay for hepatitis E virus IgG and IgM antibodies utilizing recombinant antigens and synthetic peptides. J Virol Meth 38:175–186, 1992.

6. Di Bisceglie AM, Martin P, Kassianides C, et al: Recombinant interferon alfa therapy for chronic hepatitis C: A randomized, double-blind, placebo-controlled trial. N Engl J Med 321:1506–1510, 1989.

7. Di Bisceglie AM, Shindo M, Fong T-L, et al: A study of ribavirin therapy for chronic hepatitis C. Hepatology 16:649–654, 1992.

8. Farci P, Mandas A, Coina A, et al: Treatment of chronic hepatitis D with interferon alfa-2a. N Engl J Med 330:88–94, 1994.

9. Houghton M, Weiner A, Han J, et al: Molecular biology of the hepatitis C viruses: Implications for diagnosis, development and control of viral disease. Hepatology 14:381–388, 1991.

10. Kaneko S, Miller RH, Di Bisceglie AM, et al: Detection of hepatitis B virus DNA in serum by polymerase chain reaction: Application for clinical diagnosis. Gastroenterology 99:799–804, 1990.

11. Koretz RL, Abbey H, Coleman E, Gitnick G: Non-A, non-B post-transfusion hepatitis: Looking back in the second decade. Ann Intern Med 119:110–115, 1993.

12. Krawczynski K, Bradley DW: Enterically transmitted non-A, non-B hepatitis. Identification of virus-associated antigen in experimentally infected cynomologus macaques. J Infect Dis 159:1042–1049, 1989.

13. Perrillo RP, Regenstein FG, Peters MG, et al: Prednisone withdrawal followed by recombinant alpha interferon in the treatment of chronic type B hepatitis: A randomized, controlled trial. Ann Int Med 109:95–100, 1988.

14. Seeff LB, Ruskell-Bales Z, Wright EC, et al: Long-term mortality after transfusion-associated non-A, non-B hepatitis. N Engl J Med 327:1906–1911, 1992.

15. Sherman KE, Creager RL, O'Brien J, et al: The use of oral fluid for hepatitis C antibody screening. Am J Gastroenterol 89:2025–2027, 1994.

16. Zaaijer HL, Borg F, Cuypers HTM, et al: Comparison of methods for detection of hepatitis B virus DNA. J Clin Microbiol 32:2088–2091, 1994.

17. AUTOIMMUNE HEPATITIS

Albert J. Czaja, M.D.

1. What is autoimmune hepatitis?

Autoimmune hepatitis is an unresolving inflammation of the liver of unknown cause that is characterized by at least periportal hepatitis (piecemeal necrosis or interface hepatitis) on histologic examination, autoantibodies in serum, and hypergammaglobulinemia. The disease behaves aggressively and may produce cirrhosis, portal hypertension, liver failure, and death. Because there are no pathognomonic features, the diagnosis requires the exclusion of chronic viral hepatitis, Wilson's disease, alpha-1 antitrypsin deficiency, hemochromatosis, drug-induced hepatitis, alcoholic and nonalcoholic steatohepatitis, and other immunologic conditions, such as autoimmune cholangitis, primary biliary cirrhosis, and primary sclerosing cholangitis. A careful clinical history, selected laboratory tests, and expert histologic examination establish the diagnosis in most instances.

Differential Diagnosis and Discriminative Tests

POSSIBLE DIAGNOSES	DIAGNOSTIC TESTS	DIAGNOSTIC FINDINGS
Wilson's disease	Copper studies	Low ceruloplasmin
		Low serum copper level
		High urinary copper
		Increased liver copper
	Slit lamp eye exam	Kayser-Fleischer rings
Primary sclerosing cholangitis	Cholangiography	Focal strictures intra- and/or extraheptic bile ducts
	Liver biopsy	Fibrous obliterative cholangitis
Primary biliary cirrhosis	Antimitochondrial antibodies	AMA ≥ 1:160
		Anti-pyruvate dehydrogenase-E2
	Liver biopsy	Florid duct lesion
		Increased copper stores
Autoimmune cholangitis	Liver biopsy	Cholangitis, ductopenia
Chronic hepatitis C	Viral markers	Anti-HCV/RIBA positive
		HCV RNA present
	Liver biopsy	Portal lymphoid aggregates
		Steatosis
		Bile duct damage/loss
Drug hepatitis	Clinical history	Exposure to methyldopa, isoniazid, nitrofurantoin, propylthiouracil, ethanol
Hemochromatosis	Iron/ferritin	Increased serum levels
	Liver biopsy	Iron overload
Alpha-1 antitrypsin deficiency	Phenotype	ZZ or MZ
	Liver biopsy	Hepatocytic inclusions
Nonalcoholic steatohepatitis	Clinical findings	Obesity, diabetes, drugs
	Ultrasonography	Increased echogenicity
	Liver biopsy	Fat

2. What are its predominant features?

The disease afflicts mainly women (71%). It may occur at any age (range = 9 months to 77 years) but typically is diagnosed before the fourth decade. An acute, even fulminant presentation is possible, and the disease may be mistaken for acute viral or toxic hepatitis. Concurrent immunologic diseases are present in 38% of patients. The most common are autoimmune thyroiditis, ulcerative colitis, Graves' disease, and synovitis. Unfortunately, cirrhosis is already present at accession in 25% of patients, indicating that the disease has an indolent, subclinical course. Smooth muscle antibodies (SMA) and antinuclear antibodies (ANA) are the most common immunoserolgoic markers. In 64% of patients, SMA and ANA are present concurrently, whereas 22% have only SMA and 14% have only ANA. Autoantibody titers may fluctuate, and the antibodies may actually disappear, especially during corticosteroid therapy. There is no minimal titer of significant seropositivity, but titers in adults should be ≥1:40. Serum titers >1:80 increase diagnostic confidence. Hypergammaglobulinemia, especially elevation of the serum immunoglobulin G level, is a hallmark of the disease, and the diagnosis is suspect without it. Marked cholestatic features are incompatible with the diagnosis, and a predominant serum alkaline phosphatase abnormality, pruritus, hyperpigmentation, and bile duct lesions on histologic examination suggest alternative diagnoses, such as primary biliary cirrhosis, primary sclerosing cholangitis, or autoimmune cholan-

Immunologic Diseases Concurrent with Autoimmune Hepatitis

Autoimmune thyroiditis *	Neutropenia
Dermatitis herpetiformis	Pericarditis
Erythema nodosum	Peripheral neuropathy
Fibrosing alveolitis	Pernicious anemia
Focal myositis	Pleuritis
Gingivitis	Primary sclerosing cholangitis
Glomerulonephritis	Pyoderma gangrenosum
Graves' disease *	Rheumatoid arthritis *
Hemolytic anemia	Sjögren's syndrome
Idiopathic thrombocytopenic purpura	Synovitis *
Insulin dependent diabetes	Systemic lupus erythematosus
Intestinal villus atrophy	Ulcerative colitis *
Iritis	Urticaria
Lichen planus	Vitiligo
Myasthenia gravis	

*Most common associations

gitis. Similarly, serologic evidence of active infection with hepatitis A, B, or C viruses, Epstein-Barr virus, or cytomegalovirus argues against the diagnosis.

3. What are the characteristic histologic findings in autoimmune hepatitis?
Periportal hepatitis (piecemeal necrosis or interface hepatitis) connotes disruption of the limiting plate of the portal triad by inflammatory infiltrate and is the sine qua non for the diagnosis of autoimmune hepatitis (Fig. 1). This characteristic histologic pattern is not a pathognomonic finding. Piecemeal necrosis may be found in many types of acute and chronic hepatitis, including viral-induced, drug-related, alcohol-associated, or toxic liver injuries. Lobular hepatitis, which is characterized by prominent cellular infiltrates that line sinusoidal spaces in association with degenerative or regenerative changes, is another common but nondiagnostic histologic manifestation of autoimmune hepatitis, especially in patients who relapse after corticosteroid withdrawal (Fig. 2). Marked plasma cell infiltration of the portal tracts is also a histologic change that characterizes the disease (Fig. 3). In contrast, prominent portal lymphoid aggregates and steatosis suggest the diagnosis of chronic hepatitis C (Fig. 4); ground-glass hepatocytes are characteristic of chronic hepatitis B; and marked bile duct damage or loss connotes a cholangiopathy.

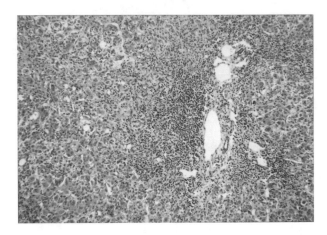

Figure 1. Piecemeal necrosis. The limiting plate of the portal tract is disrupted by inflammatory infiltrate (H & E; original magnification ×100).

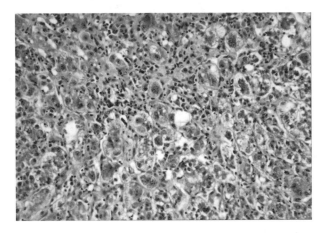

Figure 2. Lobular hepatitis. Inflammatory cells line the sinusoidal spaces in association with liver cell regenerative or degenerative changes (H & E; original magnification × 200).

4. What are the different types of autoimmune hepatitis?

Patients with autoimmune hepatitis are classified according to the species of autoantibodies associated with their disease. Patients with SMA and/or ANA seropositivity comprise the most common form of autoimmune hepatitis in the United States and western Europe. Such patients have **type 1** autoimmune hepatitis. Antibodies to actin (antiactin), a subgroup of SMA, are present in high titer and also support the designation of type 1 autoimmune hepatitis.

Patients with antibodies to liver/kidney microsome type 1 (anti-LKM1) have **type 2** autoimmune hepatitis. The antibodies to LKM1 do not coexist with SMA, ANA, or antiactin and define an immunoserologically distinct subgroup. Patients with type 2 autoimmune hepatitis are typically young (ages 2–14 years), but adults may be afflicted. They have concurrent immunologic diseases, such as autoimmune thyroiditis, vitiligo, insulin-dependent diabetes, and ulcera-

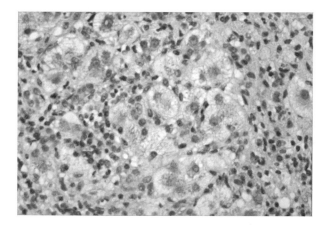

Figure 3. Plasma cell infiltration. Plasma cells infiltrate the periportal region (H & E; original magnification × 400).

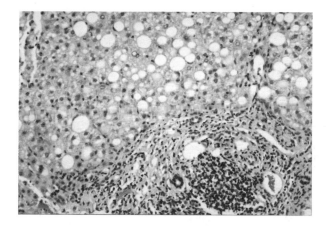

Figure 4. Chronic hepatitis C. Small lymphocytes aggregate in the portal tract and vacuoles of lipid are present within the cytoplasm of hepatocytes (H & E; original magnification × 200).

tive colitis, more commonly than counterparts with type 1 disease; they also have higher frequencies of organ-specific antibodies, such as antibodies to thyroid, islets of Langerhans, and parietal cells. Serum immunoglobulin A levels are lower in patients with type 2 disease than in those with type 1 autoimmune hepatitis, and preliminary studies suggest that they more commonly progress to cirrhosis than patients with type 1 disease. Although type 2 autoimmune hepatitis is an important diagnosis among adults in Europe, it is found in only 4% of adults with autoimmune hepatitis in the United States. In contrast, type 1 disease constitutes 80% of the cases of autoimmune hepatitis in American patients. Of importance, hepatitis C infection is found in 50–86% of patients with anti-LKM1 and only 11% of patients with SMA and/or ANA.

A **type 3** autoimmune hepatitis has been proposed based on the presence of antibodies to soluble liver antigen (anti-SLA). Eleven percent of patients with type 1 autoimmune hepatitis have anti-SLA and cannot be distinguished from seronegative counterparts. Similarly, antibodies to liver-pancreas (anti-LP) have been proposed as a marker for another type 3 autoimmune hepatitis, but these antibodies also occur in conjunction with those of type 1 disease. Consequently, it is still unclear if anti-SLA and anti-LP are variant markers of type 1 autoimmune hepatitis or mutually exclusive manifestations of distinctly different subpopulations.

Subtypes of Autoimmune Hepatitis

FEATURES	TYPE 1	TYPE 2
Characteristic autoantibodies	Smooth muscle	Liver/kidney microsome 1
	Nucleus	P450 IID6
	Actin	254-271 core motif
Associated autoantibodies	Asialoglycoprotein receptor	Asialoglycoprotein receptor
	Perinuclear antineutrophil cytoplasm	Cytosol type 1
Organ-specific autoantibodies (parietal cell)	4%	30%
Autoantigen	Unknown	Cytochrome P450 IID6
Concurrent hepatitis C virus	≤11%	50% to 86%
HLA phenotype	A1-B8-DR3 and DR4	B14, DR3, C4A-QO
Predominant age	Adult	Pediatric
Concurrent immune diseases	17%	34%
Hypergammaglobulinemia	+++	+
Low IgA	−	+
Progression to cirrhosis	45%	82%
Corticosteroid responsiveness	+++	++

5. What are the diagnostic criteria?

The diagnostic criteria for autoimmune hepatitis have been standardized by international consensus. Definitive diagnosis requires histologic evidence of piecemeal necrosis with or without lobular hepatitis or bridging necrosis and absence of biliary lesions, granulomas, copper deposits, or other changes suggestive of a different etiology. Any abnormality in serum aminotransferase activity is consistent with the diagnosis if it is a predominant abnormality. Total globulin, gamma globulin, or immunoglobulin G levels must be greater than 1.5 times the upper limit of normal, and serum titers of SMA, ANA or anti-LKM1 must be grater than 1:80. There must be no history of parenteral exposure to blood or blood products, recent use of hepatotoxic drugs, or excessive alcohol consumption (<35 gm/day in men and 25 gm/day in women). Serologic evidence of active infection with hepatitis A virus, hepatitis B virus, hepatitis C virus, Epstein-Barr virus, and cytomegalovirus must be absent, and serum levels of alpha-1 antitrypsin, copper, and ceruloplasmin must be normal. Patients with similar findings but less pronounced abnormality of serum gamma globulin level, lower titers of autoantibodies, histories of greater alcohol consumption or recent drug exposure, nondiagnostic abnormalities of serum copper and ceruloplasmin levels, or false-positive reactivities to hepatitis C virus warrant a probable diagnosis. A scoring system has been developed to balance properly all clinical, laboratory, and histologic manifestations and to provide an objective measure of the net strength of the final diagnosis. The result of corticosteroid therapy also may be scored, and the treatment response can be used to upgrade or downgrade the diagnosis. Unlike other forms of chronic hepatitis, the diagnosis of autoimmune hepatitis does not require 6 months of disease activity to establish chronicity. In recognition of its propensity for an acute presentation, autoimmune hepatitis may be diagnosed at any time in its clinical course.

Proposed Scoring System for the Diagnosis of Autoimmune Hepatitis

Clinical features		Autoantibodies	
Gender		ANA, SMA or LKM1 titers	
Male	0	>1:80	+3
Female	+2	1:80	+2
Immunologic disease(s)	+1	1:40	+1
Epidemiologic features		<1:40	0
Blood transfusions/drugs		Other markers	+2
Yes	−2	AMA	
No	+1	Present	−2
Alcohol consumption	0	Absent	0
(adjusted by amount)	−1	**Histologic features**	
	−2	Piecemeal necrosis and	
	+2	lobular hepatitis +	
IgM anti-HAV	−3	bridging necrosis	+3
HBsAg or IgM anti-HBc	−3	Piecemeal necrosis only	+2
HCV RNA	−3	Rosettes	+1
Anti-HCV and/or RIBA	−2	Plasma cells (marked)	+1
Other viral markers	−3	Bile duct changes	
No viral markers	+3	Mild	−1
Laboratory features		severe	−3
HLA B8-DR3 or DR4	+1	**Treatment response**	
Globulin, IgG or GG		Complete response	+2
x 2 normal	+3	Partial response	0
x 1.5-2 normal	+2	No response	−2
x 1-1.5 normal	+1	Relapse after therapy	+3
x <1 normal	0		
Alk phosphatase:AST			
x <3 normal	+2		
x ≥3 normal	−2		

Aggregate scores: Before treatment	After treatment
Definite diagnosis >15	>17
Probable diagnosis 10–15	12–17

6. Are SMA, ANA, and anti-LKM1 pathogenic autoantibodies?

Although SMA, ANA and anti-LKM1 are the bases for subclassifying patients with autoimmune hepatitis, they do not have pathogenic properties.

Antinuclear antibodies produce homogeneous or speckled patterns by indirect immunofluorescence on HEp-2 cell lines, but they also may be associated with diffuse granular, centromeric, nucleolar, and mixed patterns. Patients with speckled patterns of immunofluorescence are younger and have higher serum aspartate aminotransferase levels at presentation than patients with other patterns, but prognosis has not been associated with individual patterns of immunofluorescence. Indeed, it is still unclear whether the speckled pattern represents a release of nuclear material during hepatocyte destruction or an immunoreaction against a nuclear antigen that interferes with critical cell functions.

Smooth muscle antibodies reflect the presence of antibodies to actin or nonactin components (tubulin, vimentin, desmin, and skeletin). If the reactivity by indirect immunofluorescence is against actin cables in cultured fibroblasts, it has a high specificity for autoimmune hepatitis. Polymerized F-actin, the target of such reactivity, is closely associated with the hepatocyte membrane. Although antibodies to actin may promote an antibody-dependent, cell-mediated form of cytotoxicity, no direct evidence indicates that SMA induce liver cell injury.

Antibodies to liver/kidney microsome type 1 are reactive against a 50-kDa microsomal antigen in the liver and kidney that has been identified as the cytochrome monooxygenase, P450 IID6. Antibodies to LKM1 inhibit P450 IID6 activity in vitro but not in vivo, and their pathogenicity has not been established. An 8-amino acid core motif within P450 IID6, either in isolation or as part of sequences extending up to 33 amino acids, has been identified as the epitope of anti-LKM1. Reactivity at the site between amino acids 254 and 271 of recombinant P450 IID6 distinguishes patients with autoimmune hepatitis and anti-LKM1 from those with chronic hepatitis C and anti-LKM1. Antibodies to anti-LKM1 may be present in both conditions, but they are two different species of autoantibodies as defined by epitope specificity.

Autoantibodies Associated with Autoimmune Hepatitis

AUTOANTIBODY SPECIES	IMPLICATION (S)
Nuclear	Type 1 autoimmune hepatitis
	Nonspecific in low titer
	May affect nuclear functions
Smooth muscle	Type 1 autoimmune hepatitis
	Nonactin activity in viral infections
Actin	High specificity in type 1 autoimmune hepatitis
	May facilitate surface binding of antibody
LKM1	Type 2 autoimmune hepatitis
	Inhibits P450 IID6 in vitro
	Commonly accompanied by HCV infection
P450 IID6	Type 2 autoimmune hepatitis
	Recombinant antigen used in immunoassay for antibodies
254-271 core motif	Type 2 autoimmune hepatitis
	Synthetic peptides derived from P450 IID6 for immunoassay
	Not associated with HCV
Liver cytosol 1	Associated with anti-LKM1
	Infrequently found with HCV infection
	Associated with younger patients and more severe disease than anti-LKM1 only
Soluble liver antigen	Type 3 autoimmune hepatitis
	Marker of cryptogenic chronic hepatitis
	May occur in type 1 disease
Liver-pancreas	Type 3 autoimmune hepatitis
	Marker of cryptogenic chronic hepatitis
	May occur in type 1 disease
Asialoglycoprotein receptor	Autoimmune marker
	May reflect inflammatory activity
Perinuclear anti-neutrophil cytoplasmic antibodies	Present in most patients
	High titer
	IgG1 isotype
	Unknown function

7. What other autoantibodies are important?

Multiple other autoantibodies have been described in autoimmune hepatitis, but none has been shown to be pathogenic or clinically versatile. Investigational goals are to identify and characterize these autoantibodies to gain insight about candidate target autoantigens.

Antibodies to soluble liver antigen (anti-SLA) react specifically with liver cytokeratins 8 and 18. They are found only in autoimmune hepatitis but do not define a clinically distinct subgroup. Indeed, their greatest clinical value may be in the reassignment of some patients with cryptogenic chronic hepatitis to the autoimmune category.

Antibodies to liver-pancreas (anti-LP) are demonstrated in only 17% of patients with type 1 autoimmune hepatitis, 8% of patients with type 2 autoimmune hepatitis, and 3% of patients with chronic hepatitis B and C. In contrast, they are present in 33% of patients who are seronegative for all conventional liver-related autoantibodies. Antibodies to liver-pancreas, therefore, may define another subtype of autoimmune hepatitis. Assays for these antibodies may be useful in reclassifying patients with cryptogenic chronic hepatitis.

Antibodies to asialoglycoprotein receptor (anti-ASGPR) are specific for autoimmune hepatitis and directed against a putative target autoantigen. Antibodies to human anti-ASGPR are present in all types of autoimmune hepatitis, including 82% of patients with SMA and/or ANA, 67% of patients with anti-LKM1, and 67% of patients with anti-SLA. The autoantibodies are directed against a transmembrane hepatocytic glycoprotein that can capture, display, and internalize potential antigens, induce T-cell proliferation, and activate cytotoxic T-cells. Because anti-human anti-ASGPRs occur in 88% of patients with autoimmune hepatitis compared to 7% of patients with chronic hepatitis B, 8% with alcoholic liver disease, and 14% with primary biliary cirrhosis, they offer diagnostic specificity and another mechanism to monitor disease activity. Autoantibody reactivity correlates with inflammatory activity and anti-ASGPRs disappear during successful therapy. Loss of these antibodies may identify patients who are less likely to relapse after termination of treatment.

Antibodies to liver cytosol type 1 (anti-LC1) are present mainly in patients who are uninfected with hepatitis C virus and have been used mainly to discriminate anti LKM1–positive patients with and without HCV infection. They occur only in young patients, typically less than 20 years of age, and their presence has been associated with more severe disease. Antibodies to liver cytosol type 1 are detected in only 32% of anti-LKM1–positive patients who are uninfected with hepatitis C virus and therefore must be regarded as supplemental findings. In 14% of patients with autoimmune hepatitis, they are the sole marker of the disease and also may be useful in evaluating young patients who lack conventional autoantibodies

Perinuclear antineutrophil cytoplasmic antibodies (pANCA) have recently been described in patients with autoimmune hepatitis, but their significance remains uncertain. Antineutrophil cytoplasmic antibodies are directed against the cytoplasmic components of neutrophil granules and have been found in glomerulonephritis, systemic vasculitis, Wegener's granulomatosis, ulcerative colitis, primary sclerosing cholangitis and autoimmune hepatitis. In contrast to the granular, diffuse cytoplasmic pattern of immunofluorescence characteristic of Wegener's granulomatosis (cANCA), the antibodies in patients with primary sclerosing colitis and autoimmune hepatitis produce a perinuclear staining pattern (pANCA). This perinuclear pattern seems to be sensitive and specific for these liver diseases; 93% of patients with severe type 1 autoimmune hepatitis have pANCA. Of importance, pANCAs in autoimmune hepatitis differ from those in primary sclerosing cholangitis by being higher in titer and predominantly of the IgG_1 isotypes.

8. What is the significance of antimitochondrial antibodies in autoimmune hepatitis?
Antimitochondrial antibodies (AMA) can be demonstrated by indirect immunofluorescence in 20% of patients with autoimmune hepatitis, but serum titers are low (<1:160 in 88% of instances). The histologic findings in such patients are indistinguishable from those in patients without AMA, and tissue copper stains by rhodanine are negative or only mildly positive. Most importantly, such patients typically respond to corticosteroids. Patients with high AMA titers may have primary biliary cirrhosis or unrecognized anti-LKM1 seropositivity. The recognition of AMA by indirect immunofluorescence requires reactivity to the distal tubules of the murine kidney and parietal cells of the murine stomach. The recognition of anti-LKM1 requires reactivity to the proximal tubules of the murine kidney and hepatocytes of the murine liver. An exuberant reaction against the renal tubule may obscure these distinctions, and in some patients anti-LKM1 reactivity may be reported as AMA positivity. The antibodies that are specific against the mitochondrial autoantigens of primary biliary cirrhosis (the E2 subunits of pyruvate dehydrogenase and/or branched-chain ketoacid dehydrogenase) occur in only 8% of patients with autoimmune hepaitis. These autoantibodies may indicate an incorrect original diagnosis, a disorder with mixed features, or a rare instance of false seropositivity.

9. Can autoimmune hepatitis exist in the absence of conventional autoantibodies?
Thirteen percent of patients with severe chronic hepatitis lack a confident etiologic diagnosis. Such patients are now classified as having cryptogenic chronic hepatitis, but many undoubtedly have an autoimmune hepatitis that has escaped detection by conventional immunoserologic assays. Patients with cryptogenic chronic hepatitis are similar by age, gender, HLA phenotype, laboratory findings, and histologic features to patients with type 1 autoimmune hepatitis and respond

well to corticosteroid therapy, entering remission (83% vs. 78%) and failing treatment (9% vs. 11%) as commonly as patients with conventional autoimmune markers. A synonym for this condition is autoantibody-negative autoimmune hepatitis; it must be distinguished from cryptogenic chronic liver disease, which typically connotes end-stage inactive cirrhosis that has lost all distinctive features. Autoantibody-negative patients may develop SMA and/or ANA seropositivity later in their course or have the less conventional autoantibodies (anti-SLA, anti-LP, or anti-LC1). The scoring system is the best method of securing the diagnosis (see question 5), and patients with the condition should be managed in the same fashion as those with autoantibodies.

10. What are the pathogenic mechanisms?

The pathogenic mechanisms of autoimmune hepatitis are unknown, but but two theories prevail. One theory is based on an **antibody-dependent cell-mediated form of cytotoxicity** and the other presumes a **cellular form of cytotoxicity.** In the former theory, a postulated defect in the function of suppressor T-cells results in the unmodulated B-cell production of immunoglobulin G. These autoantibodies are directed against normal hepatocytic membrane proteins, and the antigen-antibody complex on the hepatocyte surface is then targeted by lymphocytes that have Fc receptors for the antibody molecule (natural killer cells). These lymphocytes do not require previous exposure to the target antigen for activation. Antigenic specificity is conferred by the antibody bound to the antigen, and the lymphocytes accomplish cytodestruction.

In the second theory, a disease-specific autoantigen is aberrantly displayed on the hepatocyte surface in association with HLA antigens. Immunocytes that are HLA-restricted are sensitized to the self-antigen, and clonal expansion of the antigen-primed lymphocytes follows. The activated immunocytes (cytotoxic T-lymphocytes) infiltrate the liver tissue and destroy the hepatocytes displaying the target autoantigen. Lymphokines facilitate cell-to-cell communication, promote neoexpression of class II HLA antigens, enhance autoantigen presentation, activate the immunocytes, and promote tissue damage by direct action. Concurrently, intercellular adhesion molecules, induced by proinflammatory cytokines, permit attachment of the effector cell to the target cell and facilitate cell destruction.

Common to both theories are a host predisposition for heightened immunoreactivity that is genetically determined and uncertainty about the nature or need of a triggering factor. Viral infections, drug exposures, and environmental factors have been evoked as triggering mechanisms that activate a final common pathway of pathogenesis. Autoimmune diseases, however, do not require a trigger, and the emergence (or persistence) of "forbidden clones" of autoreactive cells remains intrinsic to the theory of autoimmunity.

11. What are the autoantigens?

The target autoantigens of autoimmune hepatitis are uncertain, but the cytochrome monooxygenase P450 IID6 and asialoglycoprotein receptor are excellent candidates. Each is expressed on the hepatocyte surface, and each is associated with tissue-infiltrating lymphocytes reactive to that antigen in patients with the disease. Analyses of the cellular infiltrate in liver tissue samples have disclosed increased numbers of helper lymphocytes in the portal tracts and scar tissue, predominence of antigen-sensitized suppressor/cytotoxic lymphocytes in the hepatic parenchyma near areas of piecemeal necrosis, and sparsity of B-cells and natural killer cells. Such findings support a cellular immune reaction rather than an antibody-dependent, cell-mediated form of cytotoxicity and implicate the cytotoxic T-lymphocyte as the most likely effector. P450 IID6 is a 50-kDa microsomal enzyme that metabolizes at least 25 different drugs, including antihypertensive agents (debrisoquine), beta blockers, antiarrhythmic drugs, and antidepressants. It has genetic polymorphism and is absent in 10% of the population. Asialoglycoprotein receptor is a transmembrane hepatocytic glycoprotein that can process and display multiple intrinsic and extrinsic antigens.

12. Do viruses cause autoimmune hepatitis?

Autoimmune hepatitis has been reported to occur after acute infections with hepatitis A virus and hepatitis B virus; it also has been observed in patients infected with human immunodeficiency virus.

The measles virus genome has been found more commonly in the peripheral blood cells of patients with autoimmune hepatitis than in normal controls, and serological surveys in countries endemic for hepatitis C virus have described frequencies of seropositivity for antibodies to hepatitis C virus (anti-HCV) that range from 44–86% in patients with autoimmune hepatitis. The initial (first-generation) immunoassays for anti-HCV were commonly confounded by the hypergammaglobulinemia associated with autoimmune hepatitis, and false-positive results were common. Later studies using second- and third-generation immunoassays and polymerase chain reaction assays for the detection of HCV RNA in serum have disclosed lower frequencies of HCV infection in these patients, but the possibility of a viral etiology has not been excluded. Antibodies to HCV and/or HCV RNA are found in 11% of patients with type 1 autoimmune hepatitis and 50–86% of patients with type 2 disease by current assay systems. Unfortunately, it is impossible to determine whether viruses are a cause of the disease or a coexistent process, because there is no animal model for the disorder and prospective documentation of the evolution of autoimmune hepatitis from a viral infection is limited.

Currently, the definite diagnosis of autoimmune hepatitis requires the exclusion of viral infection, and patients with true infection and low-titer autoanibodies are considered to have viral disease with nonspecific features of autoimmunity. Of importance, the P450 IID6 antigen shares homologies with the genomes of hepatitis C virus and herpes simplex virus type 1. Cross-reacting antibodies may occur in patients with type 2 autoimmune hepatitis and patients with chronic hepatitis C as a result of molecular mimicry. In addition, patients with chronic viral hepatitis rarely have anti-LKM1, although patients with anti-LKM1 are commonly infected with hepatitis C virus. No evidence suggests that the strain of virus is different in these patients, and the expression of anti-LKM1 is probably related to host-determined rather than virus-associated factors.

13. Are there genetic predispositions for autoimmune hepatitis?

The human leukocyte antigens (HLA) DR3 and DR4 are independent risk factors for type 1 autoimmune hepatitis in the United States and western Europe. In Japan, the disease is associated with HLA DR4. Fifty-two percent of American patients with type 1 autoimmune hepatitis are HLA DR3-positive and 42% are HLA DR4-positive, including 11% with both HLA DR3 and HLA DR4. Human leukocyte antigen B8 is in strong linkage disequilibrium with HLA DR3 (94% cooccurrence) and is present in 47% of patients. The HLA phenotype A1-B8-DR3 is found in 37% of patients with type 1 disease and has been the classically described phenotype of this condition. In contrast, HLA B14, DR3 and C4A-QO characterize patients with type 2 autoimmune hepatitis. The frequency of HLA B14 alleles in patients with type 2 autoimmune hepatitis is 26% compared with 4% of a control population. Of patients seronegative for anti-HCV, HLA DR3 is found in 70% and C4A-Q0 is found in 90%. The HLA phenotype identifies patients with a predisposition for autoimmune hepatitis, but the phenotype itself does not predict emergence of the disease. Autoimmune hepatitis does not have a strong penetrance in families, and familial occur-

Human Leukocyte Antigen Phenotypes and Disease Expression and Behavior

FEATURES	PHENOTYPES	
	HLA DR3	HLA DR4
Higher serum AST and bilirubin levels at presentation	+	−
More frequent confluent necrosis and/or cirrhosis at presentation	+	−
Higher frequency of relapse after drug withdrawal	+	−
More commonly require liver transplantation	+	−
Higher frequency of treatment failure	+	−
Higher frequency of remission during corticosteroid therapy	−	+
Older age	−	+
More commonly women	−	+
More commonly accompanied by other immunologic diseaes	−	+
Higher serum levels of gamma globulin and immunoglobulin G	−	+
More frequently associated with high-titer antinuclear antibodies	−	+
More frequently associated with smooth muscle antibodies	−	+

rence of the disease is rare. A susceptibility gene has not been described, and data suggest that no single gene is responsible.

14. Do the HLA phenotypes influence disease expression and outcome?
In type 1 autoimmune hepatitis, both HLA DR3 and HLA DR4 have been associated with different clinical manifestations and behaviors. Patients with HLA DR3 are younger and have more active disease, as assessed by serum aminotransferase levels and histologic findings of confluent necrosis and cirrhosis, than counterparts without HLA DR3. Similarly, patients with HLA DR3 relapse more frequently after drug withdrawal than patients with other phenotypes. They also enter remission less frequently and deteriorate more commonly during corticosteroid therapy than patients with other phenotypes and more frequently require liver transplantation.

In contrast, patients with HLA DR4 are older and more commonly women than patients with HLA DR3. They also have higher serum levels of gamma globulin, a greater frequency of concurrent immunologic diseases, and a greater likelihood of entering remission during therapy. The expression of SMA and high-titer ANA also has been associated with HLA DR4. Specific alleles within the DR loci have now been linked to such manifestations. Patients with DRB1*0401, a subtype of HLA DR4, have less severe disease at presentation, relapse less frequently after drug withdrawal, and develop disease later in life than counterparts with DRB3*0101, a subtype of HLA DR3. These alleles encode specific amino acid sequences in the DR beta polypeptide that determine the ability of each class II molecule to bind and present antigens to T-cells. Therefore, they can influence the immunoreactivities of effector cells and in turn modulate the manifestations and behavior of disease.

15. What are the determinants of prognosis at presentation?
The severity of inflammatory activity, as reflected in conventional biochemical indices and histologic assessment, is the principal determinant of immediate prognosis. Sustained serum aspartate aminotransferase (AST) activity of at least 10-fold normal or more than 5-fold normal in conjunction with a hypergammaglobulinemia of at least twice normal is associated with a 3-year survival rate of 50% and 10-year survival rate of 10%. Lesser degrees of biochemical activity are associated with better prognoses. In such patients, the 15-year survival exceeds 80%, and the probability of progression to cirrhosis during this interval is less than 50%. Histologic findings at presentation also reflect disease severity and immediate prognosis. Extension of the inflammatory process between portal tracts or between portal tracts and central veins (bridging necrosis) is associated with a 5-year mortality rate of 45% and an 82% frequency of cirrhosis. Similar consequences occur in patients who have destruction of entire lobules of liver tissue at presentation (multilobular necrosis). Cirrhosis with active inflammation at accession is also associated with a poor prognosis. The 5-year mortality rate in such patients is 58%, and 20% die of variceal hemorrhage within 2 years. In contrast, patients with periportal hepatitis (piecemeal necrosis) on histologic examination have a normal 5-year life expectancy and a low frequency of cirrhosis (17%) during this interval. Of importance spontaneous resolution of inflammatory activity may occur unpredictably in 13–20% of patients, regardless of disease activity at accession, and no findings at presentation, including hepatic encephalopathy and ascites, preclude a satisfactory response to corticosteroid therapy.

16. What therapies are effective?
Multiple controlled clinical trials have proved the efficacy of prednisone in combination with azathioprine or a higher dose of prednisone alone in the management of severe autoimmune hepatitis. Both regimens are equally effective in inducing clinical, biochemical, and histologic remission and enhancing immediate life expectancy. The combination regimen is associated with a lower frequency of drug-related side effects than the regimen using higher doses of prednisone alone (10% vs. 44%); hence it is the preferred treatment in patients who can tolerate azathioprine. Postmenopausal women and patients with labile hypertension, brittle diabetes, emotional instability, exogenous obesity, acne, or osteoporosis are ideal candidates for the combination regimen.

Recommended Treatment Regimens

| INTERVAL ADJUSTMENTS | PREDNISONE (MG DAILY) | COMBINATION | |
		PREDNISONE (MG DAILY)	AZATHIOPRINE (MG DAILY)
Week 1	60	30	50
Week 2	40	20	50
Week 3	30	15	50
Week 4	30	15	50
Daily maintenance until end point	20	10	50

Indications for Corticosteroid Therapy and Criteria for Treatment Selection

INDICATIONS FOR TREATMENT	CRITERIA FOR TREATMENT SELECTION
Absolute	**Prednisone Regimen**
AST ≥10-fold normal	Severe cytopenia
AST ≥5-fold normal	Pregnancy or contemplating pregnancy
and gamma globulin ≥2-fold normal	Concurrent neoplasia
Histological findings of bridging necrosis	Short term (≤6 months) trial
or confluent necrosis	**Combination Regimen**
Incapacitating symptoms	Preferred regimen
Relative	Postmenopausal women
Relentless progression	Obesity
AST ≤10-fold normal but ≥5-fold normal	Acne
with gamma globulin <2-fold normal	Labile hypertension
Mild-moderate symptoms	Emotional lability
No indications	Osteoporosis
Minimal or no symptoms and periportal hepatitis	Brittle diabetes
AST <5 fold normal	Long-term (>6 months) treatment
Inactive or minimally active cirrhosis	
Liver failure with minimal	
or mild inflammatory activity	

Women who are pregnant or contemplating pregnancy and patients with neoplasia or severe cytopenia associated with hypersplenism are candidates for therapy with prednisone alone. Because severe corticosteroid-induced side effects typically do not develop for at least 18 months if doses of prednisone do not exceed 10 mg daily, the single-drug regimen also may be used in patients in whom a short treatment trial (6 months or less) is anticipated.

17. What are the indications for treatment?
The benefits of corticosteroid therapy have been proved only in patients with severe inflammatory activity. Therapy in patients with less active disease has an uncertain benefit-risk ratio. The absolute indications for treatment are incapacitating symptoms, bridging necrosis or multilobular necrosis on histological examination, and sustained severe biochemical abnormalities. Other findings do not compel treatment. In such instances, the treatment decision must be individualized, and therapy is frequently empiric. Treatment is not indicated in patients with inactive or minimally active cirrhosis, patients with decompensated liver disease and mild or no inflammatory activity, and patients who are asymptomatic with histological features of mild periportal hepatitis.

18. Are there any "predictors" of response to treatment?
No findings at presentation predict response to treatment and no patient with absolute indications for therapy should be denied treatment a priori, even in the presence of cirrhosis, ascites, or hepatic encephalopathy. The principal indices of response are the levels of serum aspartate aminotransferase, bilirubin, and gamma globulin. At least 90% of patients demonstrate improvement in

at least one of these parameters within 2 weeks of therapy, and such changes predict immediate survival with 98% accuracy. In contrast, failure to improve a pretreatment hyperbilirubinemia within 2 weeks of therapy in a patient with multilobular necrosis at presentation invariably augurs death within 6 months. Such patients should be considered for liver transplantation. Patients who fail to enter remission within 2 years of treatment have a 43% frequency of subsequent hepatic decompensation, and after 4 years of continuous therapy without remission the frequency of decompensation increases to 69%. Typically, the first feature of decompensation is ascites formation, which compels evaluation for liver transplantation. Long-term prognosis relates to the ability to induce remission and to prevent features of liver failure.

19. What are the results of corticosteroid therapy?

Sixty-five percent of patients achieve clinical, biochemical, and histological remission within 3 years of treatment. The average duration of therapy required to induce remission is 22 months. The probability of entering remission increases at a constant annual rate during the first 3 years of therapy, and the majority of patients who enter remission (87%) do so during this period. Patients without cirrhosis at presentation have 5- and 10-year life expectancies that exceed 90%, whereas patients with cirrhosis at presentation have a 5-year life expectancy of 80% and 10-year life expectancy of 65%. Thirteen percent of patients develop drug-related side effects that prematurely limit treatment. The most common serious complication is intolerable obesity or cosmetic change (47%). Osteoporosis with vertebral compression (27%), brittle diabetes (20%), and peptic ulceration (6%) restrict therapy less frequently. Patients with cirrhosis develop serious side effects more commonly than others. This propensity may relate to higher serum levels of unbound prednisolone that result from the prolonged hyperbilirubinemia and/or hypoalbuminemia that frequently accompanies cirrhosis. Of importance, no findings at presentation predict a serious side effect, and all previously untreated patients with absolute indications for therapy, including postmenopausal women, should be managed aggressively. Deterioration despite compliance with therapy (treatment failure) develops in 9% of patients, and an incomplete response occurs in 13%. Cirrhosis develops in 36% of patients within 6 years; 50–86% of individuals who enter remission relapse after drug withdrawal; only 14% of patients have sustained inactivity after cessation of therapy; and the risk of extrahepatic malignancy in patients receiving long-term immunosuppressive therapy is 1.4-fold greater than that in an age- and sex-matched normal population (95% confidence limits, 0.6- to 2.9-fold normal). Clearly, responsiveness to corticosteroid therapy is not universal or uncomplicated. This realization underscores the importance of adhering to rigid selection criteria for treatment.

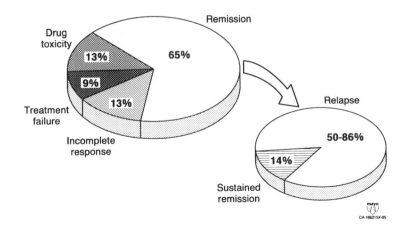

Responses to initial course of corticosteroid therapy.

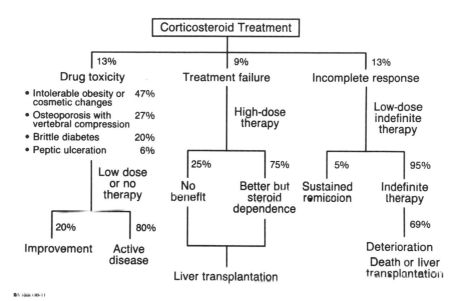

Frequency and consequences of suboptimal responses to corticosteroid therapy.

20. What are the endpoints of treatment?

Conventional treatment should be continued until remission, drug toxicity, clinical deterioration, or confirmation of an incomplete response. Remission connotes absence of symptoms, resolution of laboratory indices of active inflammation, and histologic improvement to normal, inactive cirrhosis, or features of portal hepatitis. Improvement of the serum aspartate aminotransferase level to twice normal or less is compatible with remission if the other criteria are met. Liver biopsy assessment before drug withdrawal is essential to establish remission, because histologic activity may be present in 55% of patients satisfying the clinical and laboratory requirements for remission. Typically, histologic improvement lags behind clinical and biochemical resolution by 3–6 months, and treatment should be extended for at least this period before proceeding with liver tissue examination. Treatment failure connotes progressive worsening of laboratory tests and/or symptoms, ascites formation, or features of hepatic encephalopathy despite compliance with therapy. Such changes justify an alternative treatment strategy, as do the emergence of serious drug-related complications and failure to induce remission after protracted treatment. The risk of serious drug toxicity exceeds the likelihood of inducing remission after 3 years of continuous therapy. In such patients an incomplete response is established, and a decreasing benefit-risk ratio justifies termination of conventional treatment and institution of alternative therapy.

21. Does corticosteroid treatment prevent cirrhosis?

Cirrhosis develops in 36% of patients within 6 years despite corticosteroid treatment. Typically, it eventuates during the early, most active stages of disease and is less likely after induction of remission. The mean annual incidence of cirrhosis is 11% during the first 3 years of illness and 1% thereafter, despite relapse and retreatment. Of importance, the development of cirrhosis during or after treatment does not diminish survival or increase morbidity. The 5-year life expectancy of such patients is 93%; the probability of esophageal varices is 13%; and the likelihood of upper gastrointestinal bleeding is 6%. Progression to cirrhosis undoubtedly reflects the difficulty in obtaining complete, rapid, and sustained suppression of inflammatory activity.

22. Does hepatocellular carcinoma occur?
Hepatocellular cancer may develop in patients with autoimmune hepatitis who have cirrhosis. The frequency of this occurrence in patients with cirrhosis of at least 5 years' duration is 7%; the incidence in such patients is 1 per 182 patient-years of follow-up; the probability of tumor is 29% after 13 years; and the risk is 311-fold greater than that in a normal population (95% confidence intervals, 64- to 906-fold normal). The efficacy of a surveillance program in detecting early treatable tumors is uncertain, and implementation of such a program is empiric. Of importance, 35% of all patients with severe autoimmune hepatitis have abnormal serum alpha fetoprotein levels at presentation. Such abnormalities are typically mild (range = 19.6–262 ng/ml) and commonly normalize during corticosteroid therapy. Late elevation of the serum alpha fetoprotein level suggests neoplasm, but normal levels do not exclude the diagnosis.

23. What is the most common treatment problem?
Relapse after and drug withdrawal is the most common management problem. Fifty percent of patients who enter remission relapse within 6 months after termination of treatment, and 70% relapse within 3 years. The relapse frequency may be as high as 86% and increases after each subsequent retreatment and drug withdrawal. The risk of relapse diminishes with duration of sustained remission, and a sustained remission of a least 6 months is associated with only an 8% frequency of subsequent relapse. The risk, however, is always present, and relapse may occur years later. The principal factor that contributes to relapse is premature withdrawal of medication, which usually results from anxiety about possible drug-related side effects, or reliance on clinical and laboratory indices to define the endpoint of treatment. Patients who have periportal hepatitis at termination of therapy and patients who have developed cirrhosis during treatment invariably relapse after withdrawal of medication. Patients with portal hepatitis at drug withdrawal have a 50% probability of relapse, whereas patients with normal liver tissue have a 20% likelihood of relapse. The inability to eliminate the risk of relapse probably reflects failure of corticosteroid therapy to disrupt completely or permanently the pathogenic mechanisms of the disease. Patients with the HLA A1-B8-DR3 phenotype and patients with persistence of antibodies to asialoglycoprotein receptor during treatment relapse more commonly than counterparts without such findings.

24. How should relapse be managed?
The major consequence of relapse and retreatment is the development of drug-related side effects that diminish the net benefit-risk ratio of conventional treatment. The frequency of side effects after relapse and readministration of the original treatment regimen is similar to that after initial treatment (33% vs. 29%). This frequency, however, increases to 70% after a second relapse and retreatment. In patients with multiple relapses, alternative therapies are appropriate.

Two regimens have been used in the management of such patients. The objective of **indefinite low-dose prednisone therapy** is to control symptoms and to maintain serum aspartate aminotransferase levels below 5-fold normal on the lowest dose of medication possible. Accordingly, the daily dose of prednisone is reduced by 2.5 mg each month until the goals are achieved. Eighty-seven percent of patients can be managed on 10 mg of prednisone daily or less (median dose = 7.5 mg daily). Side effects that occurred during conventional therapy improve in 85% of patients; new side effects do not develop; and mortality is similar to that of patients treated with full-dose conventional regimens (9% vs. 10%).

The objective of **indefinite azathioprine therapy** is to sustain the remission achieved by conventional corticosteroid treatment with nonsteroidal medication. This objective can be accomplished by administering a fixed daily dose of azathioprine (2 mg/kg) and withdrawing the prednisone. Cytopenia compels dose reduction in only 9% of patients; corticosteroid-induced side effects improve; and arthralgias associated with steroid withdrawal eventually resolve. Because the regimens have not been compared for efficacy, there is no valid basis for preference. Concerns about the uncertain long-term oncogenic and teratogenic consequences of indefinite azathioprine therapy, however, must be factored into the treatment decision.

25. How should treatment failure be managed?

High-dose prednisone (60 mg daily) or prednisone (30 mg daily) in conjunction with azathioprine (150 mg daily) induces clinical and biochemical remission in 75% of patients within 2 years. The doses of medication are reduced each month of clinical and biochemical improvement until conventional maintenance doses are achieved. Unfortunately, histologic remission occurs in less than 20% of patients. The majority of patients who fail treatment, therefore, become corticosteroid-dependent and remain at risk for eventual disease progression and drug-related complications. Such patients frequently become candidates for liver transplantation. Liver transplantation is an excellent treatment for patients with decompensated disease. The 5-year life expectancy after transplantation is 92%, and the autoantibodies invariably disappear within 2 years. Recurrence after transplantation has been reported in patients who are inadequately immunosuppressed and in HLA DR3-positive patients who receive HLA DR3-negative grafts.

26. What strategy is best for patients with drug toxicity or incomplete response?

Unfortunately, there are no confident treatment guidelines for patients with drug toxicity or incomplete response. Management is improvisional and empiric. The dose of medication is reduced to the lowest possible level or withdrawn fully if symptoms and inflammatory indices allow. Patients eventually may decompensate and require liver transplantation. Novel therapies, such as cyclosporine (5–6 mg/kg daily), have been used anecdotally, and results after 1 year have been encouraging. Of importance, patients subsequently become dependent on cyclosporine therapy and are at an uncertain risk for serious long-term complications from the drug. The use of cyclosporine, therefore, must be recognized as empiric and unestablished.

27. What therapy is recommended for patients with autoimmune and viral features?

Fortunately, patients with mixed autoimmune and viral features are unusual, but they do exist. If such patients have absolute indications for treatment, the regimen must be directed against the predominant manifestations of the disease. Corticosteroid therapy in patients with chronic viral

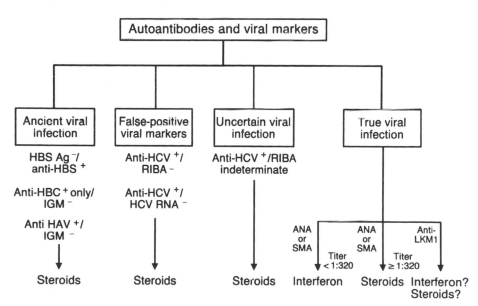

CA-166215B-14

Treatment strategies for patients with autoantibodies and viral markers.

hepatitis may enhance the viral burden, and interferon treatment in patients with autoimmune hepatitis may exacerbate the disease. Patients who have autoimmune hepatitis with false-positive viral markers or serologic findings of indeterminate viral infection should be treated with corticosteroids, as should patients with serologic features of a previous infection that is not active. Such patients respond to corticosteroid treatment as well as counterpart without viral markers, and false-positive serologic reactions may actually disappear. Patients with true viral infection and low titers of SMA and/or ANA (titers <1:320)) have viral-predominant disease with nonspecific autoimmune features; a closely monitored treatment trial with recombinant interferon is appropriate. Patients with true viral infection and high titers of SMA and/or ANA (titers ≥1:320) probably have concurrent diseases. Because interferon therapy may exacerbate the disorder, a well-monitored treatment trial with corticosteroids is appropriate. Fifty-three percent of patients treated in this fashion achieve clinical, biochemical, and histologic remission despite concurrent viral infection, and patients who do not respond tolerate the medication satisfactorily. Patients with true viral infection and anti-LKM1 may have coexistent diseases or autoimmune reactivity attributable to viral infection. The response to interferon or corticosteroids in such patients is uncertain. Recombinant interferon may be administered cautiously as initial treatment, and corticosteroids may be given later, depending on response.

28. What new therapies are promising?

Several novel immunosuppressive and cytoprotective agents have been tested or contemplated in the management of autoimmune hepatitis, but none has been established as superior to conventinal corticosteroid regimens.

Cyclosporine has been used most commonly in an empiric fashion for corticosteroid-recalcitrant disease, but the net benefit-risk ratio and indications for its use remain undefined.

Preliminary, small, open-labelled treatment trials have indicated that **FK-506** can reduce serum aminotransferase and bilirubin levels by at least 50% of baseline, but such therapy is also associated with an increase in serum creatinine level by 150% of baseline. In addition, no evidence to date indicates that FK-506 can induce clinical, biochemical, and histologic remission, and studies in animal models of liver injury suggest that it may facilitate hepatic fibrogenesis.

Ursodeoxycholic acid has a theoretical rationale for use in autoimmune hepatitis if it can alter aberrant class I HLA expression on the hepatocyte membrane and impair lymphocytokine production. Preliminary studies showing biochemical improvements in patients with chronic hepatitis may reflect such immunomodulatory actions.

Brequinar and **rapamycin** are novel immunosuppressive agents that have emerged from the transplantation arena, and they have actions of theoretical advantage to patients with autoimmune hepatitis. They have not yet, however, been submitted to clinical trial.

Thymic hormone extracts have been shown to stimulate suppressor T-cell activity and to inhibit immunoglobulin production, but an early controlled treatment trial failed to demonstrate a difference in the frequency of relapse after conventional drug withdrawal in patients receiving the extract or no therapy during the tapering process. Optimal doses, duration of treatment, and mode of administration, however, were uncertain, and the promise of such therapy cannot as yet be discounted.

Polyunsaturated phosphatidylcholine has been used successfully in conjunction with prednisone for the initial management of autoimmune hepatitis, but its role has not been established. A double-blind, controlled trial indicated that this combination reduces histologic activity better than prednisone alone, presumably by modifying the hepatocyte membrane and blocking or altering the cytotoxic attack on the liver cell. The early reported success of this regimen has not been confirmed, and the combination cannot yet be recommended as the initial approach to therapy.

Similar results have been reported in a preliminary fashion for **arginine thiazolidinecarboxylate.**

As the pathogenic mechanisms of autoimmune hepatitis are clarified, therapies can be directed against one or more of the critical steps in pathogenesis, and behavior and expression of

Promising New Therapies

AGENT	PUTATIVE ACTIONS	EXPERIENCE
Immunosuppressive drugs		
Cyclosporine	Inhibits lymphokine release Impairs effector cell expansion	Anecdotal use
FK-506	Prevents effector cell expansion Inhibits interleukin-2 receptor Impairs antibody production May facilitate fibrogenesis	Limited open-label trial
Thymic extracts	Stimulates suppressor cells Inhibits antibody production	Controlled trial
Intravenous immunoglobulin	Interferes with Fc receptors Induces suppressor cells Inhibits antiidiotypes	Anecdotal use
Brequinar	Inhibits pyrimidine synthesis Prevents lymphocyte proliferation	Hypothetical value
Rapamycin	Blocks interleukin-2 signal Prevents effector cell expansion	Hypothetical value
Cytoprotective drugs		
Phosphatidylcholine	Modifies hepatocytic membrane	Controlled trial
Thiazolidine-carboxylate	Modifies hepatocytic membrane	Anecdotal use
Ursodeoxycholic acid	Alters class I HLA expression Reduces hydrophobic bile acids Modifies hepatocytic membrane Inhibits cytokines	Anecdotal use

the disease can be more precisely modified. Such drugs will have the potential to interfere with HLA expression, lymphocyte activation, antibody production, effector cell proliferation, cytokine modulation, adhesion molecule expression, and fibrin deposition. The introduction of new drugs must not be compromised by perceptions that corticosteroids are unchallengeable. All new strategies, however, must be tested rigorously by controlled clinical trial before endorsement.

BIBLIOGRAPHY

1. Czaja AJ: Autoimmune chronic active hepatitis. In Czaja AJ, Dickson ER (eds): Chronic Active Hepatitis: The Mayo Clinic Experience. New York, Marcel Dekker, 1986, pp 105–126.
2. Czaja AJ: Diagnosis, prognosis, and treatment of classical autoimmune chronic active hepatitis. In Krawitt EL, Wiesner RH (eds): Autoimmune Liver Disease. New York, Raven Press, 1991, pp 143–166.
3. Czaja AJ: Chronic active hepatitis: The challenge for a new nomenclature. Ann Intern Med 119:510–517, 1993.
4. Czaja AJ: Clinical aspects of autoimmune hepatitis in North America. In Nishioka M, Toda G, Zeniya M (eds): Autoimmune Hepatitis. Amsterdam, Elsevier, 1994, pp 27–43.
5. Czaja AJ: Treatment of autoimmune hepatitis. In Nishioka M, Toda G, Zeniya M (eds): Autoimmune Hepatitis. Amsterdam, Elsevier, 1994, pp 283–304.
6. Czaja AJ: Autoimmune hepatitis: Current therapeutic concepts. Clin Immunother 1:413–429, 1994.
7. Czaja AJ: Autoimmune hepatitis and viral infection. Gastroenterol Clin North Am 23:547–566, 1994.
8. Czaja AJ: Autoimmune hepatitis: evolving concepts and treatment strategies. Dig Dis Sci 40:435–456, 1995.

18. PRIMARY BILIARY CIRRHOSIS AND PRIMARY SCLEROSING CHOLANGITIS

Vijayan Balan, M.D., and Nicholas F. LaRusso, M.D.

1. Define primary biliary cirrhosis and primary sclerosing cholangitis.
Primary biliary cirrhosis (PBC) and primary sclerosing cholangitis (PSC) are idiopathic cholestatic liver diseases in adults. PBC mainly affects middle-aged women and is characterized by destruction of interlobular and septal bile ducts. PSC mainly affects young men and is characterized by diffuse inflammation and fibrosis of the entire biliary tree. Both PBC and PSC eventually progress to end-stage liver disease.

2. What is the cause of PBC?
The cause of PBC is unknown; however, an autoimmune etiology has been proposed because of the following features:

1. Frequent association of PBC with other autoimmune disease, such as Sjögren's syndrome, rheumatoid arthritis, scleroderma, Raynaud's disease, thyroiditis, cutaneous disorders such as lichen planus, discoid lupus, pemphigoid, and the syndrome consisting of calcinosis, Raynaud's phenomenon, esophageal disease, sclerodactyly, and telangiectasia (CREST);

2. Presence of circulating antibodies, such as antimitochondrial antibodies, rheumatoid factor, smooth muscle antibody, thyroid specific antibodies, extractable nuclear antigen, and antinuclear antibody;

3. Hepatic histology indicative of immunologic bile duct destruction;

4. Familial clustering of PBC;

5. Increased prevalence of circulating antibodies in relatives of patients with PBC; and

6. Increased frequency of class II major histocompatibility complex (MHC) antigens, especially HLA-DRw8.

3. Is PSC an autoimmune disorder?
The evidence supporting an immunogenic origin of PSC includes:

1. Increased incidence of both PSC and chronic ulcerative colitis (CUC) in families of patients with PSC;

2. Increased frequency of human leukocyte antigen, HLA B8, DR2, DR3, and DRw52a;

3. Abnormalities in the immune system, including increased serum immunoglobulin M levels, decreased hepatic clearance of circulating immune complexes, increased complement activation, and abnormalities in lymphocyte subsets in the peripheral blood; and

4. Aberrant expression of HLA class II antigen on bile duct epithelial cells.

4. Do viral infections have a role in the development of PSC?
Viral agents such as respiratory enteric orphan (REO) virus type III and cytomegalovirus may infect the biliary tree and have been implicated in the development of PSC. Viral infections have been postulated to trigger the immune system and consequent immunologically mediated bile duct destruction. However, no direct evidence links these or other viruses to the development of PSC.

5. What are the clinical features of PBC and PSC?
The clinical presentations of both PBC and PSC may be similar, although the demographics differ. Ninety percent of patients with PBC are women, usually in the fourth to sixth decade of life. Seventy percent of patients with PSC are men with the mean age of 43 at diagnosis. Generally, both conditions present with a gradual onset of pruritus. Jaundice develops within 6 months to 2 years after the onset of pruritus. In a small number of the patients, jaundice and pruritus start si-

multaneously. In PBC jaundice before pruritus is unusual but may be the most common presenting complaint in men. Fatigue, right upper quadrant pain, and lethargy are also common presenting symptoms. Symptoms of end-stage liver disease, such as gastrointestinal bleeding, ascites, and encephalopathy, occur late in the course of both diseases. In PSC cholangitis characterized by recurrent fever, right upper quadrant pain, and jaundice occur in patients with previous reconstructive biliary surgery or a dominant stricture of the extrahepatic bile duct.

Physical examination may reveal jaundice and excoriations. Xanthelasma and xanthomas are occasionally seen about the eyes and the extensor surfaces in the later stages of both diseases, particularly PBC. Hyperpigmentation is present, especially in sun-exposed areas. The liver is usually enlarged and firm, and the spleen also may be palpable. Characteristics of end-stage liver disease, including ascites, spider angiomata, and hepatic encephalopathy, appear in the latter stages of both diseases and are rare as presenting features.

6. What diseases are associated with PBC and PSC?
Scleroderma, rheumatoid arthritis, thyroiditis, and Sjögren's syndrome are commonly associated with PBC. Chronic ulcerative colitis (CUC) and rarely Crohn's colitis are present in at least 70% of cases of PSC. CUC usually manifests before the onset of PSC but may be diagnosed simultaneously or after PSC. CUC associated with PSC is usually quiescent; in 80% of patients CUC is either asymptomatic or mildly symptomatic when PSC is diagnosed.

7. What are the abnormalities in blood chemistries in PBC and PSC?
An elevated alkaline phosphatase (3 or 4 times normal), with mild-to-moderate elevations in alanine aminotransferase (ALT) and aspartate aminotransferase (AST), are usually present. In PBC serum bilirubin values are usually initially normal. In PSC serum bilirubin values are modestly increased in one-half of patients at time of diagnosis. Tests assessing the synthetic function of the liver (serum albumin level and prothrombin time) remain normal until late in the course of the disease. Serum immunoglobulin M (IgM) is elevated in 90% of patients with PBC. Tests related to copper metabolism are virtually always abnormal in both diseases. The widespread use of automated blood chemistries has resulted in diagnosis of an increasing number of patients at the presymptomatic stage of both diseases.

8. What is the lipid profile of patients with PBC? Are they at increased risk for development of coronary artery disease?
Serum cholesterol levels are usually elevated in PBC. In the early stages, the increases in high-density lipoprotein (HDL) cholesterol exceed those of low-density lipoprotein (LDL) and very-low-density lipoprotein (VLDL). As the disease progresses, the concentration of HDLs decreases, whereas LDLs are markedly elevated. The hyperlipidemia associated with PBC does not appear to place patients at increased risk for atherosclerotic disease.

9. What autoantibodies are associated with PBC?
Circulating antimitochondrial antibodies (AMA) are found in virtually all patients with PBC. AMA, which are non–organ- and non–species-specific, are usually detected by an enzyme-linked immunsorbent assay (ELISA) and are not specific for PBC. However, antibodies (anti-M2) directed against a specific group of antigens located on the inner membrane of mitochondria designated M2 are present in 98% of patients with PBC. This subtyping of the AMA increases the sensitivity and specificity of the test.

Other AMA subtypes related to PBC react with antigens on the outer mitochondrial membrane. Anti-M4 occurs in association with anti-M2 in patients with features of both chronic active hepatitis and PBC. Anti-M8 is present in patients with anti-M2 and may be associated with a more rapid course of PBC. Anti-M9 has been seen in patients with and without anti-M2 and may be helpful in the diagnosis of early and asymptomatic PBC.

10. What autoantibodies are associated with PSC?

In PSC the presence of serum antimitochondrial, antinuclear, and antismooth muscle antibodies is infrequent. Anticolon, antineutrophil nuclear, and neutrophil cytoplasmic antibodies are present in most patients with PSC. However, these antibodies also occur in a high percentage of patients with ulcerative colitis and no evidence of PSC.

11. What are the cholangiographic features of the biliary tree in PSC?

The biliary evaluation by endoscopic or transhepatic cholangiography in PSC is diagnostic and classically demonstrates diffuse stricturing and beading of the intrahepatic and extrahepatic bile ducts. The strictures are short and annular with intermediate segments of slightly dilated bile ducts.

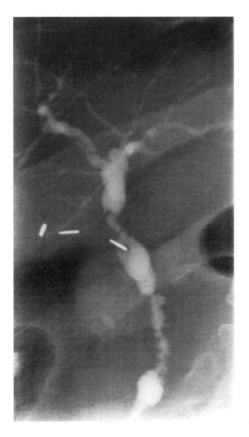

A retrograde cholangiogram exhibiting classic features of PSC, showing diffuse stricturing and beading of intra- and extrahepatic bile ducts. (Reprinted with permission from LaRusso NF, et al: Primary sclerosing cholangitis. N Engl J Med 310:899–903, 1984. Copyright 1984. Massachusetts Medical Society. All rights reserved.)

12. Is it important to evaluate the biliary tree in PBC?

In PBC an ultrasound examination of the biliary tree is usually adequate to exclude biliary obstruction. However, in patients with atypical features of PBC, such as a male gender, AMA negativity, or associated inflammatory bowel disease, an endoscopic or percutaneous cholangiography should be considered to distinguish PBC from PSC and other disorders causing biliary obstruction.

13. What are the histologic features of the liver in patients with PBC and PSC?

Histologic abnormalities found on liver biopsy are highly characteristic of both PBC and PSC early in the disease. In PBC, the diagnostic finding is the florid duct lesion (granulomatous bile duct destruction). Inflammatory cell accumulation in the portal tracts are accompanied by segmental degeneration of the interlobular and septal bile ducts (chronic nonsuppurative destructive cholangitis).

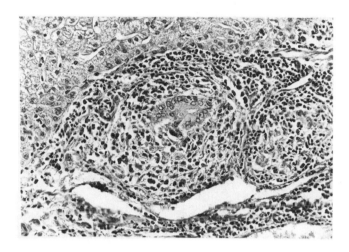

Florid duct lesion (granulomatous bile duct destruction) in PBC. A poorly formed granuloma surrounds and destroys the bile duct in an eccentric fashion.

Early histologic changes in PSC include enlargement of portal tracts characterized by edema, increased connective tissue, and proliferation of interlobular bile ducts. The diagnostic histologic abnormality in PSC is fibrous obliterative cholangitis, which results in replacement of the duct segments by fibrous chords and connective tissue and leads to complete loss of interlobular and adjacent septal bile ducts. The histologic findings at end stages of both diseases are characterized by paucity of bile ducts and biliary cirrhosis.

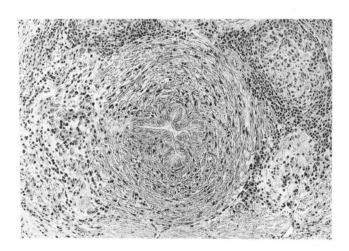

Fibrous obliterative cholangitis in PSC. The interlobular bile duct shows a typical fibrous collar and epithelium appears undamaged.

14. Do asymptomatic patients with PBC and PSC have a normal life expectancy?
Patients with PBC in the asymptomatic stage follow the same course as patients with symptoms except that mortality lags by approximately 4 years. In a Mayo Clinic study, asymptomatic patients with PBC followed for 4–6 years developed increasing serum bilirubin and decreasing serum albumin. Eighty-four percent developed symptoms related to the liver disease and had a 4-fold increase in mortality compared with the general population. The usual course of PBC is long, exceeding 10–15 years. Although some symptomatic or minimally symptomatic patients with PSC may do well for many years, the majority experience progression of disease and symptom exacerbation.

15. What is the role of statistical models of survival in patients with PBC and PSC?
Statistical models have been devised to predict the probability of survival for individual patients with PBC and PSC. They are useful in selecting and timing patients for liver transplantation, designing treatment trials, stratifying patients, and developing endpoints of treatment failure. Models for PBC developed at the Mayo Clinic rely on measures such as serum bilirubin, albumin, prothrombin time, presence or absence of peripheral edema, and patient's age. In PSC the important clinical variables predicting survival are age, serum bilirubin, hepatic histologic stage, and presence of splenomegaly.

16. What vitamin deficiencies are associated with PBC and PSC?
Patients with PBC and PSC are susceptible to fat-soluble vitamin deficiencies in the advanced stages of the disease. **Vitamin A deficiency** may lead to night blindness. **Vitamin K deficiency** leads to prolonged prothrombin time. **Vitamin E deficiency** may cause neurologic abnormalities affecting the posterior columns, characterized by areflexia or loss of proprioception and ataxia. **Vitamin D deficiency** occurs commonly in patients with marked steatorrhea, which often is related to a decrease in the concentration of bile acids in the duodenum. Vitamin D deficiency may contribute to metabolic bone disease.

17. What bone disease is associated with PBC and PSC?
Metabolic bone disease (i.e., hepatic osteodystrophy), which may lead to disabling pathologic fractures, is a serious complication of both PBC and PSC. It is related to osteoporosis and rarely to vitamin D deficiency.

18. What complications are specific for PSC?
Complications specific for PSC include recurrent bacterial cholangitis, bacteremia, dominant stricturing of the extrahepatic bile ducts, and cholangiocarcinoma. Cholangitis is frequent in patients with previous biliary surgery or dominant stricture formation of the extrahepatic bile duct.

Dominant strictures of the biliary tree occur in approximately 15–20% of patients with PSC during the course of the disease. They occur most often at the hilus and also may involve the common bile duct as well as the right and left hepatic ducts. Dominant strictures are frequently associated with the acute onset of jaundice, pruritus, and bacterial cholangitis with fever and chills.

In 10–15% of patients with PSC, **cholangiocarcinoma** develops during the course of the disease. The highest incidence apparently occurs in patients with long-standing CUC and cirrhotic-stage PSC. Because patients with PSC often have long-standing, relatively quiescent colitis, they are at risk for developing both cholangiocarcinoma and colon cancer. Unfortunately, it is difficult to diagnose cholangiocarcinoma early in patients with PSC, because fine-needle aspiration, brush cytology, and exfoliative cytology are not sensitive enough to detect bile duct cancer in the presence of PSC. A recent report suggests that the measurement of serum concentrations of the glycoprotein, CA-19-9, may be promising for the detection of cholangiocarcinoma complicating PSC.

19. What is the differential diagnosis of PBC and PSC?

The differential diagnosis of PBC and PSC includes other causes of chronic cholestatis, such as extrahepatic biliary obstruction due to biliary stones, iatrogenic strictures, and tumors. Although ultrasonography or computed tomography may suggest biliary dilation, cholangiography is the definitive diagnostic study for PSC; AMA is absent in most patients. Drug-induced cholestasis secondary to phenothiazines, estrogens, androgens, and a number of other drugs also should be considered in the differential diagnosis. Autoimmune chronic active hepatitis (AICAH) may be confused with PBC in some patients. Patients with AICAH may be positive for AMA, but usually in low titers (<1:40). Liver biopsy is helpful; bile duct abnormalities are uncommon in AICAH and characteristic in PBC. AMA subtyping, such as the finding of anti-M4, may allow differentiation between the two conditions. AICAH also may overlap with PSC. Patients with AICAH may develop a cholestatic biochemical profile, and the cholangiogram may show changes consistent with PSC. Therefore, patients with AICAH and associated CUC should have a cholangiogram to exclude PSC.

20. What is the treatment of pruritus in patients with PBC and PSC?

Cholestyramine relieves itching and lowers serum bile acids in patients with cholestasis. Cholestyramine increases intestinal excretion of bile acids by preventing their absorption. Cholestyramine is given in 4-gm doses (mixed with liquids) with meals or after breakfast for a total daily dose of 12–16 gm. Cholestyramine should be given 1 1/2 hours before or after other medications to avoid nonspecific binding and diminished intestinal absorption. Once the itching remits, the dosage should be reduced to the minimum that maintains relief.

If cholestyramine is ineffective, phenobarbital may be added in a dose of 120–160 mg/day. Rifampin, 300–600 mg/day, also has been effective in relieving pruritus, possibly due to p450 enzyme induction or inhibition of bile acid uptake. Experimental approaches include phototherapy and plasmapheresis to remove bile acids.

21. What is the treatment of osteopenia in PBC and PSC?

There is no effective therapy for the osteoporosis in patients with PBC and PSC. As mentioned earlier, the bone disease associated with PBC and PSC is due most often to osteoporosis and infrequently to osteomalacia. However, low serum vitamin D levels can be corrected by administering 50,000 units of vitamin D once or twice weekly.

Postmenopausal estrogen therapy, especially when instituted soon after menopause, has been associated with slowing of bone loss. In cholestatic patients, estrogen therapy was thought to be contraindicated, because it may contribute to intrahepatic cholestasis. However, this problem does not seem to be associated with standard estrogen replacement therapy, which was shown to improve osteoporosis in a recent retrospective study. However, it is prudent to reassess the patient clinically and biochemically within 2–3 months after starting estrogen therapy.

22. What is the treatment of fat-soluble vitamin deficiency in PBC and PSC?

Problems with night vision due to vitamin A deficiency may be alleviated by replacement therapy. Decreased serum levels can be corrected with oral administration of vitamin A (25,000–50,000 units 2–3 times/week). Excessive vitamin A intake is associated with hepatotoxicity; thus, serum levels should be monitored. Vitamin K deficiency is associated with a prolonged prothrombin time (PT). A trial of vitamin K (5–10 mg) should be given; if the PT improves, patients should be maintained on a water-soluble vitamin K replacement, 5 mg/day. In patients with low vitamin E levels, replacement therapy can be instituted with 100 mg twice daily, although replacement is not always effective.

23. Do lipid-lowering agents have a role in treatment of PBC and PSC?

Because patients with PBC and PSC do not appear to have an increased risk of atherosclerotic disease despite high serum cholesterol, lipid-lowering agents are not usually recommended. In some patients with xanthelasma, cholestyramine may stabilize or even decrease the size of cutaneous lipid deposits.

24. What is the treatment of bacterial cholangitis in PSC?
Bacterial cholangitis in PSC should be treated with broad-spectrum antibiotics. Ciprofloxacin reaches high biliary concentrations and has broad gram-negative and gram-positive bacterial coverage. Prophylactic therapy with ciprofloxacin reduces the frequency of bacterial cholangitis in patients with PSC and a history of recurrent bacterial cholangitis.

25. What are the therapeutic options for treatment of strictures of the biliary tree in PSC?
Balloon dilatation of dominant strictures by either a transhepatic or endoscopic retrograde approach may relieve biliary obstruction. Dominant strictures developing in patients with PSC often are successfully treated with percutaneous balloon dilatation and long-term stenting. Thus, biliary surgical intervention may be minimized. Balloon dilatation is most effective in patients with a recent increase in serum bilirubin levels or recent onset of bacterial cholangitis; it is less effective in patients with longstanding jaundice or a longstanding history of recurrent bouts of bacterial cholangitis.

26. What is the role of transjugular intrahepatic portosystemic shunt (TIPS) in PBC and PSC?
TIPS placement is used with increasing frequency for bleeding esophageal varices; however, its role in PBC and PSC is not defined. TIPS rapidly decompresses the portal system and in turn decompresses not only the esophageal varices but also gastric varices, which are not accessible to sclerotherapy. TIPS also may reduce ascites quite dramatically. Unfortunately, the incidence of hepatic encephalopathy may increase after TIPS.

27. What medical agents have been tried for the treatment of PBC and PSC?
A number of therapies for PBC and PSC have been tested in controlled trials. None is totally effective. Specific therapeutic agents include cupruretic, antifibrinogenic, immunosuppressive, and anticholestatic agents. Presently, ursodeoxycholic acid (UDCA) has generated considerable enthusiasm, particularly in PBC.

Medical Therapy for PBC and PSC

Immunosuppressive	Cupruritic
Corticosteroids	D-penicillamine*
Cyclosporine A*	Antifibrinogenic
FK506	Cholchicine
Methotrexate*	Choleretic
Azathioprine*	Ursodeoxycholic acid (UDCA) *

*Controlled trial performed.

28. What is the effectiveness of UDCA in the treatment of PBC and PSC?
UDCA is under evaluation in randomized, controlled trials for the treatment of PBC and PSC. Endogenous hydrophobic bile acids, some of which may be hepatotoxic, appear to be replaced with the hydrophilic, nonhepatotoxic UDCA. Alterations in the bile pool may occur by competition for ileal uptake sites or by direct action at the level of the liver. In addition, UDCA may reduce class I and class II HLA antigen expression on the hepatocytes and bile duct epithelial cells and also may decrease the number of CD8 cells surrounding bile duct epithelial cells in patients with PBC. Results from clinical trials show that UDCA reduces symptoms and improves liver tests and some histologic features. Thus far UDCA has not been shown to have an effect

on survival, need for liver transplantation, histologic progression to cirrhosis, or development of varices or ascites in patients with PBC. Nevertheless, most patients with PBC are currently treated with UDCA.

29. What is the role of reconstructive biliary tract surgery in PSC?

Choledochoduodenostomy or choledochojejunostomy for PSC are palliative measures to alleviate symptoms. Reconstructive surgery does not have a beneficial effect on the natural history of PSC, particularly in patients with cirrhotic stage disease. Furthermore, episodes of bacterial cholangitis develop postoperatively in more than 60% of patients undergoing such surgery. However, patients with severe hilar or extrahepatic biliary stricturing and persistent jaundice or cholangitis but without cirrhosis may benefit from biliary reconstruction and long-term transhepatic stenting. At most centers, however, reconstructive surgery is rarely done with PSC, because the same goal can be achieved by endoscopic or transhepatic approaches.

30. Does proctocolectomy in patients with PSC and CUC favorably affect hepatobiliary disease?

Proctocolectomy has not been shown to have any beneficial effect on clinical, biochemical, hepatic histologic, or radiologic features of PSC or on overall survival. In addition, proctocolectomy is associated with considerable morbidity from the development of peristomal varices after ileostomy. At present, proctocolectomy should not be performed simply to remove the colon in a patient with PSC in anticipation of a beneficial effect on liver disease. If carcinoma or precancerous lesions develop in the colon, a proctocolectomy is indicated. Patients who require a proctocolectomy should undergo an ileal-anal anastomosis to avoid the potential formation of peristomal varices.

31. What is the role of liver transplantation in PBC and PSC?

The treatment of choice for patients with end-stage PBC and PSC is liver transplantation. One-year survival after liver transplantation is currently about 80%, and 5-year survival is over 60%. Factors that promote consideration for liver transplantation are decreased quality of life, progressive cholestasis (bilirubin > 10 mg/dl), deteriorating hepatic synthetic function, or intractable symptoms. Disabling fatigue, pruritus, uncontrolled ascites, hepatic encephalopathy, or variceal bleeding not controlled with sclerotherapy are also indications for liver transplantation. Successful liver transplantation normally results in increased survival and dramatic improvement in the quality of life. Most patients resume normal activities after recovering from the postoperative period.

32. Do PBC and PSC recur after liver transplantation?

A positive AMA persists in the majority of patients with PBC after liver transplantation. In 7% of posttransplant patients, there is evidence of histologic recurrence of PBC (florid duct lesion) in the grafted liver. However, the presence of an isolated florid duct lesion has thus far not been of clinical significance.

There is also evidence of recurrence of PSC in the form of biliary stricturing in a small number of patients after liver transplantation. However, the bile duct strictures after liver transplantation may be attributable to low-grade bacterial cholangitis, which may be related to the Roux-en-Y biliary anastomosis that is routinely performed in patients with PSC. In addition, rejection, ischemia, ABO mismatch, and possibly cytomegalovirus or other viral infections are known to contribute to biliary stricturing after liver transplantation. Therefore, it is difficult to attribute the biliary stricturing after liver transplantation conclusively to recurrent PSC.

33. What are the complications in PSC patients after liver transplantation?

Patients with PSC seem to have an increased incidence of chronic ductopenic rejection, graft loss from rejection, and biliary stricturing.

BIBLIOGRAPHY

1. Balan V, Batts KP, Porayko MK, et al: Histologic evidence for recurrence of primary biliary cirrhosis after liver transplantation. Hepatology 18:1392–1398, 1993.
2. Batts KP, Ludwig J: Histopathology of autoimmune chronic active hepatitis, primary biliary cirrhosis, and primary sclerosing cholangitis. In Krawitt EL, Wiesner RH (eds): Autoimmune Liver Diseases. New York, Raven Press, 1991, pp 75–92.
3. Cangemi JR, Wiesner RH, Beaver SJ, et al: Effect of proctocolectomy for chronic ulcerative colitis on the natural history of primary sclerosing cholangitis. Gastroenterology 96:790–794, 1989.
4. Cotton PB, Nickl N: Endoscopic and radiologic approaches to therapy in primary sclerosing cholangitis. Semin Liver Dis 11:40–48, 1991.
5. Crippin JS, Lindor KD, Jorgensen R, et al: Hypercholesterolemia and atherosclerosis in primary biliary cirrhosis: What is the risk? Hepatology 15:858–862, 1992.
6. Dickson ER, Grambsch PM, Fleming TR, et al: Prognosis in primary biliary cirrhosis: Model for decision making. Hepatology 10:1–7, 1989.
7. Dickson ER, Murtaugh PA, Wiesner RH, et al: Primary sclerosing cholangitis: Refinement and validation of survival models. Gastroenterology 103:1893–1901, 1993.
8. Hay JE, Lindor KD, Wiesner RH, et al: The metabolic bone disease of primary sclerosing cholangitis. Hepatology 14:257–261, 1991.
9. Jahn CE, Schaefer EJ, Taam LA, et al: Lipoprotein abnormalities in primary biliary cirrhosis: Association with hepatic lipase inhibition as well as altered cholesterol esterification. Gastroenterology 89: 1266–1278, 1985.
10. Kaplan MM: Primary biliary cirrhosis. N Engl J Med 316:521–528, 1987.
11. Kaplan MM: Medical approaches to primary sclerosing cholangitis. Semin Liver Dis 11:56–63, 1991.
12. LaRusso NF, Wiesner RH, Ludwig J, MacCarty RL: Primary sclerosing cholangitis. N Engl J Med 310:899–903, 1984.
13. Lindor KD, Dickson ER, Baldus WP, et al: Ursodeoxycholic acid in the treatment of primary biliary cirrhosis. Gastroenterology 106:1284–90, 1994.
14. MacCarty RL, LaRusso NF, Wiesner RH, Ludwig J: Primary sclerosing cholangitis: Findings on cholangiography and pancreatography. Radiology 149:39–44, 1983.
15. Maddrey WC: Bone disease in patients with primary biliary cirrhosis. Prog Liver Dis 9:537–554, 1990.
16. Markus BH, Dickson ER, Grambsch PM, et al: Efficacy of liver transplantation in patients with primary biliary cirrhosis. N Engl J Med, 320:1709–1713, 1989.
17. Marsh JW Jr, Iwatsuji S, Makowka L, et al: Orthotopic liver transplantation for primary sclerosing cholangitis. Ann Surg 207:21–25, 1988.
18. Nichols JC, Gores GJ, LaRusso NF, et al: Diagnostic role of CA 19-9 for cholangiocarcinoma in patients with primary sclerosing cholangitis. Mayo Clin Proc 68:874–879, 1993.
19. Quigly EMM, LaRusso NF, Ludwig J, et al: Familial occurence of primary sclerosing cholangitis and ulcerative colitis. Gastroenterology, 85:1160–1165, 1983.
20. Rosen CB, Nagorney DM, Wiesner RH, et al: Cholangiocarcinoma complicating primary sclerosing cholangitis. Ann Surg 213:21–25, 1991.
21. Wiesner RH, LaRusso NF, Ludwig J, Dickson ER: Comparison of the clinicopathologic features of primary sclerosing cholangitis and primary biliary cirrhosis. Gastroenterology 88:108–114, 1985.

19. HEPATITIS VACCINES AND IMMUNOPROPHYLAXIS

Maria H. Sjogren, M.D., COL, MC

1. Discuss the concept of immunization (vaccination).
During the last century major progress in the control of infectious diseases has been possible by the remarkable developments in microbiology. In 1798 Edward Jenner first described his work with cowpox vaccination. He demonstrated that a person inoculated and infected with cowpox was protected against smallpox. The procedure, which he called vaccination, represented the first use of a vaccine in the prevention of disease. The word "vaccine" is derived from the Latin word for cow; cows were host to the first true vaccine virus, cowpox. The success of immunization in humans rests on one major concept: humans have specific immunologic mechanisms that can be programmed to provide a defense against infectious agents. The body's immune mechanism is stimulated by direct introduction of infectious agents or smaller components in the form of vaccines. The evolution into the golden era of vaccine development began in 1949 with the discovery of virus propagation in cell culture. Such breakthroughs made it possible to produce and license the first product developed by using the new cell culture technique: the Salk trivalent formalin-inactivated polio vaccine. Following this success, vaccines to prevent human hepatitis A and B have been developed rapidly, considering that the viral agents were recently discovered in 1973 and 1965, respectively.

2. Distinguish between active and passive immunization.
Immunization may be active or passive. Active immunization involves the introduction of a specific antigen to provoke an antibody response that will prevent disease. Passive immunization or immunoprophylaxis is the introduction of antibodies produced by immunization or prior natural infection (of a suitable animal or human host) to prevent or modify the natural infection in a susceptible individual.

3. What are the major categories of vaccines?
Classic vaccines are usually prepared by manipulating the agent in the laboratory to provide a modified product suitable for human use. Two forms are widely available: (1) the inactivated or killed vaccines, in which the product is incapable of multiplying in the host but retains antigenic properties and is capable of evoking an antibody response, and (2) live, attenuated vaccines, which are prepared with live, viable agents. Because of attenuation, however, the agents are incapable of inducing clinical disease. The end result is development of antibody and prevention of infection. The live vaccines generally contain relatively low concentrations of the infectious

Human Vaccines

LIVE ATTENUATED AGENTS	KILLED AGENTS	PURIFIED PROTEINS (OR POLYSACCHARIDES)
Smallpox (1798)	Rabies (recent)	Diphtheria toxin (1888)
Rabies (1885)	Typhoid	Diphtheria (1923)
Yellow fever (1935)	Cholera (1896)	Tetanus (1927)
Polio (Sabin)	Plague (1897)	Pneumococcus
Measles	Influenza (1936)	Meningococcus
Mumps	Polio (Salk)	*Hemophilus influenzae*
Rubella	Hepatitis A (1995)	Hepatitis B (1981)
Adenovirus		
Hepatitis A (research)		

agent. Ideally, only one single administration is required with the live vaccines, and the immunity is long-lasting. With killed vaccines, the immunologic response correlates with the concentration of the antigenic component. Inactivated vaccines commonly require a series of doses to stimulate a long-lasting immunologic response.

4. Define the concept of immunoprophylaxis.

In immunoprophylaxis or passive immunization, antibodies produced by immunization or prior natural infection of a suitable animal or human host are used to prevent or modify the natural infection in humans. Passive immunization affords a relatively brief period of protection (weeks to a few months). Before the development of hepatitis A and B vaccines, immunoprophylaxis was the mainstay to prevent infection. Passive immunization occurs naturally in humans when maternal antibodies of the immunoglobulin G class are passed to neonates. Thus, the newborn infant is provided with a number of antibodies from the mother. Such antibodies provide protection against many communicable bacterial and viral diseases for a period of months. These antibodies provide crucial protection to the infant during the period in which the immune system has not yet fully developed; they disappear within the first year of life.

At the onset of passive immunization therapy, the antibody-containing serum (e.g., horse serum) was administered directly. Recently, by means of fractionation of serum, the antibody of interest is isolated and concentrated.

Immunoglobulins Available for Human Use

PRODUCT	SOURCE	USE
Immune serum globulin	Pooled human plasma	Prevents measles Prevents hepatitis A
Measles immunoglobulin	Pooled human plasma	Prevents measles

Hepatitis B immunoglobulin	Pooled plasma donors
	  with high antibody titer
		Used in accidental needle
		  stick or sexual exposure

Rabies immunoglobulin	Pooled plasma from hyperimmunized donors	Immunotherapy of rabies
Botulism	Specific equine antibody	Treatment and prophylaxis for botulinum toxin

5. Which are the main viral agents responsible for acute and chronic viral hepatitis?

ACUTE HEPATITIS	CHRONIC HEPATITIS	MAIN ROUTE OF TRANSMISSION
Hepatitis A virus (HAV)	No	Fecal-oral
Hepatitis B virus (HBV)	Yes	Bloodborne
Hepatitis C virus (HCV)	Yes	Bloodborne
Hepatitis D virus (HDV)	Yes	Bloodborne
Hepatitis E virus (HEV)	No	Fecal-oral

6. What kind of immunoprophylaxis is available for hepatitis A?

An excellent prophylactic measure is the administration of serum immunoglobulin G (IgG). The recommended dose of IgG is 0.02 ml/kg for preexposure when the period of exposure will not exceed 3 months. If the period of exposure is prolonged, 0.06 ml/kg every 5 months is recommended. IgG affords excellent prophylaxis, but is an impractical method because protection lasts only a few months. Although considered safe, it may cause fever, myalgias, and considerable pain at injection sites.

7. Is a vaccine available for hepatitis A?

Although several experimental hepatitis A vaccines exist, data from two inactivated vaccines tested for efficacy in humans are clinically relevant. The first efficacy trial, conducted by Werzberger and colleagues, demonstrated the 100% protective efficacy provided by an inactivated vaccine administered as a single dose to people at risk. The trial included 1,037 children aged 2–16 years and took place in an upstate New York community where a 3% annual incidence of acute hepatitis A had been observed. Children were randomized to receive one intramuscular injection of a highly purified, formalin-inactivated hepatitis A vaccine (Merck, Sharp & Dohme, West Point, PA) or placebo. From day 50 until day 103 after injection, 25 cases of clinically apparent hepatitis A occurred in the placebo group. None occurred in the vaccine group (p <0.001). The vaccine gave a calculated 100% efficacy rate. The second efficacy trial, conducted by Innis and coworkers, used an inactivated hepatitis A vaccine (Havrix, SmithKline, Rixensart, Belgium) different from the one used by Werzberger. Tested against placebo in a population of more than 40,000 Thai children, the vaccine gave a calculated 97% rate of protective efficacy after subjects received three doses. This vaccine was recently approved by the Food and Drug Administration for use in special populations within the U.S. (military, international travelers). The recommended dose is 1440 EU (1.0 ml) intramuscularly (deltoid muscle) followed by a booster dose at 6 months or 1 year.

8. What is the difference between an inactivated vaccine against hepatitis A and a live, attenuated vaccine?

Hepatitis A Vaccines

	INACTIVATED (KILLED)	ATTENUATED (LIVE)
Main source	HAV cultured in vitro	HAV cultured in vitro
Attained by	Formalin-inactivation	Multiple passage in cell culture
Immunogenicity	Contains alum as adjuvant; evokes anti-HAV antibodies	Adjuvant is not needed; evokes anti-HAV antibodies
Disadvantage	Multiple doses needed	Theoretical possibility of reversal to virulence and ability to cause acute hepatitis A
Availability	Commercially available in Europe and U.S.	Still at the research level in the U.S., Asia and Europe

9. What kind of immunoprophylaxis is available for hepatitis B?

Two types of products are available for prophylaxis against hepatitis B virus infection:

1. **Active immunization:** hepatitis B vaccine, first licensed in the United States in 1981, is recommended for both pre- and postexposure prophylaxis.

2. **Passive immunization:** hyperimmune globulin (HBIG) provides temporary, passive protection and is indicated in certain postexposure situations.

10. What is the recommended dose of HBIG for adults? for children?

HBIG contains high concentrations of anti-HBs. This is a major difference from regular immunoglobulin, which is prepared from plasma with varying concentration of anti-HBs. In the United States, HBIG has an anti-HBs titer of higher than 1:100,000 by radioimmunoassay.

Hepatitis B Virus Postexposure Recommendations

Exposure	HBIG Dose	HBIG Timing	VACCINE Dose	VACCINE Timing
Perinatal	0.5 ml IM	Within 12 hours of birth	0.5 ml at birth	Within 12 hours of birth; repeat at 1 and 6 months
Sexual	0.6 ml/kg IM	Single dose within 14 days of sexual contact	Same time as HBIG	Start immunization at once

IM=intramuscularly.

11. How many hepatitis vaccines are available in the U.S.? Are they comparable?

Three vaccines have been licensed in the U.S. For practical purposes, they are comparable in immunogenicity and efficacy rates. However, the preparations are different:

1. Heptavax - B (Merck, Sharp & Dohme) became available in 1986. It consists of hepatitis B surface antigen purified from the plasma of chronically infected humans and evokes antibodies to the group *a* determinant of the HB_sAg, effectively neutralizing the various subtypes of hepatitis B virus. Abundant evidence supports its efficacy, but it is expensive to prepare and a number of physical and chemical inactivation steps are needed for purification and safety. Because of these problems, alternate approaches were developed. Chief among these developments are HBV vaccines, products of recombinant DNA technology. Each 1ml of plasma-derived vaccine has 20 µg of HB_sAg.

2. Recombivax HB became available in 1989 and is manufactured by Merck, Sharp & Dohme Research Laboratories (West Point, PA). It is a noninfectious, nonglycosylated HB_sAg hepatitis B vaccine, subtype adw, made by recombinant DNA technology. Yeast cells (*Saccharomyces cerevisiae*) expressing the HBsAg gene are cultured, collected by centrifugations, and broken by homogenization with glass beads. HB_sAg particles are purified and absorbed in aluminum hydroxide. Each 1 ml consists of 10 µg of HB_sAg.

3. Engerix-B, manufactured by SmithKline Biologicals (Rixensart, Belgium), is a noninfectious recombinant DNA hepatitis B vaccine. It contains purified hepatitis B surface antigen obtained by culturing genetically engineered *Saccharomyces cerevisiae* cells, which carry the surface antigen gene of the hepatitis B virus. This surface antigen is purified from the cells and adsorbed on aluminum hydroxide. Each 1 ml consists of 20 µg of HB_sAg.

12. What is the immunization schedule for HBV vaccine in adults? in children?

Recombivax-HB Vaccine (Merck, Sharp & Dohme)

GROUP	FORMULATION	INITIAL	1 MONTH	6 MONTHS
Younger children (birth to 10 years)	Pediatric dose: 0.5 ml			
Adults and older children	Adult dose: 10 µg/1.0 ml	0.5 ml 1.0 ml	0.5 ml 1.0 ml	0.5 ml 1.0 ml
Dyalisis patients	Special dose: 40 µg/1.0 ml	1.0 ml	1.0 ml	1.0 ml

Recommended Treatment Regimen for Infants Born to HBsAg-positive Mothers

TREATMENT	BIRTH	WITHIN 7 DAYS	AT 1 MONTH	AT 6 MONTHS
Recombivax-HB (pediatric dose)	0.5 ml	0.5 ml	0.5 ml	0.5 ml
HBIG	0.5 ml	None	None	None

Energix-B Vaccine (SmithKline Biologicals)

GROUP	FORMULATION	INITIAL	AT 1 MONTH	AT 6 MONTHS
Children (birth to 10 years of age)	Pediatric dose: 10 µg/0.5 ml	0.5 ml	0.5 ml	0.5 ml
Adults and older children	Adult dose: 20 µg/1.0 ml	1.0 ml	1.0 ml	1.0 ml
After needlestick injury		20 µg/1.0 ml	1.0 ml at 0, 1, and 2 months	
Hemodialysis patients		40 µg/ 2.0 ml	2.0 ml at 0, 1, 2, and 6 months	

13. Is a booster needed after immunization? How often?
The persistence of antibody directly correlates with the peak level achieved after the third dose. Follow-up of adults who were immunized with the plasma-derived hepatitis B vaccine demonstrated that the antibody levels had fallen to undetectable or very low levels in 30–50% of recipients. Long-term studies of adults and children indicate that protection lasts at least 9 years, despite loss of anti-HBs in serum. This statement is underscored by reports that after 9 years of follow-up, anti-HBs loss ranged from 13–60% in a group of homosexual men and Alaskan Eskimos, two groups at high risk of infection. However, vaccine recipients were virtually 100% protected from clinical illness, despite the absence of booster immunizations. It is fair to say that among individuals who completely lose detectable anti-HBs, breakthrough infections have been noted in later years, based on the detection of hepatitis B core antibody. However, clinical illness did not occur, and hepatitis B surface antigen was not detected. The infection is assumed to be without consequence and to confer permanent immunity. In light of such data, booster shots are not recommended for healthy adults or children. For immunocompromised patients (e.g., hemodialysis) a booster dose should be administered when anti-HBs levels drop to 10 mIU/ml or less.

14. Is it possible that the vaccine will not protect against HBV infection?
The major HBsAg epitope is the *a* determinant. Hepatitis B vaccines effectively evoke neutralizing antibodies to the group *a* determinant of the HBsAg. The *a* determinant is believed to be formed by the highly conformational structure between amino acids 124 and 147. Although the form is highly conserved, some diversity has been demonstrated, which probably does not affect neutralization of the HBsAg. Hepatitis B mutants have been reported; probably they arose randomly and were not corrected because of an intrinsic failure of the polymerase enzyme. Significant variants have been described in HBV vaccinees, initially in Italy but also in Japan and the Gambia. Italian investigators reported that 40/1600 immunized children showed evidence of HBV infection despite adequate antibody response to the HBV vaccine. The mutant virus had substitutions in amino acids 145 (Italy), aa 126 (Japan), and aa 141 (the Gambia). Whether HBV mutants have substantial clinical impact is not known. Large-scale epidemiologic studies of the incidence, prevalence, and clinical correlation have not been performed.

15. Is it harmful to give hepatitis B vaccine to known hepatitis B carriers?
No deleterious effects were observed in 16 chronic carriers of HB$_s$Ag who received at least 6 monthly injections of hepatitis B vaccine. The vaccine was administered in an attempt to eliminate the chronic carrier status. However, no such result was observed. None of the volunteers lost HB$_s$Ag or developed anti-HBs. This knowledge simplified the design of hepatitis B vaccination programs.

16. Is immunoprophylaxis advisable for hepatitis C?
No firm recommendation can be made for postexposure prophylaxis for hepatitis C. Results of studies of postexposure prophylaxis are equivocal. Some experts recommend administration of immunoglobulin (0.06 mg/kg) when a bona-fide percutaneous exposure has taken place. The immunoglobulin should be administered as soon as possible. However, animal work in chimpanzees has shown the lack of protectiveness when animals that received prophylaxis with immunoglobulin were challenged with the hepatitis C virus. Moreover, recent data showed that in humans the neutralizing antibody evoked after infection with hepatitis C virus is short-lived and does not protect against reinfection. Immunoprophylaxis for hepatitis C seems to be quite difficult. It is rather problematic to design a vaccine to prevent the disease because of the multiple viral genotypes. Moreover, the hepatitis C genotypes do not afford cross-protection.

17. Is it possible to immunize people simultaneously for hepatitis A and B?
In at least two studies, seronegative volunteers received hepatitis A and hepatitis B simultaneously, albeit in different injection sites. Both studies compared antibody results in volunteers to

subjects who received a single vaccine (either hepatitis B or hepatitis A vaccine). There were no deleterious effects to this regimen, and in fact one study found a higher antibody to hepatitis A vaccine with simultaneous immunization. Now, with the commercial availability of hepatitis A vaccine, these early experiences show that people can be immunized with both vaccines without serious side effects.

BIBLIOGRAPHY

1. American College of Physicians Task Force on Adult Immunization and Infectious Diseases: Guide for Adult Immunization. Philadelphia, American College of Physicians, 1994.
2. Carman WF: Vaccine Associated mutants of hepatitis B virus. In Nishioka K, Suzuki H, Mishiro S, Oda T (eds): Viral Hepatitis and Liver Disease. New York, Springer-Verlag, 1994, pp 243–247.
3. Carman WF, Zanetti AR, Karayaiannis P, et al: Vaccine-induced escape mutants of hepatitis B virus. Lancet 336:325–329, 1990.
4. Hepatitis B virus: A comprehensive strategy for eliminating transmission in the United States through universal childhood vaccination. Centers for Disease Control: MMWR 40/RR-13:10, 1991.
5. Flehmig B, Heinricy U, Pfisterer M: Simultaneous vaccination for hepatitis A and B. J Infect Dis 161: 865–868, 1990.
6. Merck, Sharp & Dohme: Recombivax-HB, package insert.
7. Parkman PD, Hopps HE, Meyer HM: Immunoprevention of infectious diseases. In Nohmias AJ, O'Reilly RJ (eds): Immunology. New York, Plenum, 1982, pp 561–583.
8. Plotkin S, Plotkin S: A short history of vaccine. In Plotkin S, Mortimer E (eds): Vaccines, 2nd ed. Philadelphia, W.B. Saunders, 1988, pp 1–7
9. SmithKline Biologicals: Engerix B, package insert, 1989.
10. Whittle HC, Inskip H, Hall AJ, et al: Vaccination against hepatitis B and protection against viral carriage in the Gambia. Lancet 337:747–750, 1991.
11. Hadler SC, Francis DP, Maynard J, et al: Long-term immunogenicity and efficacy of hepatitis B vaccine in homosexual men. N Engl J Med 315:209–214, 1986.
12. Wainright RB, McMahon B, Bulkow L, et al: Duration of immunogenicity and efficacy of hepatitis B vaccine in a Yupik Eskimo population. JAMA 261:2362–2366, 1989.

20. PREGNANCY AND LIVER DISEASE

Maria H. Sjogren, M.D., COL, MC

1. Are abnormal laboratory tests expected during pregnancy?

During pregnancy most laboratory tests, including liver function tests, remain within normal limits. The few exceptions include lower serum levels of albumin, blood urea nitrogen (BUN), and hemoglobin and increased serum levels of alpha-fetoprotein, white blood count, alkaline phosphatase, and triglycerides. These changes resolve shortly after delivery, have no long-term effect, and should not be perceived as evidence of disease.

The elevated serum levels of alkaline phosphatase may be confusing in certain situations and deserve further explanation. This abnormality usually does not exceed a fourfold increase and manifests during the third trimester of pregnancy. The origin of this enzyme is placental, and serum levels regain normal limits by the third week after delivery. It is not accompanied by abnormal aminotransferases, although slight elevation of bilirubin may be present. When an abnormal alkaline phosphatase is detected, serum levels of 5'-nucleotidase and gamma-glutamyl transpeptidase are helpful tests, because they are expected to remain normal in the absence of liver disease.

2. Do physiologic changes during pregnancy make women prone to liver disease in the future?

Certain physiologic changes during pregnancy may have long-term repercussions. Among these changes is an increased hepatic cholesterol synthesis and excretion into bile, which may lead to an increased cholesterol concentration in bile. Such changes may contribute to the development of gallstones in multiparous women.

3. Which liver diseases may be observed during the first or second trimester?
- Jaundice with hyperemesis gravidarum
- Cholestasis of pregnancy
- Dubin-Johnson syndrome

4. Which main liver diseases may be observed during the third trimester?
- Cholestasis of pregnancy
- Dubin-Johnson syndrome
- Acute fatty liver of pregnancy
- Toxemia with liver involvement
- Acute hepatic rupture
- Budd-Chiari syndrome.

5. What algorithm should a clinician use when liver disease is detected in a pregnant woman?

Several considerations need to be taken into account when liver disease is recognized in a pregnant woman. Among such considerations are the trimester of pregnancy, the degree and nature of the liver test abnormalities, the health status of the patient before pregnancy, and the epidemiologic risk factors that may play an etiologic role. This type of information may be crucial to make a presumptive diagnosis and to generate an intelligent approach to care of the patient.

In pregnant women with acute liver disease, in addition to the diagnoses listed in questions 3 and 4, the following should be considered: viral hepatitis, cholecystitis, decompensated underlying chronic liver disease, drug-induced hepatitis, or alcoholic liver disease. In reality, any liver disease may be diagnosed in a pregnant woman. However, the reverse is not true; acute fatty liver of pregnancy, toxemia of pregnancy, and intrahepatic cholestasis of pregnancy are diagnosed only in pregnant women.

6. What is the role of biochemical profile of liver tests in the differential diagnosis?

When alkaline phosphatase is the predominantly abnormal liver test in pregnant women, suspect:
- Normal pregnancy (third trimester)
- Hyperemesis gravidarum (first trimester)
- Intrahepatic cholestasis of pregnancy (third trimester)
- Cholelithiasis (anytime)
- Dubin-Johnson syndrome (second or third trimester)

When the predominant abnormality is elevation of serum level of aminotransferases, suspect:
- Fatty liver of pregnancy, viral hepatitis
- Toxemia with hepatic infarct
- Drug-induced hepatitis
- Toxemia of pregnancy
- HELLP (see question 12)
- Chronic liver disease

7. Can hyperemesis gravidarum result in abnormal liver tests?

Hyperemesis gravidarum is a rare syndrome that occurs almost exclusively in the first trimester. Bilirubin and alkaline phosphatase may be mildly elevated; aminotransferases also may be mildly abnormal. The syndrome usually recurs in subsequent pregnancies.

8. What is intrahepatic cholestasis of pregnancy?

Intrahepatic cholestasis of pregnancy (ICP) is also called cholestasis of pregnancy, benign recurrent cholestasis of pregnancy or pruritus gravidarum. The incidence appears to vary geographically. Some European countries (Sweden, Poland) and some South American countries (Chile) report a 10% incidence, whereas in other European countries, the ICP rate is estimated at 0.1–0.2%. The origin of ICP remains unknown. Although ICP typically presents during the third trimester, some cases have been described as early as 13 weeks' gestation.

The syndrome has a range of clinical presentations from mild forms, in which pruritus is the only abnormality, to profound cholestasis with vitamin K deficiency and significant postpartum hemorrhage. The condition is usually benign for the mother; however, the incidence of prematurity, fetal distress, and stillbirths is increased. ICP recurs with subsequent pregnancies and is often familial. Some studies suggest that the histocompatibility antigen HLA-BW 16 is frequently observed in women with history of ICP compared with healthy controls. The liver histologic sample shows mild focal and irregular cholestasis. There are no distinguishing features from other types of cholestasis. Treatment consists of supportive therapy; cholestyramine, 10–12 gm/day, to relieve pruritus; and vitamin K administered parenterally. Vitamin K is advocated because of the 20% increased rate of postpartum uterine bleeding, presumably due to malabsorption secondary to cholestasis.

9. What is acute fatty liver of pregnancy?

The first distinct clinical description of acute fatty liver of pregnancy is attributed to Sheehan in 1940. However, fatty liver in women dying during puerperium was first documented in 1857. The condition is rare, with an estimated rate of 1 case in 13,000 deliveries. Most cases do not have defined risk factors. In a few patients large doses of intravenous tetracycline or acute respiratory infections have preceded the syndrome. The following associations also have been observed: plural gestation, male births, first pregnancy, arterial hypertension, peripheral edema, and proteinuria.

The onset of symptoms is usually between the 30th and 39th week of pregnancy. Prominent symptoms are nausea, vomiting, and abdominal pain. Jaundice usually becomes evident 1 week to 10 days after onset of symptons. Rare patients present with coma, renal failure, or hemorrhage. Ascites may be present in 50%. Sherlock reports two laboratory distinctive features: increased serum uric acid levels (probably due to tissue injury) and giant platelets with basophilic stippling. These findings are not observed in acute viral hepatitis and may be helpful in the differential diagnosis. Patients with acute fatty liver of pregnancy may have profound hypoglycemia, high serum ammonia, and generalized hyperaminoacidemia.

A liver biopsy may be necessary to distinguish this syndrome from acute viral hepatitis. The liver is pale and small, and the hepatocytes are pale and swollen, preferentially in the pericentral areas. The periportal areas are often spared. Special fat stains reveal that the swollen hepatocytes are filled with microvesicular fat droplets. The nuclei remain centered with the cell, in contrast to syndromes with large droplet fatty deposition, and the fat vacuole pushes the nucleus to the side.

10. What is toxemia of pregnancy?

Toxemia of pregnancy is a syndrome of unknown cause that usually occurs after the 20th week of gestation. It ranges in severity from lack of clinical symptons through preeclampsia with edema, proteinuria, and arterial hypertension to eclampsia with seizures. Toxemia is reported in about 5% of gestations. Risk factors include pregnancy at a very young age or late in life, first pregnancy, plural gestation, diabetes, preexisting hypertension, and maternal history of toxemia.

Preeclampsia is a common clinical problem, and it is estimated that about 50% of patients have mild abnormalities of aminotransferases and alkaline phosphatase. Liver biopsy samples usually show minimally abnormal histology. Characteristic changes are periportal hemorrhages, scattered fibrin deposition, and subcapsular hemorrhages. Fibrin deposits occlude the hepatic sinusoids with subsequent hepatic cell necrosis in the same area. If cell necrosis is severe, areas of hepatic hemorrhage may be observed. A major differential diagnosis is diffuse intravascular coagulation syndrome. In severe cases hepatic rupture with massive intraperitoneal hemorrhage may occur.

11. What is Budd-Chiari syndrome?

Budd-Chiari syndrome is not exclusively associated with pregnancy. Indeed, it is observed with similar frequency in men and women. In women, there appears to be an association with intake of oral contraceptive pills; however, evidence to prove causation is insufficient. Although Budd-Chiari syndrome is the most frequently described vascular thrombosis in pregnancy, the true incidence is unknown.

When associated with pregnancy, Budd-Chiari syndrome usually occurs in the immediate postpartum period, although some cases have been described during the second trimester of gestation or during septic abortions. The syndrome manifests by abdominal pain and sudden onset of ascites. The hepatic veins are thrombosed with subsequent portal hypertension. The liver is often enlarged and tender.

Liver tests show modest abnormalities of the aminotransferases and alkaline phosphatase. The ascitic fluid is usually an exudate; however, low-protein content has been described in some cases. The liver-spleen scan may help the diagnosis if the caudate lobe shows intense uptake (due to spared venous outflow) with faint uptake in the remainder of the liver. A hepatic venogram shows the site of vascular occlusion, either in the inferior vena cava or hepatic vein. When available, the liver biopsy specimen shows intense congestion, particularly around the terminal hepatic veins. The sinusoids are markedly dilated with atrophy of adjacent hepatocytes. In advanced cases, thrombi may be seen in the terminal hepatic veins. The prognosis is grim; as a rule, patients with Budd-Chiari syndrome have a steady clinical deterioration until death. Mortality during the first year is 30–40%, whereas the 4-year mortality rate is approximately 85%.

Treatment with anticoagulants is of little value in well-established Budd-Chiari syndrome; however, thrombolytic treatment with agents such as streptokinase or alteplase (TPA) during acute hepatic vein thrombosis is warranted. Surgical treatment is an option, with the major goal being to decompress the congested liver, usually by constructing portosystemic shunts (portacaval or mesocaval). Several patients with Budd-Chiari syndrome have undergone successful liver transplantation. Four cases of uncomplicated pregnancy in patients with previous Budd-Chiari syndrome have been reported.

12. What is HELLP?

First described by Weinstein in 1982, the acronym stands for **H**emolysis, **E**levated **L**iver En-zymes, and **L**ow **P**latelets. The syndrome probably represents a subgroup of women with toxemia of pregnancy who also have disseminated intravascular coagulation and liver disease. Approximately 10% of women with severe preeclampsia or eclampsia have the HELLP syndrome.

13. What is the course of viral hepatitis in pregnancy?

Viral hepatitis is a necroinflammatory disease commonly caused by hepatitis A, B, C, D, or E viruses. In addition, cytomegalovirus or Epstein-Barr virus may cause acute viral hepatitis. Specific information about these viruses is widely available in the literature. It is safe to state that the clinical manifestations of viral hepatitis are the same in pregnant and nonpregnant women, with few exceptions. Collective data suggest that in some areas of the world, such as the sub-Indian continent, the Middle East, and Africa, both frequency and severity of hepatitis are greater in pregnant women than in nonpregnant women or men. The reported higher mortality rate for acute hepatitis in pregnant women in these areas may be due to epidemic non-A, non-B hepatitis (now known as hepatitis E or HEV). The hepatitis E virus has been isolated and partially characterized. Hepatitis E is usually self-limited, and chronic hepatitis has not been observed after acute illness. The liver histology in HEV-infected patients has been described by Gupta and Smetana in biopsy specimens from 78 patients, including pregnant women. Fifty-eight percent of specimens showed one or more of the following distinctive pathologic findings: (1) cholestasis, especially around the periportal areas; (2) canalicular and intracellular bile stasis in pseudoglandular structures; and (3) an increased number of acidophilic bodies.

The first large documented outbreak of HEV occurred in Delhi, India in 1955–1956. The main epidemiologic and clinical characteristics have been observed in several other reported outbreaks: association with consumption of contaminated water, higher attack rate in young adults, and high fatality rate in pregnant women. In 1978, an outbreak of epidemic non-A, non-B was reported in Kashmir, India. The attack rate was 2.8% in men, 2.1% in nonpregnant women, and 17.3% among pregnant women. Fulminant hepatitis developed in 2.8% of men, 0% of nonpregnant women, and 22% of pregnant females. Of pregnant women with fulminant hepatitis, 75% died. In 1980–1981, during a waterborne epidemic in Algeria, 788 cases of hepatitis were reported with a 100% mortality among 9 pregnant women. In contrast, reports from Europe and the United States indicate that pregnant women and their fetuses are affected more adversely by viral hepatitis other than by an increased rate of premature delivery.

14. Can hepatitis B (HBV) be transmitted to neonates of HBV-infected mothers?

Hepatitis B may be transmitted to neonates during the perinatal period. The rate of transmission from mothers to infants has been reported to be between 0% and more than 70%. Two studies have attempted to explain this wide range of transmission rate. The first study showed that no infection among infants was observed when the mother had the acute illness during the first trimester of pregnancy, whereas 25% of infants whose mothers were ill during the second trimester were infected with HBV and the infection rate increased to 70% when the mother had acute HBV during the third trimester. The incidence rose to 84% if the mothers had acute hepatitis during the first 2 months after delivery, most likely because the disease was incubating and the mother was at the peak of infectivity at delivery. The second study had remarkably similar findings: 0% infectivity during the first trimester, 6% during the second trimester, 67% during the third trimester, and 100% during the immediate postpartum period. Such statistics are staggering, particularly if one takes into account that over 90% of infected neonates become HBV carriers.

15. What is the recommended dose of hepatitis B vaccine for infants born to HBV-infected mothers?

Beasley and coworkers demonstrated that chronic HBV infection in infants born to HBV-infected mothers is prevented in 90% of cases by using a combination of hepatitis B immune globulin (HBIG) and a regular schedule of HBV vaccine inoculations. This and other studies have provided the guidelines for the prevention of maternal-infant transmission of HBV. All infants born to mothers with HBV infection should receive prophylaxis against HBV. The current recommended regimen for newborns is: HBIG, 0.5 ml intramuscularly at birth; HBV vaccine, 10 μg (0.5 ml) intramuscularly within 7 days of birth and 1 and 6 months later.

16. Can hepatitis C be transmitted to infants of HCV-infected mothers?

Approximately 50% of HCV-infected individuals have no recognized risk factor for acquiring HCV infection. This finding has prompted a search for nonpercutaneous routes of infection. Before assays for HCV were available, apparent vertical transmission of bloodborne non-A, non-B (now known as hepatitis C) was occasionally observed. Two recent studies have addressed the issue of neonatal transmission of HCV. Although both studies have an excellent design and use credible serologic markers, both also have limitations, including the small number of observed infants and the short follow-up. Reinus and associates followed 23 HCV-infected mothers and their 24 newborn infants for at least 3 months. The patients were recruited from a hospital in Westchester County, New York. In 16–23 women HCV RNA was detectable in sera, indicating high potential to transmit HCV to offspring. All infants had antibody to HCV (anti-HCV) in cord blood samples, but the antibody disappeared in subsequent samples. Only 1 cord-blood sample had detectable HCV RNA, which disappeared during follow-up. The second study is strikingly similar. Wejstal and coworkers studied 14 Swedish women and their 21 newborn infants. All mothers had detectable HCV RNA in sera, and 2 of 21 babies had persistent alanine aminotransferase elevation; however, only one became HCV RNA-positive during follow-up. The child's liver biopsy specimen was consistent with chronic hepatitis. Both studies concluded that mother-to-infant transmission of HCV infection seems to be uncommon. This conclusion is valid even in the presence of human immunodeficiency virus type 1 (HIV-1), because some of the mothers in both studies had detectable antibody to HIV-1 in sera.

17. Does chronic liver disease have an impact on the health of a pregnant woman?

Cirrhosis is an uncommon occurrence in women of childbearing age. The incidence of pregnancy in cirrhotic women is unknown, although lower fertility rates have been reported. Schreyer and coworkers studied 60 women with documented cirrhosis who had 69 deliveries. Their ages ranged between 18 and 44 years, with a mean of 40.5 years. Ten of the 60 women died during pregnancy, 7 due to massive gastrointestinal bleeding. Only 45 of 69 (65%) of the infants survived the neonatal period.

A major consideration in pregant cirrhotic women is the presence of esophageal varices. In the past, termination of pregnancy was advised in the belief that variceal rupture and fatal hemorrhage were more likely in the presence of esophageal varices. Later, cesarean section was advocated to avoid straining and provoking variceal rupture. In 1982, however, Britton reviewed 53 cirrhotic patients with 83 pregnancies and 38 noncirrhotic patients with 77 pregnancies for risk of variceal bleeding. He found that the majority of gestational hemorrhages occurred in the second trimester and that the risk of variceal bleeding was not increased during vaginal delivery. Transient varices may develop in women with liver disease during the second trimester as a result of a maximal increase in blood volume during weeks 28 to 32. In the cirrhotic group, there were 7 maternal deaths, 3 due to variceal bleeding. In the noncirrhotic group, there were 2 maternal deaths, 1 from variceal bleeding. This study indicated no significant difference between cirrhotic and noncirrhotic pregnant women with respect to variceal bleeding.

Reports of women with underlying primary biliary cirrhosis (PBC) or autoimmune chronic active hepatitis (CAH) have shown some clinical deterioration of the underlying condition during pregnancy. Four or five women with PBC had increased jaundice during pregnancy, and bilirubin remained elevated after delivery. Of 6 pregnancies in the patients with PBC, only two produced viable infants, and 3 of 5 women died within a few years after the pregnancies. A review of 30 pregnant women with autoimmune CAH found no maternal deaths and only 4 perinatal deaths. The women were treated with prednisolone while pregnant with no adverse effect to the fetuses.

In summary, pregnancy in cirrhotic women is uncommon, and the management of liver disease in these is not different from that in nonpregnant patients. Fetal wastage due to stillbirths, prematurity, or spontaneous abortion is increased in cirrhotic women.

BIBLIOGRAPHY

1. Beasley RP, Hwant LY, Lee GC, et al: Prevention of perinatally transmitted hepatitis B virus infection with hepatitis B immune globulin and hepatitis B vaccine. Lancet 2:1099–1102, 1983.
2. Belabbes El-H, Bouguermouth A, Benatallah A, et al: Epidemic non-A, non-B, viral hepatitis in Algeria: Strong evidence for its spreading by water. J Med Virol 16:257–263, 1985.
3. Britton RC: Pregnancy and esophageal varices. Am J Surg 143:421, 1982.
4. Calne RY, Williams R: Orthotopic liver transplantation: The first 60 patients. BMJ 1:471–476, 1977.
5. Centers for Disease Control: Recommendations for protection against viral hepatitis. MMWR 34:313–335, 1985.
6. Cheng Y-S: Pregnancy in liver cirrhosis and/or portal hypertension. Am J Obstet Gynecol 128:812, 1977.
7. Feingold KR, Wiley T, Moser AH, et al: De novo, cholesterologenesis in pregnancy. J Lab Clin Med 101:256–263, 1983.
8. Gerety RJ, Schweitzer IL: Viral hepatitis type B during pregnancy, the neonatal period, and infancy. J Pediatr 90:368, 1977.
9. Gupta DA, Smetana HF: The histopathology of viral hepatitis seen in the Delhi epidemic (1955–1956). Indian J Med Res 45 (Suppl):101–113, 1957.
10. Johnston WG, Baskett TF: Obstetric cholestasis: A 14-year review. Am J Obstet Gynecol 133:299–301, 1979.
11. Kern F Jr, Everson GT, DeMark B, et al: Biliary lipids, bile acids, and gallbladder function in the human female. J Clin Invest 68:1229–1243, 1981.
12. Khuroo MS, Teli MR, Skidmore S, et al: Incidence and severity of viral hepatitis in pregnancy. Am J Med 70:252, 1981.
13. Larrey D, Rueff B, Feldmann G, et al: Recurrent jaundice caused by recurrent hyperemesis gravidarum. Case report. Gut 25:1414, 1984.
14. Lunzer M, Barens P, Byth K, et al: Serum bile acid concentrations during pregnancy and their relationship to obstetric cholestasis. Gastroenterology 91:825–829, 1986.
15. Maddrey WC: Hepatic vein thrombosis (Budd-Chiari syndrome): Possible association with the use of oral contraceptives. Semin Liver Dis 7:32–39, 1987).
16. Pockros PJ, Peters RL, Reynolds TB: Idiopathic fatty liver of pregnancy findings in ten cases. Medicine 63:1–11, 1984.
17. Pritchard JA, MacDonald PC, Grant NF: Hypertensive disorders in pregnancy. In Pritchard JA, MacDonald PC, Grant NF (eds): Williams's Obstetrics, 17th ed. Norwalk, CT, Lange, 1985.
18. Reinus JF, Leikin EL, Alter HJ, et al: Failure to detect vertical transmission of hepatitis C virus. Ann Intern Med 117:881–886, 1992.
19. Reyes H: The enigma of intrahepatic cholestasis of pregnancy: Lessons from Chile. Hepatology 2:87–96, 1982.
20. Schreyer P, Caspi E, El Hindi JM: Cirrhosis—pregnancy and delivery: A review. Obstet Gynecol Surv 37:304, 1982.
21. Sherlock S: The liver in pregnancy. In Sherlock S (ed): Diseases of the Liver and Biliary System, 8th ed. Oxford, Blackwell, 1989, pp 523–532.
22. Sibai BM, Tasmini MM, El-Nazer A, et al: Maternal-perinatal outcome associated with the syndrome of hemolysis, elevated liver enzymes, and low platelets in severe preeclampsia-eclampsia. Am J Obstet Gynecol 155:501–509, 1989.
23. Sjogren MH: Hepatic emergencies in pregnancy. Med Clin North Am 77:1115–1127, 1993.
24. Steven MM, Buckley JD, Mackay JR: Pregnancy in chronic active hepatitis. Q J Med 192:519, 1979.
25. Tong MJ, Thursby M, Rakela J, et al: Studies on the maternal-infant transmission of the viruses which cause acute hepatitis. Gastroenterology 80:999–1004, 1981.
26. Viswanathan R: Infectious hepatitis in Delhi (1955–1956): A critical study: Epidemiology. Indian J. Med Res 45 (Suppl):1–30, 1957.
27. Wejstal R, Widell A, Mansson A-S, et al: Mother to infant transmission of hepatitis C virus. Ann Intern Med 117:887–890, 1992.
28. Whelton MJ, Sherlock S: Pregnancy in patients with cirrhosis of the liver. Obstet Gynecol 36:315, 1970.

21. RHEUMATOLOGIC MANIFESTATIONS OF HEPATOBILIARY DISEASES

Sterling G. West, M.D.

1. List the diseases of the liver that may present with rheumatic manifestations.
- Viral hepatitis
- Autoimmune chronic active hepatitis
- Primary biliary cirrhosis
- Hemochromatosis

2. Which viral hepatitis is most commonly associated with rheumatic manifestations?
Approximately 25% of patients develop a rheumatic syndrome related to hepatitis B antigenemia.

3. What are the most common extrahepatic rheumatologic manifestations of hepatitis B infection?
- Acute polyarthritis–dermatitis syndrome
- Polyarteritis nodosa
- Membranous glomerulonephritis
- Cryoglobulinemia

4. Describe the clinical characteristics of the polyarthritis–dermatitis syndrome associated with hepatitis B infection.
The polyarthritis is acute, severe, and symmetric, involving both small and large joints. A classically urticarial rash usually accompanies the arthritis. Both the arthritis and rash precede the onset of jaundice and/or elevated liver associated enzymes by several days. The arthritis improves with nonsteroidal antiinflammatory drugs (NSAIDs) and resolves with onset of jaundice.

5. What is the typical presentation of hepatitis B-associated polyarteritis nodosa (PAN)?
Approximately 25% of all patients with PAN have the hepatitis B antigen. They may present with a combination of fever, arthritis, mononeuritis multiplex, abdominal pain, renal disease, and/or cardiac disease. Although liver enzymes may be abnormal, symptomatic hepatitis is not a prominent feature.

6. How is PAN associated with hepatitis B antigenemia diagnosed?
The diagnosis is made on the basis of a consistent clinical presentation coupled with an abdominal or renal angiogram showing vascular aneurysms and corkscrewing of blood vessels. The gold standard is a tissue biopsy showing medium-vessel vasculitis (see figure on p. 144).

7. What is the treatment of hepatitis B-associated PAN?
Patients typically are very ill and will die without aggressive corticosteroid and cytotoxic drug therapy. Adjunctive antiviral (vidarabine) and plasmapheresis therapy may be beneficial. The overall 5-year survival rate is 50–75%.

8. What is the relationship between viral hepatitis and cryoglobulinemia?
Approximately 70% of patients with essential mixed cryoglobulinemia (type III) are positive for hepatitis B antigen, hepatitis B core antibody, and/or hepatitis C antibody. Because these antigens and antibodies are part of the cryoglobulin, they may play a role in the pathogenesis of cryoglobulinemia. Hepatitis A is rarely associated with cryoglobulinemia.

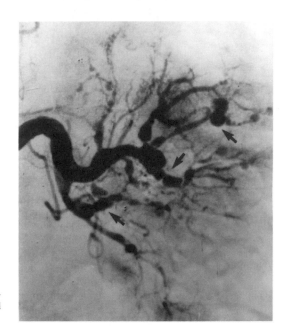

Renal angiogram showing vascular aneurysms in a patient with hepatitis B-associated polyarteritis nodosa (arrows).

9. Describe the typical clinical features of cryoglobulinemia associated with hepatitis B or C infection.

Patients present with a combination of fever, arthritis, renal disease, paresthesias, and a predominantly lower extremity petechial rash. Hepatitis is not a prominent feature. Patients have been successfully treated with combined corticosteroids, interferon, and plasmapheresis.

10. What is lupoid hepatitis?

Lupoid hepatitis is a type of autoimmune chronic active hepatitis (CAH) associated with multisystem clinical and laboratory manifestations that resemble systemic lupus erythematosus (SLE). Patients commonly have positive antinuclear antibodies (ANA), antibodies against smooth muscle antigen (F1 actin), and occasionally LE cells.

11. To what degree is lupoid hepatitis similar to SLE?

Comparison of Lupoid Hepatitis and SLE

	SLE	LUPOID CAH
Young women	+	+
Polyarthritis	+	+
Fever	+	+
Rash	+	+
Nephritis	+	-
Central nervous system disease	+	-
Photosensitivity	+	-
Oral ulcers	+	-
ANA	99%	70–90%
LE cells	70%	40–50%
Polyclonal gammopathy	+	+
Anti-Smith antibodies	25%	0
+ anti-ds DNA	70%	Rare–40%
+ anti-F1 actin	Rare	80–95%

12. What is the difference between anti-Sm and anti-SM antibodies?
Anti-Sm antibodies are antibodies against the Smith antigen, which is an epitope on small nuclear ribonuclear proteins. It is highly diagnostic of SLE. Anti-SM antibody is an antibody against the smooth muscle antigen (F1 actin). It is highly diagnostic of autoimune CAH (lupoid hepatitis).

Anti-Sm vs. Anti-SM Antibodies

	SLE	CAH
Anti-Smith (Sm) antibodies	Yes	No
Anti-Smooth muscle (SM) antibodies	No	Yes

13. List the common autoimmune diseases associated with primary biliary cirrhosis (PBC).
Up to 80% of patients with PBC have one or more of the following disorders:
- Keratoconjunctivitis sicca (Sjögren's syndrome)   66%
- Autoimmune thyroiditis (Hashimoto's disease)   20%
- Scleroderma/Raynaud's disease   20%
- Rheumatoid arthritis   10%

14. Compare and contrast the arthritis that may occur with PBC and rheumatoid arthritis.

PBC Arthritis vs. Rheumatoid Arthritis

	PBC ARTHRITIS	RHEUMATOID ARTHRITIS
Frequency in patients with PBC	10%	10%
Number of joints	Polyarticular	Polyarticular
Symmetry	Symmetric	Symmetric
Inflammatory	Yes	Yes
Rheumatoid factor	No	Yes (85%)
Erosions on radiograph	Rare	Common

15. What other musculoskeletal manifestations may occur in patients with PBC?
- Osteomalacia due to fat-soluble vitamin D malabsorption
- Osteoporosis due to renal tubular acidosis
- Hypertrophic osteoarthropathy

16. What autoantibodies commonly occur in patients with PBC?
- Antimitochondrial antibodies   80%
- Anticentromere antibodies   20%*

*Most patients also have manifestations of the CREST variant of scleroderma. (CREST = calcinosis, Raynaud's phenomenon, esophageal disease, sclerodactyly, and telangiectasia).

17. How commonly does arthritis occur in patients with hemochromatosis?
Approximately 50% of patients have a noninflammatory degenerative arthritis, most commonly involving the second and third metacarpophalangeal joints (MCPs), proximal interphalangeal joint, wrists, knees, and hips. Of importance, this arthropathy may be the presenting complaint of hemochromatosis and is frequently misdiagnosed as seronegative rheumatoid arthritis.

18. Describe the radiographic features suggestive of hemochromatotic arthropathy.
Suggestive radiographic features include subchondral sclerosis, cyst formation, irregular joint space narrowing, and osteophyte formation consistent with degenerative arthritis of involved joints. The key is finding degenerative changes in the MCP joints (typically 2nd and 3rd) with

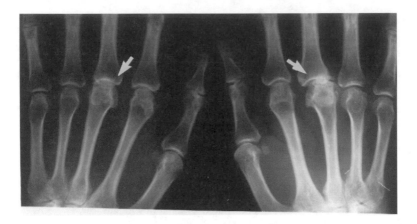

Radiograph of hands showing degenerative arthritis with hooklike osteophytes of the second and third metacarpophalangeal joints in a patient with hemochromatosis (arrows).

hooklike osteophytes. This finding is important, because the MCPs and wrists rarely develop degenerative joint disease without an underlying cause such as hemochromatosis.

19. What is the relationship between calcium pyrophosphate disease and hemochromatosis?
Chondrocalcinosis of the triangular fibrocartilage at the ulnar side of the wrist and the hyaline cartilage of the knees is seen in 50–70% of patients with hemochromatosis. Crystals of calcium pyrophosphate may shed into the joints, causing superimposed flares of inflammatory arthritis (i.e., pseudogout).

20. What human leukocyte antigen (HLA) occurs more commonly than expected in patients with hemochromatosis?
HLA-A3 occurs in 70% of patients with hemochromatosis compared with 20% of a normal healthy population. HLA-B7 and B14 are also increased. However, none of the HLA antigens predispose to developing the arthritis.

21. Compare and contrast the features of hemochromatotic arthropathy (HA) and rheumatoid arthritis (RA).

Comparison of Hemochromatotic Arthropathy and Rheumatoid Arthritis

	HA	RA
Sex	M>F (10:1)	F>M (3:1)
Age of onset	>35 years	All ages
Joints	Polyarticular	Polyarticular
Symmetry	Symmetric	Symmetric
Inflammatory signs/symptoms	Only if pseudogout attack	Yes
Rheumatoid factor	Negative	Positive (85%)
HLA	HLA-A3 (70%)	HLA DR4 (70%)
Synovial fluid	Noninflammatory	Inflammatory
Radiographs	Degenerative changes	Inflammatory, erosive disease

22. How effective is phlebotomy in halting the progression of hemochromatotic arthropathy?
Phlebotomy does not halt the progression of the arthropathy.

23. What is the correlation between the severity of arthropathy and severity of liver disease in hemochromatosis?
There is no correlation.

24. Why does hemochromatosis cause a degenerative arthritis?
The arthropathy is characterized by hemosiderin deposition in synovium and chondrocytes. The presence of iron in these cells may lead to increased production of destructive enzymes (e.g., collagenase) that cause cartilage damage. Other mechanisms also may be possible; the precise pathway by which chronic iron overload leads to tissue injury has not been fully established.

25. What other musculoskeletal problems may occur in patients with hemochromatosis?
Osteoporosis due to gonadal dysfunction from pituitary insufficiency caused by the iron overload state.

BIBLIOGRAPHY

1. Culp KS, Fleming CR, Duffy J, et al: Autoimmune associations and primary biliary cirrhosis. Mayo Clin Proc 57:365–370, 1982.
2. Duffy J: Arthritis and liver disease. In McCarty DJ, Koopman W (eds): Arthritis and Allied Conditions, 12th ed. Philadelphia, Lea & Febiger, 1993, pp 1111–1120.
3. Duffy J, Lidsky MD, Sharp JT, et al: Polyarthritis, polyarteritis, and hepatitis B. Medicine 55:19–38, 1976.
4. Ferri C, Greco F, Longombardo G, et al: Association between hepatitis C virus and mixed cryoglobulinemia. Clin Exp Rheumatol 9:621–624, 1991.
5. Hall S, Czaja AJ, Kaufman DK, et al: How lupoid is lupoid hepatitis? J Rheumatol 13:95–98, 1986.
6. Inman RD: Rheumatoid manifestations of hepatitis B infections. Semin Arthritis Rheum 11:406–420, 1982.
7. Levo Y, Gorevic PD, Kassab HJ, et al: Association between hepatitis B virus and essential mixed cryo globulinemia. N Engl J Med 296:1501–1504, 1977.
8. Makinen D, Fritzler M, Davis P, Sherlock S: Anticentromere antibodies in primary biliary cirrhosis. Arthritis Rheum 26:914–917, 1983.
9. Marx WJ, O'Connell DJ: Arthritis of primary biliary cirrhosis. Arch Intern Med 139:213–216, 1979.
10. Matthews JL, Williams HJ: Arthritis in hereditary hemochromatosis. Arthritis Rheum 30:1137–1141, 1987.
11. Nichols GM, Bacon BR: Hereditary hemochromatosis: pathogenesis and clinical features of a common disease. Am J Gastroenterol 84:851–862, 1989.
12. Baer DM, Simons JL, Staples RL, et al: Hemochromatosis screening in asymptomatic ambulatory men 30 years of age and older. Am J Med 98:464–468, 1995.
13. Khella SL, Frost S, Hermann GA, et al: Hepatitis C infection, cryoglobulinemia, and vasculitic neuropathy: Treatment with interferon alpha. Neurology 45:407–411, 1995.
14. Gumber SC, Chopra S: Hepatitis C: A multifaceted desease. Ann Intern Med 123:615–620, 1995.

22. EVALUATION OF FOCAL LIVER MASSES

Steven P. Lawrence, M.D.

1. Describe the initial work-up for a patient with a liver mass.

The first step is an accurate history and physical examination. Age, sex, and birthplace are important clues to etiology. Risk factors for viral hepatitis or a history of liver cirrhosis increases the possibility of a primary malignant process. A previously diagnosed neoplasm heightens suspicion for metastatic disease. Use of oral contraceptives or anabolic steroids, alcohol intake, and potential occupational exposure to carcinogens such as vinyl chloride should be noted. Hepatomegaly and/or splenomegaly, liver tenderness, or stigmata of chronic liver disease, such as palmar erythema or spider angiomata, may be present.

Laboratory investigations, with the exception of alpha-fetoprotein, are nonspecific and cannot narrow the differential diagnosis. Liver-associated enzymes, albumin, coagulation parameters, hepatitis B and C serologies, and iron studies may suggest an underlying chronic hepatitis, cirrhosis, or infiltrative process.

Differential Diagnosis of Focal Liver Masses in Adults

BENIGN	MALIGNANT
Epithelial tumors	
Hepatic adenoma	Hepatocellular carcinoma
Bile duct adenoma	Cholangiocarcinoma
Biliary cystadenoma	Biliary cystadenocarcinoma
	Squamous carcinoma
Mesenchymal tumors	
Cavernous hemangioma	Angiosarcoma
	Epithelioid hemangioendothelioma
Fibroma	Fibrosarcoma
Leiomyoma	Leiomyosarcoma
Lipoma	Liposarcoma
	Rhabdomyosarcoma
	Primary hepatic lymphoma
Other lesions	
Focal nodular hyperplasia	Metastatic tumors
Liver abscess	
Macroregenerative nodules in cirrhosis	
Focal fatty infiltration	
Focal sparing with diffuse fatty liver	
Simple hepatic cyst	
Microhamartoma (von Meyenburg complex)	

Modified from Kew MC: Tumors of the liver. In Zakim D, Boyer TD (eds): Hepatology: A Textbook of Liver Disease, 2nd ed. Philadelphia, W.B. Saunders, 1990, pp 1206–1239.

2. What is the most common benign cause of a focal liver lesion?

Cavernous hemangiomas are the most common benign hepatic tumor, occurring in 1–20% of the population. They occur in all age groups, more commonly in women, as a solitary (80–90%), asymptomatic mass <3 cm, usually in the posterior segment of the right hepatic lobe. The term **giant hemangioma** is used by some authors when the size exceeds 4 cm. Microscopically, hemangiomas consist of blood-filled vascular sinusoids separated by connective-tissue septae. Rarely, hemangiomas have been noted to grow during pregnancy or with estrogen use. Occasionally they are large enough to cause abdominal pain, but the risk of spontaneous rupture is minimal and does not justify surgical removal unless the patient is significantly symptomatic. Attempts to treat such lesions with radiation or embolization therapy have not been uniformly successful.

3. How are hemangiomas diagnosed radiographically?

Hemangiomas are often found incidentally during an abdominal **ultrasound** (US) or CT scan. The US characteristics of hemangiomas are variable, but the majority appear as well-defined, homogeneous, hyperechoic masses with posterior wall acoustic enhancement. This sonographic pattern may be found with many other benign or neoplastic lesions and necessitates further work-up.

If the mass is 2.5 cm or larger technetium 99m-labeled red blood cell imaging with **single-photon emission computed tomography** (SPECT) is the diagnostic modality of choice. Sluggish blood flow through the cavernous vascular channels of the hemangioma, which are supplied by normal arterial vessels, causes perfusion to blood-pool mismatch, resulting in radiotracer accumulation and increased activity on delayed images taken at 1–2 hours. Because its specificity approaches 100%, SPECT confirms the diagnosis of hemangioma. Because smaller or thrombosed or fibrotic lesions and lesions close to major intrahepatic vessels may be missed, however, its sensitivity is lower (80–90%).

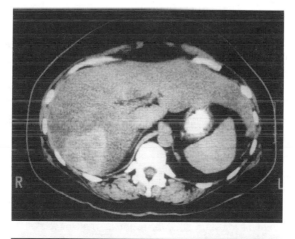

A

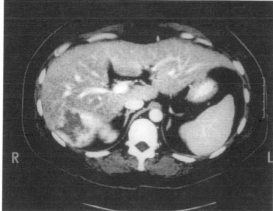

B

Unenhanced (*A*) and enhanced (*B*) CT appearance of a cavernous hemangioma in the right lobe of the liver.

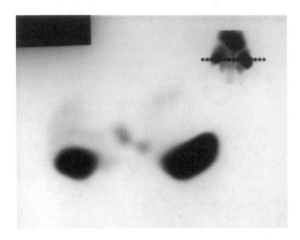

Delayed tagged-red blood cell SPECT image of the same lesion confirms the diagnosis of hemangioma. Note the increased uptake in the corresponding area seen on CT.

MRI should be used in a suspected hemangioma smaller than 2.5 cm. Hemangiomas are hypointense or isointense on T1-weighted images but show an increasingly more hyperintense (bright) signal as the image becomes more T2-weighted (the "light-bulb" sign). Hypervascular metastases from endocrine tumors, adenocarcinomas, or sarcomas occasionally cause a false-positive MRI.

Sequential dynamic-bolus **CT scanning** may be diagnostic if (1) the lesion is hypodense on unenhanced CT, (2) peripheral contrast enhancement occurs in the dynamic-bolus phase, and (3) the lesion becomes isodense or hyperdense on delayed scans. Only 55–62% of hemangiomas show this triad on CT.

Angiography is seldom necessary in view of the accuracy of noninvasive testing but characteristically shows rapid filling in the arterial phase with persistent opacification in the venous phase and no neovascularity or arteriovenous shunting.

Percutaneous biopsy, although advocated by some clinicians, is not uniformly accepted as a means to establish the diagnosis. A more reasonable approach in equivocal cases is to repeat the imaging study in 2–3 months to confirm that the lesion has not changed.

4. Why is oral contraceptive use important in the differential diagnosis of focal liver masses?

The occurrence of hepatic adenomas directly relates to the use of oral contraceptives in most cases. This benign tumor was rarely seen before oral contraceptive agents came into common usage in the 1960s. The risk of hepatic adenomas in women correlates with duration of contraceptive use: the majority of patients report continued use for more than 4–5 years. Age greater than 30 years also increases the risk. The decreased potency of the estrogen component of currently available oral contraceptives may reduce the incidence of 3–4 per 100,000 reported with long-term use in the 1970s. Men infrequently develop adenomas, although cases have been reported with anabolic steroid use.

Hepatic adenomas most commonly occur in asymptomatic young or middle-aged women. Hepatomegaly or a palpable mass may be found on examination. Approximately one-fourth of patients have abdominal pain, often as a result of hemorrhage into the tumor and subsequent necrosis. Spontaneous rupture and hemoperitoneum are not uncommon, occurring in up to 30% of cases, especially during menstruation, pregnancy or the postpartum period. The potential for catastrophic rupture and documented reports of hepatocellular carcinoma arising within the adenoma warrant surgical resection when feasible. Tumors have been known to regress or resolve with discontinuation of birth control pills, but this should not be the management of choice.

5. What are the histologic characteristics of hepatic adenomas? How do they appear on imaging studies?

Hepatic adenomas are well-demarcated, fleshy tumors with prominent surface vasculature. Most are 8–15 cm in diameter. Microscopically, they appear as monotonous sheets of normal or small hepatocytes with no bile ducts, portal tracts, or central veins. Fibrous septae and Kupffer cells are inconspicuous.

The radiographic characteristics of hepatic adenomas are varied, ranging from hypo- to hyperechoic on US and hypo- to hyperdense on CT. Contrast enhancement may occur on CT, especially around the periphery of the mass. Central areas of increased density, representing hemorrhagic foci, make the diagnosis more likely. MRI has shown similar degrees of variability and remains nonspecific.

6. What role does the technetium 99m-sulfur colloid liver scan play in the diagnosis of focal liver masses?

Most benign and malignant lesions produce a focal defect on sulfur colloid scans; because the radiotracer is taken up by Kupffer cells, the presence of normal hepatic architecture is required. The exception to this rule is seen in focal nodular hyperplasia, a rare, benign tumor thought to arise as a hyperplastic response to preexisting arterial malformation. Focal nodular hyperplasia (FNH) is a round, nonencapsulated mass usually exhibiting a central scar with blood vessels, bile ductules, and chronic inflammatory cells. Radiating from the scar in a spokelike fashion are fibrous septae containing similar histologic elements. Between the septae, hepatocytes are arranged in nodules or cords, with a microscopic picture similar to that seen in cirrhosis.

Kupffer cells within FNH take up sulfur colloid and on liver scan appear as an area of normal or increased uptake compared with the normal surrounding liver. Unfortunately, only 60–70% of FNH lesions contain enough Kupffer cells to display this scintigraphic appearance. The remainder present as a cold defect requiring further evaluation.

7. Discuss the clinical and prognostic differences between focal nodular hyperplasia and hepatic adenoma.

Like hepatic adenomas, FNH occurs more commonly in women (80%) and is usually diagnosed between 20–60 years of age. FNH tends to be a smaller lesion, often smaller than 3 cm, and is more likely to be asymptomatic. In contrast to adenomas, patients with FNH are not considered to be at risk for lesional bleeding, rupture, or neoplastic transformation. Despite speculation that estrogen may enhance growth of FNH, oral contraceptives are not considered a causative agent. Resection is not necessary once FNH is diagnosed.

8. What other radiographic features characterize FNH?

The US and CT patterns of FNH do not allow differentiation from other hepatic neoplasms. Typically, FNH is hypodense on unenhanced CT, although it may be isodense to the liver and not readily visible. Contrast produces variable degrees of enhancement, and the central scar may not be seen on CT or US. MRI may prove to be a more useful imaging modality. Recent literature suggests that MRI can establish the diagnosis of FNH when the lesion shows isointensity on T1- and T2-weighted images, homogeneous signal intensity throughout, and hyperintensity of the central scar on T2-weighted sequences. This characteristic pattern is seen in less than one-half of reported cases, and further evaluation may require angiography or wedge biopsy.

9. Do central scars occur in hepatic lesions other than FNH?

Yes. Although most frequently seen in FNH, central scars may occur in the fibrolamellar variant of hepatocellular carcinoma, hemangiomas, and hepatic adenomas. Benign lesions such as FNH show a hyperintense scar on T2-weighted MRI, reflecting vasculature. Neoplastic masses have a hypointense scar on T2-weighted sequences due to fibrosis.

10. What is the most frequent malignancy in the liver?

In the United States and Europe, metastatic disease is much more common than primary hepatic tumors. Cancers arising in the colon, stomach, pancreas, breast, and lung are the most likely to metastasize to the liver. Esophageal, renal, and genitourinary neoplasms also should be considered in searching for the primary site. Multiple defects suggest a metastatic process: only 2% present as a solitary lesion. Involvement of both lobes is most common: 20% are confined to the right lobe and 3% to the left lobe.

Hepatocellular carcinoma (HCC) predominates in Asia and Africa because of the higher prevalence of hepatitis B virus. HCC usually occurs within established cirrhosis, although this association is not mandatory. Its gross pathologic appearance is commonly described as nodular, focal (or massive), or diffuse. The nodular form is most common, consisting of one or more lesions scattered throughout the liver. Massive HCC tends to occur in younger patients as a large, solitary mass in the right lobe, often accompanied by small satellite nodules. The rarer diffuse variety may be difficult to detect on imaging studies, because minute tumor foci infiltrate a widespread area of similarly appearing cirrhotic nodules.

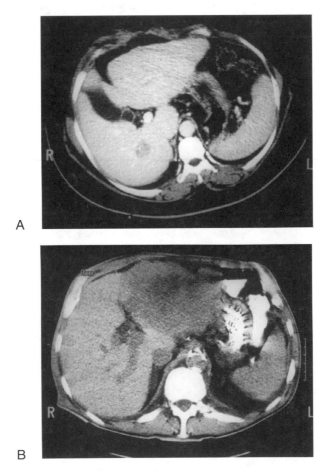

Variable CT presentations of hepatocellular carcinoma. *A* (with contrast) shows a single nodular hypodense area with some peripheral enhancement in the right lobe. *B* (non-contrast) demonstrates the massive type with replacement of the left lobe.

11. What is a hepatobiliary cystadenoma? How does it differ from a benign hepatic cyst?
Simple hepatic cysts are common, with an incidence of 2.5%, but rarely cause symptoms. They are easily diagnosed on US as a smooth, anechoic area lacking discrete walls. Volume averaging may make the CT diagnosis difficult when the cyst is smaller than 2 cm, but US is confirmatory in such situations. Hepatobiliary cystadenomas differ from benign cysts because they have thick, septated walls. This multiloculated lesion is very rare, occurring predominantly in middle-aged women, and often causes some degree of abdominal pain. Hepatobiliary cystadenomas may be several centimeters in diameter and contain a mucinous fluid. Although most are benign, up to 25% develop malignant foci (cystadenocarcinoma) if not resected. Nodular projections from the cyst wall or dense calcifications suggest malignant transformation. Complete surgical excision is the treatment of choice, even in benign lesions, because survival rates decrease dramatically when adenocarcinoma is identified. Pyogenic liver abscesses and echinococcal cysts may resemble hepatobiliary cystadenomas on imaging studies but these should be distinguishable on clinical and serologic grounds.

12. Which etiologies of cirrhosis are associated with HCC?
Autopsy studies indicate that 20–40% of patients dying with cirrhosis harbor HCC. Conversely, 56–84% of patients diagnosed with HCC have cirrhosis. The incidence is highest with hepatitis B- or C-induced cirrhosis, especially when evidence of active viral replication is present. Hemochromatosis and to a lesser extent alcoholic cirrhosis are also associated with this tumor. Alcohol may potentiate the carcinogenic risk of viral-induced liver damage.
    Geographic location influences both the age of peak occurrence (over age 55 years in the United States) and the male-to-female incidence ratios, although men are more likely to develop HCC worldwide by a factor of 4 to 1.

13. List some clinical and laboratory findings that should raise suspicion for HCC.
1. New abdominal pain or weight loss in a stable cirrhotic patient
2. Hepatomegaly
3. Hepatic bruit
4. Acute hemoperitoneum
5. Blood-tinged ascitic fluid
6. Persistent fever
7. Sudden increase in serum alkaline phosphatase
8. Increasing ratio of AST to ALT
9. Erythrocytosis or persistent leukocytosis
10. Hypoglycemia
11. Hypercholesterolemia
12. Hypercalcemia

Findings 9–12 are paraneoplastic syndromes associated with HCC.

14. How may serum alpha-fetoprotein help in the diagnosis of HCC?
Alpha-fetoprotein (AFP) is the best diagnostic marker for HCC and also plays a role in screening programs of at-risk populations. Sensitivity varies, depending on the type of assay; the radioimmune assay is the most sensitive technique available in most laboratories. AFP values above 400 ng/ml are indicative of HCC. Benign chronic liver disease may cause a nonspecific elevation in serum AFP, which is almost always below the cutoff point. AFP levels correlate with tumor size, and successful treatment should decrease or normalize the value. Not all hepatomas secrete AFP. Approximately 30% of patients have a normal AFP, especially when the tumor is smaller than 2 cm and amenable to resection.
    Screening programs with serum AFP determinations and liver ultrasonography every 3–12 months are advocated in cirrhotic patients at high risk for HCC. High-resolution US is more sensitive than AFP for early detection. Tumors as small as 1 cm may be visualized as an echolucent area surrounded by an echoic capsule. Of note, 25–65% of identified lesions are 2 cm or smaller with rigorous surveillance.

15. What primary liver tumor occurs in young adults without underlying cirrhosis?
The fibrolamellar variant of HCC is a distinctive, slow-growing subtype of hepatic neoplasm, occurring at a mean age of 26 years. Patients seldom have a history of prior liver disease. Unlike the

more common form of hepatoma, men and women are equally affected. Fibrolamellar tumors usually present with abdominal pain due to a large, solitary mass, often in the left lobe (75%) of the liver. Mild-to-moderate transaminase elevations may occur, but the AFP level is normal. The term fibrolamellar characterizes the microscopic appearance of the lesion; thin layers of fibrosis separate the neoplastic hepatocytes. A fibrous central scar may be seen on imaging studies. Recognition of this variant is important because nearly one-half are resectable at the time of diagnosis.

16. What factors predispose to the development of cholangiocarcinoma? Name the basic subtypes of this tumor.

Cholangiocarcinomas, which account for 10–20% of primary liver tumors, arise as adenocarcinomas from bile duct epithelium. Primary sclerosing cholangitis, liver fluke infection, exposure to Thorotrast, and congenital cystic liver diseases such as Caroli's disease and choledochal cysts are associated risk factors. Jaundice is the most frequent clinical feature, and the tumor markers CEA, CA 19–9, or AFP may be elevated.

Cholangiocarcinoma is divided into peripheral and hilar (Klatskin tumor) subtypes according to location. Peripheral cholangiocarcinoma resembles HCC in presentation but usually is not accompanied by cirrhosis. It tends to be hypovascular by provoking a characteristic desmoplastic reaction. The hilar type arises at the junction of the right and left hepatic ducts and is often poorly seen on imaging studies. US and CT show marked intrahepatic duct dilation in the clinical setting of obstructive jaundice. Rarer variants include cholangiolocellular carcinoma, arising from the canals of Hering, and mixed hepatocellular-cholangiocarcinoma, in which both tumor components are adjacent or admixed.

17. Describe the radiographic characteristics that help to distinguish primary hepatic tumors from metastases.

Distinguishing among various intrahepatic malignancies may be difficult on US,CT, or MRI, but some features have diagnostic relevance. A dynamic-bolus CT, preceded by unenhanced scans, is the best procedure, although some clinicians consider MRI superior for planning surgical resection.

Most metastases appear on CT as multiple, low-density (dark) areas after contrast injection, which imparts some enhancement to the surrounding normal liver tissue. They typically have irregular margins and may have darker central necrotic regions. Hypervascular metastases, such as renal-cell tumors, sarcomas, and carcinoid, tend to have early peripheral enhancement before becoming isodense and thus are indiscernible after contrast. Unenhanced scans are valuable in this setting. Colorectal metastases often show central enhancement of connective tissue surrounded by lower-density tumor on delayed CT images 3 to 5 minutes after contrast is given. This finding corresponds to the characteristic target lesion (bull's-eye) on US.

CT findings that favor a diagnosis of HCC include the presence of a capsule, bulging of tumor beyond the normal hepatic contours, or a lesion with an interior composed of several different densities. Dynamic-bolus CT yields additional information because of the hypervascular nature of HCC. Contrast injection produces an immediate, homogeneous enhancement of most hepatomas before the slower parenchymal uptake occurs. Portal vein invasion also may be seen with this technique.

Primary and metastatic hepatic malignancies have similar appearances on MRI, with low signal intensities (dark) on T1-weighted images and high signal (bright) on T2 sequences. MRI is especially helpful in the differentiation of HCC from benign hemangiomas.

The echo characteristics of intrahepatic lesions may suggest the tumor's origin, although the broad variations in sonographic appearance of a given cell type make distinction with US of limited value.

18. What hepatic neoplasm is associated with a history of vinyl chloride exposure?

Angiosarcoma is the most common primary mesenchymal malignancy in adults, although all neoplasms of this particular group are exceedingly rare. Vinyl chloride has been identified as the carcinogen most frequently associated with angiosarcoma. This tumor, derived from endothelium, is hypervascular and usually involves both hepatic lobes at diagnosis. Its rapid growth and tendency to metastasize contribute to its dismal prognosis.

19. What other mesenchymal cell malignancies may arise in the liver?

Other mesenchymal primary tumors in the liver include rhabdomyosarcoma, fibrosarcoma and leiomyosarcoma. A recently described entity most often seen in middle-aged women is the slow-growing epithelioid hemangioendothelioma.

Special mention should be made of primary hepatic lymphomas, although they are much less common than secondary liver involvement from Hodgkin's and non-Hodgkin's lymphomas. Primary lymphoma typically presents as a large, solitary mass, whereas secondary spread is characterized by multiple nodules or hepatomegaly. In one-third of secondary hepatic lymphomas the disease is so diffusely infiltrative that imaging studies appear normal.

20. What are the contraindications to surgical excision of primary cancers and colorectal metastases?

Resection remains the only curative approach to primary and metastatic liver cancers. Current data for HCC indicate that between 9% and 37% are resectable at diagnosis: 5-year survival rates in most series are approximately 30% in patients without concomitant cirrhosis. The surgical experience with metastases of colorectal origin has shown similar 5-year survival rates when curative excision is attempted. Contraindications to surgical resection include:

- Extrahepatic spread or metastases
- Involvement of hepatic nodes by tumor
- Decompensated cirrhosis (Child's C or marked ascites)
- Greater than 4 colorectal metastases in the liver
- Invasion of HCC into the inferior vena cava, portal vein, or hepatic veins
- Bilobar extension of HCC

21. What newer imaging modalities are under development for preoperative assessment of resectability?

Because successful surgical therapy depends on precise staging of tumor extent, recently developed techniques that improve sensitivity may play an important role in the future. Examples include lipiodol CT, CT-portography, and intraoperative ultrasonography. Lipiodol CT involves the injection of an iodized oil contrast medium into the hepatic artery; CT scanning is carried out several days later. Because hepatomas are unable to clear the contrast, the resolution of very small lesions is greater. CT-portography delivers conventional contrast directly into the portal vein system by way of a catheter placed in the superior mesenteric or splenic artery. Some reports indicate that this modality improves sensitivity by 30–40% over that of conventional CT, although problems with specificity (false-positive benign lesions) may limit its usefulness. Intraoperative US is considered the most accurate technique; its sensitivity exceeds 90%.

22. Describe two palliative therapies for the management of inoperable HCC.

The palliative treatment of HCC, in general, has yielded inconsistent and unimpressive results. Systemic and intraarterial chemotherapy, radiation therapy, and hepatic artery ligation do not produce favorable responses in most patients. Two newer options, which have yet to be fully evaluated, should be considered when surgical resection is not feasible. Transarterial embolization, in which feeding arteries are occluded through an angiographically guided catheter, and percutaneous intratumor ethanol injection with US localization have shown beneficial effects on survival in pilot studies. Complete assessment awaits long-term, controlled trials.

23. What benign tissue abnormalities may simulate a focal liver mass?

Focal fatty infiltration and macroregenerative nodules (also known as adenomatous hyperplasia or pseudotumors) may appear confusingly similar to the focal hepatic lesions described above.

Focal fatty liver is often seen in alcoholism, obesity, diabetes mellitus, malnutrition, cortico-steroid excess or therapy, and AIDS. The diagnosis is suggested by a well-demarcated hypere-choic area on US, lack of mass effect, and low attenuation values on unenhanced CT consistent with fat, although variable echo and CT patterns are seen. A technetium sulfur colloid liver scan often shows normal uptake in the fatty area, and hepatic imaging with xenon-133 has been used to confirm areas of fatty change. MRI characteristically shows a slightly increased signal inten-sity on T1-weighted images and a normal T2 sequence. An interesting aspect of focal fat is its rapid disappearance once the inciting disease process is corrected. Diffuse fatty infiltration of the liver with areas of focal sparing (non–fat-laden hepatocytes) may be more problematic. Echo pat-terns may be reversed, metastases may blend into the surrounding steatotic parenchyma, or fo-cally spared regions may mimic masses. A high index of suspicion, together with careful atten-tion to the overall liver attenuation, may clarify such situations.

Macroregenerative nodules ($\geq$1-cm foci of hepatocytes with intact portal tracts) are seen in up to 25% of cirrhotic livers. Although benign, they may contain dysplastic hepatocytes and are considered precancerous lesions because of their intimate association with HCC. Iron or hetero-geneous foci within a nodule suggest malignant transformation. Imaging patterns vary, but MRI may become the preferred method of differentiation from HCC, based on T2-weighted signals. Macroregenerative nodules tend to be iso- or hypointense, whereas HCC usually is hyperintense. Pitfalls make tissue diagnosis mandatory. US-guided fine-needle aspiration or biopsy, repeated if the area changes in size or texture, has its proponents, given the attendant surgical risk in patients with cirrhosis.

24. Outline a logical approach to the evaluation of a focal hepatic mass.

The work-up of a focal liver mass must occur in the context of a carefully considered differ-ential diagnosis in a given patient. Associated symptoms, presence of underlying liver disease or extrahepatic malignancy, drug and occupational exposures, and laboratory abnormalities must be assessed before proceeding with further radiographic studies. Symptomatic lesions and lesions noted incidentally are likely to have different etiologies. The patient's age and sex are important clues. Cirrhosis requires a different approach, as does the search for hepatic metastases. Knowl-edge of the variable presentations of specific lesions on imaging studies is necessary to avoid di-agnostic oversights.

Incidental lesions. Simple cysts appearing on CT or MRI may be verified with US. Heman-giomas, the most common benign lesion, may be confirmed with MRI (if <2.5 cm) or tagged red blood cell nuclear medicine study. When focal nodular hyperplasia is suspected, a radionuclide liver scan is useful.

Symptomatic lesions. Hepatic adenoma should be considered in any young or middle-aged woman with a history of oral contraceptive use, even if she is asymptomatic. Liver abscess should be excluded by US if the clinical picture of sepsis is present, although primary tumors sometimes mimic this lesion.

Neoplasms. Primary hepatic tumors are suspected on the basis of AFP determination, coex-istent liver disease, and imaging features. Unenhanced and dynamic-bolus CT should be used for evaluating metastatic disease. Hypervascular lesions may require angiography to characterize the etiology. Gallium uptake into HCC has been used in the past but is nonspecific.

Tissue diagnosis. Radiographically guided biopsy is frequently used when metastatic dis-ease is likely or cirrhosis requires exclusion of HCC. In 80–90% of cases the diagnosis of malig-nancy is obtained with fine-needle aspiration or biopsy; few complications occur when 18- to 22-gauge needles are used.

In noncirrhotic patients, directed biopsy rarely provides confirmatory diagnosis in most benign lesions and carries a potential bleeding risk in vascular or malignant tumors. Laparoscopy or lap-arotomy with wedge biopsy is often the best approach when the neoplastic status of a mass is un-clear and histologic diagnosis is deemed essential. Suitable patients may proceed directly to resec-tion at the time of laparotomy, if warranted. If the lesion is considered benign and surgery is not performed, follow-up imaging study in 2–3 months is necessary to document stability.

BIBLIOGRAPHY

1. Bennett WF, Bova JG: Review of hepatic imaging and a problem-oriented approach to liver masses. Hepatology 12:761–775, 1990.
2. Craig JR, Peters RL, Edmondson HA, Omata M: Fibrolamellar carcinoma of the liver: A tumor of adolescents and young adults with distinctive clinico-pathologic features. Cancer 46:372–379, 1980.
3. Di Bisceglie AM, Rustgi VK, Hoofnagle JH, et al: Hepatocellular carcinoma. Ann Intern Med 108: 390–401, 1988.
4. Farlow DC, Chapman PR, Gruenewald SM, et al: Investigation of focal hepatic lesions: Is tomographic red blood cell imaging useful? World J Surg 14:463–467, 1990.
5. Kerlin P, Davis GL, McGill DB, et al: Hepatic adenoma and focal nodular hyperplasia: Clinical, pathologic, and radiologic features. Gastroenterology 84:994–1002, 1983.
6. Kew MC: Tumors of the liver. In Zakim D, Boyer TD (eds): Hepatology: A Textbook of Liver Disease, 2nd ed. Philadelphia, W.B. Saunders, 1990, pp 1206–1239.
7. Kruskal JB, Kane RA: Correlative imaging of malignant liver tumors. Semin Ultrasound CT MR 13: 336–354, 1992.
8. Mahfouz AE, Hamm B, Taupitz M, Wolf KJ: Hypervascular liver lesions: Differentiation of focal nodular hyperplasia from malignant tumors with dynamic gadolinium-enhanced MR imaging. Radiology 186:133–138, 1993.
9. Mitchell DG: Focal manifestations of diffuse liver disease at MR imaging. Radiology 185:1–11, 1992.
10. Oka H, Kurioka N, Kim K, et al: Prospective study of early detection of hepatocellular carcinoma in patients with cirrhosis. Hepatology 12.680–687, 1990.
11. Okuda K, Kojiro M, Okuda H: Neoplasms of the liver. In Schiff L, Schiff ER (eds): Diseases of the Liver, 7th ed. Philadelphia, J.B. Lippincott, 1993, pp 1236–1296.
12. Reddy KR, Schiff ER: Approach to a liver mass. Semin Liver Dis 13:423–435, 1993.
13. Shamsi K, De Schepper A, Degryse H, Deckers F: Focal nodular hyperplasia of the liver: Radiologic findings. Abdom Imaging 18: 32–38, 1993.
14. Vassiliades VG, Bree RL, Korobkin M: Focal and diffuse benign hepatic disease: Correlative imaging. Semin Ultrasound CT MR 13: 313–335, 1992.
15. Yamauchi M, Nakahara M, Maezawa Y, et al: Prevalence of hepatocellular carcinoma in patients with alcoholic cirrhosis and prior exposure to hepatitis C. Am J Gastroenterol 88:39–43, 1993.

23. DRUG-INDUCED LIVER DISEASE

Peter R. McNally, DO

1. How common is drug-induced liver disease?

More than 600 medicines have been reported to cause liver injury. Drug-induced liver disease accounts for 2–5% of hospital admissions for jaundice in the United States and 10–20% of cases of fulminant liver failure.

2. What are the three patterns of drug-induced liver injury?

The three categories are typically separated by the height of elevation in alanine aminotransferase (ALT) and alkaline phosphatase (AP) levels.

Patterns of Drug-Induced Liver Disease

	ALT	AP	ALT:AP RATIO
Hepatocellular injury	≥2×	Normal	High (≥5)
Cholestatic injury	Normal	≥2×	Low (≤2)
Mixed injury	≥2×	≥2×	2–5

3. What is the typical chronologic association between drug exposure and the onset of hepatitis or cholestasis?

Typically, cholestatic or hepatocellular liver injury occurs between 5 and 90 days from the initial exposure. Upon withdrawal of the drug, biochemical improvement in hepatocellular injury is usually seen within 2 weeks, whereas cholestatic or mixed injury may not improve for 4 weeks. Persistence of abnormal liver biochemistries beyond these intervals suggests a coexistent or independent etiology of liver disease (viral or autoimmune liver disease, primary biliary cirrhosis, primary sclerosing cholangitis, etc.).

4. What is the differential diagnosis of drug-induced liver diseases?

Incrimination of a drug as the cause of liver injury requires exclusion of viral, toxic, cardiovascular, inheritable, and malignant causes of liver injury. Careful history, review of past laboratory testing, and physical examination are often helpful. When drug-induced liver injury is suspected, withdrawal of the offending agent and close observation often provide adequate circumstantial evidence for the diagnosis. Liver biopsy should be reserved for situations in which discontinuation of the medication is not followed by prompt improvement, the etiology of liver disease remains in question, or the severity necessitates intervention (organ transplantation, corticosteroids).

5. Name the two most common mechanisms of drug-induced liver injury.

- Direct or indirect toxicity to the hepatocyte (intrinsic hepatotoxin).
- Idiosyncratic stimulation of a hyperimmune reaction.

Examples of intrinsic hepatotoxins include phosphorus, carbon tetrachloride, acetaminophen, and chloroform. Intrinsic hepatotoxins cause direct damage to the liver by covalently binding to cellular macromolecules, such as hydrogen peroxide, hydroxyl radicals, or lipid peroxides. These, in turn, interrupt cell membranes or inactivate critical cellular enzyme systems.

Examples of agents causing idiosyncratic hypersensitivity injury include phenytoin, isoniazid, ticrynafen, halothane, and valproic acid. Idiosyncratic hepatotoxins are dose-independent, and hepatic injury cannot be reproduced in animal models. Clinical features of hypersensitivity (rash, fever, eosinophilia) are common. The mechanisms of injury for these toxins is poorly understood.

6. What variables appear to influence susceptibility to drug-induced hepatic injury?

Age	Young more susceptible to aspirin and valproic acid.
	Old more susceptible to isoniazid, halothane, and acetaminophen.
Sex	Women more susceptible to all drug-induced liver disease, probably due to lower body mass and susceptibility to autoimmune hepatitis (e.g., alcohol, methyldopa, nitrofurantoin, etc.).
Route of administration	Tetracycline toxicity primarily parenteral.
Drug–drug interactions	Valproic acid increases chlorpromazine-induced cholestasis.
	Rifampin potentiates isoniazid hepatotoxicity.
	Chronic alcohol ingestion potentiates acetaminophen and isoniazid hepatotoxicity.

7. Name the two most common causes of drug-induced liver disease.
Alcohol and acetaminophen.

8. How is acetaminophen toxic to the liver?
Acetaminophen is only toxic to the liver when taken in excessive doses or when the protective detoxifying pathway in the liver is overwhelmed. Accumulation of the toxic metabolite, N-acetyl-p-benzoquinone, is responsible for death of hepatocytes. Acetaminophen is the second most common cause of death from poisoning in the United States.

9. At what dose is acetaminophen toxic?
Hepatotoxicity of acetaminophen occurs in nonalcoholic patients at doses >7.5 g. A potentially lethal effect is seen with ingestion of >140 mg/kg (10 g in a 70-kg man). Chronic alcoholics are at greater risk of acetaminophen injury due to alcohol induction of the cytochrome P450 system and attendant malnutrition and low levels of glutathione. Glutathione is an intracellular protectant naturally found in the hepatocyte.

10. How is acetaminophen toxicity treated?
The Rumack-Matthew nomogram is helpful in predicting the likelihood of liver injury from acetaminophen and in recommending therapy. The antidote for acetaminophen overdose is oral administration of N-acetylcysteine (NAC), 140 mg/kg, followed by 17 maintenance doses of 70 mg/kg given every 4 hours. Ipecac is given if the time of ingestion can be verified to be <4 hours. The use of activated charcoal is controversial, since it can interfere with the adsorption of the NAC antidote.

11. What are the clinical findings of chlorzoxazone hepatotoxicity?
Chlorzoxazone (Parafon Forte) is a centrally acting muscle relaxant. Hepatotoxic effects are rare, but severe hepatitis, including fulminant hepatic failure, has been reported. Onset of injury may occur within 1 week of initiation or up to several years later. The transaminase elevation may exceed 1,000 IU/l. Most patients exhibit hyperbilirubinemia as well. Discontinuation of the medication is usually the only intervention necessary.

12. What commonly used "recreational" drug is associated with hepatotoxicity?
An estimated 30 million Americans have experimented with cocaine, and 5 million habitually abuse it. Patients suffering cocaine hepatotoxicity may present with jaundice or fatigue and generalized malaise. The aminotransferase elevations can be in the 5,000-IU/l range. Cocaine toxicity may also cause coagulopathy, rhabdomyolysis, and disseminated intravascular coagulation. The mechanism of hepatotoxicity is unknown. Liver biopsy typically shows zone III injury, suggesting ischemia is somehow related. Liver injury in these patients may be multifactorial and include coexistent viral liver disease (hepatitis B, C, and delta) and acetaminophen or alcohol use.

13. What anesthetic agents are associated with hepatocellular injury?
Halothane, enflurane, methoxyflurane, and isoflurane.

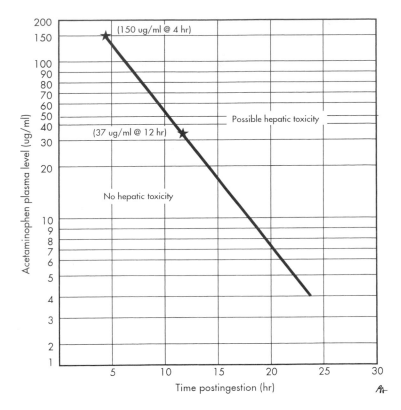

Rumack-Matthew nomogram.

Whenever hepatitis occurs postoperatively, nonanesthetic causes of hepatitis must be considered (viral hepatitis, drug-induced hepatitis, bile duct injury, cholestasis of total parenteral nutrition or sepsis, transfusion hepatitis, ischemic hepatopathy, etc.).

The risk for **halothane** hepatitis is 1/10,000 patients but increases to 7/10,000 after two or more exposures. Over 75% of patients with halothane liver injury present within 2 weeks of exposure with fever, nausea, rash, arthralgias, and diffuse abdominal discomfort. Laboratory abnormalities include eosinophilia, AST and ALT elevations in the 500–1,000-IU/l range, and alkaline phosphatase elevation (usually <2× normal). The oxidative metabolite of halothane, trifluoroacetyl halide, is felt to be responsible for the exaggerated humoral and cellular immune response seen after exposure. Prognostic factors for a poor outcome include short latent period from exposure to jaundice, obesity, age >40 years, hepatic encephalopathy, and prolongation of the prothrombin time. Corticosteroids and exchange transfusions are not helpful, and the mortality of fulminant halothane hepatitis is nearly 80% without liver transplantation.

14. Who is at risk for liver toxicity from isoniazid (INH) therapy?

INH hepatitis may present insidiously from 4–6 months after initiation of therapy. Some patients experience influenza-like symptoms. Abnormal AST and ALT elevations develop in up to 20% of patients taking INH, but aminotransferase activity usually subsides to normal spontaneously. The risk for frank hepatitis is low in the young (0.3% between 20–34 years), 1.2% at ages 35–49, and 2.3% in those >50 years old. Coadministration of rifampin increases the likelihood of INH toxicity. Acetaminophen toxicity is increased by INH owing to its induction of the cytochrome P450 enzyme system.

Current recommendations to prevent INH toxicity include screening patients for ethanol abuse and preexisting liver or renal disease. The presence of chronic liver disease is not an absolute contraindication to the use of INH, but the indications should be scrutinized and therapy monitored more closely. The American Thoracic Society recommends dispensing just 1 month's supply of INH to ensure close monitoring. Patients should be advised to report prodromal symptoms immediately. All patients >35 years should have serial monitoring of ALT, with the use of INH being reconsidered when ALT elevations persist or remain >100 IU/l.

15. Describe the clinical features of phenytoin hepatotoxicity.

Phenytoin has been shown to cause an allergic hepatitis, cholestasis, granulomatous liver disease, and even frank fulminant hepatic failure. Symptoms of hepatotoxicity usually occur within the first 8 weeks of administration. The incriminated metabolite responsible for liver injury is arene oxide. Systemic symptoms include pharyngitis, lymphadenopathy, and atypical lymphocytosis, so-called pseudolymphoma syndrome. There are some favorable reports of treating acute phenytoin hepatitis with corticosteroids.

16. What drugs have been identified to cause chronic hepatitis and cirrhosis?

Isoniazid, methotrexate, methyldopa, nitrofurantoin, oxyphenisatin, perhexiline maleate, and trazodone.

17. What are the clinical features of methyldopa (Aldomet) hepatocellular injury?

Liver injury usually occurs within 6–12 weeks of initiation of methyldopa therapy. Aminotransferase values should be obtained periodically during the first 4 months of drug administration. Females appear to be more susceptible to hepatotoxicity of methyldopa, and the clinical presentation may mimic autoimmune "lupoid" hepatitis.

18. Describe the clinical features of nitrofurantoin hepatocellular injury.

A cholestatic pattern of liver injury is usually seen with nitrofurantoin. Clinical symptoms of fever, rash, and eosinophilia are common. There are over 100 cases of chronic active hepatitis reported secondary to nitrofurantoin, with most of these cases seen in women taking the drug for >6 months. Laboratory findings consist of high aminotransferase values, increased gamma globulin, HLA-B8 histocompatibility markers, and, often, positive autoimmune markers (antinuclear antibody).

19. What laxative is associated with chronic hepatitis?

Oxyphenisatin. Laxatives containing oxyphenisatin are no longer available in the United States.

20. What antiarthritic drugs have been reported to cause liver injury?

NSAIDs Causing Hepatotoxicity

Sulindac (Clinoril)	Over 400 cases of sulindac-induced hepatitis have been reported. A cholestatic hepatitis is seen in most. Common clinical manifestations include fever, rash, and Stevens-Johnson syndrome. A "trapped" common bile duct causing cholestasis has been reported after sulindac-induced pancreatitis.
Diclofenac (Voltaren)	Uniquely, more common in females than males. The pattern of injury is primarily hepatitis. Fulminant hepatitis and death have been reported.
Phenylbutazone (Butazolidin)	An immunologic type of injury is usually seen, with fever, rash, and eosinophilia. Illness usually starts within 6 weeks of initiating the drug. The hepatic injury seen is variable, with acute hepatitis, cholestasis, and granulomatous hepatitis all reported to occur.
Ibuprofen (Motrin, Advil)	Hepatic injury due to ibuprofen is relatively uncommon. OTC doses of ibuprofen have not been reported to cause clinically apparent liver injury.
Piroxicam (Feldene)	Lethal hepatitis and cholestasis have been reported, but overall liver injury appears to be uncommon.

21. Name the two types of cholestatic drug-induced hepatic injury.
Inflammatory and bland cholestasis.

22. List the common causes of drug-induced cholestasis.

Inflammatory Cholestasis	Bland Cholestasis
Allopurinol	Anabolic steroids
Amitriptyline	Androgens
Azathioprine	Estrogens
Captopril	Oral contraceptives
Carbamazepine	Phenytoin

23. What chemotherapeutic agent is associated with a sclerosing cholangitis pattern of injury?
Floxuridine. Selective hepatic artery infusion of this agent has been associated with a large bile duct injury and cholestasis in up to 30% of patients.

24. List the drugs associated with mixed cholestatic-hepatitis type of liver injury.

Amitriptyline	Flutamide	Ranitidine
Amoxicillin	Ibuprofen	Sulfonamides
Ampicillin	Imipramine	Sulindac
Captopril	Nitrofurantoin	Toxic oil syndrome
Carbamazepine	Phenylbutazone	Trimethoprim-sulfamethoxazole
Cimetidine	Quinidine	Naproxen

25. Name the three types of drug-induced steatosis ("fatty liver"). Which drugs cause them?

Drugs Causing Steatosis

MICROVESICULAR STEATOSIS	MACROVESICULAR STEATOSIS	PHOSPHOLIPIDOSIS
Aspirin (Reye's syndrome)	Acetaminophen	4,4'-Diethylamino ethyl hexestrol
Ketoprofen	Cisplatin	Perhexiline maleate
Tetracycline	Corticosteroids	Amiodarone
Valproic acid	Methotrexate	Trimethroprim-sulfamethoxazide
Zidovudine (AZT)	Tamoxifen	Parenteral nutrition

26. How is the hepatic injury caused by amiodarone unique?
Amiodarone is an iodine-containing benzofuran used in Europe as an antianginal and antiarrhythmic agent. Amiodarone accumulates within the lysosome, where it complexes with phospholipids and inhibits lysosomal phospholipases.

27. How should patients receiving chronic methotrexate (MTX) be monitored for chronic hepatitis and cirrhosis?
Methotrexate has been used in patients with refractory psoriasis and rheumatoid arthritis. In patients with **psoriasis,** many advocate an index liver biopsy after 2–4 months of MTX therapy, then serial repeat biopsies after every 1.0–1.5 g of cumulative dose.

In patients with rheumatoid arthritis, MTX appears to be somewhat less hepatotoxic. The American College of Rheumatology, in a position paper on MTX use in rheumatoid arthritis patients, did not recommend a pretreatment liver biopsy in the absence of preexisting liver disease. Monitoring of liver-associated enzymes was recommended. MTX discontinuation was advised when AST or ALT levels exceeded three times the baseline values. Liver biopsies were advised every 2 or 3 years (or every 1.5 g of cumulative dose).

28. What are the histologic grades of methotrexate liver injury?

Histologic Grades of MTX Liver Injury

GRADE	FIBROSIS	FATTY INFILTRATION	NUCLEAR VARIABILITY	PORTAL INFLAMMATION
I	none	mild	mild	mild
II	none	moderate to severe	moderate to severe	portal expansion, lobular necrosis
IIIA	mild (septa extending into the lobules)	moderate to severe	moderate to severe	portal expansion, lobular necrosis
IIIB	moderate to severe	moderate to severe	moderate to severe	portal expansion, lobular necrosis
IV	cirrhosis			

29. Outline the recommendations for change in MTX therapy based on liver biopsy findings.

- I   Continue therapy; repeat biopsy after 1–1.5 g of cumulative dose.
- II   Continue therapy; repeat biopsy after 1–1.5 g of cumulative dose.
- IIIA Continue therapy, but repeat biopsy in 6 mo.
- IIIB No further MTX; exceptional cases need close histologic followup.
- IV   No further MTX; exceptional cases need close histologic followup.

30. What is veno-occlusive disease (VOD)? What drugs have been incriminated to cause it?

VOD is an occlusive disease that affects terminal hepatic venules and veins. Typically, patients present with hepatomegaly, ascites, weight gain, peripheral edema, jaundice, and pain from capsular distention of the liver. Aminotransferase values may be normal or modestly elevated. Liver biopsy is often required for the diagnosis and shows histologic features of perivenular sclerosis, blood-filled congested sinuses, and hemorrhagic necrosis.

Drugs Causing VOD

Vincristine	6-Thioguanine	Carmustine (BCNU)
Azathioprine	Radiotherapy	6-Mercaptopurine
Doxorubicin	Aflatoxin	Pyrrolizidine alkaloids (bush tea)

31. What drugs are associated with the development of hepatic adenomas?

Before the availability of **oral contraceptives**, hepatic adenomas were very uncommon. Since oral contraceptives were shown to be a cause of hepatic adenomas in 1970, numerous additional cases have been reported. After 5 years of oral contraceptive use, the relative risk of developing a hepatic adenoma has been estimated to increase 116-fold. Hepatic adenomas often regress when exogenous estrogen is removed and can recur during pregnancy. **Anabolic steroids** have also been reported to cause hepatic adenomas. Hepatic adenomas are usually asymptomatic but can be associated with abdominal fullness and pain, hepatomegaly, and hemorrhage.

32. What is peliosis hepatis, and what drugs are associated with this condition?

Peliosis hepatis describes small venular cavities or lakes within the liver that arise from injury to sinusoids. Generally, the condition is asymptomatic, but it may result in hemorrhage or liver failure. Anabolic steroids and oral contraceptives both have been shown to cause this disorder.

33. Which three vascular injuries to the liver can be caused by drugs?

Hepatic veno-occlusive disease	Pyrrolizidine alkaloids, antineoplastic drugs
Peliosis hepatis	Anabolic steroids, oral contraceptives
Hepatic vein thrombosis	Oral contraceptives

34. What are the three most common drug-induced hepatic neoplasms?

Hepatic adenoma	Oral contraceptives, anabolic steroids
Hepatocellular carcinoma	Anabolic steroids, oral contraceptives, thorium oxide (Thorotrast), vinyl chloride
Angiosarcoma	Thorium oxide (Thorotrast), vinyl chloride, arsenic, anabolic steroids

35. Over 50 drugs have been cited to cause hepatic granulomas. Name some of the most common ones.

Allopurinol	Phenylbutazone	Isoniazid
Chlorpromazine	Quinidine	Nitrofurantoin
Diazepam	Sulfonamides	Penicillin
Gold	Aspirin	Phenytoin
Mineral oil	Oral contraceptives	Quinine
Oxicillin	Diltiazem	Tolbutamide

36. Which drugs commonly used to treat endocrine disease have been reported to cause liver injury?

Sulfonylureas (tolbutamide, tolazamide, glipizide, acetohexamide, glyburide, chlorpropamide): The pattern of injury is cholestatic for chlorpropamide, glipizide, tolazamide, and tolbutamide, and hepatocellular or mixed with the remainder. A hypersensitivity reaction is thought to be responsible. Hypersensitivity to chlorpropamide does not predict the same for tolbutamide.

Thiourea derivatives (propylthiouracil, methimazole): May cause a hepatocellular or cholestatic injury.

Steroid derivatives (anabolic steroids, oral contraceptives, tamoxifen, danazol, glucocorticoids): Reported to cause a cholestasis or canalicular type of liver injury.

Lipid-lowering agents (niacin, HMG-CoA reductase inhibitors): A mixed cholestatic-hepatic injury is seen with niacin (nicotinic acid). Injury is more common with the sustained-release form or at doses >3 g/day for the regular-release form. Serial monitoring of liver enzymes is recommended, and drug discontinuation if elevations are detected. Lovastatin is the most commonly prescribed of the HMG-CoA reductase inhibitors used to treat hypercholesterolemia. Mild elevations in aminotransferases are common, but these usually return to normal upon drug withdrawal.

37. What commonly prescribed cardiovascular drugs have been reported to cause liver injury?

Quinidine	Liver injury has been reported after a single dose. The predominant injury is hepatocellular with focal necrosis, but diffuse granulomas have also been seen.
Procainamide	Injury to the liver is rare, but hepatocellular, cholestatic, and granulomatous injury have been reported.
Verapamil, nifedipine	Hepatitis has been reported to occur within 2–3 weeks of drug administration. Cholestatic, hepatocellular, and a mixed pattern of injury have been reported. A pseudo-alcohol pattern of steatosis and Mallory's hyaline has been reported to occur with nifedipine.
Methyldopa	Asymptomatic elevations in aminotransferases are seen in up to 5% of patients taking this drug. Women are especially susceptible. Both acute and chronic forms of hepatitis have been reported.
Hydralazine	Hepatocellular and granulomatous injury have been reported.
Captopril	Hypersensitivity symptoms usually herald jaundice. Cholestasis usually ameliorates rapidly after drug removal.
Enalapril	Scattered cases of hepatitis and cholestasis have been reported.
Ticrynafen	This uricosuric diuretic was removed from the U.S. market shortly after its introduction due to the significant number of cases. of associated liver injury. The hepatitis can be very fatal.
Amiodarone	This antianginal and antiarrhythmic drug is widely used in Europe. A characteristic injury of phospholipidosis is seen.

38. What commonly used antimicrobial agents have been shown to cause liver injury?

Tetracycline	Liver injury almost exclusively seen with parenteral administration of the drug. More common in women, especially when pregnant. Microvesicular steatosis is the characteristic histologic finding.
Erythromycin estolate	Initially thought to occur only with the estolate form, but the ethylsuccinate form has recently been incriminated to cause a cholestatic hepatitis as well. A hypersensitivity picture is usually seen within days to 2 weeks of exposure.
Chloramphenicol	Rare cases of cholestasis and jaundice have been reported.
Penicillin	Both cholestatic and hepatitis-like patterns have been seen. Hypersensitivity is the mechanism of injury.
Amoxicillin, clavulanic acid	Cholestatic hepatitis has been seen during or within weeks of administering the drug.
Sulfonamides	Causes mixed hepatocellular injury that is usually heralded by rash, fever, and eosinophilia.
Pyrimethamine-sulfadoxine	Hepatocellular pattern most common, with fulminant hepatitis and death reported.
Sulfasalazine	Used to treat inflammatory bowel disease. Same injury as the sulfonamides.
Nitrofurantoin	Hallmarks of hypersensitivity are common, with both cholestatic and hepatocellular injury reported. Chronic active hepatitis has been reported, usually in a women >40 years old with HLA-B8 histocompatibility.
Isoniazid	Age-related risk for toxicity. Fulminant hepatitis with death has been reported. (*See* Question 14.)
Rifampin	Potentiates hepatotoxicity of isoniazid, presumably due to cytochrome P450 induction. Women >50 years especially susceptible.
Griseofulvin	Hepatitis rare, but the drug can precipitate attacks of acute intermittent porphyria.
Ketoconazole	Toxic hepatitis more common in women >40 years. Fulminant hepatitis has been reported. Periodic monitoring of liver enzymes is recommended to detect early injury.
Flucytosine	Transaminase elevations are common; significant hepatitis is rare.

BIBLIOGRAPHY

1. Burgquest SR, Felson DT, Prashker MJ, Freedberg KA: The cost of liver biopsy in rheumatoid arthritis patients treated with methotrexate. Arthritis Rheum 38:326–333, 1995.
2. Kremer JM, Alaarcon GS, Lightfoot RW, et al: Methotrexate for rheumatoid arthritis: Suggested guidelines for monitoring liver toxicity. Arthritis Rheum 37:316–328, 1994.
3. Lindberg MC: Hepatobiliary complications of oral contraceptives. J Gen Intern Med 7:199–209, 1992.
4. Ranek L, Dalhoff K, Poulsen HE, et al: Drug metabolism and genetic polymorphism in subjects with previous halothane hepatitis. Scand J Gastroenterol 28:677–680, 1993.
5. Roy AK, Mahoney HC, Levine RA: Phenytoin-induced chronic hepatitis. Dig Dis Sci 38:740–743, 1993.
6. Scully LJ, Clarke D, Barr RJ: Diclofenac-induced hepatitis: Three cases with features of autoimmune chronic active hepatitis. Dig Dis Sci 38:774–751, 1993.
7. Sherlock S, Dooley J: Drugs and the liver. In Sherlock S (ed): Disease of the Liver and Biliary System, 9th ed. Oxford, Blackwell, 1993, pp 322–356.
8. Tarzi EM, Harter JG, Zimmerman HJ, et al: Sulindac-associated hepatic injury: Analysis of 91 cases reported to the Food and Drug Administration. Gastroenterology 104:569–574, 1993.
9. Zimmerman HJ, Maddrey WC: Toxic and drug-induced hepatitis. In Schiff L, Schiff ER (eds): Diseases of the Liver, 7th ed. Philadelphia, JB Lippincott, 1993, pp 707–783.

24. ALCOHOLIC LIVER DISEASE AND THE ALCOHOL WITHDRAWAL SYNDROME

John H. Bloor, M.D., Ph.D.

1. Define the three patterns of alcohol use related to development of alcoholic liver disease?

Not surprisingly, **alcohol ingestion** is a prerequisite to, and the most important etiologic factor in, the development of alcoholic liver disease (ALD). For this reason, ALD can occur in heavy drinkers, alcohol abusers, and drinkers who are alcohol-dependent.

The first group, **heavy drinkers,** comprises people who drink large amounts of alcohol — enough to cause injury to their liver and other organs — without losing control of their drinking. These people usually consider themselves social drinkers and generally have no legal and social problems related to alcohol. **Alcohol abuse** and **alcohol dependence,** in contrast, are both characterized by an inability to accomplish the activities of daily living, resulting in severe social problems such as family disruption, job loss, and legal difficulties. In addition, in drinkers who are alcohol dependent, craving, tolerance, and physical dependence contribute to their inability to exercise behavioral restraint over alcohol consumption. However, the important point is that ALD is related to the **amount of alcohol consumed** and can occur in all three groups. The behavioral patterns of alcohol abuse and alcohol dependence are not required for development of ALD.

2. What are ounce-years, and how are they calculated?

The risk of alcoholic liver disease increases with the **amount** and **duration** of alcohol consumption, and is not related to the drinking pattern or type of beverage consumed. By converting the number and type of drinks to ounces of alcohol and then multiplying by the number of years that the person has used that much alcohol, one can estimate lifetime alcohol consumption as **ounce-years,** analogous to the "pack-years" used to quantitate cigarette smoking. The following table makes the conversion to ounce-years easy — if an accurate drinking history can be obtained. The data in the table are calculated from the formula below, then rounded to the nearest ounce:

$$\text{Grams of alcohol} = \text{volume (ml)} \times \text{concentration (\% alcohol)} \times 0.00798$$
$$\text{Fluid ounces of alcohol} = \text{Grams of alcohol} \div 29.6$$

where % alcohol = proof/2; density of pure alcohol = 0.798 g/ml; and volume (in ml) = volume (in fl oz) × 29.6. By this formula, one mixed drink is equivalent (in alcohol content) to one glass of wine or one can of beer. In taking a drinking history, this quantity is referred to as "one drink."

Alcoholic Beverage Conversion Table

	ALCOHOL CONTENT	
Hard Liquor (vodka, scotch, rum, gin; ~ 80 proof or 40% alcohol)	Gm of alcohol	Fl oz of alcohol
1 Quart	302	10.2
1 Fifth	242	8.2
1 Pint	151	5.1
1 Shot or average drink (1.5 oz, 80 proof)	14	0.5
Wine (~ 12% alcohol; fortified wine is ~ 17% alcohol)		
1 Gallon	363	12.3
1 Liter	96	3.2
1 Pint	45	1.5
1 Glass (5 oz, 150 ml)	14	0.5
Beer (4.8% alcohol)		
1 Case (24 cans, 288 oz)	327	11.0
1 Gallon (128 oz)	145	4.9
1 Six pack (72 oz)	82	2.8
1 Quart (32 oz)	36	1.2
1 Pint (16 oz)	18	0.6
1 Can (12 oz)	14	0.5

3. Are there cofactors or complications to alcohol use that worsen the course of ALD?

Malnutrition: In the absence of alcohol consumption, malnutrition does not cause cirrhosis. At one time, it was thought that the poor diets of many alcoholics was the cause of their liver disease, leading to the term **nutritional cirrhosis** to describe the hepatic lesion found in these patients. It has now been clearly demonstrated that alcohol can cause liver disease in baboons and humans who are well nourished. Nevertheless, general malnutrition or deficiencies of specific nutrients may contribute to the development of liver disease. Certainly, poor nutrition complicates the course of ALD and can have specific effects on several extrahepatic organs.

Hepatitis virus infection: Hepatitis B and C viruses can both cause chronic infection, leading to chronic active hepatitis. When these occur together with ALD, progression of the liver injury is more rapid and the risk of hepatocellular carcinoma is greater than with either ALD or chronic viral hepatitis alone. Because hepatitis C virus and alcohol are both common causes of liver disease, they are often found together in the same patient. It is particularly important that persons with hepatitis infection stop all alcohol consumption, thereby removing one of the hepatotoxins.

Note that not all liver disease in drinkers is caused by alcohol. Just because ALD is common and a person gives a history consistent with alcohol abuse, do not assume that liver enzyme abnormalities are due to alcohol until other diseases have been ruled out.

4. What do you say when a family member tells you that their mother can't have liver disease because they know she never drinks?

There are at least three reasons why you may be faced with this situation.

1. Alcohol is the most common, *but not the only,* **cause of liver disease.** It is a common perception in the community—and even among health professionals—that most or all liver disease is due to alcohol. In particular, hepatitis C virus (HCV) is becoming recognized as a major cause of chronic liver disease. When the biochemical abnormalities are noted incidentally during a health screening, they are often attributed to alcohol. The patient is told to stop drinking, but there is no follow-up to determine whether the enzymes return to normal with abstinence. Prior to there being any treatment, this misdiagnosis was relatively unimportant, except that the patient was stigmatized as an alcoholic. Now that interferon is available, correct diagnosis of hepatitis C is important so that treatment can be tried if the patient wants it.

HCV has been emphasized because of its high prevalence. Coupled with the frequency of alcohol consumption, it is inevitable that many people with hepatitis C will also drink alcohol on occasion on purely statistical grounds. Similarly, the high prevalence of social alcohol consumption means that most people with liver disease of any etiology will also drink alcohol. Even with an apparently compelling history of heavy alcohol use, one must eliminate other liver diseases before settling on alcohol as the etiologic agent.

2. Drinking histories are notoriously inaccurate. According to an old-rule-of-thumb, one can accurately estimate alcohol consumption by multiplying by five the largest amount of alcohol that the patient admits to drinking. Although this is probably not very accurate either, it emphasizes how inaccurate self-reported drinking histories can be. In a patient with liver disease that appears to be ALD by objective criteria (*see* Question 7), do not eliminate ALD from the differential diagnosis just because the patient gives an apparently benign alcohol history. Talking to family, friends, and coworkers can reveal a startlingly different drinking history. However, be aware that some people you question might themselves be heavy drinkers or enablers who lie to "protect" your patient or cover their own drinking habits. Alternatively, your patient may have hidden heavy drinking even from close relatives, including spouse or children.

3. Hepatic susceptibility to alcohol can vary. Although demographic studies indicate that the risk of ALD is related to the amount of alcohol consumed, there is considerable individual variation in the toxic effects of a given amount of alcohol on the liver and other organs. Only about 10–20% of heavy alcohol users develop cirrhosis, and some individuals develop alcoholic hepatitis and cirrhosis with seemingly innocuous and socially acceptable levels of drinking. This variable susceptibility is due to genetic and environmental differences and probably other factors. Women develop ALD more rapidly than men at the same quantity and duration of alcohol consumption. The best test to determine whether hepatitis in a particular patient is due to alcohol is to have the patient remain abstinent from alcohol and see if their liver disease improves.

5. Describe the differences between fatty liver, alcoholic hepatitis, and cirrhosis.

Fatty liver, hepatitis, and cirrhosis are three types of histologic change in the liver associated with alcohol. However, none of them is pathognomonic for ALD. All three can and usually do occur simultaneously in patients with ALD, but their relative importance in the histologic appearance can be quite variable. Although they are sometimes viewed as a progression of injury, it is now clear that cirrhosis can develop without any clinical evidence of hepatitis. Furthermore, in heavy drinkers without signs or symptoms of liver disease, the liver may appear normal on biopsy.

Fatty liver (steatosis) is characterized by small (microvesicular) or large (macrovesicular) fat droplets in the cytoplasm of hepatocytes. Both can occur in ALD. If inflammation is present, the lesion is referred to as **steatohepatitis.** Fatty liver can occur after consuming as little as 10 oz (240 gm) of alcohol (15–20 mixed drinks, 3 l of wine, or 3 six-packs of beer) over a weekend and is probably present in 90–100% of heavy drinkers (>80 gm of alcohol/day for >5 yrs). It is often accompanied by fibrosis even without evidence of hepatitis. The same lesions can be caused by other diseases or toxins, including chronic active hepatitis C, diabetes mellitus, obesity, and starvation. If inflammation and fat droplets are both present but there is no history of alcohol use, the entity is referred to as **nonalcoholic steatohepatitis** (NASH). Transaminases can be increased to about 10 times the upper limit of normal in both NASH and alcoholic fatty liver.

Alcoholic hepatitis is characterized histologically by hepatocyte necrosis, inflammatory infiltrates (with a predominance of polymorphonuclear leukocytes), and fibrosis. Because *hepatitis* refers generally to liver inflammation, viruses and autoantibodies that affect the liver also cause hepatitis, but the inflammatory pattern tends to be qualitatively different than that due to alcohol. Clinically, patients with alcoholic hepatitis may be asymptomatic and anicteric, or heavily jaundiced with ascites and other evidence of severe portal hypertension. Approximately 40–50% of heavy drinkers develop alcoholic hepatitis at some time during their drinking.

Alcoholic cirrhosis, as with cirrhosis from any cause, is characterized by a diffuse destruction and regeneration of the liver, with an increase in the amount of fibrous tissue relative to the number of hepatocytes. The regeneration is nodular and disorganized, and the normal functional and vascular anatomy is lost. Alcoholic cirrhosis is usually micronodular, with the nodules <3 mm in diameter and completely surrounded by fibrous tissue. The notion of a scar on the liver is useful when describing cirrhosis to patients and their families. By the time cirrhosis develops, it is often difficult to determine the original cause of the liver injury except by history.

6. What in the world are Mallory's bodies?

Mallory's bodies, also called Mallory's or alcoholic hyaline, can occur in other types of liver disease, but they are most often seen and most abundant in ALD. They are eosinophilic, intracellular granules composed of cytokeratins, the intermediate filament proteins. Their presence is suggestive of, but not pathognomonic for, ALD.

7. How can I tell whether a patient's liver disease is caused by alcohol?

History is the most important factor in diagnosing ALD, as it is with many diseases. However, alcoholics are notoriously poor historians, and corroboration of the drinking history from family, friends, and medical records is important.

As with any new patient, you should develop a **differential diagnosis** as you interview and examine the patient, then perform tests to narrow and reorder the list. Acetaminophen in high doses can cause an acute and often fatal liver injury and should be suspected in any patient presenting with evidence of an acute hepatitis. If it is suspected, a serum acetaminophen level should be obtained, and the patient and family should be questioned concerning medications (including nonprescription ones), suicide attempts, and psychiatric illness. Other toxic exposures also need to be considered, and other common causes of liver disease, particularly those due to hepatitis B and C viruses, ruled out. Hemochromatosis is a relatively common cause of cirrhosis but usually causes little or no hepatitis.

There are a number of **objective criteria** that, when present in the proper clinical setting, strongly suggest liver disease due to alcohol. None of these is pathognomonic for ALD.

Diagnostic Features of Alcoholic Liver Disease

	FINDINGS IN ALD	COMMENTS
Biochemical/ hematologic	AST usually greater than ALT (often >2× ALT value)	Can also occur in end-stage liver diseases from other causes; ratio inverted in HCV
	GGT is often elevated	Very sensitive but not specific for alcohol, not reflective of severity of hepatic injury
	MCV often increased	Can occur in other liver diseases but is exacerbated by folate and B_{12} deficiencies often seen in alcoholics; iron deficiency plus a reason for macrocytosis can give a normal MCV.
Clinical	Signs of feminization: Spider nevi Gynecomastia Dupuytren's contractures Palmar erythema	Most frequently seen in ALD but can occur in other liver diseases. Dupuytren's contractures related to amount of alcohol consumed, not severity of liver disease. Spironolactone, used to treat ascites, also causes gynecomastia.
	Extrahepatic effects of alcohol: Skeletal muscle wasting Dilative cardiomyopathy Pancreatitis Peripheral neuropathy	All have other causes, but their occurrence in a patient with suspected ALD tends to support a history of alcohol abuse.
Histologic	Mallory's bodies	Occur in other liver disease but most frequently and most abundantly in ALD
	Fat vesicles	Useful in suspected ALD; differential Dx includes obesity, diabetes, HCV, AIDS, drugs, toxins, etc.

GGT = gamma glutamyl transpeptidase; MCV = mean corpuscular volume.

8. Can alcoholic liver disease be treated?

Yes, sort of. The best treatment for ALD is simple **abstinence** and **good nutrition.** The importance of these measures cannot be overemphasized. The trick is getting the patient to take the cure. Patients may give up alcohol for a short time, particularly after a hospitalization for acute alcoholic hepatitis or variceal hemorrhage, but many return to drinking within weeks or months. Aversive therapy with **disulfiram** or **naltrexone,** together with intensive counseling, may improve the rate of abstinence. Nevertheless, because of the high rate of recidivism, research has focused on ways to halt or reverse liver injury in patients who continue to drink, to decrease mortality in patients who already have severe acute or chronic ALD, and to treat the complications of ALD.

At present, there is no therapy having any effect on progression of ALD in patients who continue to drink heavily. If alcohol consumption is reduced but not stopped and good nutritional support is provided, partial hepatitic improvement may occur. A trial currently under way is investigating the possibility that **polyenoylphosphatidylcholine,** a polyunsaturated lecithin, can block progression of or reverse early alcoholic fibrosis. Another ongoing trial is studying the ability of **colchicine** to reduce mortality in patients with alcoholic cirrhosis. **Corticosteroids** have been studied previously, and some trials have shown a small effect on reducing the mortality of acute alcoholic hepatitis (*see* Question 10).

9. Why is the liver the only organ damaged by alcohol?

The answer is, it isn't. Although ALD is the most commonly recognized medical complication of alcohol abuse, virtually every major organ system can suffer alcohol-related injury. As with the liver, there is considerable individual variation in susceptibility of particular organs to alcohol. The liver is more sensitive to alcohol than are other organs, probably because of its central role in metabolism of alcohol to acetaldehyde, which is the compound thought to actually cause liver damage.

Effects of Alcohol on Extrahepatic Organs

ORGAN AFFECTED/INJURY	SYMPTOMS	PROGNOSIS/TREATMENT
Heart		
Alcoholic cardiomyopathy	Related to lifetime alcohol dose; not caused by thiamine deficiency; arrhythmias, dilatation of all 4 heart chambers; low output	Reversible with abstinence in about 30%; with advanced cardiomyopathy, 3-yr survival about 25%
Holiday heart	Arrhythmias occurring after a drinking binge in person with no previous history of heart disease	Reversible with abstinence but can be fatal
Hypertension	Caused by chronic consumption of >3 drinks daily	Severity related to amount of alcohol consumed; reversible after a few weeks of abstinence
Skeletal muscle		
Myopathy	Muscle swelling, tenderness, CK elevation; wasting visible in extremities, abdomen, and temples; related to amount of alcohol consumed; alcohol may be directly myotoxic	Usually reversible with abstinence
Nervous system		
Wernicke's encephalopathy	Ataxia, ophthalmoplegia, global confusion-apathy; caused by thiamine deficiency	Medical emergency; treat with thiamine, 50 mg iv plus 50 mg im; repeat im dose daily until normal diet is resumed; must give thiamine before starting iv glucose to avoid worsening symptoms
Korsakoff's syndrome	Antero- and retrograde amnesias; caused by thiamine deficiency	Often appears as Wernicke's confusion recedes; usually irreversible
Alcohol withdrawal syndrome	Caused by removal of alcohol from neurons that have developed cellular tolerance to alcohol	(*see* Question 27)
Peripheral neuropathy	Occurs in about 5–15% of alcoholics; due to thiamine deficiency and perhaps to direct neurotoxic effect of ethanol	Some symptomatic improvement with abstinence, good nutrition, and thiamine administration
Pancreas		
Acute and chronic pancreatitis	Most common cause in U.S. is alcohol; may be acute, chronic, or both; when exocrine function is <10%, maldigestion, malabsorption, and type I diabetes mellitus are often seen; due to direct toxic effect of alcohol plus probably other mechanisms	Acute pancreatitis treated with abstinence, hydration, and analgesia; chronic pancreatitis can cause chronic pain; exocrine deficiency treated with enzyme replacement; diabetes treated as usual

Effects of Alcohol on Extrahepatic Organs (Continued)

ORGAN AFFECTED/INJURY	SYMPTOMS	PROGNOSIS/TREATMENT
Pancreatic pseudocyst	Develops in setting of pancreatitis; apparently due to autodigestion of tissue; complicated by bleeding or infection	Can be drained endoscopically or surgically; often regress spontaneously with abstinence; bleeding or infection must be treated as appropriate
Reproduction		
Men	Testicular atrophy, infertility; acutely, alcohol increases libido but decreases erectile capacity	Testicular atrophy is irreversible; acute effects resolve with abstinence
Women	Amenorrhea, ovarian shrinkage, infertility, spontaneous abortion	May be partially reversible with abstinence
Fetal alcohol syndrome	Caused by drinking during pregnancy; mental retardation, heart defects, other anatomic abnormalities	Irreversible; no known treatment
Gastrointestinal		
Inflammation	Esophagitis, gastritis; gastritis most common cause of bleeding in alcoholics	Principal treatment for all alcohol-related GI disease is abstinence; acid suppression may also be helpful for gastritis and esophagitis
Small intestine	Local hemorrhage, malabsorption, diarrhea	
Malignancy	Risk of malignancy 10-fold higher in alcoholics; sites with greatest increase over expected rates are head and neck, esophagus, liver, stomach (and perhaps breast)	
Hematopoietic/Immune		
Pancytopenia	Marrow suppression by alcohol; decreased platelet survival; deficiencies of B_{12}, folate, and iron due to malabsorption, malnutrition, and chronic blood loss; hypersplenism	Reversible with abstinence; provide good nutrition; treat specific deficiencies; correct sources of blood loss
Immune deficiency	Marrow suppression; malnutrition; frequent infections; direct effects of alcohol on number and function of most types of leukocytes	Reversible with abstinence and good nutrition

10. Which patient groups can be given corticosteroids?

A number of clinical trials have investigated the use of corticosteroids (primarily prednisone or prednisolone) in treating acute alcoholic hepatitis. Use of these medications is based on the inflammatory nature of the disease and the hypothesized role of immunologic factors. Although results of individual trials are contradictory, corticosteroids do seem to reduce short-term mortality in patients with acute alcoholic hepatitis without causing significant side effects or increasing the risk of infection. The benefit is relatively small, however, and treatment should be used only for a subgroup of patients, who can be identified by an empirically derived **discriminant function:**

$$4.6 \times (PT - \text{control time}) + (\text{serum bilirubin})/17$$

where prothrombin time (PT) and control time are measured in seconds and serum bilirubin is expressed as μmol/L. (For serum bilirubin expressed in mg/dl, do not divide by 17.) Patients with a discriminant function >32 showed significantly longer survival at 1 and 6 months after treatment than did matched controls who received placebo. Some studies have also suggested that patients with portosystemic encephalopathy also benefit from treatment. Patients who were less ill, with lower discriminant functions or without encephalopathy, did no better than matched patients who received placebo. Whether long-term survival or progression of alcoholic hepatitis to cirrhosis is affected by this treatment is not known. Patients with GI bleeding or intercurrent infections should *not* be treated with corticosteroids.

Treatment consists of 40 mg of prednisolone a day orally for 4 weeks. Methylprednisolone is used at a dose of 32 mg/day because of its greater potency and molecular weight. Although prednisone is metabolized by the liver to prednisolone, the active form, this conversion is only minimally reduced even in severe liver disease. Consequently, prednisone, which is less expensive and more readily available, can be used instead of prednisolone without changing the dosing.

11. What is the role of liver transplantation in treating ALD?

Liver transplantation is the treatment of last resort for hepatic failure due to alcoholic cirrhosis. It is not appropriate for treatment of alcoholic hepatitis, which is reversible with abstinence, or for alcoholics who are actively drinking. Several studies have now shown that the short- and long-term outcomes of transplants done in patients with endstage ALD are identical to the outcomes in patients transplanted for non-ALD. Recidivism post-transplant is low and is inversely correlated with the length of time pretransplant that the patient had been abstinent from alcohol.

12. List the major complications of ALD, and describe their pathophysiology.

Much of the morbidity and mortality of ALD is caused by systemic consequences of the hepatic injury. Most complications of ALD are related to one of two mechanisms: (1) obstruction of normal blood flow through the liver resulting in **portal hypertension,** or (2) hepatocellular dysfunction and necrosis leading to the **reduction in functional hepatocyte mass.** Both can occur in either alcoholic hepatitis or alcoholic cirrhosis and in liver disease due to other causes.

Major Complications of ALD

PORTAL HYPERTENSION	REDUCED FUNCTIONAL MASS
Ascites	Hepatic (portal-systemic) encephalopathy
Spontaneous bacterial peritonitis	Coagulopathy
Esophageal and gastric varices	Hypoalbuminemia
Hypersplenism	

In alcoholic hepatitis, fibrosis around the central vein and in the hepatic sinusoids, hepatic engorgement due to inflammation, and loss of hepatocytes due to necrosis increase resistance to blood flow through the liver. In cirrhosis, intrahepatic resistance is increased by extensive disruption of normal hepatic architecture and replacement of hepatocytes by fibrous scar tissue. In either case, **portal hypertension** elevates the pressure throughout the vascular tree upstream from the portal vein, causing ascites formation and drastically increasing blood flow through alternative pathways with consequent development of esophageal and gastric varices and hypersplenism.

In alcoholic hepatitis and cirrhosis, **functional liver cell mass** is severely reduced owing to hepatocyte dysfunction caused by inflammation or to replacement of hepatocytes by fibrous tissue. Because the liver has a large functional reserve, 70–80% of the parenchymal cells must be compromised before clinical complications occur. The most important complications are hepatic encephalopathy, coagulopathy, and hypoalbuminemia.

13. How is ascites managed in ALD?

Ascites refers to the accumulation of serous fluid in the abdomen. Although the most common cause is portal hypertension, it can also result from carcinomatosis, tuberculosis, pancreatic disease, renal failure, and congestive heart failure. Alcoholics are at increased risk for all of these.

Even when the etiology seems obvious, the underlying cause must be determined, because in each case, management is different. New-onset ascites should *always* be sampled by diagnostic paracentesis to aid in determining the underlying cause. If there is a sudden increase in ascites in an otherwise well-compensated alcoholic cirrhotic, the cause should be investigated. Each time a cirrhotic patient with ascites is hospitalized, paracentesis should be done and the ascitic fluid evaluated for spontaneous bacterial peritonitis.

For control of ascites due to cirrhosis, the most important considerations are **salt restriction** and **careful diuresis.** Dietary sodium should be <1.5–2 gm/day (or less, in the hospital). Diuresis usually consists of a potassium-sparing diuretic, such as spironolactone or amiloride, together with a loop diuretic such as furosemide. Ideally, one should increase the dose of the potassium-sparing diuretic until urinary Na^+ exceeds urinary K^+ (the opposite of what is seen in normal urine), then add the loop diuretic, if necessary, until adequate diuresis is achieved. In practice, diuresis can be accomplished more rapidly by starting both diuretics simultaneously at daily doses of 100 mg of spironolactone and 40 mg of furosemide, and then increasing these to achieve adequate weight loss. If peripheral edema is present, a high rate of diuresis is safe. If there is no peripheral edema, loss of 2–3 lb of ascites per week is the maximum that should be attempted. Electrolytes must be monitored to avoid either hyper- or hypokalemia, and the ratio of the two drugs adjusted to regulate the electrolytes. The half-life of spironolactone is normally 24 hours and is prolonged in cirrhotics; thus, it is unnecessary to give the drug in divided doses, thereby improving patient compliance. Fluid restriction does not increase the rate of weight loss in patients with ascites, and patients and caretakers find it very unpleasant. Cirrhotics often have a mild hyponatremia that is well tolerated. Only if serum Na falls below 120 mEq/L should fluid restriction be instituted.

In a patient with tense ascites that is symptomatic (respiratory distress, abdominal pain, early satiety), **large-volume paracentesis** can be used to ease the abdominal distention. Although there was concern about precipitating hepatorenal syndrome, recent studies have demonstrated that removal of even 6–8 L can be done safely. Some advocate giving serum albumin or other colloid (e.g., dextran) intravenously during or after large-volume paracentesis, but data are insufficient to know whether this is necessary. If one prefers to give colloid, dextran is much less expensive than serum albumin. The biggest problem with large volume paracentesis is that the fluid usually reaccumulates within a few days or a week.

14. When is spontaneous bacterial peritonitis diagnosed?

Each time a cirrhotic patient with ascites is hospitalized, paracentesis should be done and the ascitic fluid evaluated for spontaneous bacterial peritonitis (SBP). This serious complication of ascites (mortality rate of 30–40%) is diagnosed by finding bacteria, an elevated number of polymorphonuclear (PMN) leukocytes (>250/μl), or both in ascites. Symptoms suggestive of SBP include fever, abdominal pain, and encephalopathy, but 50% of patients have no abdominal signs and up to 30% may have no signs or symptoms at all attributable to SBP. Consequently, a high index of suspicion is necessary to avoid missing the diagnosis. When bacteria are identified, it is usually a single gram-negative aerobic species of gut origin (most often *Escherichia coli* or *Klebsiella* spp.). Anaerobic, fungal, or polymicrobial infections suggest a perforated viscus or other cause of secondary peritonitis.

If the ascitic fluid PMN count is >250/μl in the proper clinical setting, and even if bacteria are not present, empiric antibiotic therapy should be initiated with **cefotaxime** or a similar **third-generation cephalosporin.** If bacteria are found, they can be tested for antibiotic sensitivity, allowing coverage to be narrowed. Treatment should be continued until the PMN count is <250/μl or a minimum of 5–7 days. Prophylactic antibiotics given to patients at high risk for initial or recurrent SBP decrease the number of infections but do not change the number of hospitalizations or mortality rate.

15. Describe the management of variceal hemorrhage complicating ALD.

Gastric and esophageal varices are caused by shunting of portal blood through low-pressure veins that normally drain into the portal vein. The reversal of and increase in flow through poorly supported veins in the gastric fundus and distal esophagus cause these veins to swell and burst, resulting in **massive, life-threatening upper GI bleeding.** Bleeding in these patients is usually complicated by coagulopathy and thrombocytopenia. The **coagulopathy** is caused by inadequate synthesis of several clotting factors due to liver disease and to vitamin K deficiency related to malnutrition. Thrombopathy or platelet dysfunction may also be present but is probably a minor factor in these bleeding disorders. **Thrombocytopenia** is due to marrow suppression by alcohol, folate deficiency, inhibition of folate utilization by alcohol, reduction of platelet half-life by alcohol, and splenic sequestration of platelets due to splenic congestion from portal hypertension. In bleeding patients who have received crystalloid, erythrocytes, and plasma but not platelets, thrombocytopenia may also be iatrogenic, due to dilution.

Variceal hemorrhage is a medical emergency that should be treated with prompt fluid resuscitation and treatment to halt the bleeding. Care should be taken not to overtransfuse these patients, because this can lead to recurrence of bleeding that may have stopped owing to the drop in blood pressure. The patient should be intubated endotracheally if they are comatose or at other risk for aspiration (e.g., heavily intoxicated or postictal). Infusion of Pitressin (a mixture of lysine- and arginine-vasopressin) should be considered if bleeding persists. Upper GI endoscopy should be performed as soon as possible to evaluate, and possibly treat, the source of bleeding. If the source is esophageal varices, sclerotherapy, endoscopic variceal ligation, or both should be used to stop the bleeding. This approach is successful in 90% of patients. If endoscopic therapy is unsuccessful, alternatives include a Sengstaken-Blakemore tube to tamponade the varices (a temporizing measure), fluoroscopic embolization of vessels feeding the varices, a portosystemic shunt to decompress the portal vein and decrease flow through the varices, or devascularization to eliminate the variceal veins and the vessels feeding them.

16. What shunt procedures are used for treatment of variceal bleeding?

A number of operations are available for surgical management of varices following failure of endoscopic treatment. The most widely used procedure is the **distal splenorenal shunt,** a partial portosystemic shunt that reduces hepatic vein pressure gradient to about 12 mm Hg (normal, ~3–7 mm Hg) while maintaining hepatic portal perfusion. The principal complications of this and other shunts are progressive loss of liver function and increased risk of encephalopathy, both of which are related to loss of hepatic portal perfusion. Perfusion is initially maintained in 90% of alcoholics treated with the distal splenorenal shunt, but it is lost in 50% within 6–12 months, often leading to the complications mentioned.

In recent years, a nonsurgical procedure, **transvenous intrahepatic portosystemic shunt** (TIPS), has proved useful in managing portal hypertension. Advantages include its safety of placement in extremely ill patients with a high surgical risk of bleeding and other complications. To place the shunt, a catheter is passed from the internal jugular vein, through the vena cava, and into the hepatic vein under fluoroscopic guidance. A needle is then pushed through the hepatic parenchyma from a branch of the hepatic vein into a branch of the portal vein, and an expandable metal mesh stent (Wall stent) is deployed along the path of the needle to maintain the fistula connecting the two circulations. The principal complications are the same as for surgical shunts. TIPS can also be used to control ascites that is refractory to diuresis, although it is not usually a permanent solution to these problems. It is useful primarily as a temporary measure for management of patients who are awaiting liver transplantation.

17. Can preventive measures be taken to avoid bleeding from varices?

Initial bleeding from varices occurs in only about 30% of patients within 2 years after identification of the varices. This rate can be reduced to 20% by treatment with nonselective β-adrenergic antagonists (β-blockers). Ideally, the dose should be adjusted to achieve a hepatic vein pressure gradient of <12 mm Hg. If this measurement is not available, a daily dose of 40 mg of propranolol is safe and efficacious.

Once bleeding has occurred, the risk of rebleeding can be as high 70%. Long-term management can be accomplished by repeated sclerotherapy or ligation until the varices are no longer evident endoscopically. Reduction of portal pressure by construction of a portosystemic shunt or by treatment with β-blockers as described for prophylaxis of variceal bleeding also reduces the risk of rebleeding.

18. Describe the pathogenesis and management of hepatic encephalopathy.

Hepatic encephalopathy refers to mental dysfunction occurring in the setting of liver disease. The most common form, portal-systemic encephalopathy (PSE), is nearly always found in patients with cirrhosis and portal hypertension and apparently is caused by accumulation in the blood and brain of nitrogenous waste (probably ammonia and amines) normally cleared by the liver. This accumulation occurs because of loss of hepatic metabolism and because of shunting of portal blood through venous collaterals into the systemic circulation, bypassing the liver. Levels of venous ammonia, although often moderately elevated, correlate poorly with the degree of mental dysfunction. Arterial or CSF ammonia concentrations or CSF glutamine levels show better correlation with the degree of CNS suppression but are often not readily measurable. For this reason, the diagnosis of PSE is best made on clinical grounds. PSE is usually precipitated by ingestion of protein(via a meal or due to GI bleeding), infections (e.g., spontaneous bacterial peritonitis), or dehydration due to overdiuresis. *Helicobacter pylori* may increase the risk of PSE because of its ability to release ammonia from urea.

Treatment of PSE consists of correcting the precipitating event and administering lactulose, a disaccharide that promotes the fecal elimination of ammonia and amines. Lactulose also lowers luminal pH, protonating and trapping ammonia and amines, and stimulates bacterial fixation of ammonia. Neomycin, an antibiotic that is not absorbed from the gut, can also be used. It works by killing the intestinal bacteria that degrade protein to ammonia and amines.

Pseudo-PSE is a mental dysfunction clinically indistinguishable from PSE. Although it can occur in the absence of liver disease, it is seen most often in cirrhotics, particularly those with portosystemic shunting. It is caused by decreased clearance of sedatives, analgesics, or tranquilizing drugs or by development of metabolic abnormalities such as alkalosis, acidosis, or hypoglycemia. Serum ammonia concentration is normal in pseudo-PSE. Treatment consists of avoiding offending medications or correcting the underlying disorder. Because pseudo-PSE occurs in the same patients who are susceptible to PSE, a mixed disorder is relatively common, and both causes for altered mental function must be treated.

19. What causes coagulopathy in ALD?

Coagulopathy results from decreased synthesis of functional clotting factors due to liver disease and vitamin K deficiency. Polypeptides for clotting factors II, VII, IX, and X are synthesized in the liver but do not become active until specific glutamate residues have been γ-carboxylated in a vitamin K-requiring enzymatic reaction. This reaction is competitively inhibited by warfarin, used to treat disorders causing hypercoagulability. In ALD, synthesis of these factors can be impaired by malnutrition (inadequate supplies of amino acids and vitamin K) or by loss of functional hepatocytes to synthesize and activate the factors and to store vitamin K.

The first step in treatment is to administer 10 mg of vitamin K subcutaneously. Administration of vitamin K allows γ-carboxylation to proceed, and there is rapid release of the factors with partial or complete correction of the coagulopathy. If this does not occur, then too little functional liver is left to synthesize the factors or malnutrition is so severe that supply of amino acids is insufficient to support peptide synthesis. Treatment consists of improvement of nutrition and elimination of alcohol from the diet. Liver transplantation may ultimately be the only way to correct the problem. In a patient who is bleeding, transfusion of fresh frozen plasma will correct the coagulopathy and may help to stop the hemorrhage. However, this is only a short-term solution because the clotting factors disappear rapidly from the circulation and the coagulopathy returns.

20. Can hypoalbuminemia complicating ALD be treated medically?

Hypoalbuminemia is due to decreased hepatic synthesis and secretion of albumin, the principal protein in serum. Because serum albumin is a key protein for maintaining serum oncotic pressure, when the albumin concentration decreases, water tends to move out of serum and into tissues (edema) or into the peritoneal space (ascites). Total serum calcium (but not ionized Ca^{2+}) also falls, as do serum concentrations of the many other substances transported bound to albumin. As with the coagulopathy associated with ALD, hypoalbuminemia is due to the loss of functional hepatic parenchyma and malnutrition. Infusion of albumin increases the serum albumin concentration and can help mobilize ascites, but the half-life of albumin is short and it is an expensive and transient therapy. Good nutrition and abstention from alcohol are the best treatments, particularly if the hypoalbuminemia is due to alcoholic hepatitis. In chronic alcoholics with endstage liver disease, liver transplantation is the only effective therapy.

21. My patient with ALD wants to know how long he has to live. What should I tell him?
The answer depends on the extent of injury and on whether the patient stops drinking and improves his diet. The most important thing to emphasize to your patient is that while no one can predict life expectancy, abstinence from alcohol is the single factor most likely to prolong his life. He needs to understand that this is not because alcohol is intrinsically bad or evil, but because it is the principal factor causing damage to the liver and other organs. Continued exposure to alcohol is associated with the progression of ALD, whereas elimination of alcohol from the diet generally arrests progression and often produces regression of ALD. Once this is understood, the question becomes one of correlating the extent of existing hepatic injury with its likely effect on lifespan (see question 22).

22. Are the histologic changes in the liver associated with ALD reversible?
    Fatty liver is completely reversible with abstinence from alcohol, and there is no good evidence that it is a precursor to more serious forms of ALD. However, fatty liver is very often accompanied by early fibrosis, which is likely to presage more advanced fibrotic changes and cirrhosis if alcohol consumption continues. Abstinence in these patients will likely allow their livers to return entirely to normal, and their life expectancy may not have been shortened.
    Alcoholic hepatitis is also generally reversible with abstinence. However, because alcoholic hepatitis can cause portal hypertension, severe coagulopathy, and other life-threatening complications, it is far from a benign lesion. In cases severe enough to require hospitalization, 1-month mortality can approach 50%, particularly if the patient continues to drink. In addition, alcoholic hepatitis is clearly a precursor to cirrhosis. Patients with alcoholic hepatitis but without cirrhosis have a very good prognosis if they survive the acute illness and do not return to drinking.
    Alcoholic cirrhosis, as with cirrhosis from other causes, is usually irreversible. In heavy drinkers, though, it often is associated with alcoholic hepatitis, which is reversible with abstinence from alcohol. If a patient with alcoholic hepatitis and cirrhosis stops drinking, the inflammatory lesion will gradually resolve, and the cirrhotic lesion will probably not progress. If this occurs while there is some residual liver function, prognosis is fairly good. In patients with alcoholic cirrhosis who have stopped drinking and who have not suffered a major complication of their liver disease (jaundice, ascites, variceal bleeding), 5-year survival is 80–90%. These patients have **compensated cirrhosis.** If a patient stops drinking after complications have occurred, the 5-year survival is reduced to about 60%. **Decompensation** is said to occur when complications develop. If this happens in a previously stable, abstinent cirrhotic, the cause for decompensation should be sought. It may be as simple as a resumption of drinking or a dietary indiscretion (consumption of a large amount of sodium or protein), but it can also be related to development of a hepatoma, portal vein thrombosis, or other unexpected events. Simultaneous infection with hepatitic C virus significantly worsens the prognosis for alcoholic cirrhosis.

23. What analgesics can safely be prescribed in patients with ALD?
Alcoholics often request analgesics for the usual aches and pains as well as for alcoholic-specific ones, such as those from falls, fights, hangovers, pancreatitis, and vague gastric and abdominal complaints. Although you may meet some of these complaints with limited sympathy and a recommendation to stop drinking, the pains are still real. Patients will use whatever they can find unless you can give them some guidelines as to what is best.

Aspirin, NSAIDs	Avoid.
Acetaminophen	Probably safe in total daily doses ≤2 gm.
Codeine, opiate agonists	Safe to use but reserved for severe cases.

24. Why is aspirin unsafe?

Aspirin and nonsteroidal anti-inflammatory drugs (NSAIDs), such as ibuprofen, can cause gastrointestinal bleeding. Because active alcoholics with or without liver disease may have a bleeding disorder, these medications should be avoided. In addition, because they reduce prostaglandin synthesis, they can decrease renal perfusion and precipitate clinical renal disease in patients with hepatic dysfunction, heart failure, or on diuretics. Some NSAIDs can also affect hepatic function. In general, patients with ALD should avoid aspirin and NSAIDs, including over-the-counter compounds that contain aspirin as one component (they need to read the label).

25. At what dose is acetaminophen hepatotoxic?

Acetaminophen in large single doses (>7.5 gm) is hepatotoxic in nonalcoholics, and doses >20 gm can cause fulminant hepatic failure and death. When large amounts of acetaminophen are ingested, a normally minor metabolite, generated by oxidation of acetaminophen by cytochrome P450 2E1, accumulates within the hepatocyte and severely depletes glutathione stores. Glutathione protects against oxidative injury, and its loss leads to hepatocellular necrosis and can cause hepatic failure and death.

Alcoholics appear to be more sensitive to acetaminophen hepatotoxicity than nonalcoholics, and relatively small (therapeutic) doses of 2–10 gm/day can cause serious liver damage or death. Reasons for the increased susceptibility may include induction of cytochrome P450 2E1 by alcohol and depletion of glutathione by poor nutrition and direct effects of alcohol metabolism. Pre-existing ALD may also increase susceptibility, although nonalcoholic liver disease does not appear to carry the same risk. Alcohol abusers should be counseled strongly not to use more than 2 gm of acetaminophen per day and to watch for over-the-counter medications that contain acetaminophen as one component. Despite these concerns, acetaminophen is probably the best analgesic for relief of minor pain or inflammation in most patients with ALD.

26. When are narcotic analgesics indicated?

Codeine and other **opiate agonists,** such as Demerol, morphine, and Dilaudid, can all be used in patients with ALD. Codeine is the mildest of the narcotic analgesics and is useful by itself or in combination with acetaminophen for relief of mild to moderate pain in these patients. Other than narcotic dependence and abuse, the principal side effects of codeine are constipation and GI distress. These problems can be very significant, however, and codeine should be reserved for situations in which acetaminophen is inadequate or unsafe. Other opiate agonists are generally much more potent and should be used only for severe pain. Because liver disease increases the half-life of these drugs, dose adjustment may be necessary. Opiate agonists are one cause of pseudo-PSE.

27. What is the alcohol withdrawal syndrome (AWS)?

Symptoms of Alcohol Withdrawal Syndrome

STAGE	PRINCIPAL SYMPTOMS	APPROX. TIME AFTER LAST DRINK THAT STAGE APPEARS
I	Insomnia, anxiety, hyperactivity, nausea	5–10 hrs
II	Constant tremor, hallucinations (auditory or visual; clear sensorium), hypertension, tachycardia, fever, tachypnea, diaphoresis	6–30 hrs
III	Withdrawal seizures—usually 1–4 seizures; develop in about 5% of untreated patients; nearly always precede DTs	8–48 hrs
IV	Delirium tremens (DTs)—delirium, clouded sensorium, disorientation, auditory and visual hallucinations, hypertension, paranoia; 5% of untreated patients have DTs; mortality is ~ 5%–15%, usually due to comorbidity.	3–5 days (up to 12 days)

AWS is a complex of symptoms associated with a sudden decrease in blood alcohol level (BAL) in a person with cellular alcohol dependence. In this group, there has been neuronal adaptation to high circulating concentrations of ethanol; the cells *require* a certain BAL to function normally. When the BAL falls too low, symptoms of AWS begin to appear. An individual patient usually does not develop all of the symptoms, and in most, the clinical course is mild. The most severe type of withdrawal symptoms are **delirium tremens,** or DTs. Cellular dependence is distinct from psychological dependence, in which the patients feels "uncomfortable" without alcohol.

Cellular dependence on alcohol depends on the amount and duration of alcohol consumption. The threshold for onset of dependence is approximately 10–12 drinks daily for 2 or 3 weeks. The severity of withdrawal increases as the number of drinks and the duration of drinking increase. Most alcoholics probably experience mild withdrawal symptoms every morning after being without alcohol overnight. An "eye-opener" drink in the morning helps to relieve these symptoms. Abstinence for 12 hours usually leads to tremor, jitters, and an intense craving for a drink. Only about 5% of alcohol abusers develop severe withdrawal symptoms, particularly DTs. Persistent withdrawal symptoms, including depression, anxiety, insomnia, and mild autonomic dysfunction, can last for several weeks or months after discontinuation of drinking; this **protracted withdrawal** may be one factor that contributes to recidivism. Cellular dependence is easily reactivated by resumption of drinking.

28. How does alcohol cause cellular tolerance?
The characteristic signs and symptoms of AWS, such as hypertension, tachycardia, sweating, and tremor, are related to autonomic nervous system hyperactivity. From this has come the concept that chronic exposure to the depressant effects of alcohol causes the CNS to adapt by increasing sympathetic output. As BAL falls, the CNS depression decreases, but the adaptations disappear more slowly, over several weeks. The unbalanced excitatory output causes the symptoms of alcohol withdrawal. Exactly what the adaptive changes are and how alcohol causes them is not completely understood. Alcohol readily dissolves in biologic membranes, and some of its effects may be due to alterations in membrane properties, causing changes in membrane proteins such as ion pumps and neurotransmitter or hormone receptors. For example, alcohol intoxication increases while withdrawal decreases the activity of GABAergic neurons, which exert an inhibitory effect in the CNS. Other excitatory and inhibitory neuronal functions also are affected. Norepinephrine release is increased by alcohol, and plasma levels of norepinephrine and its metabolites are elevated during alcohol intoxication and withdrawal.

29. Distinguish between a hangover and acute alcohol withdrawal.
Hangover is a term used to describe the post-intoxication state. It can occur in light or moderate drinkers after consumption of 5–7 drinks over 1–2 hours. The type of drink, environment, and individual factors influence whether a hangover develops. Headache followed by nausea and vomiting were the most common symptoms of hangover in the only carefully done epidemiologic study that has been published. These symptoms are less common in acute AWS, and headache, in particular, may be clinically useful for distinguishing hangover from AWS.

Acute alcohol withdrawal requires chronic alcohol consumption and is caused by alcohol withdrawal from neurons that have developed cellular tolerance. It does not depend on type of beverage or drinking pattern. Headache is an uncommon symptom in acute AWS.

30. A 55-year-old known alcoholic is admitted, comatose, to your medical service. He has a BAL of 70 mg/dl, a urine screen positive for cocaine metabolites, an AST of 224, and a cut on the forehead. Why is he comatose?
Because this is a known alcoholic, it is unlikely that he will be acutely intoxicated with a BAL of only 70 mg/dl. It is more likely that the patient is experiencing AWS, has had a seizure, and is postictal. The head wound could be the consequence of a seizure. Cardiac arrhythmias are frequent during AWS and could have caused the loss of consciousness.

In general, unconsciousness with a BAL $>\sim300$ mg/dl should suggest **acute intoxication**. If BAL is $<\sim50$, then a **complication of AWS** should be considered as the cause for the coma. These rough guidelines are most useful if it is known whether the patient is an alcohol abuser. Cellular tolerance permits a chronic drinker to be awake with a much higher BAL than is possible in a naive drinker. Clinically, symptoms of alcohol intoxication include sedation, euphoria, ataxia, memory loss, poor judgment, nausea, vomiting, and obtundation. Alcoholics who are in withdrawal are in a state of sympathetic excitation, with hypervigilance, nervousness, and hyperventilation. However, because AWS is related to a *fall* in BAL rather than its absolute value, intoxication and withdrawal in some cases can coexist.

Another possible cause for unconsciousness is that the patient may have **fallen down** while drunk and knocked himself out, with a resultant head wound. While he was unconscious, his BAL could have fallen to the observed level. Other considerations or possible causes of unconsciousness include **intracranial hemorrhage** (caused by head trauma), **hepatic encephalopathy** (due to liver disease), **drug overdose** or combined **drug-alcohol intoxication** (suggested by cocaine in the urine), **cardiac arrhythmias** or **acute myocardial infarction** (due to cocaine), **hypo- or hyperglycemia** (due to chronic alcoholism with or without diabetes), or **meningitis** (risk increased owing to immune suppression by alcohol and malnutrition). More than one of these problems may be present, and furthermore, it may be more difficult to distinguish between acute intoxication and AWS if any of these disorders is also present. Careful thought and testing are necessary to decide on appropriate management, which may make the difference between life and death.

31. What are the major medical complications of alcohol withdrawal?

Alcohol withdrawal seizures, or "rum fits," are associated with a falling or low BAL. They occur in about 5% of withdrawing alcoholics, usually starting about 8–12 hours after the last drink and peaking at 24–48 hours. Withdrawal seizures are usually generalized, and their occurrence corresponds to the peak of withdrawal-related EEG changes. Perhaps 3% of seizures evolve into status epilepticus. In addition to the usual acute dangers of any grand mal seizure, patients who have a withdrawal seizure are much more likely to progress to DTs. Withdrawal seizures usually can be prevented by benzodiazepine loading. Phenytoin by itself is not effective for preventing withdrawal seizures, but in patients with a history of epilepsy or focal seizures or if multiple withdrawal seizures or status epilepticus occurs, addition of phenytoin may be beneficial. However, the half-life of phenytoin is highly variable in alcoholics and blood levels must be monitored closely.

Delirium tremens is the least common but most dangerous form of alcohol withdrawal. The defining symptom is **delirium** (delusions, agitation, disorientation, disorganized thinking, and vivid visual, auditory, and tactile hallucinations). Autonomic hyperactivity often also is present. The first occurrence of DTs is usually in men over age 30 with a history of 5–15 years of heavy drinking. Most episodes of DTs are single and last about 2–3 days. Incidence is increased by withdrawal seizures, other illnesses (pancreatitis, infections, trauma, gastritis), and a previous history of DTs. Reported mortality from DTs in recent literature ranges from about 1%–20%, with the lower numbers for patients without other illnesses. The presence of comorbidities markedly increases the risk of death and is the major cause of mortality in patients with DTs.

32. How do you treat DTs?

As with most alcohol-related illness, abstinence, good nutrition, and supportive medical care are the most important components of treatment. However, DTs constitute a **medical emergency,** requiring hospitalization and a complete evaluation with a thorough history and physical examination. Most patients entering withdrawal are adequately hydrated or overhydrated, and intravenous fluid is not needed. Metabolic and electrolyte abnormalities should be corrected. Thiamine (50 mg intravenously and 50 mg intramuscularly) should be given immediately.

The best treatment for DTs is **prevention.** Alcoholics who have stopped drinking recently or who are in early withdrawal should be treated prospectively with a CNS depressant that replaces the depressant effects of alcohol. **Benzodiazepines** are the drugs of choice, providing the best combination of efficacy and safety. Diazepam and chlordiazepoxide are usually preferred for their long half-lives, which avoid rapid fluctuations in blood level of the drug, providing better control of withdrawal symptoms. A loading dose is administered on the first day that is sufficient to control withdrawal symptoms. For mild withdrawal, typical oral or intravenous doses are 25–50 mg of chlordiazepoxide or 5–10 mg of diazepam every 4–6 hours. Higher and more frequent doses are needed for moderate and severe withdrawal. The dose is then reduced each day until it reaches zero by day 4 or 5. Careful monitoring reduces the likelihood of complications during loading, particularly at very high doses of benzodiazepines. Although this protocol provides good control of mild to moderate AWS, data are lacking that demonstrate its efficacy in preventing DTs.

If a patient presents with DTs, the best treatment is less clear. Although large doses of benzodiazepines are usually administered, the patient may remain awake and agitated. At this point, treatment is usually given to control symptoms since there is no effective way to shorten the course of or terminate the DTs. Haloperidol is useful for sedation but should be used carefully (in conjunction with benzodiazepines) because it can lower the seizure threshold. Butyrophenone antipsychotics are helpful for controlling the thought disorders and severe agitation. Ultimately, supportive care, treatment of comorbidities, and time for the delirium to run its course are the best means to manage this serious manifestation of the AWS.

BIBLIOGRAPHY

1. Bird RD, Makela EH: Alcohol withdrawal: What is the benzodiazepine of choice? Ann Pharmacother 28:67–71, 1994.
2. Bloor JH, Mapoles JE, Simon FR: Alcoholic liver disease: New concepts of pathogenesis and treatment. Adv Intern Med 39:49–92, 1994.
3. Eighth Special Report to the U.S. Congress on Alcohol and Health. Rockville, MD, U.S. Dept. of Health and Human Services, 1993.
4. Gilbert JA, Kamath PS: Spontaneous bacterial peritonitis: An update. Mayo Clin Proc 70:365–370, 1995.
5. Henderson JM: Surgical management of portal hypertension. In Schiff L, Schiff ER (eds): Diseases of the Liver, 7th ed. Philadelphia, J.B. Lippincott, 1993, pp 974–989.
6. Imperiale TF, McCullough AJ: Do corticosteroids reduce mortality from alcoholic hepatitis? A meta-analysis of the randomized trials. Ann Intern Med 113:299–307, 1990.
7. Lieber CS: Alcohol and the liver: 1994 update. Gastroenterology 106:1085–1105, 1994.
8. Lucey MR, Merion RM, Beresford TP: Liver Transplantation and the Alcoholic Patient. Cambridge, Cambridge University Press, 1994.
9. Ramond MJ, Poynard T, Reuff B, et al: A randomized trial of prednisolone in patients with severe alcoholic hepatitis. N Engl J Med 326:507–512, 1992.
10. Romach MK, Sellers EM: Management of the alcohol withdrawal syndrome. Annu Rev Med 42:323–340, 1991.
11. Rosman AS, Lieber CS: Diagnostic utility of laboratory tests in alcoholic liver disease. Clin Chem 40:1641–1651, 1994.
12. Seef LB, Cuccherini BA, Zimmerman HJ, et al: Acetaminophen hepatotoxicity in alcoholics. A therapeutic misadventure. Ann Intern Med 104:399–404, 1986.
13. Smith CM, Barnes GM: Signs and symptoms of hangover: Prevalence and relationship to alcohol use in a general adult population. Drug Alcohol Depend 11:249–269, 1983.
14. Turner RC, Lichstein PR, Peden JG Jr, et al: Alcohol withdrawal syndromes: A review of pathophysiology, clinical presentation, and treatment. J Gen Intern Med 4:432–444, 1989.
15. Zimmerman HJ, Maddrey WC: Acetaminophen (Paracetamol) hepatotoxicity with regular intake of alcohol: Analysis of instances of therapeutic misadventure. Hepatology 22:767–773, 1995.

25. VASCULAR LIVER DISEASE

Bahri M. Bilir, M.D., and Nuray Bilir, M.D., M.S.

1. Describe the important vascular anatomy of the liver.

The liver constitutes 5% of the body weight in adults. Despite this fact, it receives 20% of the cardiac output via the hepatic artery and portal vein. The **hepatic artery** is a branch of the hepaticoduodenal artery from the celiac axis. It carries approximately 30% of the afferent flow but delivers more than 50% of the oxygen utilized at the resting state.

The **portal vein** is a valveless vein that carries 70–80% of the total liver blood flow and delivers a little less than 50% of the oxygen needed. It is formed at the level of the pancreas by the splenic veins joining the superior mesenteric vein. At the liver hilum, both the portal vein and hepatic artery divide into right and left branches and subdivide further up to the level of the porta hepatis. Both hepatic arterioles and portal venules drain into the sinusoids from this point on. At this level, hepatic arteries have sphincters that dynamically regulate the blood flow. There are also sphincters within the sinusoid that help regulate the blood flow and distribution. These sphincters are very important in the physiologic regulation of blood flow to the liver through the hepatic artery. A reduction in portal vein flow will lead to an immediate increase in hepatic arterial flow. Despite this, portal vein flow is relatively constant and is not influenced by the hepatic arterial flow.

At the end of the sinusoid, blood enters into the central venule, which forms the hepatic venule. There are three major **hepatic veins:** right, middle, and left. The branches of these three main hepatic veins have a distribution that is quite different from the distribution of the hepatic artery and portal vein. Therefore, surgical and vascular anatomy of the liver differs from the four macroscopic lobes (right, left, caudate, and quadrate lobes). Vascular anatomy, as described by Coinaud, divides the liver into eight segments (see figure below). Each of these eight segments has its own afferent and efferent blood supply. This anatomy is particularly important in the resection of liver masses. It is also important to know that the caudate lobe is drained through a variable number of small veins (dorsal hepatic veins) that directly enter into the superior vena cava. This is important in understanding the compensatory hypertrophy of the caudate lobe in Budd-Chiari syndrome.

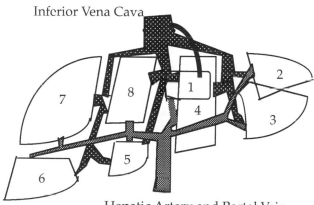

Vascular and surgical anatomy of the liver. According to Coinaud, there are eight functional segments in the liver. These segments receive blood supply via the portal vein and hepatic artery. Efferent dainage is through the right, middle, and left hepatic veins. The caudate lobe (segment 1) has a separate and direct outflow to the inferior vena cava via the dorsal hepatic veins. This vascular anatomy is particularly useful in the resection of liver masses.

2. Describe the microarchitecture of the liver, including the microcirculation.

The basic element in the liver's structure is the liver cell plate (see figure below). This plate comprises 15–20 hepatocytes that are lined up between the portal area and hepatic veins. The hepatocytes near the hepatic veins are called perivenular or pericentral hepatocytes. Perivenular hepatocytes are subject to more hypoxia than other hepatocytes because they are at the end of the unidirectional sinusoidal blood flow.

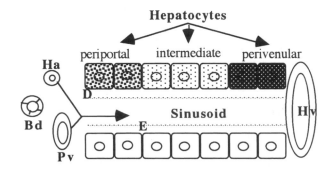

Hepatic microarchitecture. Blood from the portal vein (Pv) and hepatic artery (Ha) join and traverse the sinusoids, eventually leaving the liver from the hepatic venules (Hv). The low pressure circulation in the sinusoids allows the plasma to pass through the fenestrated endothelium (E) and reach the space of Disse (D), where, through direct contact with hepatocytes, exchange of nutrients and metabolites takes place. The hepatocytes near the portal triad are called periportal, and those near the hepatic veins are called perivenular hepatocytes.

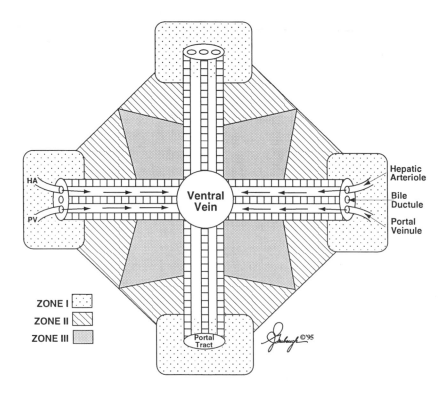

In diseases such as vaso-occlusive disease or Budd-Chiari syndrome, when the outflow tract is occluded, perivenular hepatocytes are the first to be damaged. This area is also known as Zone III in a concept of the liver lobule described by Rappaport (see figure on bottom of p. 182). Zone I hepatocytes in this model are those close to the portal tract and are also referred to as periportal hepatocytes. Zone II or intermediate hepatocytes are between the periportal and perivenular hepatocytes. There are no absolute boundaries between these zones and hepatocytes. The metabolic function of these cells, as well as their susceptibility to injury, changes only gradually depending on their position within the liver cell plate. Zone II and III hepatocytes are involved in drug metabolism and are rich in cytochrome P450 enzymes. Therefore, the toxic effects of most drugs that are metabolized by these microsomal enzymes are seen in Zone II and III hepatocytes, relatively sparing Zone I.

3. What is Budd-Chiari syndrome, and what are the predisposing conditions?

Budd-Chiari syndrome is thrombosis of the hepatic veins. The associated conditions are abdominal trauma; myeloproliferative syndromes; paroxysmal nocturnal hemoglobinuria; conditions associated with lupus, anticoagulants, antithrombin III deficiency, and protein C and S deficiency; tumors of the pancreas, adrenal glands, and kidneys; hepatocellular carcinoma; pregnancy; and drugs that cause hypercoagulability, such as oral contraceptives and dacarbazine. In 25–30% of cases, there may not be an associated cause, and these are considered "idiopathic."

4. What are the symptoms and presenting complaints in Budd-Chiari syndrome?

- **Ascites,** seen in >90% of patients, is the cardinal feature of Budd-Chiari syndrome.
- **Abdominal pain,** seen in up to 80% of patients, is localized to the right upper quadrant.
- **Hepatosplenomegaly** is a common physical finding.
- **Jaundice,** when present, is slight, and it is not a dramatic feature.
- **Hepatic encephalopathy** and **variceal bleeding** are less common (10–20% incidence) and usually are observed late in the course.

5. How is Budd-Chiari syndrome diagnosed?

The diagnosis can be made in about 75% of patients with **Doppler ultrasound** of the hepatic veins. The ultrasound may show the clot in the lumen as echogenic material, decreased or absent flow, or a hyperechogenic cord replacing one or more of the main hepatic veins. Caudate lobe hypertrophy may inaccurately be interpreted as a liver mass. **Hepatic vein catherization** and **angiography** are very sensitive and specific procedures in diagnosing this condition and are accepted as gold standards. They also allow therapeutic measures, such as the use of streptokinase, in acute Budd-Chiari syndrome. **Magnetic resonance angiography** is a research tool that may become a useful noninvasive test in the future.

6. Why do some individuals with Budd-Chiari syndrome get an enlarged caudate lobe of the liver?

Approximately half of the patients with Budd-Chiari syndrome develop a compensatory hypertrophy in the caudate lobe of the liver, because the caudate lobe has separate hepatic veins (dorsal hepatic veins) which drain directly into the inferior vena cava. If the obstruction is below the level of these veins, they remain patent, whereas the hepatic veins draining right and left lobes are thrombosed. The caudate lobe hypertrophies to compensate for the function of the failing liver. This hypertrophy may be very marked and can cause a characteristic indentation in the inferior venogram.

7. Describe the pathologic features of Budd-Chiari syndrome in liver biopsies.

In the acute event, centrilobular congestion and dilatation of the perivenular sinusoid are seen in the liver biopsy. In severe cases, Zone III necrosis may be very evident. Within 4 weeks, centrilobular fibrosis develops, and within 4 months, regenerative nodules and cirrhosis develop. Examination of the hepatic veins and inferior vena cava may show concentric thickening in the vein wall with no inflammation. Subintimal fibrosis as well as an organizing thrombus in the lumen may both contribute to the occlusion of the outflow track.

8. What is the prognosis of Budd-Chiari syndrome, and what are the treatment options?

Treatment of Budd-Chiari syndrome is very much dependent on the acuity of the onset and associated conditions. In acute presentations with clearly documented recent thrombosis (i.e., following abdominal trauma or recurrence of Budd-Chiari after liver transplantation), there is probably a place for heparinization and thrombolytic therapy. Both tissue plasminogen activator and streptokinase have been used with inconclusive results. Percutaneous transluminal and surgical angioplasty have also been tried but initial success was handicapped by a high rate of reclosure.

In patients with myeloproliferative disorders, rapid and aggressive treatments with hydroxyurea and other agents in conjunction with heparinization have provided favorable outcomes. Symptomatic treatments, such as paracentesis and diuretics, are also very useful.

Despite all of these available treatments, the long-term prognosis of Budd-Chiari syndrome remains very poor, and most patients (>90% in one study) die within 3.5 years. The only treatment modality that changed this poor outcome was liver transplantation. Even though it is still controversial, liver transplantation with post-transplant anticoagulation has been used successfully in many institutions, with a 5-year survival rate of over 60%. Some centers, however, report a 20% recurrence rate. If transplantation is not an option, surgical portocaval shunts are among the options, having similar recurrence rates.

9. What is hepatic veno-occlusive disease (VOD)?

Hepatic VOD is the nonthrombotic occlusion of small hepatic veins by connective tissue and collagen. Large-sized hepatic veins are disease-free in VOD. It is associated with centrilobular congestion with or without hepatocellular necrosis. The disease frequently progresses into extensive perivenular fibrosis, central to central bridging, and eventually to cirrhosis.

10. Name the conditions associated with hepatic veno-occlusive diseases.

Ingestion of plants containing pyrrolizidine alkaloids, cancer chemotherapy, bone marrow transplantation, hepatic irradiation, and arsphenamine and urethane therapy have been reported to cause hepatic VOD. The incidence of VOD after bone marrow transplantation varies greatly, from 2–64%, depending on the autologous or allogeneic nature of the transplant and the aggressiveness of induction chemotherapy.

11. When do you suspect hepatic veno-occlusive disease after bone marrow transplantation?

The first signs and symptoms of VOD may appear as early as the first week after exposure to the toxic insult. VOD after bone marrow transplantation presents with weight gain and ascites within the first week or two. Most cases will be diagnosed within 1–2 months. The most common features at presentation are jaundice, hepatomegaly, abdominal pain, and ascites. Transjugular biopsies at this stage are essential in the early diagnosis. The biopsy will show perivenular sinusoidal dilatation, fibrosis, Zone III necrosis, central venular occlusion, and phlebosclerosis.

12. Which cardiac conditions can cause liver dysfunction?

Hepatic congestion has been found in all forms of heart disease, both acquired and congenital, that cause congestive heart failure. Coronary artery disease, hypertension, rheumatic valve disease, cor pulmonale, congenital disease, constrictive pericarditis, scleroderma, and late syphilis have been reported to cause hepatic congestion and dysfunction. The common pathway in the pathogenesis is pump failure, resulting in stasis of flow above the level of the hepatic veins.

13. What are the clinical manifestations of hepatic congestion due to right ventricular failure?

Patients with right ventricular failure may have mild to severe RUQ discomfort and occasional mild jaundice. On physical examination, hepatomegaly with hepatojugular reflux, ascites, and peripheral edema can be found.

14. What kind of liver chemistry abnormalities are found in hepatic congestion?

In acute cardiac failure, such as shock states, the liver can be severely affected. In these cases, very high AST and ALT levels (usually the ALT is higher than AST), increased prothrombin time, and gradually rising bilirubin may be seen. Some patients with shock liver may never recover and may have full clinical and biochemical signs to acute liver failure. In chronic cardiac congestion, AST and ALT levels are slightly elevated, and bilirubin and alkaline phosphatase levels will be high

15. Describe the pathologic changes seen in liver congestion.

Centrilobular congestion manifesting as dilated central vein and sinusoids and drop out of perivenular hepatocytes are typically seen in the liver biopsies. If untreated, the stasis slowly progresses to perivenular fibrosis, bridging fibrosis between the central veins, and eventually cirrhosis. Of note, most patients die of cardiac complications before they develop complications of liver cirrhosis.

16. What is the most common vascular tumor of the liver?

Hemangiomas are the most common vascular tumors of the liver. Autopsy studies suggest that they are present in about 2–5% of the population. The incidence is similar in males and females, except sizes are greater in females, suggesting a proliferative effect of female hormones. Most patients are asymptomatic and do not require treatment. In large hemangiomas, disseminated intravascular coagulation (DIC), thrombocytopenia, and hypofibrinogenemia can occur (Kasabach-Merritt syndrome). The most specific diagnostic technique is ^{99m}Tc-labeled red blood scan, which works best if the hemangioma is >2 cm. In small hemangiomas, MRI or angiography may be helpful. Liver biopsy, unless indicated for another reason, should not be performed. Hemangiomas usually grow very little, if any, in adults. Treatment, which is usually a resection, is reserved for those cases with DIC or bleeding complications.

17. How frequently does angiosarcoma of the liver occur?

It is extremely rare—1 in 50,000 in autopsy studies. It usually occurs in the sixth or seventh decade of life and more often in men than women. Angiosarcomas originate from the endothelial lining of the sinusoid. Histologic examination reveals characteristic spindle-shaped tumor cells with hyperchromatic nuclei. Exposures to Thorotrast (thorium oxide), vinyl chloride, and arsenic are among the predisposing factors. Prognosis in angiosarcoma is dismal, and most patients die within 6 months of diagnosis.

18. Which vascular tumors of the liver synthesize factor VIII-related antigen?

Histologically, these are of two cells types: epithelioid and dendritic. These cells are located in a mixed stroma which is fibrotic and, at times, calcified. Many dendritic cells may have characteristics vacuoles that help in the diagnosis. Most patients present with constitutional symptoms (45%), anorexia, fatigue, and RUQ pain. Alpha fetoprotein is usually normal. Diagnosis is by CT and biopsy. Angiography, if performed, usually reveals a vascular mass, and ^{99m}Tc-tagged red blood cell scan is negative.

Even though in some patients the clinical course is long, it is generally accepted that these tumors, if resectable, should be treated. In nonresectable tumors, liver transplantation has been performed. Recurrence after liver transplantation has also been reported.

19. What are the common causes of portal vein thrombosis?

The most common cause of portal vein thrombosis in children is infectious thrombosis due to omphalitis. In adults, portal vein thrombosis is seen in the low-flow states such as portal hypertension in cirrhosis; hypercoagulable states that are cited in the Budd-Chiari syndrome; surrounding inflammation such as retroperitoneal infections or pancreatitis; or procedure-related traumatic complications such as postoperative or postangiography events.

In the acute phase, patients present with abdominal pain, fever, ileus, and liver failure. In the more chronic form, patients present with ascites, splenomegaly, and variceal bleeding. Portal venography is the diagnostic test of choice. Heparin and thrombolytic agents have been tried in the acute phase, but the success rate is not very good. If the portal vein thrombosis extends to the splenic or superior mesenteric veins, the transplantation becomes technically impossible and prognosis is very poor.

BIBLIOGRAPHY

1. Blendis LM: Circulation in liver disease. Transplant Proc. 25:1741–1743, 1993.
2. Chu G, Farrell GC: Portal vein thrombosis associated with prolonged ingestion of oral contraceptive steroids. J Gastroenterol Hepatol 8:390–393, 1993.
3. Dilawari JB, Bambery P, Chawla Y, et al: Hepatic outflow obstruction (Budd-Chiari syndrome): Experience with 177 patients and review of the literature. Medicine 73:21–36, 1994.
4. Gertsch P, Matthews J, Lerut J, et al: Acute thrombosis of the splanchnic veins. Arch Surg 128:341–345, 1993.
5. Glassman AB, Jones E: Thrombosis and coagulation abnormalities associated with cancer. Ann Clin Lab Sci 24:1–5, 1994.
6. MuCuskey RS, Reilly FD: Hepatic microvasculature: Dynamic structure and its regulation. Semin Liver Dis 13:1–12, 1993.
7. Panis Y, Belghiti J, Valla D, et al: Portosystemic shunt in Budd-Chiari syndrome: Long-term survival and factors affecting shunt patency in 25 patients in Western countries. Surgery 115:276–281, 1994.
8. Shulman HM, et al: Veno-occlusive disease of the liver after marrow transplantation. Histological correlates of clinical signs and symptoms. Hepatology 19:1171–1180, 1994.
9. Toledo-Pereyra LH, Suzuki S: Cellular and biomolecular mechanisms of liver ischemia. Transplant Proc 26:325–327, 1994.

26. LIVER TRANSPLANTATION

Bahri M. Bilir, M.D., and Gregory T. Everson, M.D.

PATIENT REFERRAL AND SELECTION

1. When should a patient with chronic liver disease be referred for liver transplantation?
Several factors must be considered in the timing of hepatic transplantation: the natural history of the underlying disease, effectiveness of nontransplant therapies, rate of disease progression, average waiting time on the transplant list, and availability of donor organs. One major function of the hepatologist is to estimate the patient's 1-year survival based on the known natural history of the underlying liver disease. If the estimated 1-year survival is less than the average 1 year survival after liver transplantation, it is appropriate to proceed with evaluation for transplantation.

Transplantation is indicated in virtually all patients with obvious evidence of end-state-disease (variceal hemorrhage, ascites, hepatorenal syndrome, encephalopathy, spontaneous bacterial peritonitis). Severe fatigue, inability to function, nutritional deterioration, and recalcitrant pruritus may be additional indications to proceed to transplantation. Certain indications may be disease-specific: sustained, severe hyperbilirubinemia in primary biliary cirrhosis, recurrent cholangitis unresponsive to endoscopic or radiologic intervention in primary sclerosing cholangitis, and metabolic bone disease in cholestatic liver disorders.

Donor livers are allocated on the basis of UNOS (United Network of Organ Sharing) status, ABO blood group, recipient body size, and donor liver size. The waiting period for liver transplantation is highly variable. For stable patients, the wait varies from a few months to >1 year. It is extremely important to refer patients for liver transplantation when they develop early signs of decompensation. Donor shortages and expanding waiting lists dictate that early referral will be the only way to reduce mortality in patients on waiting lists.

2. List the diseases for which transplantation is performed.

Indications for Liver Transplantation

Acute liver failure
- Viral hepatitis (A, B, non-A non-B, D, other)
- Drug-induced (acetaminophen, isoniazid, disulfiram, halothane, other)
- Metabolic liver disease (Wilson's disease, Reye's syndrome)
- Vascular (ischemic liver failure)

Chronic liver failure
- Alcoholic cirrhosis
- Post-necrotic cirrhosis (B, C, B+D)
- Chronic active hepatic necrosis (autoimmune, hepatitis C, drug-induced)
- Drug-induced cirrhosis (methotrexate, amiodarone)
- Veno-occlusive disease, Budd-Chiari syndrome
- Extensive polycystic liver disease
- Primary biliary cirrhosis (PBC)
- Primary sclerosing cholangitis (PSC)

Congenital/metabolic liver diseases
- Urea cycle enzyme deficiencies
- Glycogen storage disease
- Tyrosinemia
- Hemochromatosis
- Wilson's disease
- Alpha-1 antitrypsin deficiency
- Crigler-Najjar disease type I
- Hyperlipoproteinemias (type II)

3. A 21-year-old woman is admitted after an overdose of acetaminophen. How do you determine whether she should be referred for liver transplantation?

Acetaminophen is the most commonly diagnosed drug reaction causing severe hepatic injury. Ingestion of >15 gm in patients on no other medications or ingestion of 5–10 gm in patients on medications that induce cytochrome P450 (alcohol, barbiturates, rifampin, benzodiazepines) places the patient at high risk for severe hepatic injury. The blood level of acetaminophen relative to the time of ingestion is highly predictive of severity of injury—a plasma level >300 mg/ml 4 hours after ingestion is highly predictive of hepatic damage. N-acetylcysteine (Mucomyst, 140-mg/kg bolus followed by 70 mg/kg every 4 hours for 17 doses) is effective in preventing or decreasing the amount of hepatocellular necrosis. To be effective, N-acetylcysteine must be administered within 18 hours of the ingestion.

Certain clinical parameters on admission indicate which patients have sustained massive hepatic injury and are unlikely to recover spontaneously: arterial blood pH <7.30, creatinine >3.5 mg/dl, prothrombin time (PT) >100 sec, and grade III or IV encephalopathy. Patients fulfilling the above criteria have a <20% chance of recovery without liver transplantation. Any patient who exhibits any or all of the above signs should be transferred to medical centers capable of performing hepatic transplantation, providing the necessary critical care support, and monitoring intracranial pressure.

4. A 33-year-old man was diagnosed with acute hepatitis A 3 weeks ago. His jaundice worsened. Today, his wife found him to be mildly confused, and she brought him to the emergency room. What is the definition of fulminant hepatic failure?

Fulminant hepatic failure is defined as the onset of encephalopathy within 8 weeks of severe acute hepatic injury in a patient without preexisting liver disease. Causes include viral hepatitis, toxins or drugs, and miscellaneous cases including Budd-Chiari syndrome, hepatic ischemia, Wilson's disease, and hyperthermia. Viral hepatitis is responsible for 50–60% of the reported cases in the United States, with hepatitis A and B accounting for most of these cases. Hepatitis C is extremely uncommon. Non-A, non-B, non-C hepatitis represents 20–40% of all cases due to viral cause. Hepatitis delta and E are uncommon causes of fulminant hepatic failure in the United States.

The most important consideration in managing patients with acute hepatitis is deciding when to refer them to a liver transplant center. Any patient who has greater than grade II encephalopathy should be monitored in a setting where emergency liver transplantation is possible. Patients may progress from stage II to full coma in a matter of a few hours. The criteria commonly accepted for listing the patient for transplantation were developed by O'Grady et al., and any patient fulfilling any of these criteria is at high risk (>80% mortality) and needs to be transferred to a liver transplant center.

- Grade III or IV encephalopathy
- Prothrombin time (PT) >100 sec
- Any of the following three:
     Age <10 yr or >40 yr
     PT >50 sec
     Bilirubin >17.5 mg/dl

5. What conditions are considered to be contraindications to hepatic transplantation?
Absolute contraindications
     Extrahepatic malignancy
     Severe underlying systemic illness
     AIDS
     Uncontrolled sepsis
     Acute respiratory distress syndrome (ARDS)

Severe irreversible pulmonary hypertension
Diffuse coronary artery disease (not amenable to surgical treatment or angioplasty)
Congestive heart failure

Patients with biliary sepsis or liver abscess may be safely transplanted because the source of infection will be removed at the time of transplantation.

Relative contraindications

Elderly age (60–70 years depending on the transplant center): Patients who undergo liver transplantation are carefully screened for serious underlying illness, cardiac, or pulmonary disease. Elderly patients who are healthy, except for underlying liver disease, may do extremely well after transplantation, but elderly patients transplanted under urgent conditions (UNOS status 4) experience a poorer outcome and incur high costs. Few patients over age 70 should be considered for liver transplantation.

Portal vein thrombosis: Clot limited to the intrahepatic or main portal vein does not hamper the operation and is not a contraindication to transplantation. Clot extending into both splenic and superior mesenteric veins severely handicaps the surgical feasibility of liver transplantation.

Cholangiocarcinoma: Recurrence is nearly certain, so it is inadvisable to perform hepatic transplantation in patients with known cholangiocarcinoma. Patients who had unsuspected cholangiocarcinoma at the time of transplantation have reduced survival compared to other transplant recipients but improved rates over patients with cholangiocarcinoma treated by other means.

Fixed pulmonary hypertension: A few patients with cirrhosis have fixed pulmonary hypertension. Unlike intrapulmonary shunts, pulmonary hypertension does not reverse after transplantation.

Chronic hepatitis B: Patients who are HBeAg-positive and HBV-DNA-positive have a high rate of recurrent hepatitis B in the allograft and significantly reduced survival. Those who are HBeAg-negative and HBV-DNA-negative have excellent outcomes, as long as they are also treated with chronic hepatitis B immune globulin (HBIG). The transplantability of patients with (HBV) DNA is still controversial.

Hepatocellular carcinoma: Isolated tumors with a maximum diameter >5 cm or multicentric hepatoma are associated with high rates of recurrence in the allograft.

6. A 45-year-old man with end-stage alcoholic liver disease is presented to the Patient Selection Committee for liver transplantation. What features of the patient's psychosocial profile connote a good prognosis for continued abstinence from alcohol?

Most centers performing hepatic transplantation consider active, ongoing alcohol abuse a contraindication to transplantation. Patients with complications of Laennec's (alcoholic) cirrhosis who are abstinent from alcohol, however, may be considered for transplantation. Features correlating with successful outcome from transplantation and a low rate of recidivism to alcohol abuse include acceptance of alcoholism by the patient and family, stable occupation, stable family situation, absence of other substance abuse, presence of substitute activities, documented period of abstinence before transplantation, positive self-esteem and desire for maintaining abstinence, and willing adherence to an alcohol rehabilitation program. The length of the abstinent period does not independently correlate with low recidivism rates, but most programs insist that stable patients be monitored for at least 6 months for compliance prior to being activated for transplantation. Patients who undergo transplantation for active alcoholic hepatitis have a worse survival and a high rate of recidivism to alcoholism.

7. What factors, measured pretransplant, correlate with reduced patient survival after transplantation?

Five major variables are highly predictive of reduced post-transplant survival: UNOS status I at the time of transplantation, retransplantation, need for perioperative hemodialysis, chronic hepatitis B, and hepatobiliary carcinoma. UNOS status is the single most predictive variable. Additional predictors of reduced survival may include advanced Child's classification, elderly age, obesity, diabetes mellitus, severe metabolic bone disease, and severe nutritional deficiency. Despite these predictors of poor survival, one should remember that current results with liver transplantation are extraordinary, with a 5-year survival of 83% for patients having one liver graft and 78% for patients having two.

UNOS Status

I	Very unstable, in the ICU, intubated, on life-support systems such as hemodialysis, or life expectancy <7 days without liver transplantation
II	Unstable; cannot be discharged from the hospital owing to the complications of liver disease
III	Frequent hospitalizations due to the complications of liver disease; unable to work
IV	Stable at home; manages to perform at least part-time activity
V	Inactive

INPATIENT TRANSPLANT PERIOD (1–4 WEEKS POST-TRANSPLANT)

8. How do you regulate the dose of cyclosporine, and when is it appropriate to switch from intravenous to oral administration?

Intravenous administration of cyclosporine is begun intraoperatively, 5 mg/kg/day given in divided doses either every 8 or 12 hours. The primary mode of monitoring cyclosporine dosing is the blood or plasma level of the drug. Several methods are used to measure cyclosporine levels, including high-pressure liquid chromatography, radioimmunoassay with mono- or polyclonal antibody, and polyclonal fluorescent polarization assays. The therapeutic concentration varies between laboratories depending on which analytic technique is used. Secondary end points for adjusting cyclosporine dosage are serum creatinine, neuropsychiatric side effects, and opportunistic infection.

The patient must be able to tolerate oral intake and have an intact enterohepatic circulation in order to switch from intravenous to oral administration. The latter is essential because cyclosporine is a very lipophilic molecule, for which intestinal absorption requires the formation of bile acid micelles. Most patients are able to begin oral feedings within 2 to 3 days after transplant. The standard surgical technique of T-tube placement and external drainage of bile interrupts the enterohepatic circulation and severely impairs the absorption of cyclosporine. Oral cyclosporine may be initiated once the T-tube has been clamped. In our center, the technique of T-tube placement has been supplanted by placement of an internal draining stent that is secured to the donor duct with chromic catgut, traverses the duct lumen across the duct-to-duct anastomosis, and enters the duodenum via the papilla of Vater. Because the enterohepatic circulation is always intact in this system, one may begin oral cyclosporine as soon as the patient begins oral intake.

9. A liver transplant patient has just sustained a grand mal seizure 36 hours post-transplant. His cyclosporine level is within acceptable limits. He is postictal but has no obvious focal neurologic deficits. What factors contribute to an increased risk of seizures post-transplant?

The immunosuppressive medications cyclosporine and FK506 (tacrolimus) both have been associated with neurotoxicity. The clinical features include grand mal seizures, tremors and ataxia, delirium, paresthesia, and aphasia which is usually transient. Although the exact mechanism of this neurotoxicity is not clear, several possible explanations are proposed.

Cyclosporine and FK506 are lipophilic compounds that partition into body compartments having a rich lipid content (lipoproteins, adispose tissue, liver, brain). Bioavailability and drug distribution are best understood for cyclosporine. Whole blood cyclosporine level reflects the partition of cyclosporine between plasma, red cells, and lipoproteins. Plasma cholesterol is almost totally associated with lipoprotein particles. When plasma cholesterol is low, the lipoprotein concentration is low. Thus, plasma free cyclosporine is relatively higher in patients with hypocholesterolemia, cyclosporine will more readily cross the blood-brain barrier, and seizures are more likely to occur. Hypomagnesemia (by lowering the seizure threshhold), high plasma concentrations of drug, and rapid rates of drug infusion also favor the development of seizures.

10. A patient, 3 weeks post-transplant, is begun on erythromycin for atypical pneumonia. Does this action affect immunosuppressive therapy?
Yes. Cyclosporine is metabolized by a specific cytochrome P450 enzyme system: P450 III A. When P450 III A is inhibited, cyclosporine concentrations increase. When P450 III A is stimulated by other medications, cyclosporine concentrations decrease. Certain drugs, such as erythromycin, ketoconazole, Seldane, and calcium-channel blockers, inhibit the P450 III A system and raise cyclosporine levels, resulting in over-immunosuppression and increased susceptibility to opportunistic infections or cyclosporine toxicity (hypertension, renal failure, neuropsychiatric symptoms). Other drugs, such as phenobarbitol, rifampin, phenytoin, and carbamazepine, stimulate or induce this P450 system and lower cyclosporine levels, resulting in under-immunosuppression, rejection, and higher dosage of cyclosporine (expensive).

11. How do cyclosporine and FK506 prevent allograft rejection?
Cyclosporine A blocks the clonal stimulatory effect of interleukin-1 on both helper and cytotoxic T lymphocytes. FK506 suppresses interleukin-2-dependent reactions and has a similar effect on T cells. In addition, FK506 blocks the formation of other soluble mediators, such as interleukin-3 and gamma interferon. FK506 is approximately 100 times more potent than cyclosporine in vivo. However, in clinical studies, FK506- or cyclosporine-based regimens were very comparable in patient and graft survival. Prednisone is used as an adjunct to both cyclosporine and FK506 and blocks the synthesis of interleukin-1, thereby blocking the proliferation of antigen-specific helper and cytotoxic T lymphocytes. Azathioprine is commonly used as an adjunctive therapy because it is an antimetabolite and blocks the antigen-specific clonal proliferation of both suppressor and helper cells.

12. Are there other antirejection drugs?
OKT3 antilymphocyte globulin are two monoclonal antibodies used in severe rejections. **OKT3** is a murine monoclonal antibody that blocks the recognition of Class 1 and Class 2 antigens by helper/cytotoxic lymphocytes and interferes at the beginning of the rejection cascade. **Antilymphocyte globulin** acts in the same fashion but also directly destroys circulating helper/cytotoxic lymphocytes. Both of these agents decrease CD3 counts, which are measured during the course of the treatment.

13. A patient who had an uncomplicated operation is noted to have rising liver enzymes on day 10 after transplantation. What is the differential diagnosis, and what tests should be obtained?
A rise in liver enzymes on days 7–14 may be the first indication of a significant problem with the hepatic allograft. The single most common cause at this time is **acute allograft rejection.** Early diagnosis is critical because institution of appropriate immunosupressive treatment (bolus steroids or OKT3) will prevent graft loss. The cornerstone of diagnosing rejection is percutaneous liver biopsy. Other considerations include thrombus in the hepatic artery or portal vein, cholangitis, bile leak, drug toxicity, or opportunistic infection (unlikely this soon after transplant). Tests to rule out these possibilities include ultrasonography with Doppler cholangiography, measurement of cyclosporine (or FK506) drug levels, and cytomegalovirus (CMV) cultures of liver tissue, urine, blood monocytes, and throat washings.

14. A patient with end-stage liver disease from chronic hepatitis C undergoes liver transplantation. Ten days later, his liver enzymes increase. What are the histologic findings of acute rejection versus post-transplant hepatitis C on liver biopsy?
The histologic features of **acute cellular rejection** are (1) mixed cellular infiltrate consisting of monocytes, lymphocytes, polymorphonuclear cells, and eosinophils in the portal area; (2) inflammation of the bile duct that presents as either apoptosis or intraepithelial lymphocytes; and (3) endotheliitis of either central or portal veins. Typically, there is very little involvement of the hepatic lobule with either necrosis, inflammation, or unrest.

Recurrent hepatitis C can sometimes be distinguished from rejection. The histology may demonstrate a predominantly lymphocytic infiltrate in portal areas rather than the mixed cellular infiltrate of rejection. Lobular steatosis, lobular disarray with spotty parenchymal inflammation, and vacuolization of biliary epithelium may also be seen. In addition, Councilman's bodies are commonly seen distributed randomly throughout the lobule in hepatitis C, whereas they are rare or localized to the perivenular area in rejection. Of note, early hepatitis C is sometimes very hard to distinguish histologically, and even the most experienced hepatologist would favor antirejection treatment in these borderline cases.

15. Describe the pathophysiology of other post-transplant complications manifested by rising liver enzymes.

Patients with **hepatic artery thrombosis** typically exhibit a hectic fever pattern with the rise in liver enzymes and experience multiorganism bacteremia. The organisms found in blood mirror the organisms colonizing the extrahepatic biliary tree, and the cessation of hepatic arterial blood flow preferentially causes ischemic damage to the extrahepatic biliary tree. The latter results in breakdown of the biliary tree and development of bilomas, bile leaks, and, later, strictures. Although early hepatic artery thrombosis may be amenable to nonsurgical, radiologic intervention, in most cases retransplantation is required for successful long-term outcome.

Portal vein thrombosis may be well-tolerated and not require intervention.However, often the thrombosis is complicated by endovascular infection or compromised graft function. Percutaneous transhepatic placement of indwelling portal venous catheters, balloon angioplasty of the thrombosis, or urokinase infusion into the clot may be needed to reestablish portal circulation.

Biliary leaks are best diagnosed by either T-tube or endoscopic cholangiography. HIDA-scintigraphy may occasionally be useful in this setting. Bile leaks and bilomas occurring in the early post-transplant period are usually associated with hepatic artery thrombosis.

Certain **medications** used in the post-transplant period may cause liver abnormalities. Cyclosporine (high plasma concentrations), FK506, azathioprine, and sulfa drugs may cause a cholestatic pattern of elevation in liver enzymes. Others, such as nonsteroidal anti-inflammatory drugs, antibiotics, antiseizure medications, and antihypertensives, may cause predominantly a hepatitis-type picture.

The most common **opportunistic infection** of the hepatic allograft is cytomegalovirus (CMV) infection. Typically, the increase in liver enzymes with CMV infection usually occurs >2 weeks after surgery. One notable virus, hepatitis C virus, may recur rapidly in the hepatic allograft and cause abnormalities in liver tests as early as 1 week post-transplant. Additional infections that may be suspected after review of the histology include adenovirus, herpes viruses, and Epstein-Barr virus.

OUTPATIENT TRANSPLANT PERIOD (>4 WEEKS)

16. A patient having early allograft rejection is treated with a 10-day course of OKT3 but returns 1 week later with headache, mild fatigue, low-grade fever, and increased liver enzymes. Is this OKT3 toxicity?

This is not likely to be OKT3 toxicity. Typically, most reactions of OKT3 occur during the first 1–3 days of administration. Bronchospasm, chest and joint pains, nausea, vomiting, and diarrhea can occur during the treatment period. Rarely, aseptic meningitis may occur during or after the treatment but can present with fevers, fatigue, and severe headaches. Meningeal signs may or may not be present.

17. If it isn't OKT3 toxicity, what is the most likely diagnosis?

The most common possibilities other than OKT3 toxicity are CMV infection, incomplete treatment of rejection, postsurgical complications (hepatic artery thrombosis, hepatic abscess, bile leak), cyclosporine hepatoxicity, and other opportunistic infections, including Epstein-Barr virus, herpes simplex virus, fungal, or parasitic infections such as *Pneumocystis carinii* pneumonia.

CMV is the most likely possibility in the patient described in Question 16. Most CMV infections occur within 1–4 months after liver transplantation. It may be a primary infection in a CMV-negative recipient from a CMV-positive donor; reactivation in a CMV+-donor, CMV+-recipient situation; or superinfection of the graft in a CMV- donor, CMV+ recipient.

In all these cases, CMV usually is easily identified within 48 hours by throat, urine, blood, and/or liver tissue cultures. In addition, liver biopsy is diagnostic if the viral inclusions are seen in the hepatic parachyma and/or if immunohistochemical tests are positive. Localized collections of polymorphonuclear cells is also a very suggestive finding in the liver biopsies. Treatment of CMV infection is relatively easy with ganciclovir. Resistant cases are usually rare but can be treated with hyperimmune globulin, acyclovir, or famciclovir.

18. What are the clinical, biochemical, and histologic features of chronic rejection?

Chronic allograft rejection is a syndrome characterized by an insidious but progressive rise in alkaline phosphatase (AP) and gama-glutamyl transferase (GGT) followed by serum bilirubin in a clinically asymptomatic liver transplant recipient. Synthetic function usually stays intact until the late phases. The pathogenesis of this syndrome is still unclear, but all the evidence favors a progressive loss of bile ducts (probably immune-mediated) and development of obliterative arteriopathy in the small hepatic arteries. Histologic exam usually reveals a normal-appearing parenchyma with few mononuclear infiltrates in the portal areas but complete absence of bile ducts, in almost all the portal triads. Because of this striking loss of bile ducts, this syndrome is also referred as "vanishing bile duct syndrome." The exact time of onset is usually difficult to determine. Some groups have reported a very rapid course (3–4 weeks) of a similar clinical syndrome, naming it "acute vanishing bile duct syndrome."

Later in the course, patients develop strictures and dilatations in their larger bile ducts, eventually resembling a primary sclerosing cholangitis (PSC)-type of clinical picture. In these cases, the clinical course may be complicated by recurrent attacks of biliary sepsis. The differential diagnosis at this stage includes hepatic artery thrombosis, CMV cholangitis, anastomotic strictures of the biliary tract, and (if the patient's original disease was PSC) recurrence of PSC, which can all give the similar clinical picture.

19. How do you treat chronic rejection?

The treatment options are very limited. Symptomatic treatment and, if appropriate, retransplantation are the only options.

20. How often is it necessary to perform a second liver transplant, and for what reasons are retransplants performed?

Approximately 20–25% of the liver transplants performed in the United States are retransplants.

Early retransplants within 100 days are usually performed for primary graft failure or hepatic artery thrombosis and, very rarely, for acute rejection (an event more commonly seen in the past). Better understanding of the immunosuppressive therapies, coupled with increased surgical experience, has lowered the incidence of early retransplants.

Late retransplantations, after day 100, are usually due to recurrence of original disease (such as hepatitis B or C, primary biliary cirrhosis, primary sclerosing cholangitis, or Budd-Chiari syndrome) or due to chronic rejection. The incidence of late transplants has not changed over recent years. However, with the use of additional treatment modalities for high-risk groups (hepatitis B immune globulin for HBV+ recipients, anticoagulation for Budd-Chiari syndrome), the late retransplant rates may also improve in the future.

21. Describe the long-term metabolic complications that occur in the liver transplant recipient.

After surviving the first 6 months to 1 year after liver transplantation, patients with liver disease have a dramatic improvement in their quality of life and life expectancy. From this point on, health maintenance of these individuals becomes the most important issue. There are several metabolic complications clearly associated with the use of immunosuppressive regimens, including obesity, hypertension, renal failure, hyperlipidemia, and atherosclerosis.

Most patients gain weight rapidly after liver transplantation, in part due to prednisone and cyclosporine and in part due to their liberation from a very strict and bland pretransplant diet. Obesity, by itself, increases the risk for hypertension and cardiovascular and cerebrovascular diseases. It is therefore very important to follow a well-instructed diet and exercise schedule in post-transplant patients. Hyperlipidemia and hypercholesterolemia are almost universal in these patients and should be treated aggressively with diet and medications if serum cholesterol stays above 250 mg/dl. We prefer HMG-CoA reductase inhibitors in our patients. In addition, lowering their steroid dosages is another helpful measure.

Hypertension is mostly due to vasoconstrictive effects of cyclosporine and FK506 and due to salt and water retention caused by steroids. In addition, nephrotoxicity from these immunosuppressives will contribute. The hypertension is usually nocturnal and should be aggressively treated to prevent cardiovascular and cerebrovascular catastrophes. Calcium channel blockers or angiotension-converting enzyme inhibitors are usually first-line agents, and if not effective, alpha- and beta-adrenergic blockers and agents that work directly on smooth muscle of the vasculature may be added.

22. Are liver transplant recipients at increased risk to develop cancer?

New malignant tumors may develop after liver transplantation. Most of these tumors are of the lymphoproliferative type (mostly B-cell-type lymphomas), presumably due to Epstein-Barr virus (EBV) infections and/or immunosuppression. EBV is clearly responsible for most lymphoproliferative malignancies associated with solid organ transplantation. Examination of the tissue from these patients indicates that the EBV genome is maintained in the malignant clones, and histologically, at least three EBV transformation-associated antigens are expressed on the cell surfaces. Even though the pathogenesis is not totally clear, the development of lymphoproliferative disease appears to be due to the low level of immunosurveillance related to immunosuppression, uncontrolled clonal expansion of EBV-transformed cells, and possibly, chronic antigenic stimulation of the B cells by the allograft.

Clinical presentation includes fever in >50% of cases. In addition, lymphadenopathy, GI symptoms, tonsillitis, pharyngitis, pulmonary and CNS manifestations due to tumor invasion, and weight loss can be seen. Most of these lymphomas are non-Hodgkin type, with 65% B cell, 14% T cell, and 1% null cell types. The first line of treatment is lowering the immunosuppression. Then, ganciclovir may be used if the EBV association has been demonstrated. Surgical excision may be performed if lesions are localized and few in number. Cytotoxic and radiotherapy are rarely indicated and are usually done with the help of an oncologist.

Other tumors may be seen with an increased incidence due to immunosuppression, but this area is controversial. Nonetheless, routine screens—such as prostate-specific antigen and rectal exams in men; mammograms, breast exams, and Pap smears in women; and colon screens in patients with ulcerative colitis—should routinely be performed.

23. A liver transplant patient comes to the emergency room complaining of cough and shortness of breath. How does one suspect, diagnose, and treat *Pneumocystis carinii* infection?

Pneumocystis carinii pneumonia (PCP) is an opportunistic pulmonary infection. The clinical presentation may be highly variable, but most patients describe a rapidly progressive febrile illness characterized by dry cough and shortness of breath. If undiagnosed and untreated, patients will succumb within a few days to progressive respiratory failure and ARDS. The disease should be suspected in any immunosuppressed patient who presents with respiratory complaints or with new changes on chest x-ray. Diagnosis often requires bronchoscopy with brochoalveolar lavage. Treatment of acute PCP is with intravenous trimethoprim-sulfamethoxazole. Sulfa-allergic patients may be treated with inhalational pentamidine, but this drug is poorly tolerated in those with respiratory compromise.

24. A 23-year-old male with chronic ulcerative colitis underwent liver transplantation for primary sclerosing cholangitis. One week after discharge, he returns to the clinic complaining of bloody diarrhea. What is the likely cause of his diarrhea?
Patients who have just undergone hepatic transplantation are heavily immunosuppressed; most are discharged on moderately high doses of steroids and are taking either cyclosporine or FK506. In addition, overall immunosuppression is further increased by treatment of rejection episodes with either pulse-recycle steroids or OKT3. In this setting, it is highly unusual for patients with ulcerative colitis to experience an exacerbation of their disease. In contrast, immunosuppressed patients are susceptible to infectious colitis, in particular CMV colitis or *Clostridium difficile* pseudomembranous colitis.

The workup of this patient should include stool culture, stool O&P, *C. difficile* toxin assay, and colonoscopy with mucosal biopsies for CMV. He had negative stool cultures, O&P, and *C. difficile* toxin. Colonoscopy revealed a patchy colitis, biopsies revealed numerous epithelial and endothelial cells with CMV inclusions, and cultures of mucosal biopsies grew CMV. The patient was treated by lowering his immunosuppression and giving intravenous ganciclovir. After 5 days, he no longer had diarrhea, his appetite returned to normal, and he felt well.

25. What factors contribute to metabolic bone disease seen after transplantation?
Chronic liver diseases and cholestatic liver diseases, in particular, are associated with osteopenia. Fractures after liver transplantation tend to occur in patients whose underlying pre-transplant liver disease was either PBC or PSC. These patients appear to experience accelerated bone loss after transplantation: bone density decreases for the first 6 months and then begins to increase. Fracture risk is highest at the nadir in bone density. Two factors are highly predictive of accelerated bone loss and fracture after transplant: high dosages of steroids and prolonged periods of bedrest.

26. A patient who underwent liver transplantation for hepatitis C virus (HCV)-associated cirrhosis has persistently elevated liver enzymes. Liver biopsies reveal chronic active hepatitis but no cirrhosis. Should he be treated with interferon?
Interferon may be used after liver transplantation to alleviate the activity of chronic hepatitis C. However, there have been no reported cases in which this therapy has cleared the virus in a liver transplant recipient. HCV persists despite normalization of liver enzymes or improvement in liver histology. We currently recommend treating only patients who are at least 6 months post transplant and who have evidence of progressive liver injury. If patients do not respond by normalization or near-normalization of ALT after 4 months, then interferon should be discontinued. Patients who respond will likely need long-term maintenance therapy, but the efficacy and safety of long-term interferon treatment has not been determined. Most patients with hepatitis C do well; their 5-year survival is no different than survival rates of other liver transplant patients. It is not known whether HCV patients will experience accelerated decline in survival in later years, 10–30 years post transplant.

27. Which patients with hepatitis B virus (HBV) should undergo liver transplant?
Early experience with transplantation of hepatitis B patients suggested that recurrence was nearly uniform and that these patients experienced high rates of graft loss and diminished survival. Subsequently, European trials have shown that patients who were HBeAg and HBV-DNA-negative and who received peri- and postoperative hepatitis B immune globulin (HBIG) treatment had patient and graft survivals equivalent to those of other liver transplant patients. Additional studies have recently demonstrated that extremely high doses of HBIG allow the successful transplantation of HBeAg-positive patients. For these reasons, all patients with end-stage liver disease due to HBV may be considered candidates for liver transplantation. HBIG therapy, however, is required to achieve satisfactory results. New antiviral agents, such as famciclovir and 3-TC (lamivudine), may add further therapies against HBV.

BIBLIOGRAPHY

1. Calne RY: Immunosuppression in liver transplantation. N Engl J Med 331:1154–1155, 1994.
2. Lake JR (ed): Advances in liver transplantation. Gastroenterol Clin North Am 22(2): 1993.
3. Lucey MR, Merion RM, Beresford TP: Liver Transplantation and the Alcoholic Patient: Medical, Surgical and Psychosocial Issues. New York, Cambridge University Press, 1994.
4. Maddrey WC, Van Thiel DH: Liver transplantation: An overview. Hepatology 8:948–959, 1988.
5. Neuberger J: Liver transplantation: Indications and timing. Gastroenterology 3:402–407, 1987.
6. Phillips MG, (ed): Organ Procurement, Preservation and Distribution in Transplantation. William Byrd Press, 1991.
7. Starzl TE, Demetris AJ, Van Theil D: Liver transplantation, pts I and II. N Engl J Med 321:1014–1020, 1092–1099, 1989.
8. U.S. Multicenter FK506 Liver Study Group: A comparison of tacrolimus (FK506) and cyclosporine for immunosuppression in liver transplantation. N Engl J Med 331:1110–1115, 1994.

27. FULMINANT HEPATIC FAILURE

Paul J. Thuluvath, M.B.B.S., M.D., M.R.C.P.

1. Define fulminant hepatic failure (FHF).

The term fulminant hepatic failure (FHF) is currently used to describe rapidly progressive liver failure with onset of encephalopathy within 8 weeks of onset of symptoms in patients without previous history of liver disease. When the onset of encephalopathy is delayed more than 8 weeks but less than 6 months, the term late-onset hepatic failure (LOHF) is used. Despite suggestions that these definitions should be revised, so far there has been no consensus.

Stages of Hepatic Encephalopathy

STAGE	CLINICAL SIGNS
I	Mental slowness, slurred speech, mild confusion, euphoria
II	Inappropriate behavior, agitation, drowsiness
III	Sleeps most of the time but arousable, marked confusion
IV	Coma

2. What is the difference between FHF and LOHF?

The distinction between FHF and LOHF is clinically important, because the decision whether to transplant has to be made swiftly after the onset of encephalopathy in patients with FHF. Moreover, this distinction is diagnostically useful, because certain causes of acute liver failure are predominantly associated either with FHF or LOHF.

3. What are the common causes of FHF and LOHF?

The causes vary, depending on the country and the nature of the referral center. Acute viral hepatitis is by far the most common cause (62–68%) in the U.S. and many European countries (72% in France), but in England paracetamol (acetaminophen) overdose is the single most common cause (45–54%) of acute liver failure. Hepatitis, A, B, D, and E viruses cause predominantly FHF, whereas hepatitis C and non-A, non-B, non-C viruses cause LOHF. Acetaminophen and halothane usually result in FHF, but other drug-induced liver diseases result in LOHF.

Causes of Fulminant Hepatic Failure*

Cause	England	France	U.S.
Viral hepatitis	36	70	64
Hepatitis A	5	4	5
Hepatitis B (± HDV)	12	45	20
Undetermined (Non-A, non-B, non-C)	18	18	39
Others	1	3	—
Acetaminophen	54	2	15
Other drugs/toxins†	7	19	16
Miscellaneous	3	9	5

*Given as percent based on published studies.
†Mushroom (*Amanita phalloides*) poisoning represents about 2% of cases in France.

4. What other causes should be considered? How often is the cause not identified?

The rare causes of acute liver failure include Wilson's disease, autoimmune chronic active hepatitis, Budd-Chiari syndrome, acute fatty liver of pregnancy, diffuse malignant infiltration of liver, reactivation of HBV, and hyperthermia. Wilson's disease and autoimmune chronic active hepatitis usually present as LOHF. HEV is a rare cause of liver failure but should be considered in the differential diagnosis, especially in people from and travelers to endemic areas.

When middle-aged and older patients with no previous history of liver disease present with hepatomegaly and ascites, malignancy should be considered as a possible cause. CT scan is not often useful to make the diagnosis because the tumor spreads in an intrasinusoidal pattern. The diagnosis is frequently made after death. Amyloidosis is another rare infiltrative disorder that may present as LOHF.

Reactivation of HBV (HBV-DNA–negative to HBV-DNA–positive) usually occurs after immunosuppression or chemotherapy; rarely is it spontaneous. The extent to which mutant HBV (HbeAg-negative) causes FHF remains unknown.

In a significant number of patients (19–41%), the cause of acute liver failure remains undetermined and usually presents as LOHF. It is presumed that most of these patients have acute non-A, non-B, non-C viral hepatitis. Some may have HBV-DNA in the liver when carefully tested; however, the causative agent remains unidentified in a significant proportion of patients with FHF and LOHF.

5. Does the prognosis vary with the cause? How does one predict the prognosis?

The prognosis is better for patients with hepatitis A and acetaminophen-induced liver failure. This survival advantage was seen even in patients with coma and severe coagulopathy. The prognostic variables are similar for all causes of fulminant hepatic failure except acetaminophen toxicity. In patients with acetaminophen toxicity, severe acidosis (arterial pH <7.3) is associated with a mortality rate of approximately 95%. In the absence of severe acidosis, *presence of* all of the other three adverse factors (creatinine >3.4, INR = international normalized ratio [INR] >6.5, and stage III and IV encephalopathy) are necessary to identify patients with 95% mortality.

Prognostic indicators for non–acetaminophen-induced FHF are given in the table below. With one adverse factor, the mortality rate is around 80%; the rate increases to 95% with three or more adverse factors. However, prothrombin time >100 seconds is an absolute indication (even in the absence of other adverse factors) for liver transplantation in patients with non–acetaminophen-induced liver failure. Factor V level is an important predictor of mortality in FHF. In patients with stage III or IV coma, the chance of survival without liver transplantation is less than 10% if factor V level is less than 15–20%.

Prognosis of LOHF can be determined by the Childs-Pugh grading system, which uses ascites, albumin, bilirubin, prothrombin time, and encephalopathy as prognostic variables.

Prognostic Indicators Associated with Poor Outcome in Fulminant Hepatic Failure*

ACETAMINOPHEN-INDUCED	NON–ACETAMINOPHEN-INDUCED
Arterial pH <7.3	Non-A, non-B, non-C hepatitis, drugs, toxins
INR >6.5 or prothrombin time >100s	INR >3.5 or prothrombin time >50s
Creatinine >3.4 mg/dl	Creatinine >3.4
Stage III or IV encephalopathy	Jaundice >7 days before onset of encephalopathy
	Bilirubin >18 mg/dl
	Age <10 or >40 years

*Based on O'Grady JG, Alexander GJ, Hayllar KM, Williams R: Early indicators of prognosis in fulminant hepatic failure. Gastroenterology 97:439–445, 1989. INR = international normalized ratio.

6. What is the natural course of fulminant and subfulminant hepatic failure without liver transplantation?

The overall mortality rate, including all causes, without liver transplantation is about 70%. The mortality rate is around 50% for hepatitis A and acetaminophen-induced fulminant liver failure. Obviously such data come from referral centers; the mortality rates are likely to be higher in community hospitals. In patients with coma (stage IV hepatic encephalpathy) and severe coagulopathy or factor V level <15%, the chance of survival without liver transplantation is less than 10%.

7. What are the common complications in patients with FHF?

Although liver failure results in numerous metabolic changes, patients usually die because of increased intracranial pressure (ICP), infectious complications, or multiorgan failure. Other common complications are coagulopathy, renal failure, lactic acidosis, hypoglycemia, hypophosphatemia, hypoxemia, and hypotension, all of which are interrelated and ultimately lead to multiorgan failure.

Coagulopathy is due to a combination of reduced synthesis of clotting factors and increased peripheral consumption as a result of low-grade disseminated intravascular coagulation (DIC). Hypoglycemia is due to impaired gluconeogenesis, reduced mobilization of glycogen, and increase in circulating insulin. Lactic acidosis results from a combination of tissue hypoxia and poor hepatic uptake and metabolism of lactate.

Renal failure is seen in about 70% of patients with acetaminophen-induced FHF and about 30% with non–acetaminophen-induced FHF. The causes of renal failure include hypovolemia, acute renal tubular necrosis, and hepatorenal syndrome.

Hypotension, in the presence of adequate fluid intake, is due to high cardiac output and lowered peripheral vascular resistance. Arterial hypoxemia is seen in the presence of infection, alveolar hemorrhage, arteriovenous shunting, and adult respiratory distress syndrome (ARDS).

Because of suppression of immune function, impaired neutrophil and Kupffer cell functions, and deficiency of opsonins, patients are prone to both bacterial (gram-negative and gram-positive) and fungal (candida) infection.

Approximately 80% of patients with FHF and coma develop cerebral edema, which is perhaps the most common cause of death (brain stem or cerebellar coning is seen in 80% of patients at autopsy). The pathogenesis of cerebral edema remains poorly explained. It is presumed to be due to a combination of swelling of astrocytes (perhaps mediated by toxins) and extravasation of fluids (disruption of blood-brain barrier).

8. Is it necessary to refer patients with FHF to a tertiary center? How does one manage patients with FHF?

It is important to refer patients at an early stage to a center where they can be managed by a team with expertise. Early referral also provides adequate time to evaluate the patient for liver transplantation.

Patients with FHF should be managed in an intensive care unit by an experienced team. The cause of liver failure should be determined and treated if possible (e.g., acetaminophen toxicity). The patient is nursed with the head elevated to minimize positional influence on ICP. Sedation should be avoided if possible. Patients should have central venous pressure monitoring (Swan-Ganz catheter if necessary), and careful attention should be given to fluid replacement and correction of acidosis, electrolyte imbalances, and hypoglycemia. Arterial oxygen saturation should be monitored, and airways should be protected by endotracheal intubation in patients with stage III-IV hepatic encephalopathy. Patients should be treated with H_2 receptor antagonists as a prophylaxis against stress ulcers. Although prophylactic replacement of fresh frozen plasma does not reduce morbidity or mortality and makes it difficult to interpret the most valuable prognostic indicator, it should not be withheld in the presence of bleeding or for placement of ICP monitor. Platelets should be transfused in patients with severe thrombocytopenia.

Hypotension should be treated with adequate fluid replacement and vasopressors; however, care should be taken to avoid pulmonary edema in patients with renal failure. Continuous arteriovenous hemofiltration should be instituted in patients with uncorrected acidosis, fluid overload, hyperkalemia, and worsening creatinine levels.

No convincing evidence supports prophylactic antibacterial or antifungal treatment, but treatment should be started at the slightest suspicion of infection. It is important to culture all body fluids and catheter tips for bacteria and fungi on a daily basis. Patients with evidence of infection should be treated with antifungal agents if there is no immediate response to antibacterial treatment, especially if they have had previous antibiotics or have renal failure.

ICP monitoring is crucial in the management of patients with stage III or IV hepatic encephalopathy (see question 10). Finally, patients should undergo liver transplantation when the risk of mortality is >80%.

9. Are there any specific therapies for FHF?

Acetaminophen-induced FHF should be treated with N-acetylcysteine. Acetylcysteine has proved useful even in patients who were treated after 10 hours (but less than 36 hours), although the benefits seem to decrease with time.

Patients with signs of **autoimmune chronic active hepatitis** (e.g., high globulin levels, positive test for antinuclear antibody) should be given a trial of steroids.

Budd-Chiari syndrome may respond to decompressive surgery or transhepatic portosystemic shunting.

10. Does ICP monitoring improve the prognosis of patients with FHF? What are the goals of ICP monitoring? What are the complications?

ICP monitoring and orthotopic liver transplantation (OLT) are the two major advances in the management of FHF in the past decade. Increased ICP is seen in more than 80% of patients with FHF. Increased ICP may be recognized clinically by extensor posturing, teeth grinding, opisthotonos, impaired pupillary responses, and arterial hypertension. Initially the rises in ICP may be episodic and thus easily missed clinically. Later, when patients are paralyzed and ventilated, the clinical signs may not be available to recognize ICP. In addition, ICP may rise precipitously in some patients, making the clinical signs rather useless. Moreover, it has been shown that rises in ICP may occur without clinical signs. Other modalities, such as CT, are neither sensitive nor practical in patients with FHF.

The goal of monitoring is to maintain ICP below 15–20 mm Hg and cerebral perfusion pressure above 50 mm Hg (mean arterial pressure minus intracranial pressure). This goal may be achieved by a combination of hyperventilation, hyperosmolar mannitol, or thiopentone infusion. It is important to avoid maneuvers that may increase ICP. When mannitol is used, serum osmolality should be measured (mannitol has no benefit if serum osmolality is 320 mOsmol/L or higher). ICP monitoring is also useful intraoperatively and in the immediate postoperative period. Among patients with neurologic damage, ICP monitoring may help to select those who are likely to recover. Patients with sustained cerebral perfusion pressure below 40 mm Hg are less likely to recover after liver transplantation.

ICP monitoring may be associated with intracranial hemorrhage and infection. However, such complications are higher during the learning phase and seem to decrease with experience. Epidural transducers are the most commonly used devices (61%) in the U.S. and have the lowest complication rate (3.8%). Subdural bolts and parenchymal monitors (fiberoptic pressure transducers in direct contact with brain parenchyma and intraventricular catheters) are associated with complication rates of 20% and 22%, respectively. Fatal hemorrhages occur in 1% of patients with epidural monitoring, 5% with subdural bolts, and 4% with parenchymal monitoring.

11. What is the basis for use of prostaglandins in the management of FHF? How successful is the treatment?

The use of prostaglandin E1 (PGE1) is based on an uncontrolled study by investigators in Toronto, in which 12 of 14 patients with grade III or IV hepatic encephalopathy survived. The authors attributed the high survival rate to continuous infusion of PGE1. The rationale for this treatment in FHF remains poorly explained. Immunomodulation, improvements in tissue perfusion, and direct antiviral effects may explain the increase in survival. However, a controlled study by the same group failed to show any benefit with PGE1 therapy. Further studies are necessary before the routine use of PGE1 in patients with fulminant hepatic failure.

12. Do hepatotrophic agents have a role in the management of FHF?

Various hepatotrophic agents have been identified, but so far the clinical experience is limited to insulin and glucagon therapy. In controlled trials, insulin and glucagon therapy have failed to improve survival in patients with severe acute hepatitis. In the future other growth factors, such as transforming growth factor alpha and hepatocyte growth factor, may become available for clinical trials.

13. How successful is liver transplantation in FHF?

The experience from major centers suggests that a significant number of patients (30–40%) with FHF die without receiving liver transplantation because of either the unavailability of a suitable donor or complications that prevent OLT, such as sepsis, neurologic damage, and multiorgan failure.

The results of OLT in patients with FHF have improved significantly over the last decade, mainly because of better selection criteria and better management in intensive care. The 1-year survival rate of patients after liver transplantation for FHF is around 70% (some centers have reported survival rates as high as 90%), which is lower than the rate for non-FHF recipients. A recent study showed that FHF recipients are less likely to be matched for ABO blood type than their non-FHF counterparts, which may partly explain the survival difference. ABO mismatch and abnormal kidney function were independent predictors of adverse outcome in patients receiving liver transplantation for FHF.

14. Does artificial liver support have a role in the management of acute liver failure? Are there any other promising therapies that may be used as a bridge to OLT?

Artificial liver support is one of the most exciting areas in hepatology. OLT is a drastic and expensive procedure, but it has shown to improve survival in patients with FHF. However, many patients die because of the unavailability of a suitable donor. Liver assist devices may be useful in patients as a bridge to emergency OLT; they may help to stabilize patients with uncontrolled ICP or even negate the need for OLT if the liver is able to regenerate. Numerous such devices are currently tested in small clinical studies. Results appear promising, but controlled studies are needed.

Charcoal hemoperfusion has been used in the past, but a controlled study has shown that it does not improve survival rates. Reports of heterotrophic auxiliary liver transplantation are not encouraging, but further study is needed. Despite anecdotal reports of successful use, xenografts must be considered as an experimental procedure. Transplantation of hepatocytes is still at an experimental stage.

BIBLIOGRAPHY

1. Bernuau J, Goudeau A, Poynard T, et al: Mutivariate analysis of prognostic factors in fulminant hepatitis B. Hepatology 6:648–651, 1986.
2. Detre K, Belle S, Beringer K, Daily OP: Liver transplantation for fulminant hepatic failure in the United States: October 1987 through December 1991. Clin Transplant 8:274–280, 1994.
3. Gimson AE, O'Grady J, Ede RJ, et al: Late onset of hepatic failure: Clinical, serological and histological features. Hepatology 6:288–294, 1986.
4. Harrison, PM, Keays R, Bray GP, et al: Improved outcome of paracetamol induced fulminant hepatic failure by late administration of acetylcysteine. Lancet i:1572–1573, 1990.
5. Keays R, Harrison PM, Wendon JA, et al: Intravenous acetylcysteine in paracetamol induced fulminant hepatic failure: A prospective controlled trial. BMJ 303:1026–1029, 1991.
6. Lidofsky SD: Liver transplantation for fulminant hepatic failure. Gastroenterol Clin North Am 22:257–269, 1993.
7. Lidofsky SD, Bass NM, Pager MC, et al: Intracranial pressure monitoring and liver transplantation for fulminant hepatic failure. Hepatology 16:1–7, 1992.
8. Mortimer DJ, Elias E: Liver transplantation for fulminant hepatic failure. Prog Liver Dis 10:349–367, 1992.
9. Munoz SJ: Difficult management problems in fulminant hepatic failure. Semin Liver Dis 13:395–413, 1993.
10. O'Grady JG, Alexander GJ, Hayllar KM, Williams R: Early indicators of prognosis in fulminant hepatic failure. Gastroenterology 97:439–445, 1989.
11. Sussman NL, Gislason GT, Kelly JH: Extracorporeal liver support: Application to fulminant hepatic failure. J Clin Gastroenterology 18:320–324, 1994.

28. ASCITES

Carlos Guarner, M.D., and Bruce A. Runyon, M.D.

1. What are the most common causes of ascites?

Ascites is the accumulation of fluid within the peritoneal cavity. More than 80% of patients with ascites have decompensated chronic liver disease. However, it is important to know the other possible causes of ascites, because treatment and prognosis may be quite different. Peritoneal carcinomatosis is the second most common cause of ascites, followed by acute alcoholic hepatitis, heart failure, fulminant or subacute hepatic failure, pancreatic disease, dialysis ascites, nephrotic syndrome, hepatic vein obstruction, chylous ascites, bile ascites, and miscellaneous disorders of the peritoneum.

2. Should a diagnostic tap be performed routinely on all patients with ascites at the time of admission to the hospital?

Ascites is readily diagnosed when large amounts of fluid are present in the peritoneal cavity. If clinical examination is not definitive in detecting or excluding ascites, ultrasonography may be helpful. In addition, ultrasonography may provide information about the cause of ascites, e.g., by documenting parenchymal liver disease, splenomegaly, and an enlarged portal vein. Abdominal tap may be performed easily and safely, and analysis of ascitic fluid provides useful data for differentiating causes of ascites. Moreover, more than 30% of patients with cirrhosis and ascites have ascitic fluid infection at the time of admission to the hospital or develop it during hospitalization. As a rule, therefore, diagnostic abdominal tap should be performed routinely (1) in all patients with new-onset ascites and (2) at the time of admission in patients with ascites. In addition, it should be repeated in patients whose clinical condition deteriorates during hospitalization, especially when they develop signs or symptoms of bacterial infection.

3. How should a diagnostic paracentesis be performed?

Although paracentesis is a simple and safe procedure, precautions should be taken to avoid complications. Paracentesis should be performed under strict sterile conditions. The abdomen should be cleaned and disinfected with an iodine solution, and the physician should wear sterile gloves during the entire procedure. The needle should be inserted in an area that is dull to percussion. The midline between the umbilicus and symphysis pubis is preferable because it is avascular. Scars should be avoided, because they are often sites of collateral vessels and adherent bowel. Between 30–50 ml of ascitic fluid should be withdrawn for analysis. After paracentesis patients should recline for 10–30 minutes on the opposite side of the paracentesis to avoid leakage of ascitic fluid.

4. What tests should be routinely ordered on ascitic fluid?

Analysis of ascitic fluid is useful for the differential diagnosis of ascites. However, it is not necessary to order all tests on every specimen. The most important tests are cell count, bacterial culture, albumin, and total protein.

The **white cell count** is probably the single most important test performed on ascitic fluid, because it provides immediate information about possible bacterial infection. An absolute **neutrophil count** ≥ 250 cells/mm^3 provides presumptive evidence of bacterial infection of ascitic fluid and warrants initiation of empirical antibiotics. An elevated white blood cell count with a predominance of lymphocytes strongly suggests peritoneal carcinomatosis or tuberculous peritonitis.

Albumin concentration of ascitic fluid allows calculation of the serum-ascites albumin gradient to classify specimens into high- or low-gradient categories (see question 5).

Ascitic fluid should be cultured by inoculating blood culture bottles at the bedside. The sensitivity of this method is higher than that of the conventional technique in detecting bacterial growth. **Specific culture** for tuberculosis should be ordered when there is clinical suspicion of tuberculous peritonitis and the ascitic fluid white cell count is elevated with a predominance of lymphocytic cells.

Total protein concentration of ascitic fluid has been used to classify ascitic fluid into transudates and exudates. Presently, this classification is not particularly helpful, because >30% of cirrhotic ascites samples are exudates. Nevertheless, total protein concentration of ascites fluid should be routinely ordered, because it is useful for determining which patients are at high risk of developing spontaneous bacterial peritonitis (SBP) (total protein <1.0 gm/dl) and for differentiating spontaneous from secondary bacterial peritonitis. Measurement of **glucose** and **lactate dehydrogenase** (LDH) in ascitic fluid also has been found to be helpful in making this distinction (see question 9).

Amylase activity of ascitic fluid is markedly elevated in pancreatic ascites and gut perforation into ascites.

Gram stain of ascitic fluid is usually negative in cirrhotic patients with early SBP, but it may be helpful in identifying patients with gut perforation, in whom multiple types of bacteria are seen.

Cytology of ascitic fluid is useful in detecting malignant ascites when the peritoneum is involved with the malignant process. Unfortunately, ascitic fluid cytology is not useful in detecting hepatocellular carcinoma, which seldom metastasizes to the peritoneum.

Other analytic data proposed as helpful tests in detecting malignant ascites, such as fibronectin, cholesterol, and carcinoembryonic antigen, have limited, if any, value in ascitic fluid analysis.

5. Why is it useful to measure serum-ascites albumin gradient?

Serum-ascites albumin gradient is more useful than the total protein concentration of ascitic fluid in the classification of ascites. This gradient is physiologically based on oncotic-hydrostatic balance and is directly related to portal pressure. The serum-ascites albumin gradient is calculated by subtracting the albumin concentration of ascitic fluid from the albumin concentration of serum obtained on the same day. Patients with gradients ≥1.1 gm/dl have portal hypertension, whereas patients with gradients <1.1 gm/dl do not.

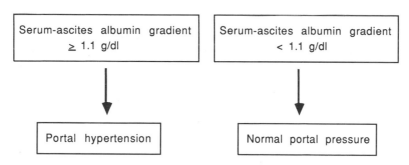

Usefulness of serum-ascites albumin gradient.

6. What are the causes of high (i.e., ≥1.1 gm/dl) serum-ascites albumin gradient?

The most common cause of a high serum-ascites albumin gradient is cirrhosis, but any cause of portal hypertension leads to a high gradient (e.g., alcoholic hepatitis, cardiac ascites, massive liver metastases, fulminant hepatic failure, Budd-Chiari syndrome, portal vein thrombosis, venoocclusive disease, myxedema, fatty liver of pregnancy, and "mixed" ascites). Mixed ascites is due to two different causes, including one that causes portal hypertension (e.g., cirrhosis and tuberculous peritonitis).

7. What are the causes of low (i.e., <1.1 gm/dl) serum-ascites albumin gradient?

Low-gradient ascites is found in the absense of portal hypertension and is usually due to peritoneal disease. The most common cause is peritoneal carcinomatosis. Other causes are tuberculous peritonitis, pancreatic disease, biliary ascites, nephrotic syndrome, serositis, and bowel obstruction or infarction.

8. What are the variants of ascitic fluid infection?

Ascitic fluid infection can be spontaneous or secondary to an intraabdominal, surgically treatable source of infection. More than 90% of ascitic fluid infections in cirrhotic patients are spontaneous. According to the characteristics of ascitic fluid culture and polymorphonuclear cell (PMN) count, three different variants of ascitic fluid infection have been described in cirrhotic patients during the last decade. SBP is defined as an ascitic fluid with PMN count ≥ 250 cells/mm^3 and positive culture (usually for a single organism). Culture-negative neutrocytic ascites (CNNA) is defined as an ascitic fluid PMN count of ≥ 250 cells/mm^3 with a negative culture. Bacterascites is defined as an ascitic fluid PMN count of <250 cells/mm^3 with a positive culture for a single organism.

9. How do you differentiate spontaneous from secondary peritonitis?

It is important to differentiate spontaneous from secondary peritonitis in cirrhotic patients, because treatment for SBP is medical, whereas treatment for secondary peritonitis is usually surgical. Although secondary peritonitis represents <10% of ascitic fluid infections, it should be con-

Variants of Ascitic Fluid Infection According to Ascitic Fluid Characteristics

	AF CULTURE	AF PMN (COUNT/MM^3)
Spontaneous bacterial peritonitis	Positive	≥ 250
Culture-negative neutrocytic ascites	Negative	≥ 250
Monomicrobial nonneutrocytic bacterascites	Positive	< 250

AF = ascitic fluid, PMN = polymorphonuclear neutrophils.

sidered in any patient with neutrocytic ascites. Analysis of ascitic fluid is helpful in differentiating the two entities. Secondary bacterial peritonitis should be suspected when ascitic fluid analysis shows two or three of the following criteria: total protein >1gm/dl, glucose <50 mg/dl, and LDH >225 mU/ml (or higher than the upper limit of normal for serum). Most of the ascitic fluid cultures in such patients are polymicrobial, whereas in patients with SBP the infection is usually monomicrobial. Patients with suspected secondary peritonitis must be evaluated by emergency radiologic techniques to confirm and localize the possible visceral perforation. In patients with nonperforation secondary peritonitis, these criteria are not as useful; however, PMN cell count after 48 hours of treatment increases beyond the pretreatment value and ascitic fluid culture remains positive. Conversely, ascitic fluid PMN cell count decreases rapidly in appropriately treated patients with SBP, and ascitic fluid culture becomes negative.

10. Who is at high risk of developing SBP?

- Cirrhotics with gastrointestinal hemorrhage
- Cirrhotics with ascites and low ascitic fluid total protein (<1gm/dl)
- Cirrhotics recovered from an episode of SBP
- Patients with fulminant hepatic failure

11. What is the pathogenesis of SBP?

Because gram-negative bacteria are normally present in the gut and are the most common causative agents isolated in bacterial infections in cirrhotic patients, the gut may be the source of the infection. Direct passage of intestinal bacteria to portal blood or ascitic fluid has not been documented in cirrhotic patients, if gut mucosa has not lost its integrity. Recently, bacterial translocation, defined as the passage of viable bacteria from gastrointestinal tract to mesenteric lymph nodes, has been demonstrated in an experimental model of cirrhotic rats with ascites. Several immune deficiencies, especially decreased activity of the reticuloendothelial system and low serum complement levels, lead to frequent and prolonged bacteremia in cirrhotic patients and to colonization of body fluids, such as ascitic fluid. The development of a bacterial infection depends on the capacity of ascitic fluid to kill the bacteria. *In vitro*, the capacity of ascitic fluid to kill a bacteria (i.e., opsonic activity) is related directly to total protein and C3 concentration of ascitic fluid. Cirrhotic patients with low ascitic fluid opsonic activity have low C3, low total protein, and thus a higher incidence of SBP. In contrast, patients with high ascitic fluid opsonic activity have high C3 and high total protein; thus bacterial colonization may resolve spontaneously.

12. What single test provides early information about the possible presence of ascitic fluid infection?

The decision to start empirical antibiotic treatment must be made as soon as possible, because the survival rate depends in part on early diagnosis and treatment. Gram stain is positive in only 5–10% of patients, and bacterial culture of ascitic fluid takes at least 12 hours to demonstrate growth. The ascitic fluid neutrophil count is highly sensitive in detecting bacterial infection of peritoneal fluid, and the result should be available in a matter of minutes. Ascitic fluid should be immediately injected into a tube containing an anticoagulant after the tap to avoid clotting of the specimen. Other single tests, such as ascitic fluid pH or its arterial gradient and ascitic fluid lactate or its serum gradient, are significantly less sensitive than ascitic fluid neutrophil count.

13. What is the treatment of choice for suspected SBP?

A relatively wide-spectrum antibiotic therapy, such as an aminoglycoside plus ampicillin, was routinely used in the past for treatment of suspected SBP. However, most cirrhotic patients treated with an aminoglycoside develop nephrotoxicity, even if serum levels are controlled. Third-generation cephalosporins cover most of the flora responsible for SBP; they are more effective than the combination of ampicillin and aminoglycoside and lack the nephrotoxicity. Cefotaxime or a similar cephalosporin should be started when SBP is suspected. Recently, it was demonstrated that 2.0 gm of cefotaxime, given intravenously every 8–12 hours, is as effective as treatment every 6 hours. The length of antibiotic therapy has recently been clarified; a short course of therapy (5 days) has been shown to be as effective as a long course (10 days).

14. When should antibiotic treatment be started in a patient with cirrhosis and suspected ascitic fluid infection?

Empirical antibiotic treatment must be started as soon as possible to improve survival. Therefore, it is important to perform routine bacterial cultures of ascitic fluid, blood, urine, and sputum as well as ascitic fluid PMN count when a hospitalized patient with ascites develops clinical signs of possible infection (fever, abdominal pain, encephalopathy) or shows deterioration in clinical or laboratory parameters. In addition, ascitic fluid and urine should be analyzed when cirrhotic patients with ascites are admitted to the hospital; about 20% are infected at this time. A high level of suspicion for bacterial infection is appropriate, because it is a reversible cause of deterioration and a frequent cause of death in patients with cirrhosis. Empirical antibiotics should be started immediately after performing cultures and ascitic fluid analysis whenever bacterial infection is suspected or ascitic fluid neutrophils are ≥250 cells/mm³ (see algorithm on next page).

15. Should the polymorphonuclear cell count in ascitic fluid be monitored during treatment of SBP?

Ascitic fluid culture becomes negative with a single dose of cefotaxime in 86% of patients with SBP. The neutrophil count also decreases rapidly to normal values during therapy in 90%. Su-

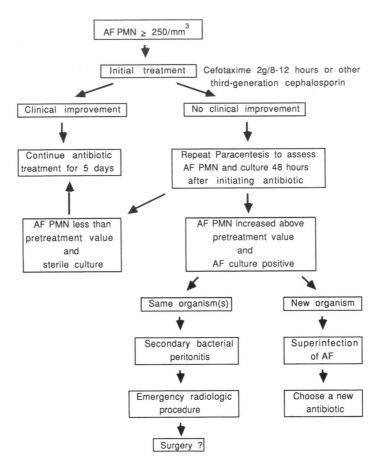

Management of spontaneous bacterial peritonitis.

perinfection or early recurrence after treatment with third-generation cephalosporins is uncommon. Repeat paracentesis is not necessary if the patient has a typical dramatic response to treatment.

16. Does bacterascites represent a real peritoneal infection? Should it be treated?

Recent studies have documented the short-term natural history of monomicrobial nonneutrocytic bacterascites. A repeat paracentesis of patients with bacterascites before starting antibiotic therapy showed that in 62–86% the episode of bacterascites resolved spontaneously. Of interest, all patients who progressed to SBP had symptoms of bacterial infection at the time of the first tap. Such data demonstrate that bacterascites is a dynamic process; its evolution may depend on several factors, including systemic and ascitic fluid defenses as well as organism virulence. According to these studies, symptomatic patients with bacterascites should be treated with antibiotics. Asymptomatic patients need not receive antibiotic treatment but should be reevaluated with a second tap. If the PMN count is ≥250/mm^3, antibiotics should be started.

17. Which subgroups of patients with liver disease should receive treatment to prevent bacterial infection?

Because enteric aerobic gram-negative bacteria are the most frequent causative agents isolated in bacterial infections in cirrhosis and because bacterial translocation seems to be an important step in pathogenesis, inhibition of intestinal gram-negative bacteria should be an effective method of preventing bacterial infections. Patients with liver disease who are at high risk of developing bacterial infection and/or SBP should be considered for selective intestinal decontamination (SID). SID consists of the inhibition of the gram-negative flora of the gut with preservation of gram-positive cocci and anaerobic bacteria. Preservation of the anaerobes is important in preventing intestinal colonization, overgrowth, and subsequent translocation of pathogenic bacteria. Several trials have shown that SID with oral norfloxacin is highly effective in preventing bacterial infections and/or SBP in cirrhotic inpatients with (1) gastrointestinal hemorrhage (400 mg twice daily) or (2) low ascitic fluid protein (400 mg/day) and (3) in patients with fulminant hepatic failure (400 mg/day). Although short-term prophylactic treatment (400 mg/day of norfloxacin) has been shown to be effective in preventing recurrence of SBP, some authors do not consider long-term therapy to be appropriate. More trials are needed. However, patients with cirrhosis recovering from an episode of SBP should be considered for liver transplantation; treatment with norfloxacin should be considered while patients await liver transplantation.

18. Why is it important to know the sodium balance in patients with cirrhosis and ascites?
Ascites formation in cirrhosis is due to renal retention of sodium and water. The aim of medical treatment of ascites in patients with cirrhosis is to mobilize the ascitic fluid by creating a net negative balance of sodium. This goal is accomplished by reducing sodium intake in the diet and increasing urinary sodium excretion. Therefore, knowledge of urinary excretion of sodium allows the clinician to plan initial treatment. In addition, urinary sodium excretion is an easily determined prognostic indicator. Patients with cirrhosis and a urinary sodium excretion <10 mEq/day have a 2-year survival rate of 20%, whereas those with sodium excretion >10 mEq/day have a 2-year survival rate of 60%.

19. Describe the initial treatment of patients with cirrhosis and ascites.
Cirrhotic patients with ascites should be treated initially by dietary sodium restriction (50–88 mEq/day) and diuretics. A more severe restriction of sodium intake may worsen anorexia and malnutrition. Water restriction is usually not necessary, if serum sodium concentration is above 120 mEq/L. In 15–20% of patients a negative sodium balance may be obtained with dietary sodium restriction in the absence of diuretics. However, because 80–85% of patients need diuretics, it is reasonable to start diuretics in all patients. The initial dose of diuretics should be 100 mg of spironolactone and 40 mg of furosemide—both orally. If the body weight does not decrease or the urinary sodium excretion does not increase after 2 to 3 days of treatment, the dose of both diuretics should be progressively increased, usually in simultaneous increments of 100 mg/day and 40 mg/day, respectively. Serial monitoring of urinary sodium excretion and daily weight is the best way to determine the optimal dose of diuretics. Doses should be increased until a negative sodium balance is obtained (i.e., urinary excretion is greater than dietary intake). The ceiling doses of spironolactone and furosemide are 400 mg and 160 mg per day, respectively. Once ascites has been mobilized, diuretic dosage should be adjusted individually to keep the patient free of ascites. Patients with tense ascites should be treated initially with a therapeutic paracentesis of 4 or more liters.

20. What is refractory ascites?
Refractory ascites is an inadequate response to salt restriction and high-dose diuretic treatment, manifested by no weight loss or development of complications of diuretics. Excessive sodium intake, bacterial infection, occult gastrointestinal hemorrhage and intake of prostaglandin inhibitors (e.g., aspirin) should be excluded before labeling patients as refractory. Less than 10% of cirrhotic patients are refractory to standard medical therapy. This small group should be evaluated for other therapeutic options, such as liver transplantation, chronic outpatient paracenteses (usually every 2 weeks), peritoneovenous shunt, TIPS.

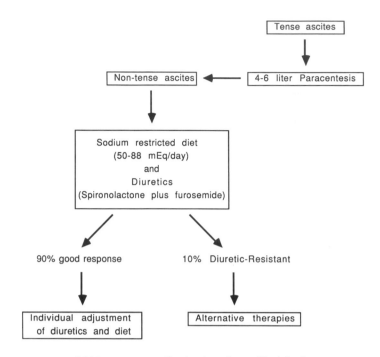

Initial management of ascites in patients with cirrhosis

21. Which patients should be treated with large-volume paracentesis?

Large-volume paracentesis is an old but safe and effective procedure to mobilize ascitic fluid in cirrhotic patients. Interest in this procedure has been renewed in the last decade. Recently, it has been shown that therapeutic paracentesis is not only safe but also may have additional beneficial effects on the hemodynamic status of patients with tense ascites. However, repeated large-volume paracenteses cause depletion of proteins and, theoretically, may predispose to SBP. Therefore, therapeutic paracentesis should not be used as a routine treatment of all cirrhotic patients with ascites and should be reserved for treating patients with tense and/or refractory ascites.

22. Is there currently any indication for peritoneovenous shunt?

Peritoneovenous shunt was introduced for the treatment of cirrhotics with refractory ascites in 1974 by LeVeen and associates. After initial enthusiasm, many complications were reported and the enthusiasm decreased progressively. The number of complications is especially high in patients with severe hepatocellular insufficiency. Peritoneovenous shunt does not reduce mortality during the initial hospitalization and does not improve long-term survival in cirrhotic patients. Therefore, peritoneovenous shunts should be considered in cirrhotic patients with refractory ascites who are not candidates for liver transplantation and in whom large-volume paracentesis is difficult.

23. Which patients with cirrhosis and ascites should be considered for TIPS?

Transjugular intrahepatic portosystemic stent shunt (TIPS) is an interventional radiologic technique that consists of creating a fistula between a hepatic vein and a portal vein and then placing an expandable metal stent in the balloon-dilated fistula to maintain patency. This technique was introduced to treat patients with recurrent variceal hemorrhage by decreasing portal pressure. Initial results show that TIPS could be useful in the treatment of cirrhotics with refractory ascites. However, the incidence of shunt dysfunction is still quite high; therefore, controlled trials are needed to establish the role of TIPS in treatment of cirrhotic patients with refractory ascites.

24. When should a patient with cirrhosis and ascites be evaluated for liver transplantation?
The probability of survival after the first episode of ascites has been estimated at 50% and 20% after 1 and 5 years of follow-up, respectively. The prognosis is even worse in patients with diuretic-resistant ascites; the 1-year survival rate is 25%. Because the 1-year survival rate after liver transplantation is >75%, patients with cirrhosis who develop ascites should be considered for liver transplantation, especially when they develop diuretic-resistant ascites. However, some alcoholic patients with diuretic-resistant ascites may become diuretic-sensitive after months of alcohol abstinence.

CONTROVERSY

25. Should volume expanders be infused after large-volume paracentesis?
Plasma volume expansion after large-volume paracentesis is controversial. Volume expanders were introduced to avoid theoretical hemodynamic disturbances that may develop in cirrhotic patients after therapeutic paracentesis of 5 or more liters of ascitic fluid. One study reported that patients receiving albumin infusion after large-volume paracentesis had less hyponatremia and azotemia than patients who did not receive albumin. However, albumin infusion did not decrease symptomatic complications or hospital readmissions or increase survival rates. Because albumin infusion is expensive, less costly volume expanders have been tried. Additional studies are needed. At this time, volume expanders should be viewed as optional until it is demonstrated that volume expansion after therapeutic paracentesis has a beneficial effect on morbidity or survival.

BIBLIOGRAPHY

1. Akriviadis EA, Runyon BA: The value of an algorithm in differentiating spontaneous from secondary bacterial peritonitis. Gastroenterology 98;127–133, 1990
2. Felisart J, Rimola A, Arroyo V, et al: Cefotaxime is more effective than is ampicillin-tobramycin in cirrhotics with severe infections. Hepatology 5:457–462, 1985.
3. Gines P, Rimola A, Planas R, et al: Norfloxacin prevents spontaneous bacterial peritonitis recurrence in cirrhosis: results of a double blind, placebo-controlled trial. Hepatology 12:716–724, 1990.
4. Gines P, Tito L, Arroyo V, et al: Randomized comparative study of therapeutic paracentesis with and without intravenous albumin in cirrhosis. Gastroenterology 94:1493–1502, 1988.
5. McHutchison JG, Runyon BA: Spontaneous bacterial peritonitis. In Surawicz CM, Owen RL (eds.): Gastrointestinal and Hepatic Infections. Philadelphia, W.B. Saunders, 1994, pp 455–475.
6. Runyon BA: Low-protein-concentration ascitic fluid is predisposed to spontaneous bacterial peritonitis. Gastroenterology 91:1343–1346, 1986.
7. Runyon BA: Ascites. In Schiff E, Schiff L (eds). Diseases of the Liver, 7th ed. Philadelphia, J.B. Lippincott, 1993, pp 990–1015.
8. Runyon BA: Refractory ascites. Semin Liver Dis 13:343–351, 1993.
9. Runyon BA: Care of patients with ascites. N Engl J Med; 330:337–342, 1994.
10. Runyon BA: Malignancy-related ascites and ascitic fluid "humoral test of malignancy" [editorial]. J Clin Gastoenterol 18:94–98, 1994.
11. Runyon BA, Canawati HN, Akriviadis EA: Optimization of ascitic fluid culture technique. Gastroenterology 95:1351–1355, 1988.
12. Runyon BA, McHutchison JG, Antillon MR, et al: Short-course vs long-course antibiotic treatment of spontaneous bacterial peritonitis: a randomized controlled study of 100 patients. Gastroenterology 100:1737–1742, 1991.
13. Runyon BA, Montano AA, Akriviadis EA, et al: The serum-ascites albumin gradient is superior to the exudate-transudate concept in the differential diagnosis of ascites. Ann Intern Med 117:215–220, 1992.
14. Soriano G, Guarner C, Teixido M, et al: Selective intestinal decontamination prevents spontaneous bacterial peritonitis. Gastroenterology 100:477–481, 1991.
15. Soriano G, Guarner C, Tomas A, et al: Norfloxacin prevents bacterial infection in cirrhotics with gastrointestinal hemorrhage. Gastroenterology 103:1267–1272, 1992.
16. Stanley MM, Ochi S, Lee KK, et al: Peritoneovenous shunting as compared with medical treatment in patients with alcoholic cirrhosis and massive ascites. N Engl J Med 321:1632–1638, 1989.

29. LIVER ABSCESS

Jorge L. Herrera, M.D.

1. What are the two major categories of liver abscess?
Pyogenic and amebic. Pyogenic abscesses usually arise from intra-abdominal infections, whereas amebic abscesses arise from colonic infection with invasive *Entamoeba histolytica*. This differentiation is important because the diagnostic approach and management differ for the two conditions.

2. Describe the clinical features of patients with liver abscess.
Pyogenic liver abscess: Most patients are middle-aged or older. The condition is equally prevalent in both sexes. The clinical findings are nonspecific and include fever, chills, right-upper-quadrant pain, malaise, and weight loss. Fever may be absent in up to 30% of cases. Abdominal pain is present in only 45% of cases. In many patients, the clinical presentation may be dominated by the underlying cause, such as appendicitis, diverticulitis, or biliary disease.
Amebic liver abscess: Patients tend to be younger (30–40 years), are more often male, have more severe right-upper-quadrant pain, and are febrile in 90% of cases. A travel history to endemic areas is commonly found in patients with amebic abscess, although it could be a remote history. Prior symptoms suggestive of previous colonic amebiasis are obtained in only 5–15% of patients. Concurrent hepatic abscess and amebic dysentery are distinctly unusual.

3. What laboratory features are distinctive in patients with liver abscess?
Results of routine laboratory tests are not diagnostic for pyogenic or amebic liver abscess. Leukocytosis is often present but may be absent in a significant number of patients. Anemia, normochromic normocytic, is present in over 70% of patients. Eosinophilia is characteristically absent in patients with amebic cysts. The erythrocyte sedimentation rate is invariably raised. Liver test abnormalities are not specific. Over 90% of the patients have elevation of alkaline phosphatase, but AST and ALT are elevated to lesser degrees. The presence of significant hyperbilirubinemia suggests that the biliary tree is the source of the abscess. Hypoalbuminemia is frequently described in these patients, and a level of <2 gm/dl carries a poor prognosis. Blood cultures are positive in 50% of patients with pyogenic abscess, and 75–90% of aspirates obtained from the abscesses are positive for bacteria.

4. What are the most common sources of pyogenic liver abscess?
Biliary tract disease is the most common source of pyogenic liver abscess, accounting for 35% of cases. Most abscesses result from cholangitis or acute cholecystitis. Malignant tumors of the pancreas, common bile duct, and ampulla account for 10–20% of hepatic abscesses originating in the biliary tree. Endoscopic or surgical intervention in the biliary tree may also result in hepatic abscess formation. Parasitic invasion of the biliary tree by roundworms or flukes can also lead to biliary infection and possible hepatic abscess.

The second most common source of pyogenic liver abscesses is **intra-abdominal infections** with bacterial seeding through the portal vein. Diverticulitis, Crohn's disease, ulcerative colitis, and bowel perforation account for 30% of pyogenic liver abscesses. Appendicitis is a rare cause of liver abscess, except in older or immunocompromised patients, in whom the diagnosis of appendicitis may be delayed. About 15% of liver abscesses arise by direct extension from a contiguous source, such as a subphrenic abscess or empyema of the gallbladder. Pyogenic infection may be carried to the liver in hepatic arterial blood flow from distant localized infections, such as endocarditis or severe dental disease.

5. List the common etiologic organisms causing pyogenic liver abscess.
Gram-negative organisms are implicated in 50–70% cases. *Escherichia coli* is the most common aerobic gram-negative organism cultured. Aerobic gram-positive organisms account for approximately 25% of the infections, and up to 50% of cases are caused by anaerobes.

Bacteriology of Pyogenic Liver Abscess

Gram-negative aerobes (50–70%)	Gram-positive aerobes (25%)	Anaerobes (40–50%)
Escherichia coli (35–45%)	*Streptococcus faecalis*	*Fusobacterium nucleatum*
Klebsiella	β-Streptococci	*Bacteroides*
Proteus	α-Streptococci	*Bacteroides fragilis*
Enterobacter	*Staphylococcus*	*Peptostreptococcus*
Serratia		*Actinomyces*
Morganella		*Clostridium*
Actinobacter		

From Frey CF, Zhu Y, Suzuki M, Isaji S: Liver abscess. Surg Clin North Am 69:259–271, 1989, with permission.

6. Do negative cultures from an abscess aspirate indicate a non-pyogenic abscess?
No. Although most cultures are positive, a negative culture may reflect improper handling of the specimen or prior antibiotic therapy. Proper collection and culture techniques are of critical importance for growing anaerobic organisms. Pus, and not swabs, should be submitted to the laboratory for cultures. Culture material should be transported to the laboratory immediately in the syringe used for aspiration to avoid exposure to air. Anaerobic organisms may require at least several days and up to a week or more for sufficient growth to establish a diagnosis. For this reason, Gram staining of the aspirate is of paramount importance. A Gram stain that demonstrates organisms with no growth in cultures after 2 or 3 days suggests an anaerobic pathogen. All aspirated material should be cultured for aerobic, anaerobic, and microaerophilic organisms.

7. What abnormalities can be detected on standard radiologic studies of patients with liver abscess?
A **chest x-ray** may be abnormal in 50–80% of patients with liver abscess. Right lower-lobe atelectasis, right pleural effusion, and an elevated right hemidiaphragm may be clues to the presence of a liver abscess. Perforation of a pyogenic liver abscess into the thoracic cavity may result in empyema. In **plain abdominal films,** air can be seen in the abscess cavities in 10–20% of cases. Gastric displacement due to enlargement of the liver may also be seen. These features are not sensitive for the diagnosis of liver abscess.

8. Which imaging studies should be obtained in evaluating a suspected liver abscess?
Ultrasonography is the initial procedure of choice in assessing a suspected liver abscess. It is noninvasive and highly accurate, with a sensitivity of 80–90% It is the preferred modality to distinguish cystic from solid lesions and is preferred to computed tomographic (CT) scanning for visualizing the biliary tree. Ultrasonography, however, is operator-dependent, and its accuracy may be affected by the patient's habitus or overlying gas. **CT scanning** may be more accurate than ultrasound in certain patients. The use of contrast material aids in the identification of smaller abscesses that could be missed on ultrasound examination; it is specially useful in the detection of microabscesses. CT scanning provides an assessment not only of the liver but also of the entire peritoneal cavity, which may provide information concerning the primary lesions causing the liver abscess.

Magnetic resonance imaging (MRI) does not add much to the sensitivity of CT scanning. **Scintigraphy** with technetium sulfur colloid is sensitive for detecting lesions >2 cm in diameter.

Gallium scanning may add to the sensitivity of technetium scanning, as pyogenic liver ab-scess avidly takes up gallium. Amebic abscesses, however, tend to concentrate gallium only in the periphery of the abscess cavity. In general, scintigraphy is the least helpful of the scanning modalities.

9. What areas of the liver are usually affected by hepatic abscess?

Right lobe only	65% of patients
Both lobes	30%
Left lobe only	5%

10. How can the location, size, and number of liver abscesses help determine the source?
Pyogenic liver abscess arising from a biliary source tends to be multiple and of small size and involves both lobes of the liver. Septic emboli from the portal vein tend to be more common in the right lobe of the liver, because most of the portal vein flow goes to the right lobe, and occa-sionally may be single. Abscesses arising from a contiguous source tend to be solitary and local-ized to one lobe only.

Amebic liver abscesses tend to be solitary and large, and most commonly they are located in the right lobe of the liver. The right lobe of the liver receives a major part of the venous drainage from the cecum and ascending colon, which are the parts of the bowel most commonly affected by amebiasis. Abscesses located in the dome of the liver or complicated by a bronchopleural fis-tula are typically amebic in origin.

11. When should a hepatic abscess be aspirated?
Hepatic abscess should be aspirated if they are thought to be pyogenic and not amebic. Patients with multiple abscesses, coexistent biliary disease, or an intra-abdominal inflammatory process are more likely to have pyogenic abscess. In these patients, aspiration under ultrasound guidance with Gram staining and culture can help guide antibiotic selection. Aspiration of amebic abscesses should be considered under the following circumstances: (1) when pyogenic abscess or secondary infection of an amebic abscess cannot be ruled out; (2) in patients who are not responding to ad-equate therapy for amebic liver abscess; or (3) in patients with a very large abscess with severe pain and evidence of impending rupture.

12. In what situation should an amebic liver abscess be treated by open surgical drainage?
When the amebic abscess is located in the left lobe of the liver, and response to therapy is not dra-matic within the first 24–48 hours, open surgical drainage should be accomplished. Complica-tions of left-lobe amebic abscess, such as cardiac tamponade, are associated with high mortality and require prompt intervention to prevent their occurrence.

13. Will aspiration of an amebic hepatic abscess yield diagnostic material in most patients?
No. Trophozoites are found in <20% of aspirates. Although classically the contents of amebic ab-scess are described as "anchovy paste" in appearance, in practice most aspirated material does not conform to this description. The contents of an amebic abscess are typically odorless. Foul-smelling aspirates or a positive Gram stain should suggest a pyogenic abscess or secondarily in-fected amebic abscess.

14. How often is the biliary tree involved in patients with amebic liver abscess?
Bile is lethal to amebae; thus, infection of the gallbladder and bile ducts does not occur. In pa-tients with a large amebic or pyogenic abscess, compression of the biliary system may result in jaundice, but cholangitis occurs only if there is secondary bacterial infection.

15. How can the diagnosis of an amebic abscess be confirmed?
Patients with amebic abscess are best differentiated from those with pyogenic abscess by **serologic tests,** including:

Hemagglutination (IHA)	Gel diffusion precipitin (GDP)
Indirect immunofluorescence (IF)	Complement fixation (CF)
Counterimmunoelectrophoresis (CIE)	Latex agglutination (LA)
Immunoelectrophoresis (IEP)	Enzyme-linked immunosorbent assay (ELISA)

Serologic tests are positive only in patients with invasive amebiasis, such as hepatic abscess or amebic colitis. They are negative in asymptomatic carriers. With the exception of CF, these tests are all highly sensitive, with reported rates of 95–99%. The IHA is extremely sensitive, and a negative test excludes the diagnosis; a titer of ≥1:512 is almost always present in patients with invasive disease. IHA, however, will remain positive for many years, and a positive titer may indicate prior infection. GDP titers usually become negative 6 months after the infection, and this is the test of choice for patients coming from endemic areas with prior exposure to amebiasis. A high GDP titer in a patient with hepatic abscess suggests an amebic abscess, even if the patient has a prior history of invasive amebiasis. In general, the choice of serologic tests used to diagnose amebic liver abscess depends on the availability of the tests and epidemiologic considerations.

16. What is the treatment for pyogenic liver abscess?

For single abscess or several large abscesses, treatment consists of antibiotics and appropriate drainage. Drainage should be achieved percutaneously whenever possible. Surgical drainage should be performed only if more conservative measures do not result in complete resolution or if surgery is needed to treat a primary intra-abdominal lesion. For multiple microabscesses, antibiotic therapy and correction of the underlying biliary abnormality may suffice. Antibiotic coverage involves a combination of antibiotics directed against anaerobes, gram negative aerobes, and enterococci. Thus, the combination of an aminoglycoside or cephalosporin for aerobic gram-negative organisms, clindamycin or metronidazole for anaerobes, and penicillin or ampicillin for enterococci is commonly employed. The antibiotic regimen may be altered as needed, depending on culture results or clinical response. Treatment should be continued for 10–14 days intravenously, or longer if drains are still in place. An additional 2 weeks of oral therapy may be added.

17. What is the treatment for amebic liver abscess?

Metronidazole is the only drug active against the extraintestinal form of amebiasis. A dose of 750 mg three times daily for 10 days is recommended for the treatment of hepatic abscess. Even at this dose, metronidazole is somewhat less effective in the intestinal form of the disease; thus, a luminal amebicide such as iodoquinol (diiodohydroxyquin), 650 mg three times daily for 20 days, should be prescribed to eradicate the intestinal form and prevent recurrence.

18. List the potential complications of pyogenic liver abscess.

Untreated, pyogenic liver abscess has a 100% mortality. Other complications include rupture into the peritoneal cavity, forming subphrenic, perihepatic, or subhepatic abscess or peritonitis. Rupture into the pleural space may cause empyema. Rupture into the pericardial sac may result in pericarditis and pericardial tamponade. Metastatic septic emboli involving the lungs, brain, or eyes may also occur.

19. List the potential complications of amebic liver abscess.

The complications of amebic liver abscess are similar to those of pyogenic liver abscess. Rupture into the pleural space results in amebic empyema. Rupture into the lung parenchyma may produce a lung abscess or bronchopleural fistula. Pericardial extension occurs in 1–2% of patients and is associated with amebic abscesses in the left lobe of the liver. A serous pericardial effusion may indicate impending rupture. Constrictive pericarditis occasionally follows suppurative amebic pericarditis. Brain abscess from hematogenous spread of the infection has also been reported.

20. What is the prognosis for patients with liver abscess?

The prognosis depends on the rapidity of diagnosis and the underlying illness. Patients with **amebic liver abscess** generally do well with appropriate treatment. Response to treatment is prompt and dramatic. Healing of the abscess leads to residual scar tissue associated with subcapsular retraction. Occasionally in patients with large abscess, a residual cavity surrounded by fibroconnective tissue may persist.

Mortality associated with **pyogenic liver abscess** has been reduced to 5–10% with prompt recognition and adequate antibiotic therapy. Mortality is highly dependent on the underlying disease process leading to the liver abscess. Morbidity remains high at 50%, primarily due to the complexity of therapy and need for prolonged drainage.

BIBLIOGRAPHY

1. Block MA: Abscesses of the liver (other than amebic). In Haubrich WS, Schaffner F, Berk JE (eds): Bockus Gastroenterology, 5th ed. Philadelphia, W.B. Saunders, 1995, pp 2405–2427.
2. Crippin JS, Wang KK: A unrecognized etiology for pyogenic hepatic abscesses in normal hosts: Dental disease. Am J Gastroenterol 87:1740–1742, 1992.
3. DeCock KM, Reynolds TB: Amebic and pyogenic liver abscess. In Schiff L, Schiff ER (eds): Diseases of the Liver, 7th ed. Philadelphia, J.B. Lippincott, 1993, pp 1320–1337.
4. Filice C, Di Perri G, Strosselli M, et al: Outcome of hepatic amebic abscesses managed with three different therapeutic strategies. Dig Dis Sci 37:240–247, 1992.
5. Frey CF, Zhu Y, Suzuki M, Isaji S: Liver abscesses. Surg Clin North Am 69:259–271, 1989.
6. Kandel G, Marcon NE: Pyogenic liver abscess: New concepts of an old disease. Am J Gastroenterol 79:65–71, 1984.
7. Knight R: Hepatic amebiasis. Semin Liver Dis 4:277–292, 1984.
8. Monroe LS: Gastrointestinal parasites. In Haubrich WS, Schaffner F, Berk JE (eds): Bockus Gastroenterology, 5th ed. Philadelphia, W.B. Saunders, 1995, pp 3123–3134.
9. Ralls PW, Barnes PF, Johnson MB, et al: Medical treatment of hepatic amoebic abscess: Rare need for percutaneous drainage. Radiology 165:805–807, 1987.
10. Teague M, Baddour LM, Wruble LD: Liver abscess: A harbinger of Crohn's disease. Am J Gastroenterol 83:1412–1414, 1988.
11. Vukmir RB: Pyogenic hepatic abscess. Ann Emerg Med 20:421–423, 1991.

30. INHERITABLE FORMS OF LIVER DISEASE

Bruce R. Bacon, M.D.

HEMOCHROMATOSIS

1. How are the various iron-loading disorders seen in humans classified?

The usual way to classify iron-overload syndromes is to distinguish hereditary hemochromatosis from secondary iron overload from parenteral iron overload.

Patients with **hereditary hemochromatosis** (HHC) have an inherited disorder that results in increased iron absorption from the gut, with preferential deposition of iron in the parenchymal cells of the liver, heart, pancreas, and other endocrine glands. In contrast, patients with **secondary iron overload** have some other stimulus to the GI tract to absorb increased amounts of iron. Thus, increased absorption of iron still occurs, but an underlying disorder causes this, so that patients are said to have iron overload secondary to some other process. Examples include ineffective erythropoiesis, chronic liver disease, and, rarely, excessive intake of medicinal iron.

In **parenteral iron overload,** patients have received excessive amounts of iron as either red blood cell transfusions or iron-dextran given parenterally. In patients with severe hypoplastic anemias, red blood cell transfusion may be necessary, but over time these patients become significantly iron-loaded. Unfortunately, some physicians give iron-dextran injections to patients with anemias that are not due to iron deficiency, and thus, patients become iron-loaded. Parenteral iron overload is always iatrogenic and should be avoided or minimized. In patients who truly need repeated red blood cell transfusions (in the absence of blood loss), a chelation program should be initiated to prevent toxic accumulation of excess iron.

2. What are neonatal iron overload and African iron overload?

There are two additional iron-overload syndromes in addition to the three major ones. **Neonatal iron overload** is a rare condition that is most likely related to an intrauterine viral infection and results in infants being born with increased amounts of hepatic iron. These infants do very poorly and, in general, die without liver transplantation. **African iron overload,** previously called Bantu hemosiderosis, was thought to be a disorder in which excessive amounts of iron were ingested from alcoholic beverages brewed in iron drums. Recent studies have suggested that this disorder may have a genetic component distinct (i.e., not HLA-linked) from the genetic disorder found in HHC. The implication for this in North America is that African-Americans may be at risk for developing iron overload from a genetic disease.

3. How much iron is usually absorbed per day?

A typical Western diet contains approximately 10–20 mg of iron. This is usually found in heme-containing compounds. Normal daily iron absorption is approximately 1–2 mg, representing about a 10% efficiency of absorption. Patients with iron deficiency, HHC, or ineffective erythropoiesis absorb increased amounts of iron upward to 3–6 mg/day.

4. Where is iron normally found in the body?

The normal adult male contains about 4 gm of total body iron. This is roughly divided between the 2.5 gm of iron found in hemoglobin in circulating red blood cells, 1 gm of iron found in storage sites in the reticuloendothelial system of the spleen and bone marrow and the parenchymal and reticuloendothelial system of the liver, and 200–400 mg in myoglobin in skeletal muscle. Additionally, all cells contain some iron because mitochondria contain iron both in heme, which is the central portion of cytochromes involved in electron transport, and in iron sulfur clusters, which are also involved in electron transport. Iron is bound to transferrin in both the intra- and extravascular compartments. Storage iron within cells is found in ferritin and, as this amount increases, in hemosiderin. Serum ferritin is proportional to total body iron stores in patients with iron deficiency or uncomplicated HHC and is biochemically different from tissue ferritin.

5. What is the genetic defect found in patients with HHC?

The specific genetic defect in HHC is unknown, but it appears that patients with HHC have a defect resulting in increased mucosal transfer of iron at the serosal surface of the enterocyte. Through linkage studies, the abnormal gene is known to be close to the HLA-A locus of the histocompatibiity complex on the short arm of chromosome 6. The gene frequency is estimated at 5%. Homozygote frequency in North America ranges between 1/220 and 1/500. The disease is usually quoted to be found in 1 in 250–300 individuals. The heterozygote frequency ranges between 1/8 to 1/12 individuals.

6. What are the usual toxic manifestations of iron overload?

In chronic iron overload, an increase in oxidant stress results in lipid peroxidation to lipid-containing components of the cell, such as organelle membranes, causing organelle damage. By unknown mechanisms, this seems to result in stimulation of increased collagen synthesis by hepatic lipocytes, the cells responsible for hepatic fibrogenesis.

7. What are the most common symptoms in patients presenting with HHC?

Currently, most patients are identified by abnormal iron studies on routine screening chemistry panels or by screening family members of a known patient. When identified in this manner, patients typically do not have any symptoms or physical findings. Nonetheless, it is useful to be aware of the symptoms that patients with more established HHC can exhibit. These are typically nonspecific and include fatigue, malaise, and lethargy. Other more organ-specific symptoms are arthralgias and those related to complications of chronic liver disease, diabetes, and congestive heart failure.

8. Describe the most common physical findings seen in patients with HHC.

As mentioned earlier, the way in which patients come to medical attention will determine whether or not they have physical findings. Thus, patients identified by screening tests have no abnormal physical findings. In contrast, physical findings may be seen in patients with advanced disease. These include a grayish or "bronzed" skin pigmentation, typically in sun-exposed areas; hepatomegaly with or without cirrhosis; arthropathy with swelling and tenderness over the second and third metacarpophalangeal joints; and other findings related to complications of chronic liver disease.

9. How is the diagnosis established in a patient suspected of having hemochromatosis?

Patients who are found to have abnormal iron studies on screening blood work, individuals who have any of the symptoms and physical findings of hemochromatosis, and individuals with a positive family history of hemochromatosis should have blood studies of iron metabolism either repeated or performed for the first time. These studies include a serum iron, total iron-binding capacity (TIBC) or transferrin, and serum ferritin. The transferrin saturation should be calculated from the ratio of iron to TIBC or transferrin. These studies are drawn in the fasting state to minimize the possibility of false-positives. If the transferrin saturation is >55% or if the serum ferritin is elevated, hemochromatosis should be strongly considered, especially if there is no evidence of other liver disease (e.g., chronic viral hepatitis, alcoholic liver disease, nonalcoholic steatohepatitis) known to have abnormal iron studies in the absence of significant iron overload. The next step is to perform a percutaneous liver biopsy to obtain tissue for routine histology, including Perls' Prussian blue staining for storage iron, and for biochemical determination of hepatic iron concentration. From the hepatic iron concentration, the hepatic iron index can be calculated and a specific recommendation as to the presence or absence of HHC can be made.

10. How commonly do abnormal iron studies occur in other types of liver disease?

In various studies, approximately 30–50% of patients with chronic viral hepatitis, alcoholic liver disease, and nonalcoholic steatohepatitis have abnormal serum iron studies. Usually, the serum ferritin is abnormal. In general, an elevation in transferrin saturation is much more specific for HHC. Thus, if the serum ferritin is elevated and the transferrin saturation is normal, another form of liver disease may be responsible for elevating the ferritin. In contrast, if the serum ferritin is normal and the transferrin saturation is elevated, then the likely diagnosis is hemochromatosis, particularly in young patients.

11. Is computed tomography (CT) or magnetic resonance (MR) imaging useful when considering the diagnosis of hemochromatosis?

In massively iron-loaded individuals, CT scans and MR images show the liver to be white or black, respectively, consistent with the kinds of changes that occur with increased iron deposition. In more subtle and earlier cases, there is tremendous overlap, and these studies are not useful. Thus, in very heavily iron-loaded individuals, the diagnosis is usually apparent without these imaging tests, and in the mild or subtler cases, they are unhelpful. The only utility of CT scanning or MR imaging is in the patient who is likely to have severe iron overload but for whom a liver biopsy is either unsafe or refused.

12. On a liver biopsy, what is the typical cellular and lobular distribution of iron in HHC?

In early HHC in young individuals, iron is entirely in hepatocytes and in a periportal (zone 1) distribution. In heavier iron-loading in older patients, iron is still predominantly hepatocellular, but some may be in Kupffer cells and bile ductular cells. The periportal to pericentral gradient is maintained but may be less distinct in more heavily loaded patients. When patients develop cirrhosis, it is typically micronodular, and regenerative nodules may have less-intense iron staining.

13. How useful is the hepatic iron concentration?

Whenever HHC is considered, the quantitative hepatic iron concentration should be obtained. Typically, in symptomatic HHC patients, the hepatic iron concentration is >10,000 μg/gm. The iron concentration threshold for the development of fibrosis is ~22,000 μg/gm. Lower iron concentrations can be found in cirrhotic HHC when there is a coexistent toxin, such as alcohol or hepatitis C or B. Young individuals with early hemochromatosis may have only moderate increases in hepatic iron concentration, but nonetheless they have HHC. These discrepancies in iron concentration with age are clarified by use of the hepatic iron index.

14. How is the hepatic iron index used in diagnosing hemochromatosis?

The hepatic iron index (HII) was introduced in 1986 and is based on the observation that the hepatic iron concentration increases progressively with age in individuals who have homozygous HHC. In contrast, in patients with secondary iron overload or in heterozygotes, there is no progressive increase over time. Therefore, the HII can distinguish patients with homozygous HHC from those with secondary iron overload and heterozygotes. The HII is calculated by taking the hepatic iron concentration (in μmol/gm) and dividing by the patient's age (in years). A value >1.9 is consistent with homozygous HHC. A value <1.5 should not be due to homozygous HHC. A value between 1.5 and 1.9 can be difficult to interpret, and it is necessary to evaluate these patients relative to family studies and to use good clinical judgment. The HII is not useful in parenteral iron overload.

15. How do you treat a patient with HHC? What kind of a response can you expect?

Treatment of HHC is relatively straightforward and includes weekly or twice-weekly phlebotomy of 1 unit of whole blood. Each unit of blood contains about 200–250 mg of iron. Therefore, a patient who presents with symptomatic HHC and who has up to 20 gm of excess storage iron will require removal of over 80 units of blood, taking close to 2 years at a rate of 1 unit of blood per week. Patients need to be aware that this treatment can be tedious and take a long time.

Some patients cannot tolerate removal of 1 unit of blood per week, and occasionally schedules are adjusted to remove only one-half unit every other week. In contrast, young patients who are only mildly iron-loaded may have their iron stores depleted quickly and require only 10–20 phlebotomies. The goal of initial phlebotomy treatment is to reduce the hematocrit to <35%. Once the ferritin is <50 ng/ml and the transferrin saturation <50%, the majority of excess iron stores has been successfully depleted, and most patients can then go into a maintenance phlebotomy regimen (1 unit of blood removed every 2–3 months).

Many patients feel better after phlebotomy therapy has begun, despite their being asymptomatic prior to treatment. Their energy level may improve, with less fatigue and less abdominal pain. Liver enzymes will typically improve once iron stores have been depleted. Increased hepatic size will diminish. Cardiac function may improve, and about 50% of patients with glucose intolerance will be more easily managed. Unfortunately, advanced cirrhosis, arthropathy, and hypogonadism do not improve with therapy.

16. What is the prognosis for a patient with hemochromatosis?
Patients who are diagnosed and treated before the development of cirrhosis can expect a normal lifespan. The most common causes of death in hemochromatosis are complications of chronic liver disease and hepatocellular cancer. If patients are diagnosed and treated early, they should not experience any of these complications.

17. Because hemochromatosis is an inherited disorder, what is my responsibility to family members once an individual has been identified?
Once a proband has been fully identified, all first-degree relatives should be offered screening with a transferrin saturation and ferritin. If either of these tests is abnormal, a percutaneous liver biopsy should be obtained for biochemical iron determination and routine histologic evaluation. HLA studies are most useful when evaluating siblings of a proband; if siblings are HLA-identical to a proband, then they, too, are homozygous for the disease. Liver biopsy is usually not performed on the basis of HLA studies alone, and iron studies should be abnormal before performing a liver biopsy. It is hoped that eventually a specific genetic test will be developed to establish the diagnosis.

α_1-ANTITRYPSIN DEFICIENCY

18. What is the function of α_1-antitrypsin in normal individuals?
α_1-Antitrypsin (α_1-AT) is a protease inhibitor synthesized in the liver that is responsible for inhibiting trypsin, collagenase, elastase, and proteases of polymorphonuclear neutrophils. In patients deficient in α_1-AT, the function of these proteases is unopposed. In the lung, this can lead to a progressive decrease in elastin and the development of premature emphysema. In the liver, there is a failure to secrete α_1-AT, and aggregates of the defective protein are found, leading by unclear means to the development of cirrhosis. Over 75 different protease inhibitor (Pi) alleles have been identified. Pi MM is normal, and Pi ZZ results in the lowest levels of α_1-AT.

19. How common is α_1-antitrypsin deficiency?
α_1-AT deficiency occurs in approximately 1 in 2,000 individuals.

20. Where is the abnormal gene located?
The gene is located on chromosome 14 and results in a single amino acid substitution (replacement of glutamic acid by lysine at the 342 position), which causes a deficiency in sialic acid.

21. What is the nature of the defect that causes α_1-antitrypsin deficiency?
α_1-AT deficiency is a protein-secretory defect. In normal individuals, this protein is translocated into the lumen of the endoplasmic reticulum, interacts with chaperone proteins, folds properly, is transported to the Golgi complex, and then exported out of the cell. In affected individuals,

the protein structure is abnormal, due to the deficiency of sialic acid, and the proper folding in the endoplasmic reticulum occurs for only 10–20% of the molecules, with resultant failure of export via the Golgi and accumulation within the hepatocyte.

In one detailed Swedish study, α_1-AT deficiency of the Pi ZZ type caused cirrhosis in only about 12% of patients. Chronic obstructive pulmonary disease (COPD) was present in 75% of patients, and of these, 59% were classified as having primary emphysema. It is unknown why some patients with low levels of α_1-AT develop liver disease (or lung disease) and others do not.

22. Describe the common symptoms and physical findings for patients with α_1-antitrypsin deficiency.

In adults with liver involvement, there may be no symptoms until they develop signs and symptoms of chronic liver disease. Similarly, children may not have any specific problems until they develop complications from chronic liver disease. In adults with lung disease, there are typical findings of premature emphysema, which can be markedly exacerbated by smoking cigarettes.

23. How is the diagnosis of α_1-antitrypsin deficiency established?

It is useful to routinely order α_1-AT levels and phenotype in all patients being evaluated for chronic liver disease because there are no particular presenting signs or symptoms to suggest the diagnosis by clinical presentation alone (apart from premature emphysema). It must be remembered that certain heterozygous states can result in chronic liver disease; for example, SZ as well as ZZ patients can develop cirrhosis. MZ heterozygotes usually do not develop disease unless there is some other liver condition, such as alcoholic liver disease or chronic viral hepatitis. Liver disease due to other causes may progress more rapidly in individuals who have an MZ phenotype.

24. What histopathologic stain is used by pathologists to diagnose α_1-antitrypsin deficiency?

Periodic acid–Schiff–diastase. Periodic acid Schiff (PAS) stains glycogen as well as α_1-AT globules a dark, reddish-purple color, and diastase digests the glycogen. Thus, when a PAS diastase stain is used, the glycogen has been removed by the diastase, and the only positively staining globules are those due to α_1-AT. In cirrhosis, these globules characteristically occur at the periphery of the nodules and can be seen in multiple sizes within the hepatocyte. Immunohistochemical staining can also be used to detect α_1-AT globules, and electron microscopy can show characteristic globules trapped in the Golgi apparatus.

25. Is there any effective treatment for α_1-antitrypsin deficiency?

The only treatment for α_1-AT-related liver disease is symptomatic management of complications and liver transplantation. With liver transplantation, the phenotype becomes that of the transplanted liver.

26. What is the prognosis for patients with α_1-antitrypsin deficiency? Should family screening be performed?

The prognosis depends entirely on the severity of the underlying lung or liver disease. Typically, patients who have lung disease do not have liver disease, and those who have liver disease do not have lung disease, although some patients can have both organs severely involved. In patients with decompensated cirrhosis, the prognosis relates largely to the availability of organs for liver transplantation, and these patients typically do fine. Family screening should be performed with α_1-AT levels and phenotype. This screening is largely for prognostic information since definitive therapy for liver disease, other than liver transplantation, is not available.

WILSON'S DISEASE

27. How common is Wilson's disease?

Wilson's disease is an autosomal recessive disorder with an estimated prevalence of 1 in 30,000 individuals.

28. Where is the Wilson's disease gene located?
The abnormal gene responsible for Wilson's disease is located on chromosome 13 and recently has been cloned. The gene has homology for the Menke's disease gene, which also results in a disorder of copper metabolism. The Wilson's disease gene codes for a P-type ATPase which is a membrane-spanning copper-transport protein. The exact location of this protein within hepatocytes is not definite, but it most likely causes a defect in transfer of hepatocellular lysosomal copper into bile. This defect results in gradual accumulation of tissue copper with subsequent hepatotoxicity.

29. What is the usual age of onset of Wilson's disease?
Wilson's disease is characteristically a disease of adolescents and young adults. Clinical manifestations of the disease have not been seen before the age of 5 years. By 15 years of age, almost half of the patients will have some clinical manifestations of the disease. Rare cases of Wilson's disease have been identified in patients in their 40s or 50s.

30. Name the organ systems involved in Wilson's disease.
The liver is uniformly involved. Patients who have neurologic abnormalities due to Wilson's disease all have liver involvement. Wilson's disease can also affect the eyes, kidneys, joints, and red blood cells. Thus, patients can have cirrhosis, neurologic deficits with tremor and choreic movements, ophthalmologic manifestations such as Kayser-Fleischer rings, psychiatric problems, nephrolithiasis, arthropathy, and hemolytic anemia.

31. What are the different types of hepatic manifestations in Wilson's disease?
The usual patient who presents with symptoms from Wilson's disease already has cirrhosis. However, patients can present with chronic hepatitis, and all young individuals with chronic hepatitis should have a serum ceruloplasmin level performed as a screening test for Wilson's disease. Rarely, patients present with fulminant hepatic failure, which is uniformly fatal without successful liver transplantation. Finally, patients can present early in the disease with hepatic steatosis. As with chronic hepatitis, young patients with fatty liver should be screened for Wilson's disease.

32. Once considered, how is a diagnosis of Wilson's disease established?
Initial evaluation should include measurement of **serum ceruloplasmin** and, if abnormal, a **24-hour urinary copper level.** Approximately 85–90% of patients with Wilson's disease have depressed serum ceruloplasmin levels, but a normal level does not rule out the disorder. If the ceruloplasmin is decreased or the 24-hour urinary copper level is elevated, then a **liver biopsy** should be performed for histologic interpretation and quantitative copper determination. **Histologic changes** can include hepatic steatosis, chronic hepatitis, or cirrhosis. Histochemical staining for copper with rhodamine is not particularly sensitive. Usually, in established Wilson's disease, **hepatic copper concentrations** are >250 μg/gm (dry wt) and can be as high as 3,000 μg/gm. Although elevated hepatic copper concentrations can occur in other cholestatic liver diseases, the clinical presentation allows for an easy differentiation between Wilson's disease and primary biliary cirrhosis, extrahepatic biliary obstruction, and intrahepatic cholestasis of childhood.

33. What forms of treatment are available for patients with Wilson's disease?
The mainstay of treatment has been the copper-chelating drug **D-penicillamine.** However, D-penicillamine is frequently associated with side effects, and so **trientine** also has been used for the treatment of Wilson's disease. Trientine is equally efficacious to D-penicillamine in the induction of negative copper balance, and it most likely has fewer side effects. Maintenance therapy with **dietary zinc supplementation** has also been used. Neurologic disorders can improve with therapy. Individuals who present with complications of chronic liver disease or with fulminant hepatic failure should be quickly considered for **orthotopic liver transplantation.**

34. Is it necessary to perform family screening in Wilson's disease?

Wilson's disease is an autosomal recessive disorder and, yes, all first-degree relatives of the patient should be screened. If the ceruloplasmin level is reduced, then a 24-hour urinary copper level should be obtained, followed by a liver biopsy for histology and quantitative copper determination.

35. Compare and contrast Wilson's disease and hereditary hemochromatosis.

Both disorders involve abnormal metal metabolism and are inherited as autosomal recessive disorders. The mechanism of tissue damage is probably related to metal-induced oxidant stress for both disorders. In HHC, the gene is on chromosome 6, whereas in Wilson's disease the abnormal gene is on chromosome 13. HHC occurs in approximately 1 in 250 individuals, but Wilson's disease only occurs in about 1 in 30,000 individuals. The inherited defect in HHC appears to be in the intestine, resulting in increased absorption of iron, with the liver being a passive recipient of the excess absorbed iron; in contrast, the inherited defect in Wilson's disease is in the liver, resulting in decreased hepatic excretion of copper with excess deposition and subsequent toxicity. While the liver is affected in both Wilson's disease and HHC, the other organs affected are quite variable. In hemochromatosis, the heart, pancreas, joints, skin, and endocrine organs are affected; in Wilson's disease, the brain, eyes, red blood cells, kidneys, and bone are affected. Both disorders are fully treatable if diagnosis is made promptly, prior to the development of end-stage complications.

BIBLIOGRAPHY

1. Bacon BR: Causes of iron overload. N Engl J Med 326:126–127, 1992.
2. Bacon BR, Britton RS: The pathology of hepatic iron overload: A free radical-mediated process? Hepatology 11:127–137, 1990.
3. Bacon BR, Tavill AS: Hemochromatosis and the iron overload syndromes. In Zakim D, Boyer TD (eds): Hepatology: A Textbook of Liver Disease, 3rd ed. Philadelphia, W.B. Saunders, 1996.
4. Bassett ML, Halliday JW, Ferris RA, Powell LW: Diagnosis of hemochromatosis in young subjects: Predictive accuracy of biochemical screening tests. Gastroenterology 87:628–633, 1984.
5. Bassett ML, Halliday JW, Powell LW: Value of hepatic iron measurements in early hemochromatosis and determination of the critical iron level associated with fibrosis. Hepatology 6:24–29, 1986.
6. Crystal RG: α_1-Antitrypsin deficiency, emphysema, and liver disease: Genetics and strategies for therapy. J Clin Invest 85:1343–1352, 1990.
7. Edwards CQ, Griffen LM, Goldgar D, et al: Prevalence of hemochromatosis among 11,065 presumably healthy blood donors. N Engl J Med 318:1355–1362, 1988.
8. Eriksson S, Calson J, Veley R: Risk of cirrhosis and primary liver cancer in alpha$_1$-antitrypsin deficiency. N Engl J Med 314:736–739, 1986.
9. Hill GM, Brewer GJ, Prasad AS, et al: Treatment of Wilson's disease with zinc: I. Oral zinc therapy regimens. Hepatology 7:522–528, 1987.
10. Hodges JR, Millward-Sadler GH, Barbatis C, Wright R: Heterozygous MZ alpha$_1$-antitrypsin deficiency in adults with chronic active hepatitis and cryptogenic cirrhosis. N Engl J Med 304:557–560, 1981.
11. Larsson C: Natural history and life expectancy in severe alpha$_1$-antitrypsin deficiency, Pi Z. Acta Med Scand 204:345–351, 1978.
12. Niederau C, Fischer R, Sonnenberg A, et al: Survival and causes of death in cirrhotic and noncirrhotic patients with primary hemochromatosis. N Engl J Med 313:1256–1262, 1985.
13. Perlmutter DH: The cellular basis for liver injury in α_1-antitrypsin deficiency. Hepatology 13:172–185, 1991.
14. Powell LW, Jazwinska E, Halliday JW: Primary iron overload. In Brock JH, Halliday JW, Powell LW (eds): Iron Metabolism in Health and Disease. London, W.B. Saunders, 1994, pp 227–270.
15. Scheinberg IH, Jaffe ME, Sternlieb I: The use of trientine in preventing the effects of interrupting penicillamine therapy in Wilson's disease. N Engl J Med 317:209–213, 1987.
16. Schilsky ML: Identification of the Wilson's disease gene: Clues for disease pathogenesis and the potential for molecular diagnosis. Hepatology 20:529–533, 1994.
17. Sternlieb I: Perspectives on Wilson's disease. Hepatology 12:1234–1239, 1990.
18. Stremmel W, Meyerrose KW, Niederau C, et al: Wilson's disease: Clinical presentation, treatment, and survival. Ann Intern Med 15:720–726, 1991.

31. LIVER HISTOPATHOLOGY

George H. Warren, M.D.

LIVER MICROANATOMY AND INJURY PATTERNS

1. Many of my liver biopsy reports say that the basic architecture is intact, and then list a string of abnormalities. What is the basic architecture?

The basic anatomy has three most obvious compartments: portal tracts, liver cell cords, and sinusoids and central veins. The portal tracts contain interlobular bile ducts, small hepatic arteries, small portal veins, and fibrous stroma with scant numbers of mononuclear cells. The lobules are formed by cords of hepatocytes, which are one cell layer thick. The row of hepatocytes immediately adjacent to the portal tract is termed the limiting plate. The liver cells are separated by vascular sinusoids lined by endothelial cells and Kupffer cells, the latter having macrophage function. Central veins, also called terminal hepatic venules, collect the circulating blood after it percolates through the lobules and then carry the blood to larger hepatic veins.

2. Are there geographic differences in pathology between portions of lobules?

Yes. Some disorders preferentially affect one area of the lobule over others. For example, because the centrilobular area is relatively hypoxic compared to the periportal area, hypoxic conditions such as heart failure will cause centrilobular necrosis of hepatocytes.

3. What is meant by distortion of the hepatic architecture?

Usually, it is fibrosis and regenerative nodules of hepatocyes, which alter the relationships of central veins, portal tracts, and hepatic cords.

4. How are degrees of fibrosis designated?

The pathologist indicates how generalized scarring is, how much collagen is present, whether anatomic structures such as portal tracts and central veins are connected by scar (bridging fibrosis), and whether the scarring has altered the architecture into nodules of hepatocytes (cirrhosis).

5. What criteria are used to define the presence of cirrhosis.

To prove that cirrhosis is present, three criteria must be met:
1. There needs to be fibrosis.
2. The scarring needs to be diffuse throughout the liver.
3. There needs to be nodular transformation of the architecture.

Therefore, focal scarring, even if significant and associated with nodules, is not cirrhosis because the process is not diffuse.

6. If cirrhosis is present, can it always be proved by a needle biopsy specimen?

No. **Micronodular cirrhosis** (nodules ≤3 mm), most often due to ethanol injury, is very uniform throughout the liver, and nodules are usually clearly defined on a needle specimen. **Macronodular cirrhosis** (nodules >3mm), due to chronic viral hepatitis among other conditions, is less uniform, and one sometimes sees relatively sparse fibrosis in a needle specimen, with some fairly normal lobules noted, even when cirrhosis is present. By the nature of the biopsy technique, the softer lobular tissue may come out in the needle more easily than the fibrous tissue, and scarring can be underrepresented.

7. What types of liver cell injury are seen on needle specimens, and what causes each type?

The difficulty in determining a specific etiology for liver injury reflects that although a lot of diseases affect the liver, there are relatively few ways for liver cells and bile ducts to express injury. So, in a number of diseases, very similar cellular injuries are present.

Types of Liver Cell Injury

TYPE	ETIOLOGIES
Fatty change	Ethanol, obesity, diabetes, drugs
Councilman bodies (acidophilic bodies)	Viral hepatitis, drugs, nonspecific reaction
Mallory bodies (hyaline)	Ethanol, obesity, diabetes, drugs, Wilson's disease
Hydropic change (ballooning degeneration)	Viral hepatitis, drugs, cholestasis
Cholestasis	Duct obstruction or injury, drugs, viral hepatitis
Interlobular duct injury	Primary biliary cirrhosis, primary sclerosing cholangitis, hepatitis C
Piecemeal necrosis	Viral hepatitis, primary biliary cirrhosis, drugs
Increased iron stores	Hemochromatosis, transfusions, hemolysis
Granulomas	Tuberculosis, fungi, drugs

8. What, in addition to biopsy findings, is needed to determine the etiology of an injury?
History, history, history. Laboratory evaluations should include AST, ALT, alkaline phosphatase, serum gamma-glutamyl transferase, protein, bilirubin, iron, total iron-binding capacity, ferritin, and, if indicated, infectious serologies, autoimmune serologies, and cultures. Special laboratory tests might include quantitative liver iron or copper, ceruloplasmin, and α_1-antitrypsin levels. Radiologic changes should be assessed by endoscopic retrograde cholangiopancreatography (ERCP), ultrasound, and computed tomography (CT). Liver pathology cannot be done in a clinical vacuum.

FATTY METAMORPHOSIS AND STEATOHEPATITIS

9. Acute and chronic ethanol injury is one of the most common insults to the liver. Describe the major characteristics of mild and severe injury.
In **mild ethanol injury,** fatty metamorphosis is seen with the cytoplasm of hepatocytes scattered throughout the lobules showing macrovesicular droplets. This can involve a few cells to almost every liver cell.
In more **severe acute injury,** "alcoholic hepatitis," or steatohepatitis, is characterized by fatty change, neutrophils surrounding injured cells, Mallory bodies or alcoholic hyaline in scattered liver cells, and some degree of hydropic change and necrosis of the most severely injured cells.

10. What is hyaline?
Hyaline is composed of irregular, ropelike strings of eosinophilic material in the cytoplasm, which represent aggregates of microfilaments. Although the fat and neutrophils can resolve relatively quickly after alcohol abstinence, hyaline can take up to 6 weeks to disappear.

11. How does scarring progress with alcohol injury?
Many patients with ethanol injury show initial scarring around central veins with delicate fibrosis along the sinusoids. Eventually, bridging fibrosis connects central veins and portal tracts and adjacent portal tracts. When cirrhosis is fully developed, most of the native central veins have been obliterated.

12. Is alcoholic cirrhosis micronodular or macronodular?
Micronodular, because the scarring is relatively uniform throughout the liver and because individual lobules have been subdivided by the portal-central bridging fibrosis. With complete alcohol abstinence, these nodules can regenerate and produce nodules >3 mm, but the central veins are decreased in number and the nodules themselves lack multiple portal tracts. One usually sees central veins and portal tracts in some nodules of a macronodular cirrhosis, e.g., those from viral hepatitis.

13. Sometimes a biopsy shows "alcoholic hepatitis," but the patient denies drinking ethanol at all. Is the pathologist's diagnosis incorrect, or is there a differential diagnosis for alcoholic hepatitis?

There is a differential diagnosis, and an important one. First, steatohepatitis is the better term to describe the pattern of liver cell injury known as alcoholic hepatitis. There are now over 20 conditions that can show hyaline on biopsy, and several of these can show full-blown steatohepatitis. Clinicopathologic correlation is required to determine the cause of the injury.

Partial List of Disorders Resembling Alcohol-related Liver Injury

Obesity	Wilson's disease
Diabetes mellitus	Vitamin A toxicity
Drugs (including glucocorticoids and amiodarone)	Prolonged cholestasis (e.g., primary biliary cirrhosis)
Jejunal-ileal bypass or gastric stapling	

Most of these conditions can be detected by history-taking. The common ones to consider are obesity and diabetes mellitus. These individuals, on occasion, show pathologic changes very similar to alcoholic liver disease, including fat, hyaline, and sinusoidal scarring (see figure below). In the patient under 40 years old, and particularly those under 30 years old, Wilson's disease needs to be excluded by multiple laboratory tests and quantitative liver copper analysis. Hyaline can be present in primary biliary cirrhosis, but it is characteristically limited to the periportal zone. Of the drugs, amiodarone is particularly serious because the drug may have a half-life up to 3 months, and injury may lead to death in that time. Clinical history of drug and toxin exposure is critical in liver disease. When all choices in the differential are exhausted, you should recognize that many alcoholics are exquisitely good at keeping their drinking a secret. The biopsy may confirm the nature and degree of injury, but it will be the history-taker who solves the case.

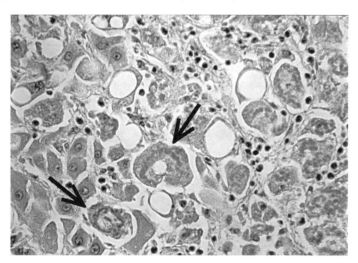

Alcoholic hepatitis with prominent hyaline (hematoxylin-eosin stain).

VIRAL HEPATITIS

14. Is a liver biopsy necessary in every patient who has viral hepatitis?

No. The diagnosis is usually recognized clinically and confirmed serologically, and the clinician is the authority in most cases, not the pathologist. This is especially true now that good serologic tests for hepatitis C virus are available.

A biopsy is needed when the differential diagnosis extends beyond the serologically established hepatitides A, B, and C (or D); when there is a second process; or when one is trying to establish the severity of the process, its chronicity, activity, or degree of irreversible fibrosis or cirrhosis.

15. When, if ever, is a biopsy ordered for a person with hepatitis A? When for hepatitis B and C?

Hepatitis A does not cause chronic liver disease, and therefore biopsy is rarely needed. Biopsies may be ordered to distinguish severe cholestasis in hepatitis A from large duct obstruction, or to determine if bridging necrosis or the rare fulminant necrosis is present (although many of the latter patients are too sick to biopsy). Usually, if a patient is positive for anti-hepatitis A, IgM type, there is no need for biopsy.

In patients with **hepatitis B or C,** if biopsy is done before 6 months of illness, it is usually to evaluate unusually severe cholestasis or severe injury. After 6 months or a year of illness, biopsy may be ordered to show if significant activity is present or, if fibrosis is developing, to consider interferon therapy.

16. What distinguishes chronic persistent from chronic active hepatitis?

These terms have been replaced by "mild" and "moderate or severe" chronic activity. In **mild chronic injury,** the lobular infiltrate is sparse, and the lymphocytes are predominantly in portal zones with minimal or no disruption of the limiting plates. **Moderate or severe activity** shows more inflammation, more necrotic liver cells, and portal inflammation that pours out of the portal tracts and obscures or irregularly breaks up the limiting plates (so-called piecemeal necrosis). A key part of the pathologist's evaluation is to state clearly whether fibrosis is present or absent; whether fibrosis is bridging portal tracts; and whether cirrhosis is present. The biopsy establishes that the injury is compatible with viral hepatitis and how active, severe, and irreversible the injury is.

17. What liver changes seen on biopsy mandate treatment?

Severe fibrosing injuries suggest the need to stop or decrease the inflammatory process, and hence require treatment. Mild, minimally fibrosing injury is a difficult problem, because treatment may be ineffective or incompletely effective and carries side effects. In both severe and mild injury, there is a role for rebiopsy to follow progression of disease and effect of treatment.

18. What do liver biopsies show in hepatitis B and C?

Active hepatitis shows lobular injury similar to acute hepatitis. Liver cords show disarray with regenerating cords more than one cell layer thick. Hepatocytes may be swollen (ballooning, hydropic change), show degeneration, single-cell necrosis (Councilman or acidophilic bodies), or associated cholestasis, and have an associated mononuclear, predominantly lymphocytic, inflammation (see figure on p. 226). Severe injuries show zonal necrosis, which may bridge central or portal zones. The portal tracts also show a significant lymphocytic or plasma cell infiltrate.

19. Can chronic viral hepatitis be confused with other injuries?

Autoimmune chronic active hepatitis looks very similar to chronic viral hepatitis, but plasma cells are more prominent in the autoimmune injury, and some serologic tests are available that can detect autoimmunity. Some drug injuries, primary biliary cirrhosis, primary sclerosing cholangitis, and other disorders can be difficult diagnostic problems. Some cases of α_1-antitrypsin deficiency can show piecemeal necrosis, but in this case, a periodic acid–Schiff–diastase strain will show numerous red cytoplasmic globules in hepatocytes.

CHOLESTASIS

20. In a patient with acute or chronic cholestasis, will the liver biopsy resolve the differential diagnosis?

Maybe. Diagnosing cholestasis requires evaluation of the many causes systematically: increased production of bilirubin, decreased excretion of bilirubin, and liver cell injuries. Hemolysis typically causes only mild hyperbilirubinemia. Extrahepatic obstruction is typically diagnosed

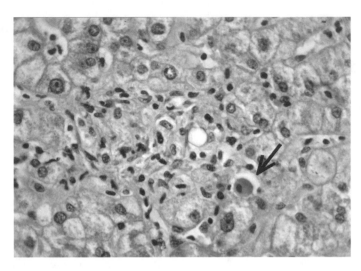

Biopsy, ordered to investigate fever of unknown origin, shows hepatitis with disorganized hepatocytes, lymphocytic infiltrate, and Councilman body (*arrow*) (hematoxylin-eosin stain).

by tests other than liver biopsy. Therefore, cases coming to liver biopsy are the difficult cases to solve, with the clinical and radiologic findings having solved the easy cases.

To solve the differential, the pathologist must ask, is there associated inflammation, or is it noninflammatory, "bland" cholestasis? Are there clues to suggest that large duct obstruction or an interlobular duct inflammatory injury are to blame? Subtle lesions in the head of the pancreas and ampulla of Vater can be missed. A stone may be missed. Is there hepatitis? Has a viral injury been excluded? What are the toxic exposures at work, home, or hobby? Has every drug been sought and disclosed? Are granulomatous causes excluded?

DRUG INJURY

21. When a careful clinical evaluation fails to disclose the cause of elevated liver function tests or cholestasis, drug or toxin injury is often considered as an etiology. When does one biopsy?
Biopsy when other approaches are exhausted.

22. What are the histologic changes that suggest drug or toxin liver injury?
Three findings should make a pathologist press the clinician to "find the drug":

1. Significant fatty change, which, after all, is most often related to toxic ethanol injury.

2. A liver biopsy that shows features of a hypersensitivity reaction. These cases will resemble viral hepatitis, with an abundance of eosinophils present. Eosinophils can also be present nonspecifically with viral hepatitis, connective tissue disorders, and some neoplasms (usually an infiltrate of Hodgkin's disease), but when eosinophils are a *striking* feature, the clinician should return for a drug or toxin search (see figure on p. 227).

3. A liver that looks like it is recovering from a one-point-in-time injury, featuring lots of liver cell mitotic figures. These findings suggest that a single or short episode of drug or toxin exposure might be to blame.

Finally, lacking other obvious cause, one might add granulomas to the list. Otherwise, the answer lies in a very good history, repeatedly taken, to generate a list of possible agents. This list is

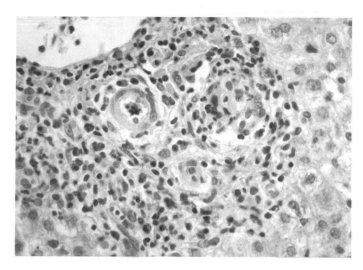

Nitrofurantoin hepatitis with prominent eosinophils (hematoxylin-eosin stain).

supplied to the pathologist, who will evaluate if the observed changes can be caused by one of these exposures. Then, one needs a good literature source.

BILE DUCT DISORDERS

23. In a patient with large duct obstruction, conjugated hyperbilirubinemia, an ultrasound showing bile duct stones, and clinical cholangitis, what would a biopsy show?
In this clinical situation, it is unusual that a liver biopsy would be necessary. If done, such a biopsy would show centrilobular cholestasis, portal tract edema, and neutrophils within portal tract stroma and within bile duct epithelium and lumens. One needs to remember that neutrophils within edematous portal stroma are a feature of large duct obstruction, even when frank cholangitis is not present.

24. When is primary biliary cirrhosis (PBC) diagnosed?

When there is an elevated serum alkaline phosphatase, modest transaminase elevation, initially mild or no hyperbilirubinemia, and the right clinical setting—a middle-aged woman, who may be itching—PBC would be a consideration. If there is obvious bile duct epithelial injury (florid duct lesion) and if the serum antimitochondrial antibody is positive, the diagnosis is made (see figure on p. 228).

However, if the duct epithelium is only mildly injured, and if the antimitochondrial antibody is negative, this dilemma may require time and re-biopsy to decide. More subtle clues of PBC include portal foamy macrophages, granulomas, periportal cholestasis, and increased periportal copper accumulation. The first task, however, is to establish that this is a portal-biliary inflammatory process and not hepatitis. If there is mild duct injury and hepatitis, hepatitis C should be suspected. If viral serology is negative and the patient has features of chronic active hepatitis, which PBC can resemble, the problem becomes more difficult. The diagnostic duct changes of PBC are focal and can be missed on any single biopsy.

25. When is primary sclerosing cholangitis (PSC) diagnosed?

PSC can be an even tougher problem to diagnose than PBC. First, does the clinical setting suggest PSC? Is there associated inflammatory bowel disease or a suggestion of large duct obstruc-

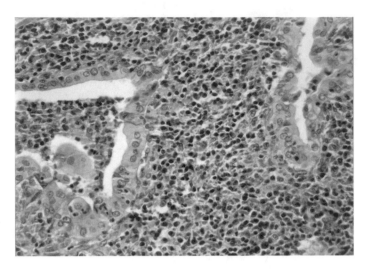

Primary biliary cirrhosis, with a florid duct lesion (hematoxylin-eosin stain).

tion? Again, it must be established that this is a bile duct problem and not hepatitis. In PSC, the inflammation will be predominantly mononuclear and in portal tracts. In some cases, the inflammation is comparatively mild, and the injury is predominantly periductal fibrosis, which "squeezes out" interlobular ducts. In a few cases, the fibrosis is laid down in a periductal, onionskin fashion. The end result is a decreased number of ducts and portal fibrosis or cirrhosis. A major goal of the biopsy interpretation is to consider PSC and then to suggest ERCP to confirm the diagnosis.

GRANULOMATOUS INFLAMMATION

26. What is a granuloma?
A granuloma is a sharply defined, or fairly sharply defined, aggregate of histiocytes.

27. Of the serum liver function tests, which one or ones raise the possibility of granulomatous inflammation?
A prominence or elevation of alkaline phosphatase or serum gamma-glutamy transferase (SGGT), over the transaminases.

28. How does one determine if an elevated alkaline phosphatase is of liver or bone origin?
Although bone alkaline phosphatase is more sensitive to deterioration by heat than is hepatic alkaline phosphatase, this is an imprecise method to separate these two isoenzymes. It is easier and faster to see if the SGGT is elevated to support a liver source for an elevated alkaline phosphatase.

29. What causes granulomas in the liver?
Infections, sarcoidosis, and drug reactions are the most common culprits, but granulomas can also be seen as a minor component of disorders such as primary biliary cirrhosis.

30. In a case of fever of unknown origin, if stains for fungi and acid-fast bacilli are negative, is infection excluded?
Not at all. Cultures for these organisms are more sensitive than special histologic stains. If infection is a possibility, a core of liver should be submitted with sterile precautions, *without fixative,*

to the microbiology laboratory, and a section sent to histology in formalin for microscopic sections.

31. Are acid-fast bacilli hard to identify on biopsy?

In *Mycobacterium tuberculosis* infection, there may be very few organisms detected in the sections. Usually, stains are negative but cultures are positive. With *M. avium-intracellular* (MAI) in AIDS, the bacilli are usually numerous. With MAI, the histiocytes may form less sharply defined granulomas, with sheets of infected histiocytes, or with organisms filling numerous Kupffer cells along sinusoids.

32. Are the granulomas of sarcoidosis characteristic?

No. Sarcoid granulomas usually show no associated necrosis, but they can be identical to infectious granulomas. A diagnosis of sarcoid requires the exclusion of other causes of granulomas and a supporting pattern of other organ involvement, clinical findings, and laboratory tests.

33. How often are liver granulomas secondary to a drug reaction?

In granulomatous liver reactions, perhaps one-third are caused by drugs.

Selected Drugs That Can Cause Liver Granulomas

Allopurinol	Nitrofurantoin
Alpha-methyldopa	Phenylbutazone
Carbamazepine	Procainamide
Diphenylhydantoin	Quinidine
Isoniazid	Sulfanilamide

IRON-OVERLOAD DISORDERS

34. If the serum iron/total iron-binding capacity (TIBC) ratio and serum ferritin are significantly elevated, is a liver biopsy indicated?

Yes. Diagnosis of iron overload is a tissue diagnosis.

35. Are the histologic findings characteristic and sufficient to make the diagnosis of genetic hemochromatosis?

Characteristic, yes. Sufficient, no. In genetic hemochromatosis, hepatocytes, and to a lesser degree, Kupffer cells and bile duct epithelium, contain increased stainable iron. This may be associated with no fibrosis, bridging fibrosis, or cirrhosis at the time of biopsy. The degree of iron deposition is qualitatively graded from 1+ to 4+.

36. If the laboratory tests are supported by 4+ iron deposition, is this sufficient evidence to diagnose genetic hemochromatosis?

Some patients do not have as much iron in their livers as suggested by the stained sections. This can be detected by comparing the stain to a quantitative iron measurement or to the results of multiple therapeutic phlebotomies.

37. What disorders are problematic in the clinical differential diagnosis of hemochromatosis?

Chronic alcoholic liver disease. Chapman and Sherlock studied several groups of patients and suggested cut-offs of quantitative iron amounts between normals, alcoholic liver disease, and hemochromatosis.

38. How does age affect the interpretation of quantitative iron results?

Among those with hemochromatosis, young patients have accumulated less iron than older patients, and menstruating females have less iron than males. The hepatic iron index (HII) takes age into account:

$$HII = \frac{\text{Hepatic iron concentration } (\mu mol/gm \text{ liver dry wt})}{\text{Patient age (yrs)}}$$

Patients with genetic homozygous hemochromatosis characteristically show an HII >2.0, whereas those with other causes of iron overload, including chronic alcoholic liver disease, show an HII <2.0.

39. How is quantitative iron measured?

A portion of fresh liver biopsy sample, measuring at least 0.5 cm in length, handled by a wooden applicator stick rather than by metal forceps, is sent without fixative in a plastic vial to a reference laboratory that performs the test. If fresh tissue was not set aside, the assay can be done on a sample from the paraffin block. The laboratory will report a result of quantitative iron in micromoles per gram of liver dry weight, and this result is then compared to the literature on hemochromatosis to calculate the hepatic iron index. In the past, there were difficulties in separating some patients with hemochromatosis from those with alcoholic levels, but today, additional genetic testing is becoming available to resolve this issue. This is an important group of patients to identify. Hemochromatosis is one of the most common genetic disorders, and the condition is treatable.

NEOPLASMS

40. What is the role of liver biopsy in diagnosing neoplasms?

First, an adequate sample of neoplasm must be obtained. One can confirm a metastasis to the liver from a known primary tumor. Most metastatic disease will not be curable, and it is appropriate to make the diagnosis with the minimally invasive technique of liver needle biopsy. Some biopsies will show tumor that is likely metastatic but for which there is no known primary. In these, the biopsy findings can guide the further workup, but it may not be possible to identify the primary from the needle specimen. A needle specimen may be used to diagnose or stage malignant lymphoma.

41. What is the role of biopsy in diagnosing primary liver tumors?

For vascular tumors, radiologic methods might be used rather than biopsy, but there are three types of liver masses that deserve special consideration: hepatocellular carcinoma, liver cell adenoma, and focal nodular hyperplasia. Each of these diagnoses may be suggested on needle biopsy samples, but definitive diagnosis can frequently be difficult or impossible in some cases without larger samples or complete resection of the mass.

Higher grade **hepatocellular carcinomas** are usually straightforward (see figure on p. 231). Low-grade hepatocellular carcinomas can be very difficult to distinguish from normal or from a regenerative nodule in cirrhosis. **Liver cell adenomas** in women on oral contraceptives can show characteristic features, but occasionally very well-differentiated hepatocellular carcinomas can resemble liver cell adenomas. **Focal nodular hyperplasia** is a localized lobulated nodule of hyperplastic liver cells surrounding a central scar. This condition can be confused with macronodular cirrhosis on a needle biopsy specimen (or even a wedge biopsy specimen), and the definite classification may require excision of the nodule.

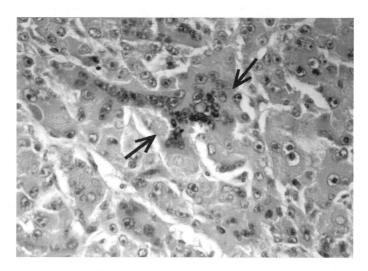

Hepatocellular carcinoma with prominent tumor giant cell (hematoxylin-eosin stain).

42. Can the clinical laboratory help in classifying tumors?

Marked elevation of serum α-fetoprotein levels in hepatocellular carcinomas or similar markers for other tumors can be a great help.

PATHOLOGIC CONSULTATION

43. Are there hepatic disorders for which biopsy interpretation should be referred to pathologists who specialize in liver pathology?

Slides can be express mailed to experts more easily than patients can be referred, and some rare disorders obviously need to be seen by specialists. Pediatric pathology is a very specialized field. Several disorders of extrahepatic and intrahepatic cholestasis in children and inherited metabolic disorders are appropriately referred to pediatric pathologists. With these disorders, the specialist should be consulted before doing the biopsy to determine if special handling of the specimen is necessary. Liver transplantation is becoming more frequent and successful, but the general pathologist usually has not seen the range of disorders in these cases to resolve diagnostic questions rapidly. Some vascular and cystic disorders deserve consultation. Drug and toxin exposure cases may warrant more than one opinion. Bile duct injury and neoplasms may need consultation. Finally, extremely difficult cases of any type deserve to be shared.

BIBLIOGRAPHY

1. Bassett ML, et al: Value of hepatic iron measurements in early hemochromatosis and determination of the critical iron level associated with fibrosis. Hepatology 6:24–29, 1986.
2. Chapman RW, et al: Hepatic iron stores and markers of iron overload in alcoholics and patients with idiopathic hemochromatosis. Dig Dis Sci 27:909–916, 1982.
3. Klatskin G, Conn HO: Viral hepatitis. In Histopathology of the Liver, vol 1. New York, Oxford University Press, 1993, pp 79–110.
4. Ludwig J, et al: Non-alcoholic steatohepatitis. Mayo Clin Proc 55:434–438, 1980.
5. Peters RL, Craig JR: Liver Pathology. New York, Churchill-Livingstone, 1986.
6. Poulsen H, Christoffersen P: Atlas of Liver Biopsies. Philadelphia, J.B. Lippincott, 1981.
7. Zimmerman HJ, Maddrey WE: Toxic and drug-induced hepatitis. In Schiff L, Schiff ER (eds): Diseases of the Liver. Philadelphia, J.B. Lippincott, 1993, pp 707–783.

32. HEPATOBILIARY CYSTIC DISEASE

Randall E. Lee, M.D.

1. Describe the five major classes and subtypes of bile duct cysts.

The classification of bile duct cysts by Todani et al. is commonly cited in the medical literature:

Type Ia: Choledochal cyst
Type Ib: Segmental choledochal dilatation
Type Ic: Diffuse or cylindrical duct dilatation
Type II: Extrahepatic duct diverticula
Type III: Choledochocele
Type IVa: Multiple intra- and extrahepatic duct cysts
Type IVb: Multiple extrahepatic duct cysts
Type V: Intrahepatic duct cysts (Caroli's disease and Caroli's syndrome)

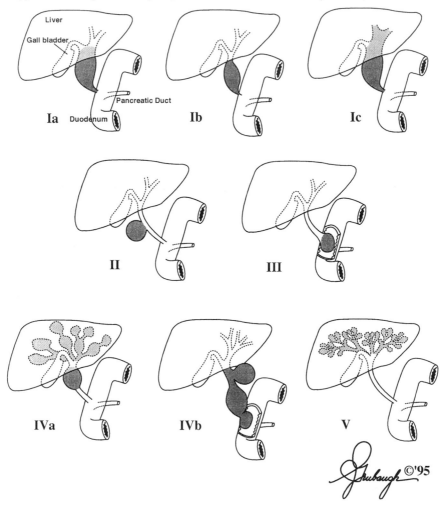

Classification of bile duct cysts.

2. What is the incidence of cancer within a bile duct cyst?
2–15%. Many of these cases occurred in patients who had undergone an internal drainage procedure rather than excision of the cyst prior to 1980.

3. What is the typical clinical presentation of a bile duct cyst?
The classic clinical presentation of a bile duct cyst includes a symptom triad of abdominal pain, jaundice, and an abdominal mass. Typically, however, only one or two of these symptoms are present at any one time. Many reports describe fever as a presenting symptom.

4. What is the preferred treatment for patients with bile duct cyst disease?
The preferred treatment is complete surgical excision of the cyst, rather than an internal drainage procedure. Postoperative complications, such as stricture formation, recurrent jaundice, and cholangitis, occur in about 8% of those undergoing complete excision of a bile duct cyst. The corresponding complication rate for those undergoing an internal cyst drainage procedure is about 50%. In addition, the risk of bile duct cancer is reduced with complete excision.

Unilobar intrahepatic cyst disease is usually treated by resection of the affected lobe. There is at least one case report of unilobar type V (Caroli's) disease treated by endoscopic retrograde cholangiopancreatography (ERCP), sphincterotomy, and ursodiol.

5. What is the role of ERCP in the evaluation of a patient with bile duct cyst disease?
Patients with extrahepatic bile duct cysts have an increased incidence of an anomalous pancreaticobiliary junction. Identification of the pancreatic duct insertion is critical to the planning of an extrahepatic bile duct cyst excision.

6. Compare the main features of Caroli's syndrome and Caroli's disease.
Initially described by Caroli in 1958, both of these clinical entities are characterized by congenital dilatations of the intrahepatic bile ducts. Patients usually become symptomatic as adults, presenting with abdominal pain and hepatomegaly. The mode of inheritance is autosomal recessive.

In **Caroli's syndrome**, the cystic dilatations are distributed along the portal tract. This distribution is believed to result from a ductal plate malformation that affects bile ducts at all levels, including the smaller interlobular ducts. Caroli's syndrome is associated with congenital hepatic fibrosis. Consequently, patients often have manifestations of portal hypertension, such as splenomegaly and esophageal varices.

Patients with **Caroli's disease** have cystic dilatations limited to the larger intrahepatic bile ducts. Some reports of Caroli's disease describe lesions in only one of the hepatic lobes. The cystic dilatations of the larger intrahepatic bile ducts predispose affected patients to recurrent intrahepatic calculi and cholangitis.

7. Describe some of the main nonhepatic manifestations of autosomal dominant polycystic kidney disease (ADPKD).
ADPKD is characterized by both kidney and liver cysts. In addition, there are strong associations between ADPKD and the presence of intracranial saccular aneurysms (berry aneurysms), mitral valve prolapse, and colonic diverticula. In whites, ADPKD occurs in about 1 in 400 to 1 in 1,000 individuals. Most families affected by ADPKD have a genetic defect located on the short arm of chromosome 16 (ADPKD1). Slightly less than one-half of ADPKD patients will develop end-stage renal disease.

8. What are the risk factors for cystic liver disease in patients with ADPKD?
Liver cysts are the most common extrarenal manifestation of ADPKD. The presence and severity of liver cyst disease in individuals with ADPKD increase with age, female gender, number and frequency of pregnancies, and severity of renal disease.

9. What are the clinical manifestations of complicated cystic liver disease?
The common complications of liver cyst disease include mass effect and cyst infection. Compression of adjacent structures by large cysts or by massive involvement may be manifest by

chronic pain and/or by obstructive jaundice. Clinical cues to the presence of a cyst infection include fever, right-upper quadrant abdominal pain, and leukocytosis. A definitive diagnosis of cyst infection usually requires percutaneous computed tomography (CT)- or ultrasound-guided fine-needle aspiration.

10. How does the presence of liver cysts affect hepatic function?

Hepatic function usually is not affected by liver cysts. In the absence of complications, the serum aminotransferase, bilirubin, and alkaline phosphatase levels typically are within the normal range or only slightly elevated. In patients with ADPKD, serum chemistry abnormalities generally reflect the degree of renal dysfunction.

11. What are the treatment options for ADPKD patients with symptomatic liver cysts?

Symptomatic liver cysts may be treated either percutaneously or surgically. Simple ultrasound- or CT-guided percutaneous aspiration of symptomatic liver cysts usually results in rapid reaccumulation of the cyst fluid. The rate of cyst recurrence is greatly reduced by instilling a sclerosing agent, such as absolute ethanol, at the time of aspiration. Patients treated in this manner may experience a low-grade fever and transient pain, as well as ethanol intoxication! Percutaneous sclerosis of a liver cyst is contraindicated when the cyst communicates with either the biliary system or peritoneal cavity.

Infected cysts will not resolve with systemic antibiotic therapy alone; antibiotic therapy should be combined with either percutaneous or surgical drainage.

12. What is the significance of a simple hepatic cyst?

Simple hepatic cysts (often referred to as solitary hepatic cysts) are benign fluid collections usually surrounded by a thin columnar epithelium. They are frequently noted as an incidental finding on hepatic ultrasonography or CT scanning. Simple hepatic cysts are not associated with cystic disease in other organs, and there is no genetic transmission. Many, but not all, simple hepatic cysts are solitary, and most are asymptomatic. Treatment is indicated if symptoms develop. Cyst-related symptoms include abdominal pain, increasing abdominal girth, infection, and obstructive jaundice.

13. What are the ultrasound characteristics of a simple hepatic cyst?

No internal echoes, a smooth margin with the surrounding parenchyma, and no appreciable wall. The absence of any of these characteristics should make one suspect a complication, such as a cyst infection, or another diagnosis, such as a hydatid cyst.

14. What are the characteristics of a simple hepatic cyst on CT and magnetic resonance imaging (MRI)?

A simple hepatic cyst appears on CT as a thin-walled lesion that does not enhance with iodinated intravenous contrast agents. The density of the lesion is that of water. On MRI, a simple hepatic cyst is a homogeneous, very low intensity lesion on T1-weighted scans, and a discrete high-intensity lesion on T2-weighted scans.

15. What is *Echinococcus granulosus*?

E. granulosus is a small tapeworm responsible for unilocular hydatid cyst disease. The adult worm is 2–8 mm long and consists of a bulbous scolex with four suckers and a coronet of hooklets, followed by three or four body segments called proglottids. The last proglottid is typically gravid with hundreds of eggs. Each egg measures only about 30 μm in diameter.

16. Describe the life cycle of *Echinococcus granulosus*.

The adult worm lives in the intestinal lumen of the definitive host, usually a predator such as a dog, fox, or cat. Eggs discharged from the gravid proglottid segment leave the definitive host in the feces. These eggs then are ingested by an intermediate host, such as a rabbit or sheep, through contaminated food or water. Ingested eggs hatch in the duodenum, and the larvae penetrate the

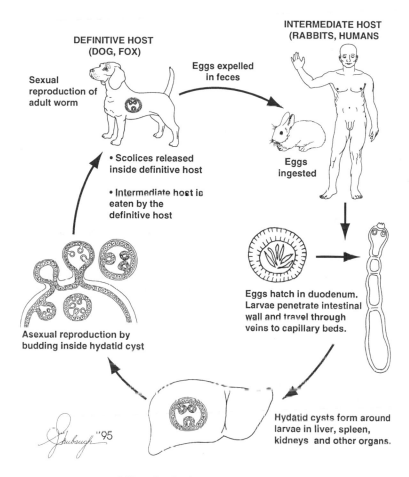

Life cycle of *Echinococcus granulosus*.

intestinal mucosa to be carried by the circulatory system to the capillary beds of distant organs. As a defense mechanism, the intermediate host lays down layers of connective tissue around each larva, thus forming the hydatid cyst. The liver is affected most commonly, but hydatid cysts also occur in the spleen, kidneys, lungs, heart, and brain. New scoleces bud from the inner wall of the cyst. Over time, daughter cysts may form within the original cyst. When the infected viscera are eaten by a predator, the scoleces develop into adult worms.

17. Where and how does *Echinococcus granulosus* infect humans?

Human infection by *E. granulosus* occurs throughout the world, including Alaska, Canada, and the western United States. Infections occur most commonly in sheep- and cattle-raising areas. Humans are usually infected as intermediate hosts when they ingest contaminated food or water. Additionally, children are commonly infected by allowing dogs to lick them in the mouth.

18. What is the typical clinical presentation of hepatic hydatid cyst disease?

Hydatid cysts grow at a rate of about 1–5 cm/yr, and thus many patients unsuspectingly harbor the infection until they present with a palpable abdominal nodule or other symptoms. The symptoms of hydatid cyst disease are related primarily to the mass effect of the slowly enlarging cyst: abdominal pain from the hepatic capsule stretching, jaundice from compression of the bile duct, or portal hypertension from portal vein obstruction. Approximately 20% of patients have cysts that communicate with the biliary tree and may have symptoms similar to those of chole-docholithiasis. Leakage of a cyst into the peritoneal cavity may cause an intense antigenic response, resulting in eosinophilia, bronchial spasm, or anaphylactic shock.

19. What is *Echinococcus multilocularis*?

E. multilocularis is the small tapeworm responsible for alveolar echinococcal disease. Its distribution is limited primarily to regions of Alaska, Siberia, Switzerland, France, and southern Germany. The developing scolices of *E. multilocularis* do not become encysted like those of *E. granulosus,* but instead they invade adjacent tissue by exogenous budding. Surgical resection of the infested tissue is the only chance for cure. Those patients with unresectable alveolar echinococcosis have a 10-year mortality of >90%. Chemotherapy with mebendazole or albendazole may reduce the amount of infested tissue and may prolong survival. Long-term albendazole therapy has been associated with bile duct strictures similar to those seen in primary sclerosing cholangitis.

20. How does one diagnose suspected echinococcosis?

Confirming a diagnosis of echinococcosis usually requires a combination of diagnostic imaging and serologic tests. CT scans may show the hydatid cyst as a sharply defined, low-density lesion with spoke-like septations. The presence of a calcified rim or daughter cysts greatly enhances the specificity of the CT scan.When viewed by ultrasound, the hydatid cyst appears as a complex mass with multiple internal echoes from debris and septations. Enzyme-linked immunosorbent assay or indirect hemagglutinin serologic assays for echinococcal antibodies are positive in about 85–90% of patients with hepatic hydatid cyst disease. Recovery of scolices from a suspected hydatid cyst by percutaneous needle aspiration is diagnostic; however, this technique must be used with extreme caution due to the risk of spilling scolices into the peritoneal cavity.

21. What are the treatment options for hepatic hydatid cyst disease?

The primary therapy for hepatic hydatid cyst disease is surgical excision of the cyst. Medical therapy with albendazole combined with percutaneous drainage has also been effective therapy. The instillation of a scolicidal solution into the cyst is controversial, with reports of sclerosing cholangitis associated with this practice.

BIBLIOGRAPHY

1. Ammann RW, Ilitsch N, Marincek B, et al: Effect of chemotherapy on the larval mass and the long-term course of alveolar echinococcosis. Hepatology 19:735–742, 1994.
2. Behrns KE, Van Heerden JA: Surgical management of hepatic hydatid disease. Mayo Clinic Proc 66:1193–1197, 1991.
3. Bernardino ME, Galambos JT: Computed tomography and magnetic resonance imaging of the liver. Semin Liver Dis 9:32–49, 1989.
4. Cheng TC: General Parasitology. New York, Academic Press, 1973, pp 510–516.
5. D'Agata IDA, Jonas MM, Perez-Atayde AR, Guay-Woodford LM: Combined cystic disease of the liver and kidney. Semin Liver Dis 14:215–227, 1994.
6. Dumont JA, Fields MS, Meyer RA, et al: Alcohol sclerosis for polycystic liver disease and obstructive jaundice: Use of a nasobiliary catheter. Am J Gastroenterol 89:1555–1557, 1994.
7. Gabow PA: Autosomal dominant polycystic kidney disease. N Engl J Med 329:332–342, 1993.
8. Igidbashian VN, Liu J, Goldberg BB: Hepatic ultrasound. Semin Liver Dis 9:16–31, 1989.
9. Khuroo MS, Dar MY, Yattoo GN, et al: Percutaneous drainage versus albendazole therapy in hepatic hydatidosis: A prospective randomized study. Gastroenterology 104:1452–1459, 1993.
10. Que F, Nagorney DM, Gross JB, Torres VE: Liver resection and cyst fenestration in the treatment of severe polycystic liver disease. Gastroenterology 108:487–494, 1995.
11. Telenti A, Torres VE, Gross JB, et al: Hepatic cyst infection in autosomal dominant polycystic kidney disease. Mayo Clinic Proc 65:933–942, 1990.
12. Todani T, Watanabe Y, Narusue M, et al: Congenital bile duct cysts: Classification, operative procedures, and review of thirty-seven cases including cancer arising from choledochal cyst. Am J Surg 134:263–269, 1977.

33. GALLBLADDER DISEASE

Roshan Shrestha, M.D., and Gregory T. Everson, M.D.

1. Who is at increased risk to develop gallstones?

Epidemiologic data suggest that as many as 20 million Americans have gallstones. Over 500,000 cholecystectomies are performed annually in the United States, at an estimated cost of over $5 billion. Most gallstones are composed predominantly of cholesterol; their prevalence increases with age, female gender, use of exogenous estrogen or contraceptive steroids, pregnancy, obesity, and rapid weight loss in obese subjects. Gallstones are highly prevalent in Hispanic populations and in native American populations of the southwestern states; for example, as many as 90% of Pima Indian women older than age 65 have gallstones. Additional risk factors for gallstones include use of fibric acid derivatives (clofibrate), prolonged total parenteral nutrition, ileal resection or jejunoileal bypass, ileal disease (e.g., Crohn's disease), celiac disease (gluten-sensitive enteropathy, nontropical sprue), vagotomy, spinal cord injury, diabetes mellitus, chronic hemolysis (sickle cell disease, thalassemia), and cirrhosis.

2. What are the types of gallstones?

One classification, which is based on chemical composition, delineates three types of gallstones: cholesterol, black pigment, and brown pigment. **Cholesterol gallstones** are defined as gallstones that are more than 50% cholesterol by weight. Cholesterol gallstones are not made of pure cholesterol, but salts of calcium, pigments, and glycoprotein may be found in their center, in radiating spikes, or in concentric rings within the stone. Pigment gallstones are poor in cholesterol and contain carbonate, phosphate, calcium salts of bilirubin, and palmitate distributed throughout the stone material. **Black pigment stones** are composed almost entirely of salts of bilirubin, occur in the setting of chronic hemolytic disease, and are formed in the gallbladder under sterile conditions. **Brown pigment stones** are soft and amorphous, contain bilirubin salts, but also have a number of other components. They are the main type of primary bile duct stones and tend to form in the setting of infection.

3. How do gallstones form?

Three processes may be required: secretion of "lithogenic" bile by the liver, nucleation of molecules to initiate crystal formation, and stasis of bile in the gallbladder to allow crystals to elongate and agglomerate to form stones.

• **Secretion of lithogenic bile by the liver:** The secretion of bile that is supersaturated with cholesterol is a prerequisite for cholesterol gallstone formation. Supersaturation may result from either enhanced cholesterol secretion (obesity, pregnancy, contraceptive steroids, estrogens) or reduced bile acid secretion (fasting, ileal disease or resection, rapid weight loss). The initial secretion of cholesterol by hepatocytes into bile is tightly coupled to phospholipid secretion in the form of unilameller vesicles. When bile is unsaturated, bile acid enhances the disappearance of vesicles as cholesterol is transferred to cholesterol/bile acid/phospholipid micelles. When bile is saturated, the unilameller vesicles aggregate into large, cholesterol-rich, multilamellar vesicles, which favors nucleation of cholesterol molecules to form crystals and, ultimately, gallstones.

• **Nucleation of molecules to initiate crystal formation:** Gallbladder mucin and other glycoproteins secreted by the liver and, possibly, gallbladder mucosa have been proposed as pronucleation factors. These glycoproteins promote the formation of cholesterol crystals from saturated biles and often are found in the core matrix of both cholesterol and pigmented gallstones. In contrast, antinucleation factors (apoproteins A1 and A2) found in nonlithogenic bile may prevent the formation of cholesterol crystals from vesicular aggregates.

• **Stasis of bile allowing crystal formation and stone agglomeration:** The healthy gallbladder prevents formation of gallstones by acidifying bile, concentrating bile, and vigorously expelling crystals and sludge during contractions. Cholesterol nucleation takes place over days; if the gallbladder empties vigorously several times daily, removing mucus and bile from the gall-bladder, crystal formation and development of gallstones may not occur. Gallbladder hypomotil-ity may influence formation of gallstones during total parenteral nutrition, rapid weight loss, pro-longed fasting, pregnancy, celiac disease, massive small bowel resection, and biliopancreatic bypass procedures for treatment of obesity.

4. What abdominal complaints should be evaluated for gallstones?

Most patients with gallstones are asymptomatic. Symptoms clearly associated with gallstones include biliary colic and those symptoms that occur once a gallstone has been evacuated from the gallbladder and enters the common bile duct (jaundice, cholangitis, pancreatitis). Biliary colic is defined as pain localized to either the right upper quadrant of the abdomen or epigastrium and is characterized by a short crescendo period of increasing pain (5–15 minutes), a plateau of steady pain (15 minutes to several hours), and a decrescendo period of decreasing pain and resolution (15 minutes to 2 hours). Patients are asymptomatic between attacks of colic. Nonspecific symp-toms that do not correlate well with gallstones include nausea, vomiting, dyspepsia, diarrhea, weight loss or gain, and heartburn.

Elderly, diabetic, and immunocompromised patients may present with serious complications of gallbladder disease (gangrenous gallbladder, empyema of the gallbladder, perforation of the gallbladder, suppurative cholangitis) and exhibit few or no localizing abdominal complaints or findings on physical examination. Elderly patients may present for evaluation of fever, altered mental status, loss of appetite and weight loss, or sepsis. Rarely, a large gallstone in the gallblad-der will erode through the gallbladder wall into an adjacent viscus (usually duodenum), traverse the bowel, impact at a point of narrowing (usually the terminal ileum), and cause bowel obstruc-tion or gastric outlet obstruction (Bouveret's syndrome).

5. Do gallstones ever spontaneously disappear?

In general, most gallstones do not dissolve spontaneously or exit the gallbladder asymptomati-cally. In the National Cooperative Gallstone Study, 1% of patients experienced spontaneous clear-ance of gallbladder stones over a period of 2 years while taking placebo. Even this low rate of clearance was questioned, as the technique used to detect gallstones was oral cholecystography, which is much less sensitive than the currently recommended method of realtime ultrasonogra-phy (98% sensitivity and specificity). In contrast, two recent ultrasonographic studies suggest that one-third of cholesterol gallstones that develop during pregnancy may dissolve. Small stones (<0.5 cm), which are composed predominantly of cholesterol, are more likely to dissolve in the postpartum period. In general, calcified stones, pigment stones, and stones that have persisted over several years are not likely to dissolve spontaneously. Gallstones that are symptomatic are not likely to disappear spontaneously.

6. A 42-year-old woman was noted to have gallstones when she underwent abdominal ul-trasonography to evaluate ovarian cysts. The gallstones are asymptomatic. A surgeon rec-ommended that she undergo laparoscopic cholecystectomy. She wants to know, "Should I have my gallbladder removed?"

Most patients with gallstones are asymptomatic and will remain so for several years. One study of the natural history of truly asymptomatic gallstones indicates that only 20% of these patients will develop symptoms when followed up to 25 years. Thus, it has been suggested that the asymp-tomatic gallstone population really comprises two populations: those who ultimately become symptomatic (usually within the first 5 years of follow up), and those who never develop symp-toms. The risk of developing symptoms is 1–3% per year for the first 5–10 years but then drops to 0.1–0.3% with prolonged observation. The risk of developing serious complications from gall-stones (acute cholecystitis, cholangitis, pancreatitis, sepsis, gangrenous gallbladder) is low, only about 0.1% per year. In the most comprehensive long-term study of natural history, biliary colic always preceded any serious complications by several months. Given the costs associated with cholecystectomy, the relatively benign natural history of gallstones, and the fact that biliary colic nearly always precedes more serious complications, prophylactic cholecystectomy is not recommended for asymptomatic patients. However, prophylactic cholecystectomy may be considered in some circumstances: large ileal resections, a patient with known gallstones who will be traveling or working in remote regions of the world, and certain populations or medical conditions associated with high rates of complications or cancer (Pima Indians, calcified gallbladder, porcelain gallbladder, gallstones associated with sickle cell disease). A recent clinical decision analysis suggests that patients with diabetes mellitus do not benefit from prophylactic cholecystectomy.

7. What is Murphy's sign?

Murphy's sign is a valuable indication of acute cholecystitis also known as "inspiratory arrest." The patient is asked to take deep inspiration while the examiner holds his or her fingers under the liver border, usually around the tip of ninth rib where the gallbladder may descend upon them. Inspiration is arrested in midcycle by pain on contact with the fingers. Carcinoma of the gallbladder may produce a similar sign when it has invaded through the gallbladder wall and involves the serosa or visceral peritoneum overlying the gallbladder.

8. What is Courvoisier's sign?

A palpable, distended, nontender gallbladder. The etiology of this finding is usually a malignant obstruction of the bile duct. It is uncommon with choledocholithiasis. One reason for the lack of distention of the gallbladder with common duct stones is that the gallbladder, which is the source of the gallstone, is also likely to be a victim of chronic cholecystitis. Fibrosis and scarring render the organ nondistensible.

9. A 62-year-old man recently underwent coronary artery bypass surgery. On this morning's rounds, he was noted to have a low-grade fever and mild right-upper-quadrant abdominal pain. What is acalculous cholecystitis, and what are the risk factors for its development?

Acalculous cholecystitis, inflammation in the absence of gallstones, represents 2–5% of cases of proven acute cholecystitis. The pathogenesis is unknown. Risk factors include prior surgical procedure (nonbiliary), severe trauma, burn, total parenteral nutrition, multiorgan failure, immunocompromised host (AIDS, cancer chemotherapy, leukemia/lymphoma, uremia),and elderly age.

10. What tests are useful in diagnosing acalculous cholecystitis?

One may be nearly certain of the diagnosis in the appropriate clinical situation when the following are present: leukocytosis, fever, and right-upper-quadrant tenderness to palpation. In the absence of these findings, one must rely on imperfect confirmatory radiologic studies (ultrasonography, HIDA-scintigraphy).

On **HIDA-scintigraphy,** a positive scan for acute cholecystitis is characterized by normal uptake and clearance of HIDA by the liver, rapid excretion into the biliary system, visualization of the extrahepatic bile ducts, appearance of HIDA in the intestine, but no visualization of the gallbladder. False-positive scans may occur in patients on parenteral nutrition, alcoholics, or those who have had a prolonged fast or recent meal. In addition, in acalculous cholecystitis, the cystic duct may be patent and allow entry of radionuclide into the gallbladder lumen, resulting in a false-negative scan.

Positive findings on ultrasonography or HIDA-scintigraphy need to be assessed carefully before proceeding to cholecystectomy.

11. What is gallbladder sludge? Is it a risk factor for development of gallstones?

Sludge refers to gallbladder mucin with entrapment of particulate matter nucleated from bile. Sludge formation occurs within the gallbladder when gallbladder emptying is slow and incomplete. It is often associated with prolong fasting or lack of stimulation of intestinal release of cholecystokinin. Although sludge is a reversible stage in gallstone pathogenesis, gallstones may develop in a large percentage of patients, leading to symptomatic biliary tract disease. Sludge is a risk factor for gallstones, but it may be evacuated from the gallbladder, and gallstone formation may be prevented.

12. What is Mirizzi's syndrome?

It is a clinical syndrome of cholecystitis and jaundice that develops when a stone impacts in the cystic duct. The resulting inflammation compresses and obstructs the common hepatic or common bile duct. Obstruction of the bile duct further promotes the development of cholangitis. The stenosis of the bile duct can mimic a malignant stricture. Acute cholecystitis is often associated with mildly abnormal liver tests, but a serum bilirubin >5 mg/dl strongly suggests common duct obstruction. If untreated, the stone may erode into the common bile duct and create a biliobiliary fistula. Management involves drainage of the biliary system, antibiotic therapy, intravenous fluids, and cholecystectomy.

13. A 30-year-old woman with insulin-dependent diabetes mellitus has symptomatic gallstones (biliary colic only), but she is reluctant to have surgery because her mother, who was also diabetic, died after ulcer surgery just 3 years ago. What is the likelihood that patients with symptomatic stones will continue to have symptoms?

Biliary colic. The best data addressing this question are from the National Cooperative Gallstone Study. Patients entering the trial had a history of biliary colic and were then randomized to receive one of two doses of chenodeoxycholate or placebo; 305 patients were enrolled in the placebo arm and were followed clinically. Patients with frequent attacks of biliary-type pain 12 months prior to entry into the trial continued to experience frequent attacks of pain, some developed complicated biliary disease, and many required cholecystectomy. In contrast, those who had infrequent attacks of pain continued to have few attacks, experienced a lower complication rate, and had lower rates of cholecystectomy. In general, patients with biliary colic can expect to continue experiencing biliary colic in follow up. The severity of the attacks is highly variable but may be relatively consistent within a given individual. Patients with frequent, severe episodes may be at greatest risk for complicated gallbladder disease.

Acute cholecystitis. Patients with acute cholecystitis should be treated with cholecystectomy. Early surgery is rapidly curative, complications such as empyema and perforation are prevented, and the patient can rapidly recover and return to work. Several prospective studies have shown that early surgery is associated with few technical complications, few deaths, and quick recovery.

Cholangitis/gallstone pancreatitis. Recurrence rates of cholangitis or gallstone pancreatitis differ depending on whether the patient has a retained bile duct stone. In most cases of cholangitis, the bile duct stone is too large to pass spontaneously, and recurrence of cholangitis is predicted if the stone is not removed. In contrast, as many as 90% of bile duct stones may pass into the intestine in the setting of gallstone pancreatitis. Nonetheless, the existence of residual stones in the bile duct or gallbladder is sufficient to ensure recurrence. One study of recurrence rates in gallstone pancreatitis suggested that as many as 60% of patients will experience recurrent pancreatitis within 6 months of the initial episode. Endoscopic retrograde cholangiopancreatography (ERCP) with sphincterotomy is recommended early for severe biliary pancreatitis and allows for removal of impacted common duct stones.

14. Why not treat her pain with analgesic medication and recommend a "wait-and-see" approach?

Chronic use of analgesics in the treatment of biliary pain is discouraged because it merely masks symptoms and may increase the likelihood that the patient will only present later with more serious biliary complications of the disease. "Wait and see" is the preferred recommendation only for patients with asymptomatic gallstones. Most clinicians recommend therapy for symptomatic disease based on the high likelihood of recurrent symptoms and the risk of developing serious complications once colic has occurred. Diabetic patients may be at particularly high risk for complications compared to nondiabetics. Complications include either severe cholecystitis, gangrenous gallbladder, empyema of the gallbladder, or perforated gallbladder. The operative mortality with emergency surgery for acute complications of gallstones in diabetic patients has been reported to be as high as 15–20%, or 4–5 times higher than for matched groups of nondiabetic patients.

15. Do diabetics have higher operative mortality rates after cholecystectomy?

Stable diabetics who undergo elective cholecystectomy have no major increase in expected operative mortality. In contrast, diabetics who are poorly controlled and who undergo cholecystectomy for complicated biliary tract disease do experience increased morbidity and mortality. For these reasons, the development of biliary colic in a diabetic patient with gallstones is an indication for early elective cholecystectomy.

16. What medical therapies for gallstones are available for patients who refuse surgery or who have a prohibitive operative risk?

- Oral bile acids (chenodeoxycholate, ursodeoxycholate)
- Methyl-*tert*-butyl-ether (MTBE)
- Extracorporeal shock-wave lithotripsy (ESWL)
- Endoscopic sphincterotomy

17. Describe the indications and disadvantages of oral bile acid therapy.

Two dihydroxy bile acids, chenodeoxycholate (chenodiol, CDCA) and ursodeoxycholate (UDCA), have proven effective in dissolving gallstones in randomized controlled trials. **Criteria for use** of these agents are radiolucent gallstones on plain film of the abdomen (or CT scan), a functioning gallbladder by oral cholecystography or HIDA-scintigraphy, and an intact enterohepatic circulation. **Contraindications** include calcified stones, which are insoluble; lack of a functioning gallbladder, which prevents the bile acids from entering or concentrating within the gallbladder; and ileal disease or resection, which prevents absorption of the orally administered bile acids. Because CDCA and UDCA reduce biliary cholesterol by different but complementary mechanisms, most investigators in the field recommend using both agents simultaneously: CDCA, 8 mg/kg/day, plus UDCA, 8 mg/kg/day.

The overall **success** of dissolving radiolucent gallstones varies from 15–50%. Small stones (<5 mm) are more successfully dissolved than large stones (gallstones >2 cm rarely dissolve). The success rate of treating small stones (1–3 mm) that float within gallbladder bile is as high as 80%. **Disadvantages** of oral bile acid therapy include that it has slow rates of dissolution, it is most effective in a minority of patients (nonobese patients, <5 mm solitary stone, radiolucent), and its recurrence rates are high even with effective dissolution (10% per year for the first 5 years). Patients with multiple stones before dissolution have a higher risk of recurrence than those with single stones.

18. How is methyl-*tert*-butyl-ether (MTBE) used?

MTBE is 50-fold more potent than oral bile acid in dissolving cholesterol, but like oral bile acids, it is only effective against radiolucent gallstones. MTBE treatment requires percutaneous puncture of the gallbladder, placement of an indwelling gallbladder catheter, continuous infusion of MTBE into the gallbladder and aspiration, and close monitoring of the patient. Most cholesterol gallstones may be dissolved by one or two treatment sessions. Despite the effectiveness of MTBE in dissolving the cholesterol component of the stone, a pigmented or calcified shell or collection of debris often persists that serves as a nidus for future stone formation, resulting in high rates of stone recurrence. **Criteria for use** of MTBE are radiolucent gallstone, functioning gallbladder or patent cystic duct, and patient tolerance of percutaneous transhepatic puncture of the gallbladder. **Disadvantages** include spillage of MTBE into the duodenum, which can cause severe duodenitis, systemic absorption resulting in anesthesia of the patient, and risks associated with percutaneous puncture of the gallbladder. In general, MTBE treatment is performed only in specialized centers and only for patients with prohibitive operative risk.

19. Extracorporeal shock-wave lithotripsy (ESWL)?

ESWL is effective in fragmenting gallstones within both the gallbladder and common bile duct. ESWL of gallstones is always done with concomitant use of oral bile acids and is restricted to use in patients with a functioning gallbladder. ESWL reduces larger stones to smaller stones, increasing total surface area of stones, which then increases the success rate of oral bile acids in dissolving the stones. The combination of lithotripsy and bile acid therapy is 40–50% effective (stone- and fragment-free at 6 months) when used on single gallstones of <30 mm diameter. The advantages of litotripsy are its low morbidity, lack of general anesthesia, outpatient setting, and minimal interruption of lifestyle. The main disadvantages are the lack of efficacy in patients with multiple stones and the high recurrence rate once oral bile acid therapy is stopped (10% per year for at least 5 years).

20. When is endoscopic sphincterotomy indicated in gallstone disease?
Endoscopic sphincterotomy is not recommended in the treatment of cholelithiasis or acute chole-cystitis. If the patient's gallstone disease is complicated by choledocholithiasis (jaundice, cholan-gitis, or pancreatitis), then endoscoic sphincterotomy may be all that is required to maintain the patient. Numerous studies of endoscopic sphincterotomy for choledocholithiasis have verified its efficacy at nearly eliminating the risk of subsequent complications from passage of additional bile duct stones. In contrast, the risk of acute cholecystitis in patients who have had endoscopic sphinc-terotomy but whose gallbladder has been left in place is 5–20% during a 3–5-year follow up.

21. What is Charcot's triad?
Biliary pain, jaundice, and fever (with chills and rigors) occurring together constitute Charcot's triad, which indicates acute cholangitis. The triad occurs in 70% of cases of acute cholangitis and is the most common complication of choledocholithiasis.

22. What is Raynold's pentad?
Refractory sepsis manifested by hypotension and mental confusion in a patient with Charcot's triad constitutes Raynold's pentad. Only 10% of patients with acute suppurative cholangitis pre-sent with all five of these features.

23. You are called to the emergency department to see a patient who has acute cholangitis. After confirming the diagnosis, what is the best therapeutic approach to the patient?
Acute cholangitis results from impaction of a gallstone in the bile duct and ascending infec-tion behind the obstruction. If untreated, patients develop rapidly progressive biliary infection, jaundice, and sepsis. Therapy for cholangitis should be individualized because of the wide spec-trum of severity of illness. Antibiotic therapy and intravenous hydration should be initiated

Morbidity and Mortality after Surgery or Endoscopic Biliary Drainage
in 82 Patients with Severe Acute Cholangitis

	SURGERY (n = 41)	ENDOSCOPIC DRAINAGE (n = 41)
Complications		
Heart failure	1	3
Bronchopneumonia	15	7
Wound dehiscence	1	0
Wound infection	7	1
GI bleeding	2	0
Renal dysfunction	11	7
Bleeding after papillotomy	0	1
Disseminated intravascular coagulopathy	2	0
TOTAL	27	14 $p < 0.05$
Causes of death		
Heart failure	2	0
Bronchopneumonia	2	2
Renal failure	1	0
Multiorgan failure	4	2
Sepsis	3	0
Cerebellar hemorrhage	1	0
TOTAL	13	4 $p < 0.03$

Lai ECS, Mok FPT, Tan ESY, et al: Endoscopic biliary drainage for severe acute cholangitis. N Engl J Med 326:1582–1586, 1992.

promptly on an empiric basis. About 70% of patients will respond appropriately. Patients failing to respond to empiric therapy within 24 hours should be considered for immediate biliary decompression. The latter may be accomplished by endoscopic sphincterotomy and removal of the impacted stone, endoscopic placement of nasobiliary drainage tube, percutaneous transhepatic drainage (radiologic intervention), or cholecystectomy plus common bile duct (CBD) exploration or placement of T-tube. The choice of these modalities depends on the expertise of the available specialists, the patient's condition, and estimated operative risk. In general, either endoscopic or surgical treatment is recommended. Radiologic placement of drainage catheters is usually used only when endoscopy is unsuccessful.

Several trials have examined the role of urgent endoscopy versus early surgery. In general, these studies demonstrate that ERCP, done early in the course of acute cholangitis, is safe and effective in controlling biliary tract sepsis. It is unclear yet whether outcome is superior with the combination of early ERCP, sphincterotomy, CBD stone extraction, and drainage of the biliary system followed by elective laparoscopic cholecystectomy compared to urgent cholecystectomy, CBD exploration, and T-tube placement. There have been no critical evaluations of costs associated with these two approaches.

24. What surgical options are available for patients with symptomatic gallstones?

Elective cholecystectomy is the preferred treatment for symptomatic cholelithiasis. There are two basic techniques: open laparotomy or laparoscopy. **Open laparotomy and cholecystectomy,** until recently, were the standard surgical methods against which all other therapies were judged. In 1988, Dubio et al. demonstrated that the gallbladder could be safely and effectively removed by **laparoscopy.** Since this initial experience, most surgeons performing cholecystectomy have switched from the open to the laparoscopic technique, and several studies have compared results with the two methods. Grace et al. demonstrated a significant advantage for laparoscopic cholecystectomy in complication rate, hospital stay, and hospital costs.

Advantages of laparoscopic cholecystectomy include short hospital stay, early return to home and job, high patient acceptance, and low rate of complications. Disadvantages include higher risk of major morbidity (when the surgery is done by technically inexperienced surgeons), potential to convert an elective cholecystectomy to an urgent cholecystectomy if complications occur, and higher rate of serious bile duct injuries. Open cholecystectomy may still be the preferred approach to patients with complex gallbladder disease, such as empyema, infarction, perforation causing generalized peritonitis or subphrenic abscess, biliary-enteric fistula leading to bowel obstruction (gallstone ileus), and bacterial cholangitis.

Complications of Cholecystectomy

	LAPAROTOMY (n = 25)	LAPAROSCOPY (n = 44)	TOTAL (n = 69)
Pulmonary embolism	1 (4)	0 (0)	1 (1)
Urinary tract infection	3 (12)	0 (0)	3 (4)
Atelectasis	1 (4)	0 (0)	1 (1)
Jejunal perforation	0 (0)	1 (2)	1 (1)
Bile leak	0 (0)	2 (5)	2 (3)
Jaundice	0 (0)	1 (2)	1 (1)
Total no. of patients with complications (%)	4 (16)	4 (9)	8 (12)

Grace PA, Quereshi A, Coleman J, et al: Reduced postoperative hospitalization after laparoscopic cholecystectomy. Br J Surg 78:160–162, 1991.

25. Are there specific features of gallstone pancreatitis that suggest this diagnosis over other causes of pancreatitis?

Although alcohol is the commonest cause of pancreatitis, gallstones are responsible for 25–40% of cases. Impaction of a gallstone at the ampulla of Vater causes hypertension in the pancreatic duct, which initiates the inflammation. Impaction may be more frequent in patients with high basal pressures in the sphincter of Oddi or in patients whose sphincter fails to relax in response to physiologic stimuli. Clinical clues that suggest gallstones as the etiology include significant abnormalities in liver tests, cholelithiasis on ultrasonography, amylase level >1500 IU/l, or rapid rise and fall in amylase levels. However, clinical features of gallstone pancreatitis may be indistinguishable from those of other forms of pancreatitis.

26. How great is the risk to develop gallbladder carcinoma in patients with gallstones?
There is an association between chronic cholecystitis and gallbladder malignancy. The incidence of carcinoma increases with age and with gallstones >3 cm in diameter. Approximately 0.1–3% of gallbladders removed for symptomatic cholelithiasis or cholecystitis, especially in the elderly, contain adenocarcinoma. Pima Indians, who have an extremely high prevalence of gallstones, also have the highest rate of gallbladder cancer and mortality in the United States. Calcified (porcelain) gallbladders pose an extreme risk for development of carcinoma, as high as 25%. Most tumors are adenocarcinomas and are locally very aggressive. A tumor that extends beyond the gallbladder wall has a poor prognosis.

27. Which antibiotics are preferred in the treatment of ascending cholangitis?
Antibiotics are tailored to the types of organisms associated with acute cholangitis, which include *Escherichia coli, Klebsiella pneumoniae, Streptococcus faecalis, Pseudomonas aeruginosa,* and *Bacteroides fragilis.* In the elderly or immunocompromised patients, anaerobic coverage is necessary because these patients are at increased risk to develop suppurative cholangitis. Effective antibiotic regimens include ampicillin (or amoxicillin) plus aminoglycoside, piperacillin alone, or fluoroquinolones. In cases in which *Bacteroides* is suspected, the addition of metronidazole is recommended. Sulfa drugs and cephalosporins are not recommended for acute cholangitis. Remember that antibiotics are viewed as adjuncts to the primary therapy, duct drainage.

28. A 28-year-old woman who underwent laparoscopic cholecystectomy for RUQ abdominal pain 6 months ago returns to your clinic complaining of continuing symptoms. What clinical features would suggest a retained common bile duct stone, and what is the preferred treatment for retained stones?
Most patients with cholelithiasis are cured by cholecystectomy, although a few may have residual stones within the bile duct. The incidence of retained bile duct stones increases with increasing age and is more likely in patients with multiple gallstones. The diagnosis of a retained stone is suggested by recurrence of biliary colic, abnormal liver tests, acholic stool, dark urine, and dilatation of the bile duct on ultrasonography. However, retained stones may be present without dilatation of the common duct or abnormal liver tests. The diagnosis is established by cholangiography. ERCP is the preferred diagnostic test, as the retained stone may also be treated easily via the same modality.

29. If the ERCP is negative for retained stone and no other diagnosis is apparent, what else can cause biliary-type pain after cholecystectomy?
Approximately 5% of patients will have persistence or recurrence of nonspecific symptoms after cholecystectomy. Most commonly, patients complain of dyspepsia or upper abdominal pain. The differential diagnosis is extensive and includes recurrent or retained calculi in cystic or common bile duct, pancreatitis, cholangitis, papillary stenosis, or operative injury to the biliary tree.
Once anatomic or mechanical factors have been eliminated, one needs to consider the possibility of disordered biliary motility, **biliary dyskinesia,** as the basis for pain. Biliary dyskinesia implies a disorder of the normal contraction of the gallbladder or altered function of the sphincter of Oddi. After removal of the gallbladder, the source of biliary dyskinesia is limited to the sphincter of Oddi. The latter may be responsible for postcholecystectomy syndrome in 5–15% of patients. The diagnosis of sphincter of Oddi dysfunction is dependent upon accurate measurement of the basal pressure of the sphincter via biliary manometry at ERCP. Patients with basal sphincter pressures >40 mm Hg experience relief of their pain after endoscopic sphincterotomy. Patients

with lesser basal pressures do not respond to sphincterotomy. Sphincterotomy should not be routinely performed on all patients with postcholecystectomy pain but limited to those with high basal sphincter pressure.

30. What features, other than a basal sphincter pressure >40 mm Hg, support the diagnosis of sphincter of Oddi dysfunction?

The most specific finding for sphincter of Oddi dysfunction is an elevated basal sphincter pressure >40 mm Hg. Additional features that support the diagnosis are dilated common bile duct, abnormal liver tests, and prolonged retention of contrast in the biliary system at ERCP.

BIBLIOGRAPHY

1. Boender J, Nix GAJJ, de Ridder MAJ, et al: Endoscopic sphincterotomy and biliary drainage in patients with cholangitis due to common bile duct stones. Am J Gastroenterol 90:233–238, 1995.
2. Boey JH, Way LW: Acute cholangitis. Ann Surg 191:264–270, 1980.
3. Cooper AD: Pathogenesis and therapy of gallstone disease. Gastroenterol Clin North Am 20:1–234, 1991.
4. Deitch EA, Engel JM: Acute acalculous cholecystitis: Ultrasonic diagnosis. Am J Surg 142:290–292, 1981.
5. Geenen JE, Hogan WJ, Dodds WJ, et al: The efficacy of endoscopic sphincterotomy after cholecystectomy in patients with sphincter of Oddi dysfunction. N Engl J Med 320:82–87, 1989.
6. Glenn F: Acute acalculous cholecystitis. Ann Surg 189:458–465, 1979.
7. Grace PA, Quereshi A, Coleman J, et al: Reduced postoperative hospitalization after laparoscopic cholecystectomy. Br J Surg 78:160–162, 1991.
8. Gracie WA, Ransohoff DF: The natural history of silent gallstones: The innocent gallstone is not a myth. N Engl J Med 307.798–800, 1982.
9. Grimaldi CH, Nelson RG, Pettitt DJ, et al: Increased mortality with gallstone disease: Results of a 20 year population-based survey in Pima Indians. Ann Intern Med 118:185–190, 1993.
10. Herlin P, Ericsson M, Homin T, et al: Acute acalculous cholecystitis following trauma. Br J Surg 69:475–476, 1982.
11. Howard RJ: Acute acalculous cholecystitis. Am J Surg 141:194–198, 1981.
12. Kern F Jr: Epidemiology and natural history of gallstones. Semin Liver Dis 3:87–96, 1983.
13. Lai ECS, Mok FPT, Tan ESY, et al: Endoscopic biliary drainage for severe acute cholangitis. N Engl J Med 326:1582 1586, 1992.
14. Kee SP, Maher K, Nicholls JF: Origin and fate of biliary sludge. Gastroenterology 94:170–176, 1988.
15. Long TN, Heimbach DM, Carrico CJ: Acalculous cholecystitis in critically ill patients. Am J Surg 136:31–36, 1978.
16. Lowenfels AB, Walker AM, Althaus DP, et al: Gallstone growth, size, and risk of gallbladder cancer: An interracial study. Int J Epidemiol 18:50–54, 1989.
17. McSherry CK, Ferstenberg H, Calhoun WF, et al: The natural history of diagnosed gallstone disease in symptomatic and asymptomatic patients. Ann Surg 202:59–63, 1985.
18. Murthy GD: Bouveret's syndrome. Am J Gastroenterol 90:638 639, 1995.
19. Neoptolemos JP, Carr Locke DL, Fraser I, et al: The management of common bile duct calculi by endoscopic sphincterotomy in patients with gallbladders in situ. Br J Surg 71:69–71, 1984.
20. Ohara N, Schaefer J: Clinical significance of biliary sludge. J Clin Gastroenterol 12:291–294, 1990.
21. Polk HC Jr: Carcinoma and the calcified gallbladder. Gastroenterology 50:582–585, 1966.
22. Ramanna L, Brachman MB, Tanasescu DE, et al: Cholescintigraphy in acute acalculous cholecystitis. Am J Gastroenterol 79:650–653, 1984.
23. Ransohoff DF, Gracie WA: Treatment of gallstones. Ann Intern Med 119:606–619, 1993.
24. Schoenfield LJ, Lachin MJ, et al: Chenodiol (chenodeoxycholic acid) for dissolution of gallstones: The National Cooperative Gallstone Study. Ann Intern Med 95:257–282, 1981.
25. Stephens CG, Scott RB: Cholelithiasis in sickle cell anemia: surgical or medical management. Arch Intern Med 140:648–651, 1980.
26. Thistle JL, Cleary PA, Lachin MJ, et al: The natural history of cholelithiasis: The National Cooperative Gallstone Study. Ann Intern Med 101:171–175, 1984.
27. Weiss KM, Ferrell RE, Hanis CL, et al: Genetics and epidemiology of gallbladder disease in new world native peoples. Am J Hum Genet 36:1259–1278, 1984.

34. SPHINCTER OF ODDI DYSFUNCTION

Milton T. Smith, M.D.

1. What is the sphincter of Oddi?

The sphincter of Oddi is a fibromuscular sheath that encircles the terminal portion of the common bile duct, pancreatic duct, and common channel as they traverse the wall of the duodenum. Smooth muscle fibers in the sphincter are arranged in both a circular and longitudinal fashion. Although the choledochal sphincter was recognized in 1681 by Francis Glisson, it was subsequently named after Ruggero Oddi, who published his morphologic observations of the sphincter in 1887, as a medical student at the University of Perugia, Italy.

2. Name the major components of the sphincter of Oddi.

The sphincter of Oddi is composed of three contiguous segments (*see* figure):
- The sphincter choledochus, which surrounds the distal common bile duct,
- The sphincter pancreaticus around the duct of Wirsung, and
- The sphincter ampullae which encircles the common channel.

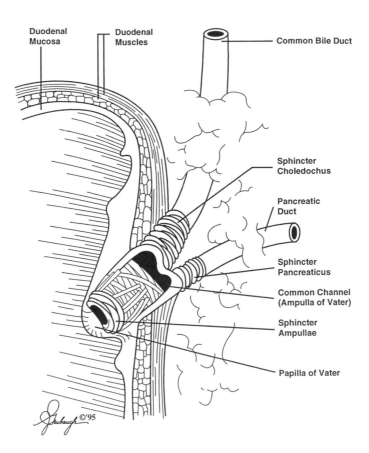

Anatomic drawing showing the three components of the sphincter of Oddi, duodenal wall, common channel, and papilla of Vater.

Manometric studies have shown that the length of the physiologic sphincter zone is approximately 8–10 mm, which may be shorter than its actual anatomic length.

3. What are the normal functions of the sphincter of Oddi?

There are three major functions: (1) regulation of bile flow (and pancreatic juice) into the duodenum, (2) prevention of reflux of duodenal contents into the bile ducts and pancreas, and (3) promotion of gallbladder filling with hepatic bile. All three functions appear to be related to the sphincter's ability to regulate the pressure gradient between the ductal systems and duodenum. Reciprocal contractile activity between the gallbladder and sphincter of Oddi promotes gallbladder filling during the interdigestive period.

4. Describe the physiologic characteristics of the sphincter of Oddi.

The physiologic control of the sphincter of Oddi appears to be multifactorial. Motor activity of the sphincter is coordinated with motility of the remainder of the GI tract and with the migrating motor complex during fasting. The sphincter is also responsive to multiple neurologic and hormonal stimuli and may be modulated, via reflex mechanisms, by other areas in the pancreaticobiliary tree. The sphincter receives both sympathetic and parasympathetic innervation, and its activity is increased by cholinergic stimulation. Cholecystokinin appears to be the major hormonal regulator and causes sphincter of Oddi inhibition with a reciprocal effect (i.e., contraction) on the gallbladder. The physiologic role of other GI hormones, such as gastrin and secretin, is less clear.

5. What is sphincter of Oddi dysfunction (SOD)?

Sphincter of Oddi dysfunction refers to the clinical condition in which there is benign, noncalculous obstruction to the flow of bile or pancreatic juice occurring at the level of the pancreaticobiliary junction. In clinical terms, the entity remains ill-defined and has been the source of considerable controversy. Patients with suspected SOD typically present with unexplained abdominal pain, with or without associated elevations in liver enzymes. SOD also may be found in a small percentage of patients with "idiopathic" pancreatitis. When the cause of a patient's symptoms is thought to be at the level of the sphincter of Oddi, the term *sphincter of Oddi dysfunction* is preferred over other terminology (e.g., papillary stenosis, biliary dyskinesia, postcholecystectomy syndrome).

6. What causes sphincter of Oddi dysfunction?

SOD is thought to be an acquired condition in which partial obstruction of the sphincter segment occurs on either an organic (i.e., structural) or functional (i.e., dysmotility) basis. As a result, patients may be subdivided into those with **sphincter stenosis** versus **sphincter dyskinesia.** True structural stenosis of the sphincter and papillary orifice is felt to be due to inflammation and fibrosis or possibly mucosal hyperplasia. Conditions that may contribute to the inflammatory/fibrotic process include the passage of small common bile duct stones and, possibly, recurrent episodes of pancreatitis. The etiology of functional SOD is unknown. It is usually difficult to separate patients who have organic versus functional stenosis, and overlap in etiologies almost certainly exists.

7. When should a diagnosis of SOD be considered?

A biliary motility disturbance should be considered in three main clinical settings:

1. Postcholecystectomy abdominal pain. Most studies have focused on SOD in these patients. In this setting, other etiologies of upper abdominal pain should be considered and are often easier to rule out. The differential diagnosis of postcholecystectomy pain is extensive (*see* table).

2. Idiopathic recurrent pancreatitis. The relationship between idiopathic pancreatitis and SOD has been reported recently. These studies have been delayed mainly due to concern over sphincter of Oddi (SO) manometry-related pancreatitis. SO manometry may reveal an elevated basal sphincter pressure in 15–57% of these patients.

Potential Etiologies of Postcholecystectomy Abdominal Pain

Musculoskeletal origin—secondary to trauma, muscular spasm/strain

Esophageal origin—esophageal spasm, gastroesophageal reflux

Pleural/pulmonary origin—pleural effusion, lower lobe pneumonia

Cardiac origin—coronary artery disease, pericarditis

Luminal GI tract origin—peptic ulcer disease, gastritis, duodenitis, obstruction, irritable bowel syndrome

Neoplasm—esophageal, gastric, pulmonary, biliary, pancreatic, papillary, other intra-abdominal tumors

Nonneoplastic intra-abdominal processes—Fitz-Hugh–Curtis syndrome, endometriosis

Narcotic withdrawal

Pancreaticobiliary origin—Residual or recurrent stones, strictures, tumors, chronic pancreatitis, pseudocyst, expanding hepatic mass/cyst, sphincter of Oddi dysfunction

---

3. Episodic gallbladder-like pain but negative diagnostic tests (including abdominal ultrasound and gallbladder ejection fraction). In patients with in-situ gallbladders and biliary-type pain, the gallbladder is usually the focus of evaluation. Recent studies suggest that some of these patients may also have SOD and abnormal SO manometry. The optimal management for this group of patients awaits further study.

8. Describe the clinical classification used for patients with sphincter of Oddi dysfunction.
Patients presenting with SOD may be divided into two broad categories based on clinical presentation. Most will have **biliary-type abdominal pain,** and a smaller group will have symptoms more referable to the **pancreas.** To deal with the different etiologies and overlap in clinical presentations, an SOD classification system was developed, based on clinical history, laboratory evaluation, and the results of diagnostic endoscopic retrograde cholangioancreatography (ERCP), that subdivides patients with the **biliary-type pain** into three groups:

Criteria
   a. Typical biliary-type pain
   b. Abnormal liver enzymes (AST and/or alkaline phosphatase >2 × normal on at least two occasions)
   c. Delayed drainage of ERCP contrast (>45 min)
   d. Dilated common bile duct (>12 mm)

Classification
   Biliary type I-meets all criteria above (*a, b, c,* and *d*).
   Biliary type II—typical biliary-type pain (*a*) plus one or two of *b, c,* and *d.*
   Biliary type III—biliary-type pain only (*a*).

In terms of etiology, type I patients are felt likely to have a true structural stenosis of the sphincter, type II may be structural or functional, and type III is usually functional. Some experts have found this classification system useful in determining which patients are likely to have abnormal findings on SO manometry as well as predicting which patients will respond to endoscopic sphincterotomy.

A similar classification scheme for patients with SOD and predominant **pancreatic symptoms** has been described.

9. Describe the nature of the pain episodes experienced by patients with suspected SOD.
Most patients presenting for evaluation of suspected SOD have undergone a prior cholecystec-tomy. Most patients experience improvement in pain after cholecystectomy but develop recurrent abdominal pain after surgery. Others do not benefit or are even made worse by cholecystectomy, presumably relating to removal of a volume reservoir. Recurrent attacks of pain often develop within 3–5 years postoperatively. The pain is usually similar in character to the pain prior to chole-cystectomy. It is typically located in the right upper quadrant of the abdomen or epigastrium, with or without radiation toward the right shoulder, scapula, or back, and is usually steady and non-colicky.

In most patients, episodes of pain initially occur infrequently, lasting several hours, followed by pain-free intervals. In some patients, the frequency and severity of attacks progress over time such that a chronic baseline pain syndrome develops with intermittent acute episodes.

The relationship of pain episodes to meals is also variable. The onset of pain within 2–3 hours postprandially is common, and many patients can identify certain foods (such as fatty or spicy foods) that seem to precipitate attacks. Unfortunately, other attacks of pain seem to have no con-sistent relationship to meals or types of food. A subset of patients appear to have a sensitivity to opiate-containing medications, which cause exacerbations of abdominal pain.

10. Describe the physical and laboratory findings in patients presenting with suspected SOD.
The majority of patients presenting for evaluation of suspected SOD are women, typically aged 30–50, who have undergone a prior cholecystectomy. The reason for the female predomi-nance is unclear but may simply reflect the higher incidence of gallstones and subsequent chole-cystectomy in women.

The **physical examination** between pain episodes is normal. During an attack of pain, the patient is distressed but afebrile. The abdominal examination is usually significant only for non-specific tenderness. Fever, palpable organomegaly, and definite signs of peritonitis are absent (i.e., excluding patients with pancreatitis).

Laboratory tests obtained during or immediately after a pain episode may be helpful. Dur-ing an acute attack, some patients have transient elevations of liver (AST, alkaline phosphatase) and/or pancreatic enzymes (amylase, lipase). Repeated evaluation of enzymes may be helpful be-cause these elevations are characteristically episodic. In most patients seen for suspected SOD, these tests as well as the white blood cell count are normal.

11. How is a diagnosis of sphincter of Oddi dysfunction established?
The diagnosis of SOD is initially based on clinical suspicion. Several diagnostic tests have been reported to be helpful in defining SOD, although none of the currently available tests are ideal and their value is controversial.

Diagnostic Tests Used in Sphincter of Oddi Dysfunction

Noninvasive diagnostic tests
    Liver and/or pancreatic enzymes during pain
    Pain provocation tests (Nardi test)
    Fatty-meal ultrasonography
    Secretin ultrasoography
    Quantitative hepatobiliary scintigraphy

Invasive diagnostic tests
    Endoscopic retrograde cholangiopancreatography (ERCP)
    Endoscopic sphincter of Oddi manometry

12. Does sphincter of Oddi dysfunction occur in association with other conditions?
An interesting feature of SOD is the common association with other smooth muscle disorders of the gut, including nonspecific esophageal dysmotility, delayed gastric emptying, and irritable bowel-type complaints. These associations suggest that some patients with SOD may have a more generalized dysmotility syndrome and that therapy directed solely at the sphincter of Oddi may not totally alleviate the patient's symptoms.

13. Describe the usefulness of the noninvasive diagnostic tests.
Transient elevation of **liver or pancreatitic enzymes** (>2 × upper limits of normal) during an attack of pain supports the presence of ductal outflow obstruction but is not specific for sphincter dysfunction. Other causes of obstruction, such as choledocholithiasis, should be ruled out.

Pain provocation tests, such as the morphine-Prostigmin (Nardi test), have been used to support the diagnosis of SOD. Patients are observed after administration of these drugs to see if pain is provoked and enzyme (liver and/or pancreatic) abnormalities develop. Morphine is given to increase sphincter resistance, and Prostigmin (neostigmine, an anticholinesterase inhibitor) to increase pancreatic juice flow. Unfortunately, the test is not sufficiently sensitive or specific.

Other noninvasive tests involve the use of ultrasound to determine common bile duct and/or pancreatic duct diameter before and after the administration a provocative agent. **Fatty-meal ultrasonography** involves administering fat (Lipomul 1.5 ml/kg; Mead-Johnson Laboratories, Evansville, IN) to stimulate endogenous cholecystokinin release and enhance biliary flow. Bile duct diameter is measured at 15-minute intervals for 60 minutes. A normal response is either no change or a decrease in duct diameter. An increase by ≥2 mm from baseline suggests partial biliary obstruction but does not distinguish SOD from other causes of obstruction (e.g., stones, stricture, tumor).

Secretin ultrasonography similarly involves measuring the pancreatic duct diameter before and after administering secretin (1 mg/kg) to stimulate pancreatic juice flow. The ductal diameter may increase normally due to enhanced flow but returns to baseline within 30 minutes. An exaggeration of this response suggests outflow obstruction (e.g., pancreatic duct dilation to 2 mm above baseline that persists after 30 minutes). The sensitivity and specificity of this test are uncertain.

Quantitative hepatobiliary scintigraphy involves determining the hepatic uptake and hepatobiliary clearance of an injected isotope. Although delayed uptake and clearance may be found in patients with SOD, this technique is also nonspecific and may be abnormal in patients with mechanical common duct obstruction or parenchymal liver disease. Quantitative criteria are inaccurate if the gallbladder is still present. Investigators from Johns Hopkins have reported a method of calculating a "scintigraphic score" that combines quantitative and visual criteria for interpreting hepatobiliary scans. Initial results suggest a high sensitivity and specificity but awaits confirmation by others.

14. How is ERCP used in diagnosing sphincter of Oddi dysfunction?
Endoscopic retrograde cholangiopancreatography (ERCP) is helpful in ruling out other pancreaticobiliary conditions that may cause similar pain, such as retained stones, strictures, papillary tumors, and chronic pancreatitis. It also allows for accurate measurement of ductal diameters and biliary and/or pancreatic drainage times. Reproduction of the patient's pain during contrast injection into the biliary tree has not been shown to be a reliable marker of SOD.

15. How is endoscopic sphincter of Oddi (SO) manometry performed?
Endoscopic SO manometry is currently considered by many to be the most reliable method of studying sphincter function. It involves directly measuring sphincter pressure with a triple-lumen water-perfused catheter that is passed through the duodenoscope into the bile duct or pancreas. The proximal end of the catheter is connected to external transducers and a paper recording device. The technology is virtually identical to systems used for esophageal manometry, except the catheter is miniaturized to permit passage through the operating channel of the duodenoscope and papillary orifice. Sphincter pressures are recorded as the catheter is slowly withdrawn from the

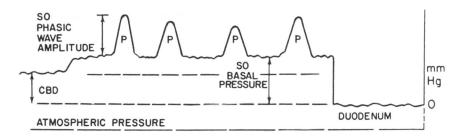

Sphincter of Oddi (SO) manometry tracing demonstrating basal sphincter pressure with superimposed phasic waves (P). CBD = common bile duct. (From Venu RP: The role of the endoscopist in sphincter of Oddi manometry. Gastrointest Endosc Clin North Am 3:77, 1993; with permission.)

duct and stationed within the sphincter zone (station pull-through technique). Duodenal pressure is taken as the zero reference point when measuring ductal and sphincter pressures.

Several aspects of sphincter motor activity can be measured with endoscopic manometry (*see* figure above). First, the sphincter exhibits a resting basal tone that is usually 10–30 mm Hg above duodenal pressure. In addition, superimposed phasic pressure waves are also seen. The amplitude, frequency, and propagation direction of phasic waves are recorded.

SO motor activity is influenced by several pharmacologic and hormonal agents. The endoscopist must therefore avoid using agents during manometry that are known to affect the sphincter (e.g., glucagon, atropine, morphine). Similarly, medications affecting the sphincter should be discontinued prior to manometric study, if possible (e.g., opiate analgesics, smooth muscle relaxants). The usual narcotics and antiperistaltic agents (e.g., glucagon, atropine) used for routine ERCP are withheld if SO manometry is to be performed, and only diazepam or midazolam is used for sedation. This often makes the procedure quite demanding for the patient and physician because of suboptimal sedation and movement of the papilla during attempts to cannulate. Recent studies have shown that meperidine (Demerol) may not affect SO basal pressure, as was previously assumed.

16. What manometric abnormalities are used to diagnose sphincter of Oddi dysfunction?

1. Elevated basal sphincter pressure
2. Increased frequency of phasic waves
3. Increased proportion of phasic waves propagated in the retrograde direction
4. Paradoxical sphincter response to cholecystokinin-octapeptide (CCK-OP) injection.

Some patients will have more than one of these findings, although there is no evidence that multiple abnormalities increase the specificity of the test. **Elevated basal sphincter pressure** is the most widely agreed upon abnormality and the finding most often used to make clinical decisions in patients with suspected SOD. Studies vary regarding the normal range for basal sphincter pressure, but values exceeding 40 mm Hg (using duodenal pressure as the zero reference) are generally considered abnormal. Elevated basal sphincter pressure may be seen in both structural stenosis of the sphincter and dyskinesia. Some investigators have attempted to distinguish these entities based on the response to pharmacologic agents such as amyl nitrite or CCK-OP; these agents have no effect on the elevated pressure in patients with stenosis but may transiently lower basal pressure and abolish phasic waves in patients with dyskinesia.

Although **increased frequency of phasic waves** (tachyoddia) and excessive **retrograde propagation of phasic waves** (i.e., >50%) are observed in some patients, most experts consider the basal sphincter pressure to be more important. The significance of other miscellaneous findings, such as increased phasic wave amplitude and low basal pressure, is also unclear.

CCK-OP is sometimes given to patients whose baseline manometric study is normal to create a situation that more closely resembles the fed state. Some patients with SOD appear to have a "paradoxical response" to intravenously administered CCK-OP with elevation of basal sphincter pressure. Although conceptually attractive, the paradoxical response to CCK-OP is infrequently observed and thus has limited usefulness.

17. What are the major problems associated with SO manometry?

Problems Associated with Endoscopic Sphincter of Oddi Manometry

Difficult for endoscopist to perform
Often poorly tolerated by patients
Performed in the fasting state
Short duration of study
Lack of uniform method for interpreting tracings
Risk of postmanometry pancreatitis

18. What steps can be taken to minimize the risk of post-SO manometry pancreatitis?

A major disadvantage in using SO manometry is the increased risk for procedure-related pancreatitis, especially if prolonged or repeated measurements are taken in the pancreatic duct. The true frequency of postmanometry pancreatitis is difficult to ascertain because many patients have manometry, ductography, and sphincterotomy performed in the same session. Pancreatitis resulting from SO manometry can be severe and occasionally may result in phlegmon or pseudocyst formation. Patients should be advised of the potential risks, and preventive measures must be taken when possible.

Preventive measures that may reduce the risk of manometry-related pancreatitis include:

1. Avoidance of trauma to the papilla by using gentle cannulation techniques;
2. Avoidance of pancreatic manometry when possible;
3. Limiting the time of pancreatic manometry when performed;
4. Recannulation and drainage of the pancreatic duct after manometry (shown effective in one study but awaiting confirmation);
5. Limiting catheter perfusion rate to 0.25 ml/lumen/min or less;
6. Sterilization of accessories and periodic culturing of ERCP endoscopes and manometry equipment;
7. Use in catheters with built-in microtransducers (not currently commercially available) rather than water-perfusion systems;
8. Use of the aspiration-type manometry catheter when measuring pancreatic sphincter pressure.

The aspiration catheter uses two channels for pressure measurements while aspirating infused fluid and pancreatic juice from the third channel. This device can significantly reduce the frequency of postmanometry pancreatitis.

19. Should patients with suspected SOD be evaluated for "microlithiasis" or subtle gallbladder disease?

Patients with biliary-type pain and intact gallbladder, but no demonstrable gallstones on ultrasound or ERCP, may have a more subtle form of gallbladder disease. Two tests may be helpful in this setting: (1) hepatobiliary cholescintigraphy with cholecystokinin administration to determine gallbladder ejection fraction (GB-EF%), and (2) microscopic examination of gallbladder bile for the presence cholesterol or calcium bilirubinate crystals.

An abnormally **low GB-EF%** implies impaired gallbladder emptying of bile and has been used to identify patients with acalculous biliary pain who may respond to cholecystectomy. Gallbladders removed from such patients often show chronic cholecystitis and/or a narrowed cystic duct.

Microscopic examination of gallbladder bile for the presence of crystals is most useful in patients with idiopathic recurrent pancreatitis (IRP). Bile is aspirated from the duodenum or directly from the bile duct at ERCP after cholecystokinin administration to induce gallbladder contraction. The presence of cholesterol or bile pigment crystals is generally accepted as evidence of gallstone disease (i.e., microlithiasis). Patients with microlithiasis and IRP frequently respond to standard therapy, such as cholecystectomy or an oral dissolution agent (Actigall), if cholesterol crystals are found.

20. What is the relationship between sphincter of Oddi dysfunction and pancreatitis?
SOD has been implicated in the pathogenesis of both idiopathic recurrent pancreatitis (IRP) and chronic pancreatitis. Although controversy exists regarding its significance, investigators have reported finding elevated basal sphincter pressure in 15–57% of patients with IRP. Most studies report favorable results of sphincter ablation in these patients, although additional outcome studies are needed. Medical therapy for SOD in this setting has not been sufficiently evaluated.

Abnormal SO manometry studies are occasionally found in patients with chronic pancreatitis. Whether this finding is a cause or result of the chronic fibrosis process is unclear.

21. Is sphincter of Oddi manometry always necessary to confirm a diagnosis of sphincter of Oddi dysfunction prior to treatment?
No. SO manometry is not essential for all patients with suspected SOD prior to institution of therapy. The decision to perform SO manometry is usually based on the severity of the patient's symptoms, response to conservative therapy, and classification according to the previously described criteria (*see* Question 8).

Virtually all patients, including those with more severe symptoms, should first be given a trial of medical therapy to determine response. Patients with more severe symptoms, particularly if unresponsive to conservative treatment, are potential candidates for SO manometry to confirm the diagnosis prior to more aggressive therapies. Classification of patients with suspected biliary pain into biliary groups I, II,and III is also helpful in that it may predict the likelihood of an abnormal manometric study and response to sphincter ablation.

SO manometry is considered unnecessary for patients who meet the criteria for **biliary type I** SOD. These patients are very likely to have abnormal manometry (approx 80–90%) and will have a favorable response to endoscopic sphincterotomy in over 90% of cases, even if SO manometry results are normal. By contrast, SO manometry is considered by some experts to be mandatory for **biliary type II** patients, because only approximately 50% of these patients will have elevated basal sphincter pressure. In a prospective randomized trial by Geenen et al., the response rate to endoscopic sphincterotomy was significantly higher (94% at 4 years) in type II patients with elevated sphincter pressure compared with only a placebo effect in those with normal manometry. The decision to perform ERCP and SO manometry in **biliary type III** patients who have abdominal pain but no objective evidence of partial biliary obstruction is more difficult. These patients are less likely to have any abnormality found and are at greater risk for endoscopic sphincterotomy-related pancreatitis in the setting of nondilated bile ducts.

22. Is manometry of both biliary and pancreatic duct sphincters necessary?
This question is important because of evidence suggesting that the incidence of pancreatitis from biliary manometry alone is minimal compared to studies involving the pancreatic sphincter. However, if only biliary manometry is performed, no information is obtained about the pancreatic portion of the sphincter. Studies have shown that elevated sphincter pressure may indeed be isolated to one portion of the sphincter. Silverman et al. prospectively evaluated a group of 88 patients undergoing biductal manometry in the same session. They found concordance of the two ducts (i.e., both normal or both abnormal) in 85% of patients. The remaining 15% had only one segment abnormal.

A reasonable approach is to attempt to study the bile duct sphincter first; if this is abnormal, proceed with therapy. If the bile duct sphincter is normal and the patient has IRP, or if the pancreas is cannulated first, the pancreatic sphincter can be evaluated with an aspiration catheter.

23. Are the results of sphincter of Oddi manometry reproducible?
Most studies indicate that SO manometry results are reproducible on separate measurements. In a study of type II patients who underwent baseline SO manometry followed by sham therapy and repeat manometry in 1 year, Geenen et al. found no significant changes in pressure between the

two measurements. Of 24 patients who were classified as normal ($n = 12$) or abnormal ($n = 12$) at baseline, no patient's classification changed at the end of 1 year.

24. What are the treatment options for SOD?

Proposed Treatment Strategies for Sphincter of Oddi Dysfunction

> Noninvasive treatments
>   Low-fat diet
>   Analgesics
>   Nitrates
>   Calcium channel antagonists
>   Anticholinergics (e.g., dicyclomine)
> Invasive treatments
>   Endoscopic balloon dilation
>   Injection of botulinum toxin
>   Temporary stenting (biliary or pancreatic)
>   Sphincter ablation
>   Endoscopic sphincterotomy
>   Surgical sphincteroplasty

Surprising few data are available regarding the efficacy of medical therapies in patients with manometrically documented SOD. As an initial approach, patients should be given a course of **medical therapy,** including a trial of a low-fat diet, antispasmodics, and nonaddictive analgesics. Sublingual nitroglycerin, nifedipine, and dicyclomine are variably effective and appear to work best for patients with mild, infrequent symptoms. None of these agents is specific for the sphincter of Oddi, and their use is often limited by side effects.

Invasive treatment modalities may be necessary for patients with more severe symptoms who fail conservative measures. Endoscopic balloon dilation and temporary stenting are alternatives to sphincter ablation. Hydrostatic balloon dilation has yielded varied results and may carry a substantial risk of pancreatitis when performed for SOD. More recent studies using balloon dilation of the sphincter for removing small common duct stones have not shown the rate of pancreatitis to be high. Although some patients appear to have benefited from balloon dilation in uncontrolled reports, its value in treating SOD patients has not been demonstrated satisfactorily, and presently the technique has little role in management. Temporary biliary or pancreatic stenting is also conceptually attractive in view of the difficulty in predicting which patients will respond to sphincterotomy and the potential risk of pancreatitis in patients with nondilated bile ducts. Very limited data are available regarding "trial" stenting for SOD. Simple stenting is also not without risks.

Intrasphincteric injection of botulinum toxin, a potent inhibitor of acetylcholine release from nerve endings, has recently been proposed as a method of lowering sphincter pressure in patients with SOD. There is no current clinical role for this approach.

25. When is sphincterotomy indicated in SOD?

Most patients failing noninvasive measures will be considered for **endoscopic sphincterotomy.** Stratification of patients according to the Milwaukee biliary classification (*see* Question 8) is helpful, because biliary type I patients will have a favorable response to endoscopic sphincterotomy in over 90% of cases. Geenen et al. have also shown in a prospective randomized study that biliary type II patients have a very good response to sphincterotomy (92%) when elevated basal sphincter pressure is documented by SO manometry. The frequency of abnormal SO manometry in biliary type III patients varies among series from 7–55%. Limited data suggest that only approximately half of the type III patients are improved after biliary sphincterotomy.

Surgical ablation of the sphincter of Oddi (**sphincterotomy** or **sphincteroplasty**) has mainly been used in patients with gallstones. Reports describing the use of these procedures in patients with postcholecystectomy pain have shown good results in 43–68% of patients who had long-term follow-up (2–4 years). Patients with recurrent pancreatitis due to pancreatic sphincter stenosis may also be candidates for surgical sphincteroplasty.

26. Is there a risk of restenosis following endoscopic sphincterotomy?
The overall risk of restenosis following endoscopic sphincterotomy appears to be low. Manoukian et al. reported a restenosis rate of 4.7% among 85 patients who underwent endoscopic sphincterotomy for biliary type II SOD and were followed for 7 ± 3 years. A similar rate of restenosis has been found among patients who had endoscopic sphincterotomy performed for choledocholithiasis.

27. Why do some patients with suspected SOD not respond to sphincter ablation?
The finding of abnormal SO manometric results in a symptomatic patient does not prove a cause-effect relationship. It has been suggested that in some patients, elevated sphincter pressure may be the consequence, rather than the cause, of disease. Potential reasons for residual or recurrent symptoms following biliary sphincterotomy include undetected stones, restenosis, incomplete sphincterotomy, strictures, pancreatic parenchymal disease or pseudocyst, or another disease accounting for the patient's symptoms that is unrelated to the biliary tree or pancreas.

BIBLIOGRAPHY

1. Cotton PB: Unexplained RUQ abdominal pain—Possible biliary dyskinesia? Contemp Gastroenterol (May/Jun).23–28, 1990.
2. Elta GH, Barnett JL: Meperidine need not be proscribed during sphincter of Oddi manometry. Gastrointest Endosc 40:7–9, 1994.
3. Goff JS: Common bile duct sphincter of Oddi stenting in patients with suspected sphincter dysfunction. Am J Gastroenterol 90:586–589, 1995.
4. Hawes RH, Lehman GA: Complications of sphincter of Oddi manometry and their prevention. Gastrointest Endosc Clin North Am 3:107–118, 1993.
5. Hogan WJ (ed): The sphincter of Oddi primer for the pancreaticobiliary endoscopist. Gastrointest Endosc Clin North Am 3:1–178, 1993.
6. Hogan WJ, Geenen JE: Biliary dyskinesia. Endoscopy 20:179–183, 1988
7. Hogan WJ, Geenen JE, Dodds WJ: Dysmotility disturbances of the biliary tract: Classification, diagnosis, and treatment. Semin Liver Dis 7:302–310, 1987.
8. Komorowski RA: Anatomy and histopathology of the human sphincter of Oddi. Gastrointest Endosc Clin North Am 3:1–11, 1993.
9. Kozarek RA: Biliary dyskinesia: Are we any closer to defining the entity? Gastrointest Endosc Clin North Am 3:167–178, 1993.
10. Lans JL, Parikh NP, Geenen JE: Application of sphincter of Oddi manometry in routine clinical investigations. Endoscopy 23:139–143, 1991.
11. Rolny P, Geenen JE, Hogan WJ: Post-cholecystectomy patients with "objective signs" of partial bile outflow obstruction: Clinical characteristics, sphincter of Oddi manometry findings, and results of therapy. Gastrointest Endosc 39:778–781, 1993.
12. Sand J, Nordback I, Koskinen M, et al: Nifedipine for suspected type II sphincter of Oddi dyskinesia. Am J Gastroenterol 4:530–535, 1993.
13. Schmalz MJ, Geenen JE, Hogan WJ, et al: Pain on common bile duct injection during ERCP: Does it indicate sphincter of Oddi dysfunction? Gastrointest Endosc 36:458–461, 1990.
14. Sherman S, Troiano FP, Hawes RH, et al: Sphincter of Oddi manometry: Decreased risk of clinical pancreatitis with use of a modified aspirating catheter. Gastrointest Endosc 36:462–466, 1990.
15. Sostre S, Kalloo AN, Spiegler EJ, et al: A noninvasive test of sphincter of Oddi dysfunction in postcholecystectomy patients: The scintigraphic score. J Nucl Med 33:1216–1222, 1992.
16. Steinberg WM: Sphincter of Oddi dysfunction: A clinical controversy. Gastroenterology 95:1409–1415, 1988.
17. Toouli J, Roberts-Thomson IC, Dent J, Lee J: Manometric disorders in patients with suspected sphincter of Oddi dysfunction. Gastroenterology 88:1243–1250, 1985.
18. Venu RP: The role of the endoscopist in sphincter of Oddi manometry. Gastrointest Endosc Clin North Am 3:67–80, 1993.
19. Venu RP, Geenen JE, Hogan WJ, et al: Idiopathic recurrent pancreatitis: An approach to diagnosis and treatment. Dig Dis Sci 34:56–60, 1989.
20. Wiedmeyer DA, Stewart ET, Taylor AJ: Radiologic evaluation of structure and function of the sphincter of Oddi. Gastrointest Endosc Clin North Am 3:13–40, 1993.

IV. Pancreatic Disorders

35. ACUTE PANCREATITIS

Brett R. Neustater, M.D., and Jamie S. Barkin, M.D.

1. What are the causes of acute pancreatitis?

Biliary stone disease and **ethanol use** combine to account for 60–80% of cases of acute pancreatitis. Their relative ranking as either the leading or second leading etiology depends upon the geographic location as well as that population's demographics. Idiopathic acute pancreatitis ranks as the third leading etiology and is generally believed to represent 10–15% of attacks. Recently, however, several studies have demonstrated microlithiasis in two-thirds to three-quarters of these patients. Other etiologies include hypertriglyceridemia, trauma, pancreatic tumors, and infection.

Among the **infectious etiologies,** several viruses have been implicated, including mumps, coxsackie, cytomegalovirus, and hepatitis A, B, and non-A/non-B viruses. Infection by bacteria, including *Mycoplasma, Legionella,* and *Mycobacterium tuberculosis,* as well as several parasitic infections, most notably ascariasis and clonorchiasis, have also been associated. In AIDS patients, the incidence of infection-related acute pancreatitis is increased compared to the general population, with *Cryptococcus, Toxoplasma, Cryptosporidium,* and *Mycobacterium avium* complex also responsible for illness.

Many **drugs** have been linked to acute pancreatitis, including azathioprine, mercaptopurine, thiazides, valproic acid, tetracyclines, furosemide, sulfonamides, sulindac, didanosine (DDI), acetaminophen, salicylates, erythromycin, pentamidine, and estrogens.

Less common etiologies include hypercalcemia, choledochocele, periampullary diverticuli, hypertensive sphincter of Oddi, Crohn's disease, ischemia, and scorpion venom.

2. What is the pathophysiology of acute pancreatitis?

The pathogenesis of acute pancreatitis is still a matter of debate. There is likely a disturbance of the intracellular secretion and transport of enzymes along with intra-acinar activation of the zymogens by hydrolases. The activation of trypsinogen to trypsin is thought to be a primary event in the cascade. The release of trypsin activates kinin and complement which, along with the release of various other toxins into the systemic circulation, may lead to the complications of multiorgan failure.

Although **alcohol** may cause acute pancreatitis in the absence of underlying chronic disease, the usual situation is that of acute inflammation superimposed on chronic pancreatitis. Proposed etiologies include a direct toxic effect on the pancreas and the creation of proteinaceous plugs that clog smaller pancreatic ducts.

Pancreatic ductal occlusion and increased intraductal pressure are the likely events leading to **gallstone-induced pancreatitis,** although this has not been proven conclusively.

3. What is pancreas divisum? Does it cause acute pancreatitis?

Pancreas divisum is a congenital variant of pancreatic ductal anatomy that occurs in approximately 5–7% of the population. The duct of Wirsung, which is larger and drains the ventral pancreas, does not fuse with the smaller duct of Santorini (which drains the dorsal pancreas), resulting in the majority of the pancreas draining via the smaller accessory papilla. It has been proposed that, at least in certain individuals, the duct and papilla are not large enough to accommodate this large volume of secretions, and along with a degree of ductal stenosis, this condition can result in pancreatitis. Support for this proposal comes from a recent prospective, randomized, controlled trial that demonstrated significant improvement in a group of patients with pancreas divisum (all other causes of pancreatitis were excluded) and acute recurrent pancreatitis who underwent either endoscopic dilation and stenting of the minor papilla or surgical papillotomy.

4. How is the diagnosis of acute pancreatitis made?
The diagnosis of acute pancreatitis is generally accepted when the **acute onset of abdominal pain** is accompanied by at least a threefold elevation in **serum amylase** and/or **serum lipase**.

5. How reliable is serum amylase as a diagnostic marker for acute pancreatitis?
Serum amylase is a sensitive marker of disease when the patient presents within several hours of the onset of abdominal pain but becomes less sensitive than serum lipase if the patient presents later. However, not all patients with abdominal pain and elevated amylase will have pancreatitis, as hyperamylasemia often arises from various nonpancreatic sources, such as the salivary glands, lungs, fallopian tubes, ovarian cysts, gallbladder, small bowel, and metabolic acidosis. Hyperamylasemia may also result from various malignancies, including those arising from the pancreas, colon, lung, and ovary and in thymoma, pheochromocytoma, and multiple myeloma. Approximately 30% of patients who have undergone cardiac surgery have demonstrated hyperamylasemia, with about 50% secondary to salivary-type amylase.

It has been reported that amylase levels tend to be lower in patients with alcoholic pancreatitis than in those with a nonalcoholic etiology. In addition, 10% of chronic alcoholics have *salivary-derived* hyperamylasemia due to the damaging effects of ethanol on the salivary glands. These abnormalities can lead to diagnostic confusion when an alcoholic patient presents with nonspecific or atypical abdominal pain and a mildly elevated serum amylase level.

6. Do pancreatic enzymes other than serum amylase have a role in the diagnosis?
Serum lipase activity has been shown to have greater sensitivity and specificity than amylase, especially after the first hospital day. Lipase is not completely specific for the pancreas, as lingual, gastric, intestinal, and hepatic isolipases have been isolated. **Serum trypsin** is more specific for the pancreas than either amylase or lipase, but it is measured only by a radioimmunoassay which is not generally available. The **urinary amylase clearance to creatinine clearance ratio** has not been shown to be very useful, with the exception of a very low ratio indicative of macroamylasemia. In the setting of renal failure, all pancreatic enzymes are elevated owing to their diminished clearance, thus making the diagnosis of pancreatitis more difficult in patients with abdominal pain and hyperamylasemia.

7. What imaging studies are useful in diagnosing acute pancreatitis?
Contrast-enhanced **computed tomography** (CT), especially when performed with incremental dynamic contrast bolus, is the best imaging study of the pancreas. It can reliably predict the severity of inflammation, evidence of pancreatic necrosis, or complications such as pseudocysts and pancreatic abscesses. With mild disease, however, the CT scan may be completely normal in 15–30% of patients.

Ultrasonography is the most sensitive method of evaluating the biliary tree. Unfortunately, overlying bowel gas can compromise its ability to visualize the pancreas in up to 30% of patients.

Endoscopic retrograde cholangiopancreatography (ERCP) is useful when a definite cause of the pancreatitis has not been identified after a thorough evaluation. It may reveal ductular abnormalities such as strictures of the pancreatic duct, biliary disease such as gallstones and choledochoceles, and small pancreatic tumors.

Prognostic Factors in Acute Pancreatitis

ETHANOL-ASSOCIATED (RANSON'S CRITERIA)		BILIARY (MODIFIED GLASGOW)
At admission	**Within 48 hrs of admission**	**During initial 48 hr**
Age >55 yr	Hct decrease of >10%	Age >55 yr
WBC >16,000/mm^3	BUN increase of >5 mg/dl	WBC >15,000/mm^3
Glucose >200 mg/dl	Calcium <8 mg/dl	Glucose >180 mg/dl
LDH >350 IU/l	PaO$_2$ <60 mm Hg	LDH >600 U/l
AST >250 U/l	Base deficit >4 mEq/L	Albumin <3.3 g/dl
		PaO$_2$ <60 mm Hg
		Calcium <8 mg/dl
		BUN >45 mg/dl

8. Describe the two major prognostic scoring systems for acute pancreatitis.

The most commonly utilized criteria for establishing the severity of acute pancreatitis are Ranson's and the APACHE-II (Acute Physiology And Chronic Health Evaluation) grading systems. **Ranson's signs** comprise five laboratory and clinical indices available on admission and another six that are assessed after 48 hours (see table above). When there are fewer than three positive signs, the patient has mild disease with a mortality rate that is near zero. This rate increases to 10–20% with three to five signs and to >50% with six or more signs (severe acute pancreatitis). Obviously, 48 hours following admission are required to fully assess the patient's disease severity.

The **APACHE-II score** has the advantage of being available at the time of admission and consists of a system in which points are awarded based on age, chronic illness, and various physiologic variables (see table below). A score of ≤7 is predictive of a mild attack, whereas higher scores correspond to greater severity of disease.

APACHE II Scoring System for Severity of Acute Pancreatitis

Age: > 45 years of age assigned ascending points to age 75 (6 point maximum)
Acute physiology score: Points are assigned for abnormal values (50 points maximum).
  Vital signs
  Arterial blook gases
  Electrolytes
  Glasgow coma scale (actual number)
Chronic health points: (2 points each)
  Liver—cirrhosis
  Lung—severe chronic obstructive pulmonary disease
  Renal—on dialysis
  Heart—congestive heart failure or angina at rest
  Immunocompromise—on chemotherapy, radiation therapy, or diagnosis of AIDS

9. How useful are other prognostic indicators in acute pancreatitis?

Clinical signs, such as respiratory failure, peritonitis, and shock, are as good as most prognostic criteria in determining the severity of disease. A **single serologic test** available on admission for the diagnosis and assessment of severity of acute pancreatitis is appealing but thus far elusive. Those proposed have included serum phospholipase A$_2$, C-reactive protein, leukocyte elastase, and trypsinogen-activated peptide, although measurements of these are not widely available in the United States. Single or multiple organ system failure is also a poor prognostic indicator. Organ failure is defined as shock (systolic blood pressure <90 mm Hg), pulmonary insufficiency (PaO$_2$ ≤60 mm Hg), renal failure (creatinine >2 mg/dl after rehydration), and GI bleeding (>500 ml/24 hrs) and is the most important indicator of severity. **Local complications,** including pseudocyst, abscess, and pancreatic necrosis if present, are also indicators of severe disease, especially in the setting of organ failure or increased Ranson's signs or APACHE-II score. In addition, **obesity** has been associated with a higher incidence of organ failure and mortality.

10. Describe the CT severity index for assessing acute pancreatitis.

A grading system based upon findings of a standard CT scan may be helpful in assessing prognosis in acute pancreatitis.

Grade A—normal-appearing pancreas

Grade B—pancreatic enlargement

Grade C—peripancreatic and peripancreatic fat inflammation

Grade D—enlarged pancreas with fluid in the anterior pararenal space

Grade E—fluid collections in at least two compartments

Mortality and disease severity are mild with grade A, B, or C but much higher with grade D or E (overall 15% mortality). Patients with grade D or E findings on CT also have a 30–50% risk of infection. The presence of infection is more likely in those with greater amounts of necrosis seen on rapid-bolus CT.

11. How is acute pancreatitis classified?

A number of classification systems have been proposed, but the most widely accepted is based on the collaborative efforts of 40 international experts on acute pancreatitis who established a clinically based system during a 3-day symposium in Atlanta in 1992. The first distinction made is between **severe** and **mild acute pancreatitis.** This distinction can be based on the Ranson's criteria (>3), APACHE-II score (≥8) (*see* Question 8), or the presence of organ failure or local complications (pancreatic necrosis, abscess, or pseudocyst).

A distinction must also be made between **interstitial pancreatitis** and **necrotizing pancreatitis** based on the findings of an incremental dynamic contrast CT. The overall mortality rate for interstitial pancreatitis is <2%, whereas that with sterile necrosis is approximately 10% and that with superimposed bacterial invasion resulting in infected necrosis is 30%. The diagnosis of pancreatic necrosis is made by CT when there are focal or diffuse, well-marginated zones of nonenhanced pancreatic parenchyma >3 cm or involving >30% of the pancreatic area. The overall accuracy of dynamic CT in this case is greater than 90%. Patients with evidence of pancreatic necrosis have a 30–50% chance of developing infection of the necrosis. Infection is diagnosed by percutaneous aspiration followed by Gram stain and culture of the aspirate. At present, infected necrosis is always an indication for surgery; however, the role of antibiotics has not been adequately evaluated.

12. How are patients with acute pancreatitis treated?

The treatment of acute pancreatitis depends on the severity of disease as well as the presence of any complications. Patients with **mild disease** are treated supportively with intravenous hydration, parenteral analgesics, and are kept NPO. Nasogastric suction may provide symptomatic relief in patients with an ileus or recurrent emesis but has not been demonstrated to shorten the hospital stay.

If the pancreatitis is **severe,** the patient should be admitted to an intensive care unit for close hemodynamic monitoring and treatment of any possible systemic complications. Trials of various therapies for severe acute pancreatitis have been performed, with most yielding disappointing results. Recently, however, there has been evidence that the empiric use of **imipenem** in patients with necrotizing pancreatitis may significantly decrease the incidence of pancreatic sepsis. In another study, Ranson studied the use of 7-day **peritoneal lavage** in patients with severe acute pancreatitis and found a significant reduction in both the frequency of septic complications and mortality.

There is general agreement that patients with **infected pancreatic necrosis,** as demonstrated by CT-guided percutaneous aspiration for Gram's stain and culture, should undergo **surgical debridement.** The debridement may be performed in conjunction with external drainage, continuous local lavage, or closed packing. On the other hand, there is no clear consensus on the best therapy for **sterile necrotizing pancreatitis.** No studies have clearly demonstrated an advantage for surgical debridement, although some anecdotal reports seem to favor this approach in the most severely ill patients with evidence of organ failure.

13. What organisms are associated with infected pancreatic necrosis?
A CT-guided aspirate of pancreatic necrosis, when Gram stained and cultured, will almost always yields organisms if present. Infected necrosis may be due to a single organism or polymicrobial infection. The most commonly isolated organism, *Escherichia coli,* is cultured in 51% of cases. Others isolated, in decreasing order of frequency, are *Enterococcus, Staphylococcus, Pseudomonas, Proteus, Klebsiella, Streptococcus faecalis,* and *Bacteroides* species. The organisms are believed to reach the pancreas by local lymphatic spread following translocation across the colonic wall.

14. When should a CT scan be obtained?
A CT scan should be obtained when severe pancreatitis is suspected because of (1) the presence of organ failure, (2) failure of the patient to improve clinically, or (3) suspicion of infected necrosis (fever >101° F, increasing pain, leukocytosis, tachycardia, or hypotension). CT-guided percutaneous aspiration of any visualized areas of necrosis should also be performed in patients with suspected infected necrosis in order to diagnose bacterial or fungal infection.

15. What is the role of therapeutic ERCP in acute biliary pancreatitis?
Biliary sepsis can have a clinical picture similar to that of acute necrotizing pancreatitis and a mortality rate approaching 50%. Unfortunately, studies examining the *surgical* removal of gallstones early in the course of acute biliary pancreatitis have failed to demonstrate any improvement in patient outcome.
ERCP can be safely performed early in the course of acute pancreatitis. The basis for its use is that the early removal of biliary stones may decrease the mortality rate for patients with acute biliary pancreatitis. Recently, a prospective, randomized trial evaluated early ERCP and demonstrated a significant decrease in biliary sepsis both in patients with mild or severe acute biliary pancreatitis who underwent early (within 24 hr) ERCP with or without endoscopic papillotomy. This study, along with another smaller trial of urgent ERCP and sphincterotomy in patients with biliary pancreatitis, has led to the recommendation that early ERCP be performed in patients with severe pancreatitis in whom there is clinical suspicion of biliary obstruction, sepsis, or evidence of worsening organ dysfunction.

16. What are some local complications of acute pancreatitis?
1. **Acute fluid collections** occur in 30–50% of patients with severe acute pancreatitis and occur during the first 4 weeks of illness. They lack a well-defined wall and regress spontaneously about half the time.
2. An acute **pseudocyst** is enclosed by a well-formed wall of fibrous or granulation tissue and takes at least 4 weeks to develop.
3. A **pancreatic abscess** is a circumscribed intra-abdominal collection of pus, usually located in or near the pancreas. This also includes a pus-containing pseudocyst, which had formerly been referred to as an **infected pseudocyst**. It is a late event in acute pancreatitis, occurring at least 4 weeks into the illness and is often accompanied by systemic signs of infection. It is distinct from pancreatic necrosis in that, by definition, little or no necrosis is present. This distinction is critical, as the mortality rate for pancreatic necrosis is twice that of pancreatic abscess, and the treatment may be different.

17. Name the major systemic complications of acute pancreatitis.
In addition to the local complications of acute pancreatitis, many systemic complications can develop. Effects on other organ systems are likely the result of the release of potent vasoactive substances, enzymes, and hormones into the circulation.
Hypotension complicated by cardiovascular collapse may occur as the result of significant "third-space" loss of fluids, peripheral vasodilatation, and possibly depressed left ventricular function. Close hemodynamic monitoring, with the assistance of a central venous catheter or pulmonary artery catheter, is indicated in the management of these patients.

Impaired renal function, in part due to renal hypoperfusion, can develop in up to 25% of patients and portends a mortality rate of up to 50% in some studies.

Pulmonary complications can range from early arterial **hypoxia,** present in more than half of patients, to the **adult respiratory distress syndrome** (ARDS), which is seen in up to 20% of patients with severe acute pancreatitis. **Pleural effusions** are common, usually left-sided, exudative, and have a markedly elevated amylase level.

GI bleeding complicating pancreatitis usually occurs from **peptic ulcer disease, gastritis,** or **varices** (occasionally gastric varices as a consequence of splenic vein thrombosis complicate acute pancreatitis). GI bleeding may also occur as the result of a **pseudocyst** rupturing into the GI tract or the **erosion** of the inflamed pancreatic mass into a major artery, with blood draining into the bowel via the pancreatic duct (hemosuccus pancreaticus).

Pancreatic **ascites** is characterized by a very high amylase content and complicates anterior rupture of the pancreatic duct or a pseudocyst. Therapy consists of bowel rest, parenteral hyperalimentation, and surgical repair if the patient does not respond to conservative management. Somatostatin or its longer-acting analogue octreotide has demonstrated effectiveness.

Metabolic complications include **hypocalcemia** due to saponification of calcium salts, **hypoalbuminemia,** transient **hyperglycemia,** and **hypertriglyceridemia.**

Less commonly, sudden blindness (referred to as **Purtscher's angiopathic retinopathy**) and **skin rash** resembling erythema nodosum due to fat necrosis may be seen.

BIBLIOGRAPHY

1. Banks PA: The role of needle-aspiration bacteriology in the management of necrotizing pancreatitis. In Bradley EL III (ed): Acute Pancreatitis: Principles and Practice. New York, Raven Press, 1993, pp 99–104.
2. Banks PA: Acute pancreatitis: Medical and surgical management. Am J Gastroenterol 89:S78–S85, 1994.
3. Block S, Maier W, Bittner R, et al: Identification of pancreas necrosis in severe acute pancreatitis: Imaging procedures versus clinical staging. Gut 27:1035–1042, 1986.
4. Bradley EL III: A clinically based classification system for acute pancreatitis: Summary of the international symposium on acute pancreatitis, Atlanta, GA, September 11–13, 1992. Arch Surg 128: 486–490, 1993.
5. Fan ST, Lai EC, Mok FP, et al: Early treatment of acute biliary pancreatitis by endoscopic papillotomy. N Engl J Med 328:228–232, 1993.
6. Forsmark CE, Grendell JH: Complications of pancreatitis. Semin Gastrointest Dis 2:165–176, 1991.
7. Grendell JH: Idiopathic acute pancreatitis. Gastroenterol Clin North Am 19:843–848, 1990.
8. Imrie CW, Whyte AS: A prospective study of acute pancreatitis. Br J Surg 62:490–494, 1975.
9. Karimgani I, Porter KA, Langevin RE, et al: Prognostic factors in sterile pancreatic necrosis. Gastroenterology 103:1636–1640, 1992.
10. Lans JI, Geenen JE, Johnson JF, Hogan WJ: Endoscopic therapy in patients with pancreas divisum and acute pancreatitis: A prospective, randomized, controlled clinical trial. Gastrointest Endosc 38:430–434, 1992.
11. London NJ, Neoptolemos JP, Lavelle J, et al: Contrast-enhanced abdominal computed tomography scanning and prediction of severity of acute pancreatitis: A prospective study. Br J Surg 76:268–272, 1989.
12. Neoptolemos JP, Carr-Locke DL, London NJ, et al: Controlled trial of urgent endoscopic retrograde cholangiopancreatography and endoscopic sphincterotomy versus conservative treatment for acute pancreatitis due to gallstones. Lancet 2:979–983, 1988.
13. Pederzoli P, Bassi C, Vesentini S, et al: A randomized multicenter clinical trial of antibiotic prophylaxis of septic complications in acute necrotizing pancreatitis with imipenem. Surg Gynecol Obstet 176:480–483, 1993.
14. Pieper-Bigelow C, Strocchi A, Levitt MD: Where does serum amylase come from and where does it go? Gastroenterol Clin North Am 19:793–811, 1990.
15. Ranson JHC, Berman RS: Long peritoneal lavage decreases pancreatic sepsis in acute pancreatitis. Ann Surg 211:708–716, 1990.
16. Steer ML: Classification and pathogenesis of pancreatitis. Surg Clin North Am 69:467–481, 1989.
17. Steinberg W, Tenner S: Acute pancreatitis. N Engl J Med 330:1198–1210, 1994.
18. Thomson SR, Hendry WS, McFarlane GA, Davidson AL: Epidemiology and outcome of acute pancreatitis. Br J Surg 74:398–401, 1987.
19. Toskes PP: Biochemical tests in pancreatic disease. Curr Opin Gastroenterol 7:709–713, 1991.

36. CHRONIC PANCREATITIS

Sal Senzatimore, M.D., and Jamie S. Barkin, M.D.

1. Describe the classification system for chronic pancreatitis.
In acute pancreatitis, lesions regress when the etiologic causes are removed, but with chronic pancreatitis (CP), persistent or progressive inflammatory disease remains even with removal of the initiating lesion. CP is classified as obstructive, calcifying, or inflammatory. **Obstructive CP** demonstrates glandular changes, including uniform fibrosis, ductal changes with dilatation, and acinar atrophy, all of which may improve when obstruction of the pancreatic duct is removed. **Calcifying CP** displays irregular fibrosis of the gland as well as intraductal stones and is most commonly caused by alcohol abuse. **Inflammatory CP** is the "waste basket" for patients with disease not fitting the above catagories and is characterized histologically by mononuclear cell infiltration with associated fibrosis.

2. What causes chronic pancreatitis?
Approximately 70% of cases of CP in western societies are caused by **prolonged alcohol intake,** although a range of individual thresholds for alcohol toxicity is noted. Epidemiologic studies suggest that a diet high in fat and protein may increase the relative risk of CP associated with prolonged alcohol use. Patients with low-threshold alcohol-induced CP may be difficult to distinguish from those with idiopathic CP. **Idiopathic CP** is diagnosed by exclusion of other causes, including hypercalcemia, cystic fibrosis (considered even in adults without lung disease), trauma with residual duct injury, and ampullary and duodenal diseases that cause obstructing chronic pancreatitis.

3. Are there nutritional causes of chronic pancreatitis?
Tropical or nutritional pancreatitis is an important cause of CP in African and Asian countries, where it usually affects young adults in their teens. The pathophysiology of this form of CP is thought to involve nutritional antioxidant deficiencies, such as zinc, copper, and selenium, which leaves free radical injury from dietary cyanogens (e.g., cassava) unopposed. These patients exhibit severe chronic calcific pancreatitis with large endoductal calcified stones.

4. Are there genetic factors that influence CP?
Hereditary pancreatitis has been described in families from different areas of the world. It typically appears by age 10 or 12, affects both sexes equally, and is inherited through an autosomal dominant gene. These patients have an increased incidence of pancreatic carcinoma.

5. What is the usual presenting symptom in patients with chronic pancreatitis?
Pain is the most common presenting symptom of patients with CP. The pain is epigastric in location and is described as dull and radiating to the back. Initially it is intermittent, but then may become constant. It may be exacerbated by the intake of food or alcohol. Pain relief is the goal in caring for these patients, which occasionally results in narcotic addiction. The causes of pain of CP are presumed to include nerve entrapment with associated inflammation and increased intraductal pressures. Pain in CP patients may also relate to complications, such as pseudocysts, common bile duct obstruction, and/or duodenal obstruction. Approximately 15% of CP patients are pain-free and present solely with exocrine and/or endocrine insufficiency.

6. Are there other presenting symptoms of chronic pancreatitis?
Other presenting symptoms can relate to the endocrine/exocrine dysfunction of the pancreas. Although digestive enzymes produced by the pancreas are necessary for fat and protein absorption and are decreased in CP, malabsorption of fat and protein is not noticed until pancreatic enzyme

output is reduced to approximately 10%. Therefore, the malabsorption of fat resulting in **steatorrhea** is a relatively late symptom in the course of CP. With malassimilation, there is an associated decreased absorption of fat-soluble vitamins (A, E, D, K). Thus, easy **bruisability, bone pain,** and **decreased night vision** are not unusual clinical symptoms. Supporting laboratory data include prolonged prothrombin time, hypocalcemia, and uncontrolled diabetes. The causes of **weight loss** in patients with CP include (1) sitophobia, or fear of eating (as the pain increases with eating, there is decreased caloric intake); (2) malassimilation, secondary to pancreatic insufficiency; and (3) loss of calories secondary to diabetes mellitus.

7. How does one diagnose CP?

CP is usually diagnosed as a result of worsening abdominal pain in patients with chronic alcohol abuse or other historical causes of CP. An abdominal x-ray may reveal pancreatic calcifications in the pancreatic ducts, confirming the diagnosis. However, further radiographic studies usually are required, including ultrasound, computed tomography (CT), or endoscopic retrograde cholangiopancreatography (ERCP).

Ultrasound findings having a high sensitivity and specificity for CP include pancreatic ductal dilatation and the parenchymal changes of increased echogenicity with irregular gland contour. Abdominal CT findings include pancreatic duct dilatation, calcifications, and cystic lesions. Other findings include heterogeneous density of the pancreatic gland with atrophy or enlargement. CT is more sensitive and specific than ultrasound in the diagnosis of CP.

8. Do serum pancreatic enzymes have a role in the diagnosis of CP?

Overall, serum amylase and lipase levels are not helpful in diagnosing CP. These pancreatic enzyme levels can be elevated (as in patients with CP who have a superimposed acute pancreatitis), normal, or low. When low levels are found, they can be suggestive of CP.

9. Are there any specialized tests to diagnose CP?

Indirect tests to diagnose pancreatic exocrine dysfunction are not useful in detecting early CP, because these tests have low sensitivity and/or are difficult to perform. One such test, the bentiromide test, exploits the lack of the digestive enzyme chymotrypsin in CP. As CP progresses, the sensitivity of the bentiromide test for diagnosing CP also increases. The most commonly used tests involve measurement of pancreatic bicarbonate **output** subsequent to secretin stimulation or measurement of pancreatic enzyme production after stimulation with cholecystokinin. Both of these tests allow direct assessment of pancreatic function. Bicarbonate levels <50 meq are indicative of chronic pancreatitis. However, these tests require placement of a duodenal tube for secretion collection.

10. What is the role of ERCP in diagnosing chronic pancreatitis?

Endoscopic retrograde cholangial pancreatography (ERCP) allows one to assess the ductular changes that occur in CP. These changes include irregularity, dilatation, tortuosity, stenosis, and the presence of cysts and intraductal stones. Interestingly, a small group of patients with CP, demonstrated by abnormal secretory tests, have normal-appearing pancreatic ducts. The most frequent role of ERCP with pancreatic duct visualization is to exclude a pancreatic neoplasm.

11. Name the common complications seen in patients with chronic pancreatitis.

The complications of CP are local and systemic. The former include jaundice, splenic vein thrombosis, and pseudocysts, whereas the latter result from malassimilation with nutritional sequelae. Jaundice can result from extrahepatic compression of the pancreas on the common bile duct or associated hepatocellular disease, i.e., toxins (alcohol) or associated viral hepatitis. Common bile duct compression occurs because of entrapment of the distal duct within the pancreatic parenchyma or via compression of the duct by a pancreatic pseudocyst, thus resulting in obstructive jaundice.

Splenic vein thrombosis occurs in approximately 5% of patients with CP and results from a combination of peripancreatic inflammation and the close anatomic relationship between the pancreas and splenic vein. The resulting thrombosis causes backflow of blood into the short gastric veins and formation of gastric varices. Massive GI bleeding from these gastric varices can occur.

12. What are pseudocysts?
Pseudocysts develop in up to 25% of all patients with CP. These fluid-filled cystic structures are called pseudocysts because they do not have a cell-lined wall. Instead, the wall is made up of a fibrous membrane produced by a reaction of local mesothelial cells.

13. Name the complications of pseudocysts.
Pseudocysts may become secondarily infected, as they are warm and wet. Clinically, patients with an **infected pseudocyst** manifest a wide variety of symptoms suggestive of an intra-abdominal abscess (e.g., temperature, abdominal pain). Diagnosis is established by Gram stain and culture of the needle aspirate.

Also, the pseudocyst may invade an adjacent vessel and be converted into a **pseudoaneurysm.** Erosion into adjacent blood vessels can result in GI bleeding (pancreatic hemosuccus) if this fluid-filled cavity communicates with the pancreatic duct.

A third complication is **pancreatic ascites,** which results from chronic leakage of pancreatic fluid from a pseudocyst or disrupted pancreatic duct. Clinically, the patient has symptoms only from increasing intra-abdominal fluid. This complication must be distinguished from ascites secondary to cirrhosis, which can be done be detecting the presence of levels of ascitic pancreatic enzymes that are higher than serum levels of amylase. The initial approach is to document the source of the leak. Treatment includes supportive measures to improve nutrition, somatostatin administration, and possible surgical intervention.

14. How is pain managed in patients with CP?
The treatment of patients with CP involves symptomatic treatment of pain as well as correction of pancreatic insufficiency. A correctable source of pain (pseudocyst, pancreatic duct obstruction) should be sought. Alcohol should be avoided if this is the etiology. Medical treatment with simple analgesics, such as acetaminophen and salicylates, can control mild pain, but in severe cases, narcotics may be needed. Secondary addiction is a risk. Nerve blocks placed under radiologic guidance into the celiac ganglion have been used, but unfortunately, they last only for months, even when initial pain relief is achieved. Thus, repeat procedures are usually needed for recurrent pain.

Pancreatic enzymes may be used for pain control in a subgroup of patients. Their mechanism is inhibition of cholecytokinin release from the duodenum, which normally stimulates pancreatic secretion. The theoretical reduction in pancreatic enzyme secretion decreases the pain responses. Pancreatic enzymes are useful in decreasing chronic pain in patients with mild disease (women with nonalcoholic, noncalcific CP). The second mechanism by which pancreatic enzymes may decrease pain is by eliminating malassimilation, with the resulting abdominal distention and diarrhea. Therefore, pancreatic enzyme replacement is a mainstay of treatment for chronic pancreatitis.

Surgery offers longer-lasting pain control. The principles of surgical intervention in patients with CP and pain is to drain the dilated, high-pressure pancreatic duct or pseudocyst when present (segmental or total) or to resect diseased pancreatic tissue when small pancreatic diffuse duct disease is present (as demonstrated at ERCP). Pain relief can be achieved with surgery in up to 50–80% of CP patients.

15. How can steatorrhea be treated in CP?
Commercially available pancreatic enzyme preparations are used to treat pancreatic exocrine dysfunction by orally supplementing digestive enzymes. They must be given in sufficient amounts or in a protected form to prevent gastric acid/pepsin inactivation, and enough should be given to replace at least 10% of pancreatic enzyme output. The dosing of pancreatic enzyme supplements

can be titrated according to the patient's clinical response, which is assessed by their decrease in steatorrhea and abdominal distention. Antisecretory medications can be added to decrease the destruction of enzyme supplements by acid and may increase efficacy of the drug.

BIBLIOGRAPHY

1. Comfort NW, Steinberg AG: Pedigree of a family with hereditary chronic relapsing pancreatitis. Gastroenterology 21:54, 1952.
2. Durbel JP, Sarles H: Multicenter survey of etiology of pancreatic disease: Relationship between the relative risk of developing chronic pancreatitis and alcohol, protein and lipid consumption. Digestion 18:337,1978.
3. Kalthoff L, Layer P, Calin JE, DiMagno EP: The course of alcoholic and non-alcoholic chronic pancreatitis. Dig Dis Sci 29:553, 1984.
4. Karimgoni I, Porter KA, Langevin RE, Banks PA: Prognostic factors in sterile pancreatic necrosis. Gastroenterology 103:1636–1640, 1992.
5. Pitchumoni CS: Special problems in tropical pancreatitis. Clin Gastroenterol 13:941, 1984.
6. Pitchumoni CS, Thomas E: Chronic cassava toxicity: Possible relationship to chronic pancreatic disease in malnourished populations. Lancet 2:1397, 1973.
7. Rossi RL, Heiss FW, Braasch JW: Surgical management of chronic pancreatitis. Surg Clin North Am 65:79, 1985.
8. Sarles H: Alcoholism and pancreatitis Scand J Gastroenterol 6.193, 1971.
9. Sarles H, Adler G, Dani R, et al: The pancreatitis classification of Marseilles-Rome 1988. Scand J Gastroenterol 24:641, 1929.

37. PANCREATIC CANCER

John Deutsch, M.D.

1. Is drinking coffee associated with developing pancreatic cancer?
This issue has not been resolved. Some studies suggest a small risk, but others suggest no risk. Tobacco, on the other hand, increases the risk of pancreatic cancer about fourfold.

2. Is there a geographic variation in the incidence of pancreatic cancer?
Pancreatic cancer appears to be more common in countries where there is high fat intake. In contrast to gastric cancer, but similar to colon cancer, the incidence of pancreatic cancer is higher in the United States than in Japan.

3. Is there a sexual or racial predilection for pancreatic cancer?
Pancreatic cancer occurs more commonly in males, and it is more common in African-Americans than in European-Americans.

4. What cell types are found in pancreatic tumors?
Most pancreatic cancers arise from the exocrine ductal epithelium and glands. Rare tumors arise from the endocrine cells of the pancreas and include insulinomas, glucagonomas, VIPomas, and gastrinomas.

5. What genetic alterations are associated with pancreatic tumors?
Mutations in the K-*ras* oncogene are very common in pancreatic cancers and have been identified in over 80% of adenocarcinomas that arise there. Mutations of the tumor-suppressor genes do not appear to be important in the development of pancreatic cancer.

6. Can pancreatic cancer be diagnosed through the use of a serum test?
The cancer antigen CA 19-9 is elevated in almost 75% of patients with pancreatic adenocarcinomas. CA 19-9 also can be elevated in benign inflammatory conditions of the pancreas, such as chronic pancreatitis. If the CA 19-9 level is markedly elevated (>10 times the upper limits of normal), this is good presumptive evidence for pancreatic cancer. Likewise, if the CA 19-9 level is rising over time, this is also presumptive evidence of pancreatic cancer. However, CA 19-9 can rise with biliary obstruction, so the diagnosis of pancreatic cancer relies on histologic confirmation.

7. What are the common locations for a gastrinoma?
The pancreas or the wall of the duodenum.

8. Why should serum calcium be measured in patients diagnosed with gastrinoma?
Gastrinoma occurs in two general circumstances: sporadically, or as part of a multiple endocrine neoplasia syndrome (MEN-1), which is familial. In addition to pancreatic islet cell tumors, pituitary tumors and parathyroid hyperplasia or adenomas also occur in MEN-1, leading to hypercalcemia.

9. How do pancreatic cancers present?
Pancreatic cancers usually present with unexplained weight loss or abdominal pain. Some cancers in the head of the pancreas present with obstructive jaundice and an enlarged gallbladder. Round cell (islet cell) tumors, such as gastrinoma, usually present either due to excessive hormone output or with bulky disease. Patients who appear to be relatively healthy but have a massive amount of metastatic tumor in the liver often turn out to have a nonfunctioning islet cell tumor of pancreatic origin.

10. Which islet cell tumor is most likely to be benign?
Generally, islet cell tumors types, including gastrinoma, somatostatinoma, and VIPoma, exhibit malignant behavior in over 50% of cases. An exception is **insulinoma,** where 80–90% of the tumors are benign.

11. What are the most sensitive methods of locating an islet cell tumor in the pancreas?
Functioning islet cell tumors can be small and below the resolution of usual diagnostic methods, such as CT scans. Endosonic ultrasonography is probably the most sensitive, nonincisional method to locate pancreatic round cell tumors. Surgical exploration with intraoperative ultrasonography of the pancreas is probably the most sensitive method to locate small islet cell tumors.

12. How is the secretin test used in diagnosing gastrinoma?
Secretin is a peptide hormone that stimulates the normal pancreas to produce a bicarbonate-rich fluid. Secretin does not stimulate normal gastrin-producing cells to increase their output, but aberrant gastrin-producing tumors will usually produce gastrin following secretin stimulation. Therefore, if someone has an elevated serum gastrin level, one administers secretin. If the gastrin level rises by 50% or >200 pg/ml in the first 5 minutes, it is presumed that the gastrin is from an islet cell tumor.

13. When should patients with pancreatic adenocarcinoma undergo resection for cure?
Pancreatic cancer is almost never curable. However, tumors in the head of the pancreas can sometimes obstruct the common bile duct when the tumors are relatively small (<2 cm across), leading to their early detection. These patients can occasionally be cured with surgery. However, patients with tumors >4 cm in diameter are rarely cured. Patients presenting with symptoms other than obstructive jaundice, such as back pain, are almost never cured with surgery.

14. How do you evaluate patients to assess whether curative resection should be attempted?
The staging of pancreatic cancer for cure includes assessments to determine the resectability of the primary tumor and to determine whether metastatic disease is present. All patients should undergo a computed tomographic (CT) scan of the abdomen to determine the size of the tumor and the presence of metastatic disease. Further workup is directed somewhat by the clinical situation. Some recommend an arteriogram, because vascular encasement precludes resection. If there is no evidence of vascular invasion, laparoscopy could be performed to look for peritoneal spread. Alternatively, if the patient is to have a surgical procedure anyway (e.g., to relieve biliary obstruction), assessment of resectability for cure can be made at the time of laparotomy. If the tumor is found to be unresectable, a definitive palliative procedure can then be performed. Even with the best preoperative assessments, most patients resected for "cure" die of pancreatic cancer.

15. Should all patients with pancreatic cancer have palliative biliary and duodenal bypass surgery?
Tumors in the head of the pancreas frequently obstruct the common bile duct, and bypass surgery can provide excellent palliation, should this occur. Likewise, 20% of tumors in the head of the pancreas will obstruct the duodenum. However, prophylactic intestinal bypass surgery is unnecessary in most patients with pancreatic cancer. Furthermore, in many patients, biliary obstruction can be managed endoscopically, although stents tend to become infected and may become plugged with sludge. Randomized trials suggest a benefit for some patients who are managed endoscopically compared to surgically, but the choice of surgical or endoscopic management of patients depends on many factors, including the local expertise and the projected life expectancy of the patient. A team approach to individualize therapy usually provides the best palliation in any individual case.

16. What is the response rate of pancreatic adenocarcinoma to chemotherapy?
Most chemotherapeutic regimens have <10% partial responses to pancreatic cancer.

17. Does chemotherapy have any role in treating pancreatic cancer?
Chemotherapy combined with radiation therapy has been shown to minimally improve survival in patients with pancreatic cancer and can be useful in alleviating pain.

18. What is the role of octreotide in the therapy of islet cell tumors of the pancreas?
Octreotide is a long half-life somatostatin analog that can be used in the therapy for functioning islet cell tumors. In general, octreotide decreases hormone output and alleviates symptoms associated with hormone excess. In a small percentage of cases, octreotide actually leads to tumor regression.

BIBLIOGRAPHY

1. Baghurst PA, McMichael AJ, Slavotinek AH, et al: A case-control study of diet and cancer of the pancreas. Am J Epidemiol 134:167–179, 1991.
2. Bueno de Mesquita HB, Maisonnueve P, Moerman CJ, et al: Lifetime consumption of alcoholic beverages, tea and coffee and exocrine carcinoma of the pancreas: A population-based case-control study in the Netherlands. Int J Cancer 50:514–522, 1992.
3. Castillo CF, Warshaw AL: Diagnosis and preoperative evaluation of pancreatic cancer, with implications for management. Gastroenterol Clin North Am 19:915–933, 1990.
4. DeCarpio JA, Mayer RJ, Gonin R, et al: Fluorouracil and high dose leucovorin in previously untreated patients with advanced adenocarcinoma of the pancreas: Results of a phase II trial. J Clin Oncol 9:2128–2133, 1991.
5. Douglass HO Jr, Tepper J, Leichman L: Neoplasms of the exocrine pancreas. In Holland JF, Frei E III, Bast RC Jr, et al (eds): Cancer Medicine, 3rd ed. Philadelphia, Lea & Febiger, 1993.
6. Lemoine NR, Jain S, Hughes CM, et al: Ki-ras oncogene activation in preinvasive pancreatic carcinoma. Gastroenterology 102:230–236, 1992.
7. Lyon JL, Mahoney AM, French TK, et al: Coffee consumption and the risk of cancer of the exocrine pancreas: A case-control study in a low risk population. Epidemiology 3:164–170, 1992.
8. Masson P, Andren-Sandberg A: Crude isolation of DNA from unselected human pancreatic tissue and amplification by the polymerase chain reaction of Ki-ras oncogene to detect point mutations in pancreatic cancer. Acta Oncol 31:421–424, 1992.
9. Mojimoto K, Urano T, Nagata Y, et al: Mutations in the Kirsten-ras oncogene are common but lack correlation with prognosis and tumor stage in human pancreatic carcinoma. Am J Gastroenterol 86:1784–1788, 1991.
10. Molina LM, Diez M, Cava MT, et al: Tumor markers in pancreatic cancer: A comparative clinical study between CEA, CA 19-9 and CA 50. Int J Biol Markers 5:127–132, 1990.
11. Rosch T, Braig C, Gain T, et al: Staging of pancreatic and ampullary carcinoma by endoscopic ultrasonography: Comparison with conventional sonography, computed tomography, and angiography. Gastroenterology 102:188–199, 1992.
12. Rosch T, Lightdale CJ, Botet JF, et al: Localization of pancreatic endocrine tumors by endoscopic ultrasonography. N Engl J Med 326:1721–1726, 1992.
13. Rosch T, Lorenz R, Braig C, et al: Endoscopic ultrasound in pancreatic tumor diagnosis. Gastrointest Endosc 37:347–352, 1991.
14. Satake K, Chung YS, Umeyama K, et al: The possibility of diagnosing small pancreatic cancer (<4.0 cm) by measuring various serum tumor markers: A retrospective study. Cancer 68:149–152, 1991.
15. Tada M, Omata M, Ohto M: Clinical application of ras gene mutation for diagnosis of pancreatic adenocarcinoma. Gastroenterology 100:233–238, 1991.
16. Vinik AI, Thompson NW, Averbuch SD: Neoplasms of the gastroenteropancreatic endocrine system. In Holland JF, Frei E III, Bast RC Jr, et al. (eds): Cancer Medicine, 3rd ed. Philadelphia, Lea & Febiger, 1993.
17. Warshaw AL, Castillo CF: Pancreatic carcinoma. N Engl J Med 326: 455–465, 1992.

38. CYSTIC DISEASE OF THE PANCREAS

Randall E. Lee, M.D.

1. What is the difference between a true pancreatic cyst and a pancreatic pseudocyst?
A true pancreatic cyst is lined by epithelium. A pancreatic pseudocyst is lined by inflammatory and scar tissue. True pancreatic cysts account for only 10–15% of all cystic lesions of the pancreas.

2. Provide a differential diagnosis for a cystic pancreatic lesion.

Differential Diagnosis of Cystic Pancreatic Lesions

Pancreatic pseudocyst	Mucinous cystic pancreatic neoplasm
Pancreatic abscess	Benign cysts associated with von Hippel–Lindau disease
Cystic necrosis of pancreatic adenocarcinoma	Benign cysts associated with polycystic kidney disease
Serous (microcystic) cystadenoma	Macrocystic changes of cystic fibrosis

3. Describe the pathogenesis of a pancreatic pseudocyst associated with acute pancreatitis.
An acute pseudocyst develops within 6 weeks of an attack of acute pancreatitis. This collection of high-amylase fluid usually is located in the peripancreatic tissues and is believed to arise from disruption of a pancreatic duct or from fluid exuded from the inflamed surface of the pancreas. Acute pancreatic pseudocysts spontaneously resolve in 25–40% of cases.

4. How does the pathogenesis differ in a pancreatic pseudocyst associated with chronic pancreatitis?
A chronic pseudocyst usually is located within the pancreas. It is believed to arise from slow blockage of a pancreatic duct by fibrosis, a protein plug, or calculus. Chronic pseudocysts also may arise in association with an exacerbation of chronic pancreatitis.

5. Explain the pathogenesis of a pancreatic pseudocyst that is associated with blunt abdominal trauma.
A traumatic pseudocyst is believed to develop when blunt trauma to the pancreas disrupts a pancreatic duct or ductule. The resulting pseudocyst contains a fluid with a high content of amylase. Patients afflicted with a traumatic pseudocyst typically present with abdominal pain, elevated serum amylase, and abdominal mass 1–2 weeks after receiving blunt, upper abdominal trauma.

6. What is the typical clinical presentation of a pancreatic pseudocyst associated with acute pancreatitis?
Formation of a pancreatic pseudocyst should be suspected if a patient with acute pancreatitis develops any of the following:
- Failure of acute pancreatitis symptoms to resolve after about 7–10 days
- Recurrence of acute pancreatitis symptoms after an initial improvement
- Epigastric abdominal mass
- Persistently elevated serum amylase
- Obstructive jaundice

7. What criteria suggest that a pseudocyst will not resolve spontaneously?
A pancreatic pseudocyst has a low probability of spontaneous resolution if any of the following criteria are present:
- Pseudocyst persists for >6 weeks
- Pseudocyst diameter >6 cm
- Concurrent evidence of chronic pancreatitis

- Thick pseudocyst wall
- Pancreatic duct abnormality other than communication with the pseudocyst
- Pseudocyst size increases on serial imaging studies

8. When should a pseudocyst be drained?

Elective surgical drainage of an acute pseudocyst should be postponed for about 4–6 weeks after the time of diagnosis. This delay allows for thickening and maturation of the pseudocyst wall, thus increasing the holding power of sutures.

A pseudocyst should be drained urgently if it is causing critical compression of an adjacent structure, such as the bile duct, or if it shows evidence of infection. Urgent drainage of a noninfected pseudocyst may be performed percutaneously with computed tomography (CT) or ultrasound guidance. An infected pseudocyst (pancreatic abscess) should be drained surgically.

9. What are three methods for draining a pancreatic pseudocyst?
1. Surgical drainage
2. CT- or ultrasound-guided percutaneous drainage
3. Transpapillary, transgastric, or transduodenal endoscopic drainage

10. How do the methods for draining a pancreatic pseudocyst compare with each other?

Surgical pseudocyst drainage has a reported morbidity of 30–40% and a mortality of 2–10%. The recurrence rate is 0–15%.

For percutaneous pseudocyst drainage, the reported morbidity and mortality rates are 0–30% and 0–10%, respectively. The recurrence rate is 0–30%.

Endoscopic pseudocyst drainage has a reported morbidity rate of 0–16%, a mortality rate of 0–6%, and a recurrence rate of 0–12%. The common complications are bleeding, infection, and perforation.

11. What criteria suggest that a pancreatic pseudocyst may undergo successful endoscopic drainage?

A pancreatic pseudocyst may undergo successful endoscopic drainage if it has one of the following criteria: (1) endoscopic retrograde cholangiopancreatography (ERCP) demonstrates a communication between the pseudocyst and the main pancreatic duct; or (2) the pseudocyst impinges upon the stomach or duodenum, creating an endoluminal bulge. Additional imaging with CT, endoscopic ultrasonography, or endoscopic injection of contrast is recommended to confirm close contact between the pseudocyst and adjacent gastric or duodenal wall prior to attempting transgastric or transduodenal endoscopic drainage.

12. How does a pancreatic abscess appear on a CT scan?

A pancreatic abscess may appear as an ill-defined, nonenhancing fluid collection of mixed densities. Unfortunately, this CT appearance may be confused with a noninfected pseudocyst or phlegmon. The presence of gas within the cystic area strongly suggests infection by gas-forming organisms.

13. What clinical criteria suggest the development of a pancreatic abscess?

A pancreatic abscess typically develops from secondary bacterial infection of necrotic pancreatic tissue during an episode of acute pancreatitis. The abscess often causes temperatures >38.5°C, leukocytosis >10,000 cells/mm^3, and increasing abdominal pain. Unfortunately, all these signs also may be found in a noninfected patient who has severe pancreatitis. Percutaneous needle aspiration of the area may help to confirm the diagnosis of a pancreatic abscess.

14. What is a serous (microcystic) cystadenoma?

A serous (microcystic) cystadenoma is an uncommon pancreatic neoplasm characterized by numerous cysts filled with a glycogen-rich serous fluid and lined by flat or cuboidal epithelium. The cysts usually are <20 mm in diameter, hence the modifier "microcystic." Fibrous septa radiating out from the tumor's center separate the cysts. This neoplasm is benign and may remain asymptomatic. Symptoms are usually a direct result of mass effect.

15. What is a mucinous cystic pancreatic neoplasm?

A mucinous cystic pancreatic neoplasm is an uncommon neoplasm characterized by large cysts filled with mucin and lined by a columnar epithelium. The cysts are usually >20 mm in diameter. This neoplasm occurs more often in women and usually is located in the body or tail of the pancreas. The most frequent presenting symptoms are epigastric pain and an enlarging abdominal mass. Jaundice is very rare.

This tumor may be subclassified as either a benign mucinous cystadenoma or a malignant mucinous cystadenocarcinoma. However, the distinction is often difficult to establish, as histologic studies reveal the frequent occurrence of both benign and malignant epithelium within the same tumor. Many authors now regard all mucinous cystic neoplasms as malignant.

The treatment of choice for a mucinous cystic pancreatic neoplasm is complete surgical resection. The survival rate for patients with this neoplasm is much higher than that for patients with pancreatic ductal adenocarcinoma.

16. List the common manifestations of von Hippel–Lindau disease.

Multiple pancreatic cysts, retinal angiomas, CNS hemangioblastomas, renal cysts, renal cell carcinoma, and islet cell tumors are the common manifestations of von Hippel–Lindau disease. The mode of inheritance is autosomal dominant. The pancreatic cysts may precede other manifestations of the disease by several years and may be the only abdominal manifestation. Abdominal ultrasound or CT scanning is recommended for individuals with a family history of von Hippel–Lindau disease.

17. What is the clinical significance of the pancreatic cysts in von Hippel–Lindau disease?

In a study of patients with von Hippel–Lindau disease who had pancreatic cysts, the cysts did not progress or cause any major clinical symptoms over a follow-up of 5 years. Nevertheless, there are several reports of these cysts causing obstructive jaundice by compression of the common bile duct.

18. Describe the pancreatic abnormalities caused by cystic fibrosis that are demonstrable by CT.

Most commonly, the pancreatic parenchyma is replaced by fatty tissue. The transformation of the pancreas into a mass of macroscopic cysts occurs with less frequency.

BIBLIOGRAPHY

1. Compagno J, Oertel JE. Microcystic adenomas of the pancreas (glycogen-rich cystadenomas). Am J Clin Pathol 69:289–298, 1978.
2. Compagno J, Oertel JE: Mucinous cystic neoplasms of the pancreas with overt and latent malignancy (cystadenocarcinoma and cystadenoma). Am J Clin Pathol 69:573–580, 1978.
3. Grace PA, Williamson RCN: Modern management of pancreatic pseuodocysts. Br J Surg 80:573–581, 1993.
4. Hough DM, Stephens DH, Johnson CD, Binkovitz LA: Pancreatic lesions in von Hippel–Lindau disease: Prevalence, clinical significance, and CT findings. AJR 162:1091–1094, 1994.
5. Howard JM: Cystic neoplasms and true cysts of the pancreas. Surg Clin North Am 69(3): 651–665, 1989.
6. Howell DA, Holbrook RF, Bosco JJ, et al: Endoscopic needle localization of pancreatic pseudocysts before transmural drainage. Gastrointest Endosc 39:693–698, 1993.
7. Huibregtse K, Smiths ME: Endoscopic management of diseases of the pancreas. Am J Gastroenterol 89:S66–S77, 1994.
8. Lawson JM, Baillie J: Endoscopic therapy for pancreatic pseudocysts. Gastrointest Endosc Clin North Am 5(1):181–193, 1995.
9. Neumann HP, Dinkel E, Brambs H, et al: Pancreatic lesions in the von Hippel–Lindau syndrome. Gastroenterology 101:465–471, 1991.
10. Thoeni RF, Blankenberg F: Pancreatic imaging, computed tomography and magnetic resonance imaging. Radiol Clin North Am 31(5):1085–1113, 1993.

V. Small Bowel Disorders

39. CELIAC DISEASE, TROPICAL SPRUE, WHIPPLE'S DISEASE, LYMPHANGIECTASIS, AND NSAIDs

Tuanh Tonnu, M.D., and Ingram M. Roberts, M.D.

1. What is the best screening test for fat malabsorption?

Microscopic examination of stool using Sudan stain to detect fat is the best screening test for fat malabsorption. This test has a 100% sensitivity and 96% specificity as a screening test for malabsorption. A stool sample is smeared on a microscope slide and mixed with ethanolic Sudan III and glacial acetic acid. The slide is covered, heated just until boiling, and then examined for the presence of fatty acid globules. The presence of >100 globules larger the 6 μm in diameter per high-powered field ($\times$430) indicates a definite increase in fecal fat excretion. The number of globules correlates well with the quantitative amount of fecal fat present.

2. What is the best quantitative test for fat malabsorption?

The 72-hour stool fat collection. The patient is given a diet consisting of 60–100 gm of fat per day. Stool is then collected, usually for 72 hours. The normal coefficient for absorption is approximately 93% of ingested fat. Consequently, if 100 gm of fat is digested, 7 gm or less of fat should appear in stool over a 24-hour period. If >7 gm of fecal fat is present, steatorrhea secondary to malabsorption is confirmed.

There are several physiologic conditions where fecal fat excretion is increased:

- when the diet is high in fiber (>100 gm/day);
- when dietary fat is ingested in solid form, such as whole peanuts; and
- in the neonatal period, when intraluminal levels of pancreatic lipase and bile salts are low.

3. What is the best test to differentiate mucosal disease from pancreatic insufficiency?

D-Xylose test is one of the best tests to differentiate mucosal disease from pancreatic insufficiency as the cause of malabsorption. D-Xylose is absorbed and excreted in an unchanged form. A 25-gm dose of D-xylose is given orally after an overnight fast, and urine is then collected for 5 hours. Normal urine excretion should be >5 gm of D-xylose. One-hour serum collection is also helpful but not as sensitive as urine collection. Normal serum levels 1 hour after ingestion are >20 mg/dl.

Several conditions that may cause false-positive findings in the D-xylose test include:

- Delayed gastric emptying
- Vomiting
- Renal disease
- Myxedema
- Ascites

4. What is the GSE panel?

Gluten-sensitive enteropathy panel (GSE) is a serologic test for celiac sprue that is being used with increasing frequency. The panel consists of anti-gliadin antibodies (AGA), IgA anti-reticulin (R1-ARA), and IgA anti-endomysial antibodies (IgA-EmA). These antibodies are directed against the connective tissue (reticulin-like structures) or surface component of smooth muscle fibrils.

IgA-EmA has 100% specificity for celiac disease, whereas its sensitivity is 85% and 90%, respectively, for untreated adult and childhood celiac disease. It can persist in low titer in 10–25% of celiac patients on a gluten-free diet despite normal histology.

AGA has fairly good sensitivity (68–76%), but it can also be found in 10–20% of patients with other diseases that affect the small intestinal mucosa. AGA is a helpful test in monitoring GSE, as it always becomes negative with the regrowth of jejunal villi in celiac patients after a gluten-free diet.

RI-ARA has a higher specificity than AGA in celiac children but a relatively low sensitivity (<40–50%).

5. Name the conditions to consider in celiac spruc if a previously responsive patient begins to deteriorate.

Noncompliance with gluten-free diet is the most common cause of deterioration in a previously responsive patient.

Lymphoma is the most common malignancy complicating celiac disease, especially that of mucosal T cell origin. Diagnosis of lymphoma requires a high index of suspicion because onset can be insidious or abrupt, and the histologic appearance can be indistinguishable from that of celiac sprue. A careful search for lymphoma is needed in patients with celiac sprue who do not respond to gluten withdrawal or in patients with recurrent weight loss and malabsorption despite strict adherence to a gluten-free diet. Computed tomographic (CT) scan and exploratory laparatomy may be necessary to establish the diagnosis.

Refractory sprue has clinical features and mucosal lesions indistinguishable from celiac sprue, but these patients do not respond to a gluten-free diet, either from the onset of diagnosis or subsequent to becoming refractory to dietary therapy. Some of these patients may respond to corticosteroids or other immunosuppressive drugs, such as azathioprine, cyclophosphamide, or cyclosporine. Others do not respond to any treatment, and they face a dismal prognosis. Absence of Paneth cells on small bowel biopsy is felt to be a poor prognostic sign.

Collagenous sprue is a subset of refractory sprue. It is characterized by the progressive development of a thick band of collagenlike material beneath the basement membrane of epithelial cells. It is usually refractory to all forms of treatment other than parenteral alimentation.

6. Describe the manifestations of Whipple's disease.

Whipple's disease is a chronic systemic illness with various potential manifestations. The most common presentation includes weight loss (90%), diarrhea (>70%), and arthralgias (>70%). Arthralgias can exist for many years before the diagnosis of Whipple's disease. Cardiac involvement includes congestive heart failure, pericarditis, and valvular heart disease (30%). Lymphadenopathy and hyperpigmentation are frequent findings on physical examination. Hematochezia is very rare, but occult bleeding has been detected in up to 80% of Whipple's patients. The most common CNS manifestations (5%) are dementia, ocular disturbances, meningoencephalitis, and cerebellar symptoms including ataxia and mild clonus.

7. What is the differential diagnosis of an increased macrophage infiltrate in the lamina propria of the small bowel?

1. Whipple's disease: Inclusions are rounded or sickle-shaped.
2. *Mycobacterium avium-intracellulare:* Inclusions contain acid-fast bacilli. This condition is commonly seen in AIDS patients with small bowel involvement.
3. Histoplasmosis or cryptococcosis: Inclusions contain large, round, encapsulated organisms.
4. Macroglobulinemia: No inclusions are seen, and there are only faintly staining, homogeneously periodic acid–Schiff (PAS)-positive macrophages.

5. Miscellaneous disease: PAS-positive macrophages are frequently present in the normal gastric and rectal mucosa, and these can be lipid-containing or mucin-containing macrophages, respectively.

8. What causes Whipple's disease?
The Whipple's disease bacillus is known to cause this disease in humans but cannot be cultured in vitro. Recently, the organism was identified by direct amplification of a 16S rRNA sequence from a microbial pathogen in tissue. According to phylogenetic analysis, this bacterium is a gram-positive actinomycete that is not closely related to any known genus. It has been named *Tropheryma whippelii*. Prolonged treatment with antibiotics (for up to 6 months) is often required to eradicate the organism.

9. What are the complications of the enteropathy induced by nonsteroidal anti-inflammatory drugs (NSAIDs)?
NSAID-induced enteropathy is associated with intestinal bleeding, protein loss, ileal dysfunction, and malabsorption. There is no close relationship between upper endoscopic finding and evidence of intestinal bleeding in NSAID-treated patients, even when blood loss has led to an iron-deficiency anemia. Chronic blood loss and protein loss seem to occur from the inflammatory site. Protein loss can result in insignificant hypoalbuminemia. Ileal dysfunction can lead to bile acid malabsorption, but a very small portion of patients have mild vitamin B12 malabsorption. The malabsorption is often mild. However, mefenamic acid and sulindac have been implicated in severe malabsorption with subtotal villus atrophy resembling celiac disese.

10. Does scleroderma produce any manifestations in the small bowel?
Patients with scleroderma may have small bowel dysfunction due to absent cycling of the normal contractile pattern, known as the migrating motor complex. Small bowel motility studies reveal markedly diminished amplitude in all phasic pressure waves. This may be manifested clinically as intestinal pseudo-obstruction and bacterial overgrowth. Patients may suffer from nausea, vomiting, abdominal pain, diarrhea, and malabsorption. Small bowel radiographic series may show megaduodenum and dilated loops of jejunum.

11. How does octreotide affect intestinal motility and bacterial overgrowth in scleroderma?
Octreotide evokes alternating phase 1 and phase 3 activity in normal subjects and patients with scleroderma. These complexes propagate at the same velocity and have two-thirds the amplitude of the spontaneous complexes in normal subjects. This effect is independent of motilin because octreotide inhibits motilin release. Octreotide may retard gastric antral motility, however, in contrast to erythromycin, which markedly stimulates gastric antral motor activity.

12. Describe the different forms of lymphangiectasia.
Congenital intestinal lymphangiectasia (Milroy's disease) results from a malformation of the lymphatics. Many areas in the body can be affected. Patients with congenital disease present at any time, from childhood to adulthood, and usually have asymmetric lymphedema. Secondary lymphangiectasia results from a disease that blocks the intestinal lymph drainage at some level. Causes of secondary lymphangiectasia include extensive abdominal or retroperitoneal carcinoma, lymphoma, retroperitoneal fibrosis, chronic pancreatitis, mesenteric tuberculosis or sarcoidosis, Crohn's disease, chronic congestive heart failure, and even constrictive pericarditis.

13. What are the clinical manifestations of abetalipoproteinemia?
Abetalipoproteinemia is an autosomal recessive condition that is characterized by the inability to form chylomicrons and very-low-density lipoprotein particles by the enterocytes due to abnormal apoprotein B. Most patients suffer severe fat malabsorption and retardation and rarely survive the third decade. The largest series of patients has been studied at the National Intitutes of Health.

14. What are the different clinical presentations of eosinophilic gastroenteritis?

Eosinophilic gastroenteritis is characterized by eosinophilic infiltration in the GI tract. Clinical features and severity depend on the layer and location of involvement. **Mucosal** involvement leads to protein-losing enteropathy, fecal blood loss, and malabsorption. Involvement of the **muscle layer** often causes obstruction of gastric or small bowel. **Subserosal** involvement causes ascites, pleural effusion, or, on occasion, pericarditis.

15. How are patients with eosinophilic gastroenteritis treated?

The mainstay of treatment for eosinophilic gastroenteritis is corticosteroids, even though no controlled trials have been performed. The recommended dosage of prednisone is usually 20–40 mg/day for treatment of the initial episode and relapses, and 5–10 mg/day for maintenance. Some patients responded to a short course of treatment but may suffer from relapse. Others may require long-term maintenance therapy. The course of disease may wax and wane in severity but is rarely life-threatening. The therapeutic effect of oral sodium cromoglycate is controversial. Trial elimination diets have occasionally been successful, but relapse is common.

16. What are the common causes of diarrhea in a patient with Crohn's disease with ileal resection?

When ileal resection is <100 cm, diarrhea commonly occurs due to malabsorption of conjugated bile acids with decreased dehydroxylation by colonic bacteria, serving as secretory agents. Bile-salt diarrhea is typically watery, may not start until a normal diet is resumed after surgery, is precipitated by a meal (typically after breakfast when a large amount of bile is stored in the gallbladder), and does not lead to weight loss. These patients would benefit from an empirical trial of cholestyramine. When ileal resection is >100 cm, diarrhea results from fat malabsorption, which is markedly impaired due to deficient intraluminal micellar dispersion of digested lipids and decreased mucosal surface area. The bile acid pool is depleted, and the liver is unable to compensate adequately. These patients would benefit from a low fat diet or supplement of medium chain triglyceride.

17. Where are the endemic areas for tropical sprue?

Tropical sprue is endemic in Puerto Rico, Cuba, the Dominican Republic, and Haiti, but not in Jamaica or the other West Indies. It is found in Central America, Venezuela, and Columbia. Sprue is common in the Indian subcontinent and the Far East, though there is little information from China. Sprue has been reported among several visitors to countries in the Middle East. It is rare in Africa, although the occurrence of sprue among populations living in the central and southern parts is now well established.

18. How is tropical sprue treated?

The most effective therapy for tropical sprue in returning travelers or expatriates is a combination of folic acid and tetracycline. Folic acid should be given in a dosage of 5 mg/day orally, and tetracycline in a dosage of 250 mg four times a day. Vitamin B12 should be given parenterally, in addition to the above combination, if deficiency of this vitamin is also discovered. Treatment should be continued for at least several months or until intestinal function is returned to normal. Treatment with folic acid alone may be effective in reversing small bowel abnormalities or even in curing the acute illness, but not the chronic form. On the other hand, long-term treatment with tetracycline alone may result in cure of both acute and chronic forms of sprue.

19. How is bacterial overgrowth diagnosed?

The gold-standard test for the diagnosis of bacterial overgrowth is the demonstration of increased concentrations of bacteria ($>10^5$ colony-forming units/ml) in fluid that is obtained from the intestine during duodenal intubation. If quantitative culture of the small bowel aspirate is not possible, the diagnosis can be made with various breath tests. In the lactulose-hydrogen breath test, a rise in breath hydrogen level of 12 ppm from baseline values is taken as diagnostic for bacterial overgrowth. The ^{14}C-glycocholate and ^{14}C-D-xylose breath tests detect the release of the radiolabeled CO_2 as the result of bacterial deconjugation of bile acid and metabolism of xylose. Normalization of the Schilling test after treatment with antibiotics is highly suggestive of bacterial overgrowth.

20. What is the mechanism of hyperoxaluria in short bowel syndrome?

One mechanism of hyperoxaluria in short bowel syndrome is the formation of insoluble calcium soaps in the presence of unabsorbed fatty acids, which allow oxalate to remain in solution and thus available for absorption. The other mechanism proposes that unabsorbed fatty acids and bile salts increase the permeability of the colon to oxalate. Therefore, hyperoxaluria appears to depend on the presence of an intact colon. To prevent calcium oxalate nephrolithiasis in patients with bowel disease, a low-oxalate and low-fat diet should be recommended.

BIBLIOGRAPHY

1. Bjarnason I, Hayllar J, Macpherson AJ, Russell AS: Side effects of nonsteroidal antiinflamatory drugs on the small and large intestine in humans. Gastroenterology 104:1832–1847, 1993.
2. Fleming JL, Wiesner RH, Shorter RG: Whipple's disease: Clinical, biochemical, and histopathologic features and assessment of treatment in 29 patients. Mayo Clin Proc 63:539–551, 1988.
3. Hofmann AF, Poley R: Role of bile acid malabsorption in pathogenesis of diarrhea and steatorrhea in patients with ileal resection: I. Response to cholestyramine or replacement of dietary long chain triglyceride by medium chain triglyceride. Gastroenterology 62:918–934, 1972.
4. Klipstein FA: Tropical sprue in travelers and expatriates living abroad. Gastroenterology 80:590–600, 1981.
5. Relman DA, Schmidt TM, MacDermott RP, Falkow S: Identification of the uncultured bacillus of Whipple's disease. N Engl J Med 327:293–301, 1992.
6. Roberts IM: Workup of the patient with malabsorption. Postgrad Med 81:32–42, 1987.
7. Soudah HC, Hasler WL, Owyang C: Effect of octreotide on intestinal motility and bacterial overgrowth in scleroderma. N Engl J Med 325:1461–1467, 1991.
8. Talley NJ, Shorter RG, Phillips SF, Zinsmeister AR: Eosinophilic gastroenteritis: A clinicopathological study of patients with disease of the mucosa, muscle layer, and subserosal tissues. Gut 31:54–58, 1990.
9. Trier JS: Celiac sprue. N Engl J Med 325:1709–1719, 1991.
10. Volta U, Molinaro N, Fusconi M, et al: IgA antiendomysial antibody test: A step forward in celiac disease screening. Dig Dis Sci 36:752–756, 1991.
11. Yamada T, Alpers DH, Owyang C, et al (eds): Textbook of Gastroenterology, 2nd ed. Philadelphia, J.B. Lippincott, 1995.

40. CROHN'S DISEASE

John W. Singleton, M.D.

1. Describe the physical findings in a patient presenting with suspected Crohn's disease.

Initial Symptoms of Crohn's Disease

SYMPTOM	PREVALENCE IN NEW-ONSET DISEASE
Diarrhea	92%
Pain	95%
Bleeding	41%
Weight loss	85%
Perianal disease	35%
Arthritis/arthralgia	22%

The diagnosis of Crohn's disease is often delayed for months or years because the symptoms are so varied and often insidious. Persistent abdominal pain with diarrhea in a person in the second or third decade should suggest Crohn's disease. However, not every patient presents with diarrhea, and patients with disease confined to the terminal ileum are sometimes even constipated. Pain is most frequently felt in the lower abdomen, related temporally to meals or bowel movements. Right-lower-quadrant pain that occurs within 0.5 hour of meals and recurs 3 to 4 hours later suggests terminal ileum disease; this pain is symptomatic as a result of the gastro-ileal reflex and again when activated by chyme reaching the terminal ileum. Pain preceding and following bowel movements suggests a colonic location of disease. Diarrheal bowel movements in Crohn's disease tend to be of large volume and relatively infrequent, reflecting the small bowel location of disease and rectal sparing.

Physical examination of the patient with Crohn's disease may demonstrate a right lower quadrant mass or tenderness, HemOccult-positive stools, or any of several extraintestinal manifestations of Crohn's disease (see Question 12). The presence of edematous, usually painless, perianal skin tags alerts the clinician to the possibility of Crohn's disease.

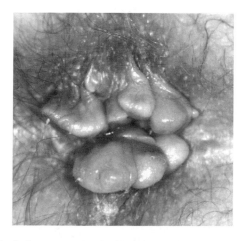

Photograph of edematous perianal skin tags in a patient with Crohn's disease.

2. How is the diagnosis of Crohn's disease established?

Unfortunately, there is no pathognomonic laboratory test for Crohn's disease. Among the acute phase reactants, quantitative C-reactive protein is the most specific for Crohn's disease and is useful in distinguishing Crohn's disease from functional bowel syndromes.

The definitive diagnosis of Crohn's disease is most often made by radiographic visualization of the terminal ileal lesion, either by reflux on barium enema or by antegrade small bowel series. **Colonoscopy** is the procedure of choice for documenting colonic involvement. The earliest endoscopic lesion of Crohn's colitis is the aphthous ulcer, although this lesion is not pathognomonic. Later, edema, erythema, and deeper, serpiginous ulcers occur. Lesions are patchy, leaving areas of near-normal mucosa adjacent to ulcerated mucosa. The rectum is often spared. Endoscopic biopsy of suspicious lesions should be done, although the likelihood of finding a granuloma, and thus clinching the diagnosis, is <10%.

3. What differential diagnoses should be considered in a patient with suspected Crohn's disease?

Because Crohn's disease shows a minor peak of age incidence in the sixth and seventh decades, in the older patient, diverticular disease and colon cancer are important differential diagnostic considerations for colonic Crohn's disease. In the developing world and in HIV-positive individuals, mycobacterial enteritis is a more likely diagnosis than Crohn's disease.

Irritable bowel syndrome is the most frequent alternative diagnosis for younger patients with Crohn's disease. The presence of weight loss, anemia, HemOccult-positive stools, night sweats, or elevated sedimentation rate or C-reactive protein should suggest Crohn's disease.

4. How can I tell Crohn's colitis from ulcerative colitis?

Symptoms: Ulcerative colitis is more likely than Crohn's disease to present as bloody, frequent, urgent diarrhea, because it routinely involves the most distal colon, if any part of the colon is involved. Crohn's colitis is more likely to be painful, with more voluminous diarrheal episodes accompanied by pain. Extraintestinal manifestations of arthritis, erythema nodosum, pyoderma gangrenosum, iritis/uveitis, and stomatitis occur in both types of colitis. Crohn's colitis is much more likely to be accompanied by significant perianal disease, and the presence of perianal skin tags or a fistula strongly favors Crohn's disease.

Endoscopy: Crohn's colitis tends to be patchy, with "skip areas" of relatively normal mucosa; it often spares the rectum and gives rise to deep, serpiginous ulcers and, later, strictures and asymmetric involvement of the bowel wall. Ulcerative colitis causes diffuse edema, friability, and granularity of the mucosa, without intervening skip areas, and always involves the rectum, unless the patient has been treated with topical rectal medications.

Radiography: If the terminal ileum shows typical lesions of Crohn's disease, the colitis is Crohn's. Crohn's disease involvement of the colon often shows stricturing, asymmetric bowel involvement, deep ulcers with intervening islands of edematous mucosa, and relative rectal sparing. In ulcerative colitis, the mucosal folds are blunted or absent, haustral markings disappear, and the ulcers are tiny, giving a granular "ground-glass" appearance to the mucosa. Involvement is always worst in the distal colon, frequently with preservation of normal haustrae and mucosal appearance in the right colon. Strictures in ulcerative colitis must always be suspected of harboring malignancy. Stricturing is more common in Crohn's disease and is usually a benign result of fibrosis and smooth muscle hypertrophy.

Severe disease: When either type of colitis is severe, the appearance of the two diseases, endoscopically and radiographically, tends to converge, so that it may be difficult or impossible, even with the resected colon in hand, to decide which disease is present. In severe colitis of either type, ulcers are deep and serpiginous, separating islands of edematous mucosa. Mucosa may be absent altogether, leaving a raw, bleeding, ulcerated surface of submucosa. Crohn's colitis, like ulcerative colitis, can progress to toxic megacolon and the risk of free perforation.

5. Who gets Crohn's disease?

Crohn's disease has been described in all ethnic groups and races. However, its incidence is highest in whites who live in the temperate zones, both north and south. North American and Western European Jews (Ashkenazi Jews) have the highest incidence of both Crohn's disease and ulcerative colitis, four- to sixfold higher than that in non-Jewish whites and higher than that in Sephardic Jews. Peak age of onset is the teens and 20s, but there is a secondary peak in late middle age. No age group is exempt—Crohn's disease has been described in neonates and nonagenarians. The sexes are equally susceptible. Crohn's disease shows a higher familial predisposition than ulcerative colitis, with approximately 20% of Crohn's patients having an affected first-degree relative.

6. Why do patients with Crohn's disease have pain?

Pain in Crohn's disease is most often due to partial obstruction of the movement of chyme through the intestine. This obstruction usually results from disturbance of normal neuromuscular function by the transmural edema and inflammation that accompanies the mucosal lesions of Crohn's disease. Fibrous stricturing usually is not present. Most episodes of partial bowel obstruction in Crohn's disease respond rapidly to high-dose glucocorticoids. When the serosal surface of intestine is inflamed, steady, aching pain occurs along with localized tenderness. Swollen, edematous, inflamed mesentery also gives rise to persistent pain. Formation of an extraintestinal abscess may also cause steady pain.

7. Why do patients with Crohn's disease have diarrhea?

Diarrhea in Crohn's disease can be due to a wide variety of mechanisms. Partial obstruction and neuromuscular incoordination probably account for much diarrhea. Bacterial overgrowth in relatively amotile, obstructed small bowel can cause bile salt deconjugation, fat malabsorption, and diarrhea. Inflamed, ulcerated terminal ileum and colon fail to reabsorb fluid and electrolyte and may actually contribute to luminal fluid by exudation. Failure of bile salt absorption by diseased or surgically absent terminal ileum leads to so-called choleric diarrhea, as unabsorbed dihydroxy bile acids stimulate water and chloride secretion by the colon. All of these mechanisms are subject to medical intervention.

8. What is likely to happen to my patient with Crohn's disease?

Prognosis for patients having a single recurrence of Crohn's disease symptoms is excellent—over 90% of such episodes subside with medical therapy. Long-term prognosis for Crohn's disease is good, with minimal decrease in life expectancy. A population-based study in Copenhagen, by Munkholm et al., showed that the 20-year survival of patients did not differ significantly from that of the background population (see figure on next page).

9. Is there any way to anticipate a flare-up of Crohn's disease before it happens?

No simple characteristic serves to identify an impending flare-up of Crohn's disease, as studies have shown. Brignola and colleagues have described a prognostic index that predicts occurrence of a flare-up with 85% accuracy. The index is composed of the serum values for three acute-phase reactants (ESR, acid alpha-1 glycoprotein, and alpha-2 globulin). Patients with an index value greater than +0.35 showed a cumulative relapse rate of 100% in 18 months, whereas the relapse rate of those with an index value less than +0.35 was only 18% in the same time interval. These authors found, as have others, that the longer patients remain in remission, the longer they are likely to remain so. Those in remission less than 12 months showed a 65% rate of relapse in the subsequent 18 months, whereas only 20% of those in remission for 12 months or more relapsed in the subsequent 18 months.

10. How likely is it that my patient's child will get Crohn's disease?

The best estimates of lifetime risk for relatives of Crohn's patients developing either Crohn's disease or ulcerative colitis come from the work of Dr. Jerry Rotter and colleagues in Los Angeles (see table on next page). Similar data have come from the University of Chicago. The lifetime risk of development of Crohn's disease for the sibling of a patient with Crohn's disease is estimated at 17% for Jews and 7% for non-Jews. Risk for other first-degree relatives (parents and offspring) is less, as is the risk if the index case has ulcerative colitis.

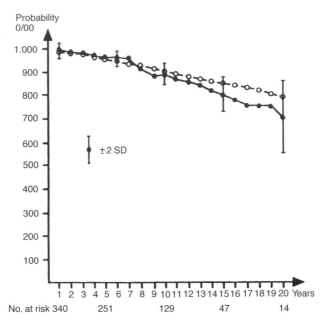

Cumulative survival of patients with Crohn's disease compared with the expected survival of the background population of same age and sex. (*Solid circles* = observed cases; *open circles*-expected cases.) (From Munkholm P, Langholz E, Davidsen M, Binder V: Intestinal cancer risk and mortality in patients with Crohn's disease. Gastroenterology 105:1716–1723, 1993, with permission.)

Lifetime Risk for Inflammatory Bowel Disease in First-Degree Relatives of Patients with Inflammatory Bowel Disease

	SIBLINGS	PARENTS	OFFSPRING
Jewish probands affected with:			
Crohn's disease	16.8%	3.8%	7.4%
Ulcerative colitis	4.6%	4.1%	7.4%
Non-Jewish probands affected with:			
Crohn's disease	7.0%	4.8%	0%
Ulcerative colitis	0.9%	1.2%	11%

From Yang H, McElree C, Roth M-P, et al: Familial empiric risks for inflammatory bowel disease: Differences between Jews and non-Jews. Gut 34:517–524, 1993, with permission.

11. Are barium x-rays useful in making the diagnosis of Crohn's disease, or should I just ask for endoscopy?

Barium x-ray visualization of the terminal ileum remains the procedure of choice in diagnosing Crohn's disease of the small bowel. In the United States, only 10–15% of patients have disease limited to the colon; all the rest have either small bowel disease alone (35%) or ileocolitis (50%). Involvement of the stomach or duodenum by Crohn's disease is uncommon (<5%), and such involvement without concomitant distal bowel lesions is extremely rare. The enteroclysis technique (small bowel enema) offers sensitivity superior to that of the small bowel follow-through for stricturing lesions of the small intestine.

Colonoscopy is certainly the method of choice for documenting location and severity of colonic involvement. Its sensitivity for the early lesions of Crohn's disease (aphthous ulcers, patchy edema, and erythema) is much greater than that of double-contrast barium enema.

12. What are the extraintestinal manifestations of Crohn's disease?

Classification of Extraintestinal Manifestations of Crohn's Disease

According to the location of intestinal inflammation:	
Colitis-related	Skin, joint, eye, mouth, hepatobiliary
Small intestine-related	Nutritional deficiency, nephrolithiasis, gallstones, hydronephrosis
Nonspecific	Amyloidosis, osteoporosis, anemia
According to degree of activity of intestinal inflammation:	
Activity-related	Arthritis, erythema nodosum, iritis/uveitis, anemia
Intermediate	Pyoderma gangrenosum
Unrelated	Sclerosing cholangitis, ankylosing spondylitis, sacroiliitis

Apart from perianal disease (not really extraintestinal), the most common extraintestinal manifestation is **joint involvement,** occurring in approximately 20% of Crohn's patients. Two distinct types of joint involvement occur. **Axial arthropathy,** consisting of sacroiliitis and ankylosing spondylitis, occurs in five-fold excess in patients with Crohn's disease, as a result of linkage of genetic susceptibility of Crohn's disease and spondylitis. Such patients are usually HLA-B27 positive. The symptoms of axial arthropathy tend to occur without relationship to the presence or absence of bowel symptoms. The nonsteroidal anti-inflammatory drugs that relieve joint symptoms often cause worsening of the inflammatory bowel disease. The other type of joint involvement is **peripheral arthropathy,** which tends to accompany flares of the bowel disease but rarely, if ever, becomes deforming.

Less common extraintestinal phenomena, all of which presumably share an **autoimmune etiology** and tend to precede or accompany flares of bowel disease, are iritis and episcleritis, aphthous stomatitis, vasculitis (most commonly phlebitis), and skin involvement (erythema nodosum and pyoderma gangrenosum). Sclerosing cholangitis, unlike the other autoimmune manifestations, tends to progress without relationship to the severity of the bowel disease.

Nonautoimmune phenomena include kidney stones (resulting from dehydration and increased oxalate absorption) and gallstones (resulting from bile salt depletion). Oxalate kidney stones are particularly common in patients with disease or absence of the terminal ileum and consequent fat malabsorption. Fatty acids remaining unabsorbed in the bowel lumen bind calcium as insoluble soaps and thus prevent the usual calcium binding to dietary oxalate. Free oxalate is absorbed by the colon, excreted in the urine, and precipitates with urinary calcium as calculi. The principal source of oxalate in the American diet is cola drinks (spinach, chard, and chocolate are also sources), which should be eliminated from the diet of such patients. Ileal disease or surgical absence also leads to bile salt malabsorption, depletion of the bile salt pool, and insufficient concentration of bile salts in the bile to maintain cholesterol in solution, leading to cholelithiasis.

13. How should I treat the first episode of Crohn's disease?

The drugs that deliver **5-aminosalicylate** (5-ASA) to the bowel mucosa are the first line of therapy for Crohn's disease of mild and moderate severity. The choice of drug depends on the location of disease. For disease of both ileum and colon, mesalamine (Pentasa and Asacol) is the best choice, because it releases active 5-ASA in both the small intestine and colon. For disease confined to the colon, sulfasalazine or olsalazine (Dipentum) should be selected, because release of 5-ASA from these drugs depends on the hydrolytic activity of colonic bacteria. For disease confined to the small bowel, Pentasa is best. Toxicity of 5-ASA itself is minimal. Dipentum use is associated with a somewhat higher incidence of diarrhea than the other 5-ASA drugs. The sulfapyridine moiety of sulfasalazine makes that drug considerably more toxic than the other 5-ASA drugs, which do not contain a sulfa moiety.

Antibiotics are certainly useful in Crohn's disease. Metronidazole is an alternate first-line drug to 5-ASA in mild-to-moderate Crohn's disease of both small bowel and colon. Metronidazole is sometimes almost miraculously effective in perianal Crohn's disease; unfortunately this response occurs in only about 25% of patients, with another 50% of patients showing some improvement and a final 25% none at all. Alternative antibiotics are sulfamethoxazole/trimethoprim and ciprofloxacin. Anecdotal evidence suggests that all three antibiotics are useful adjuncts to prednisone in maintaining remission of Crohn's disease.

For patients with moderately severe symptoms of Crohn's disease and systemic manifestations of fever, night sweats, arthralgias, and weight loss, **prednisone** is the most effective therapy. An initial dose of 40 to 60 mg/day can be tapered asymptotically when maximum benefit is obtained. Unfortunately, two-thirds of patients, once started on prednisone, cannot be withdrawn from it without a flare of disease. However, many patients can be maintained in good remission on minimal doses of prednisone, usually along with a 5-ASA drug and perhaps an antibiotic.

There is good evidence that long-term use of 5-ASA drugs helps to maintain remission in Crohn's disease. Consequently, patients should be continued on one of these drugs indefinitely, once an acute flare-up is brought under control.

14. How should I treat a recurrent flare-up of Crohn's disease?

Mild to moderate recurrent flares of Crohn's disease sometimes respond to increased doses of the suppressant **5-ASA** drug. More often, a short, tapering course of **prednisone** is required to bring the disease under control again. Addition of an **antibiotic** to the regimen should also be considered.

Recurrent episodes of Crohn's disease activity tend to be increasingly resistant to drug treatment, requiring higher doses of prednisone and eventually becoming unresponsive to prednisone alone. In this situation, the immunosuppressants **azathioprine** and **6-mercaptopurine** have proven useful. Up to 75% of patients with steroid-dependent or steroid-resistant disease improve or remit on 6-mercaptopurine. Unfortunately, these drugs act slowly, averaging over 3 months to show a beneficial effect. Also, for maximum effectiveness, 6-mercaptopurine and azathioprine must be given in doses approaching bone-marrow toxicity, which is a concern with long-term use.

15. Is there any way to keep my Crohn's disease patient in remission once it is achieved?

The 5-ASA drugs have been shown to be at least partially effective in mantaining a remission in Crohn's disease, as they are in ulcerative colitis. Doses approximating one-half the acute dose can be safely continued long-term. The immunosuppressant drugs azathioprine and 6-mercaptopurine are also useful in this setting. Once remission is achieved on the combination of prednisone and azathiprine, however, the azathioprine must be continued indefinitely to maintain remission; when azathioprine is stopped, 70% of patients relapse within 1 year.

16. When should I call the surgeon?

Indications for Surgery in Crohn's Disease

Failure of medical therapy		
Recurrent partial obstruction (3 episodes)		
Growth retardation in children		
Complications		
Small bowel (abscess, fistula, obstruction, rare perforation)	Colonic (massive bleeding, obstruction, rare perforation)	Anorectal (perirectal abscess, rectovaginal fistula, major perianal fistula)

The most common situation requiring surgery is **recurrent small bowel obstruction** that finally becomes resistant to medical therapy. Patients with recurrent episodes of obstruction should always have their small bowel visualized by careful small bowel barium follow-through or enteroclysis. One or more very localized strictures may be remedied by surgery (so-called stricture-plasty) without sacrifice of useful bowel and with good symptomatic relief. More extensive stricturing require resection.

An **abscess,** either perianal or intraabdominal, always requires drainage. Intra-abdominal abscesses due to Crohn's disease requires surgical drainage with resection of the fistula that led to the abscess; percutaneous drainage rarely leads to a satisfactory cure. Perianal abscesses should be drained with as little damage to the anal sphincter as possible.

The presence of a **fistula** is not necessarily an indication for surgery. Enteroenteric fistulae are often asymptomatic and may respond to medical therapy. Perianal fistulae sometimes close with metronidazole or other medical therapy, and surgical attack often leads to nonhealing and sphincteric injury. Enterovaginal fistulae are notoriously difficult to heal by surgical means and often can be kept minimally symptomatic on medical therapy. Enterocutaneous fistulae similarly are often minimally symptomatic but, if operated on, require resection of the fistulizing bowel, which sometimes results in formation of more fistulae. Enterourinary fistulae usually require surgical resection.

17. How likely is recurrence after the surgeon has removed all grossly observable disease?

Several careful endoscopic studies following resection of ileo-colonic Crohn's disease indicate that endoscopically diagnosable recurrence is present in over 70% of patients within 1 year after surgery. Symptomatic recurrence is less frequent and more delayed but reaches 35% by 3 years after surgery. Symptomatic recurrence after partial colonic resection of disease confined to the colon approximates 40% at 5 years.

Prospective controlled studies have shown that mesalamine (both Asacol and Pentasa) are effective in delaying recurrence after surgery. Current practice favors placing patients on one of these drugs for an indefinite period following resective surgery.

18. How should I treat perianal Crohn's disease?

Very carefully! Perianal Crohn's disease can vary in severity from an asymptomatic edematous skin tag or tiny fistula to severely painful, open, draining, "watering can" perineum. Local therapy is almost always indicated: sitz baths, apply heat, encourage drainage, and keep the perineal area clean. Hydrocortisone cream and suppositories may decrease anal inflammation and soreness. Metronidazole, 1–1.5 gm/day, should be tried and is often effective. Ciprofloxacin is an alternative antibiotic. If the area is too painful to examine, even with intravenous analgesia, examination under general anesthesia by a knowledgeable surgeon may be indicated to rule out a perianal or perirectal abscess. A pelvic CT scan may also reveal an abscess that requires drainage. Whatever surgery is done should be very conservative, lest anal sphincter function be impaired. Perianal surgery in Crohn's disease often leads to nonhealing, chronically open, draining wounds.

19. What is the risk that a patient with Crohn's disease will develop cancer of the intestine?

This is a controversial area. Small bowel cancer, though it is increased in incidence in the Crohn's population, is still extremely rare. The reason small bowel cancer favors bypassed loops is that bypassed loops are the site of longest duration Crohn's involvement, as well as being relatively unlikely to cause early obstructive symptoms. Estimates of the relative risk of colon cancer in Crohn's disease, compared with that in the normal population, vary from no increase to an 18-fold excess. Data from a recent comparative study in Copenhagen, Denmark suggest that the time-dependent risk of cancer in Crohn's colitis is no less than that in ulcerative colitis.

Estimate of Cancer Risk in Crohn's Disease vs Ulcerative Colitis

SITE	RELATIVE RISK	CONFIDENCE LIMITS
Ulcerative colitis (extensive)	19.2	12.9–27.5
Crohn's colitis (extensive)	18.2	7.8–35.8

From Munkholm P, Langholz E, Davidsen M, Binder V: Intestinal cancer risk and mortality in patients with Crohn's disease. Gastroenterology 105:1716–1723, 1993, with permission.

Colonoscopic surveillance in Crohn's colitis is much more difficult than in ulcerative colitis because of the mucosal morphology of Crohn's disease, which is typically lumpy with multiple discrete ulcers and frequent stricture formations, any one of which could harbor dysplasia or frank cancer. "Dysplasia-associated lesion or mass" (DALM), the signal lesion in ulcerative colitis, is impossible to recognize in Crohn's colitis. Whether such surveillance should be undertaken in Crohn's colitis is one of the most controversial issues in gastrointestinal practice.

20. Is Crohn's disease infectious?

In a clinical sense, the answer is clearly no. In tens of thousands of couples, one member of which has Crohn's disease, there are only a handful of reports of acquisition of Crohn's disease by the unaffected member. In an etiologic sense, however, the question remains open. Despite multiple negative attempts to detect antibodies, cellular immunity, and histologic evidence of mycobacterial infection, the possibility that Crohn's disease is caused by *Mycobacterium paratuberculosis* or a related organism is still open. Sophisticated molecular biologic techniques have offered sporadic reports of tantalizingly positive findings. The most recent infectious organism nominated as a cause of Crohn's disease is the measles virus. The most widely held view at present is that an autoimmune attack on the intestinal mucosa may be triggered by a variety of foreign antigens, some of which could be from infectious organisms. However, the basic defect lies in the defective immune system rather than the trigger antigen.

21. What is the role of enteral and parenteral nutrition in treating Crohn's disease?
Both enteral nutrition, with elemental or polymeric diets, and parenteral nutrition are useful in treating patients with Crohn's disease. Growth failure in children can be reversed and catch-up growth promoted with enteral or parenteral nutrition that provides the large amount of calories and protein needed for growth. Several controlled trials prove that both enteral and parenteral nutrition as the exclusive source of nutrition can induce clinical remission of Crohn's disease symptoms as completely and almost as rapidly as high-dose steroid therapy. However, the long-term effect of nutritional therapy is not as satisfactory as that of steroids, with over 70% of patients suffering relapse of symptoms with reintroduction of regular food. This relatively transient effect, the expense and poor patient acceptance of elemental diets, and the necessity, therefore, of nasogastric intubation for their administration combine to limit the usefulness of this therapy except in compliant children.

22. When should immunosuppressant drugs be considered in treatment of Crohn's disease, and how should they be used?
At this time, immunosuppressant drugs are not considered first-line therapy for Crohn's disease. Rather, they are principally used to augment the effect of steroids to bring about remission of active Crohn's disease and to allow reduction or elimination of steroids in management of chronic active disease. Azathioprine and 6-mercaptopurine are most frequently used for these purposes, having proven effective in controlled clinical trials. These drugs characteristically take 3–4 months to show therapeutic effect. Methotrexate and cyclosporine are less well documented as effective in Crohn's disease. Cyclosporine acts quickly, within a week or two, to induce improvement, but patients regularly have relapse when it is withdrawn, and its long-term toxicity has limited its use to clinical trial protocols. Methotrexate was shown to be superior to placebo in a very recent Canadian trial, but its role in management of Crohn's disease remains unclear.

BIBLIOGRAPHY

1. Brignola C, Campieri M, Bazzocchi G, et al: A laboratory index for predicting relapse in asymptomatic patients with Crohn's disease. Gastroenterology 91:1490–1494, 1986.
2. Feagan BG, Rochon J, Fedorak RN, et al: Methotrexate for the treatment of Crohn's disease. N Engl J Med 332:292–297, 1995.
3. Gillen CD, Walmsley RS, Prior P, et al: Ulcerative colitis and Crohn's disease: A comparison of the colorectal cancer risk in extensive colitis. Gut 35:1590–1592, 1994.
4. Munkholm P, Langholz E, Davidsen M, Binder V: Intestinal cancer risk and mortality in patients with Crohn's disease. Gastroenterology 105:1716–1723, 1993.
5. O'Donoghue VP, Dawson AM, Powell-Tuck J, et al: Double-blind withdrawal trial of azathioprine as maintenance treatment for Crohn's disease. Lancet 2:955–957, 1978.
6. Present DH, Korelitz BI, Wisch N, et al: Treatment of Crohn's disease with 6-mercaptopurine: A long term randomized double-blind study. N Engl J Med 302:981–987, 1980.
7. Rutgeerts P, Geboes K, Vantrappen G, et al: Predictability of the postoperative course of Crohn's disease. Gastroenterology 99:956–963, 1990.
8. Wakefield AJ, Pittilo RM, Sim R, et al: Evidence of persistent measles virus infection in Crohn's disease. J Med Virol 39:345–353, 1993.
9. Yang H, McElree C, Roth M-P, et al: Familial empiric risks for inflammatory bowel disease: Differences between Jews and non-Jews. Gut 34:517–524, 1993.

41. ULCERATIVE COLITIS

John W. Singleton, M.D.

1. How can ulcerative colitis be distinguished from acute infectious colitis?
Ulcerative colitis (UC) usually has a gradual onset over several weeks, with progressively more severe diarrhea and increasing amounts of blood and mucus in the stool. However, a fairly common presentation is continuing diarrhea after what appeared to be an acute infectious diarrhea. The sigmoidoscopic appearance of UC may be indistinguishable from that of acute infectious diarrhea caused by *Entamoeba histolytica, Campylobacter jejuni, Shigella, Neisseria gonorrhoeae,* or enteroinvasive *Escherichia coli.* However, the histologic appearance differs from these infectious colitides in that the mucosa of UC shows crypt distortion and a more chronic inflammatory reaction. The diagnosis of UC can never be made with certainty until stool culture and examination for ova and parasites have been found negative. Table 1.

Infectious Causes of Diarrhea Simulating Ulcerative Colitis

ORGANISM	FEATURES
Shigella	Fever, dysentery, culture +
Campylobacter	Fever, pain, culture +
Clostridium difficile	Antibiotic history, endoscopic appeareance, toxin assay
Neisseria gonorrhoeae	Homosexual, culture +
Entamoeba histolytica	Serology, ova and parasites exam
Chlamydia trachomatis	Homosexual, nodes, serology
Cytomegalovirus	HIV +, biopsy

+ = positive

2. Who gets ulcerative colitis?
The peak age for onset of UC is the second and third decades. However, a secondary peak is seen in late middle-age, and new-onset cases may occur in the eighth and even ninth decades of life. Sex incidence is equal. The disease is probably more prevalent in whites than in non-whites, and Jewish populations show a two- to fivefold greater incidence than non-Jewish whites depending on geographic location. Heredity is clearly important in determining the risk of acquiring UC; approximately 10% of patients with UC have a first-degree relative with the disease (*see* Question 5).

3. What is the range of severity of ulcerative colitis?
The severity of UC depends on both the extent and severity of colonic involvement. UC can involve only a few centimeters of the most distal rectum, the entire colon from pectinate line to and including the appendix, and any extent in between. The disease is almost always most severe in the rectum, lessening in severity in more proximal colon. Topical treatment of rectal disease can

Classification of Severe and Fulminant Ulcerative Colitis

SEVERE	FULMINANT
≥9 Movements/day	≥9 Movements/day
Abdominal tenderness	Abdominal tenderness
Pulse >100 bpm or temp >37.5°C	Temp >38°C or colonic dilatation (>6 cm)

From Meyers S, Sachar DB, Goldbert JD, Janowitz HD: Corticotropin vs hydrocortisone in the intravenous treatment of ulcerative colitis: A prospective, randomized, double-blind clinical trial. Gastroenterology 85:351–357, 1983, with permission.

alter this relationship. Patients with UC limited to the rectum and sigmoid rarely have systemic signs of fever, weight loss, and toxicity, whereas pancolitis is often manifest as systemic illness.

The mildest colonic involvement with UC may be totally asymptomatic, as evidenced by histologic changes typical of UC in some patients with the extraintestinal complication of sclerosing cholangitis. At the other end of the scale is toxic megacolon, a life-threatening complication of fulminant colitis.

4. What can my patient with new-onset ulcerative colitis expect for the future?

Prognosis in UC has been carefully analyzed in a prospective, population-based study in Copenhagen by Binder and colleagues. After the first year of disease, approximately 40% of patients will be in remission each year. In the second to fourth years of disease, 40–50% of patients experience activity of disease each year, but that proportion falls to about 30% by year 10 of disease. Approximately 20% of patients will undergo colectomy within 10 years, and 30% within 25 years. About one-fourth of patients experience only a single episode of disease. The cumulative probability of continuously active disease is only about 1% after 5 years, and the longer a patient goes without experiencing a relapse, the less likely a subsequent relapse becomes.

Continuous prophylactic therapy with 5-aminosalicylate drugs (sulfasalazine, olsalazine, mesalamine) has been shown to maintain remission in UC. A recent study has demonstrated that azathioprine is effective in maintaining a remission induced by combination steroid-azathioprine therapy. A similar effect of azathioprine in Crohn's disease was demonstrated over 15 years ago by O'Donoghue et al.

5. Should patients be concerned that their disease will be passed on to their children?

Lifetime Risk of IBD in First-Degree Relatives of Patients with UC

RELATIVE	SIBLINGS (%)	PARENTS (%)	OFFSPRING (%)
Jewish			
UC	4.6	4.1	7.4
Crohn's disease	16.8	3.8	7.4
Non-Jewish			
UC	0.9	1.2	11.0
Crohn's disease	7.0	4.8	0

From Yang H, McElree C, Roth M-P, et al: Familial empiric risks for inflammatory bowel disease: Differences between Jews and non-Jews. Gut 34:517–524, 1993, with permission.

The table presents estimates of the lifetime risk of acquiring an inflammatory bowel disease (IBD, ulcerative colitis or Crohn's disease) for the first-degree relatives of patients with UC. Risk data for individual ethnic groups other than Jews have not been estimated, and the data given here must be regarded as preliminary. However, these data are useful in counseling and reassuring patients.

6. What is the relationship between smoking and ulcerative colitis? Should a patient with ulcerative colitis take up smoking?

Data from population-based surveys in many countries have established that patients with UC are less likely to smoke cigarettes than matched controls from the general population. The relative risk of developing UC for current smokers (compared with matched nonsmokers) is about 40%. Even more striking, former smokers are approximately 1.7 times more likely to develop UC than never smokers. Numerous anecdotal reports document improvement in active UC when former smokers resume smoking. The active ingredient of cigarette smoke with regard to UC has not been identified. However, a recent controlled trial of nicotine patch therapy for UC suggests that nicotine may play a role.

Patients whose UC began or flared noticeably when they gave up smoking might be tempted to resume smoking. Certainly, more conventional and proven therapies should be tried first. The controlled trial of nicotine patch therapy demonstrated significant symptomatic benefit in the treated group, but a high proportion of nonsmokers experienced unacceptable side effects from the patches.

7. How is ulcerative proctitis best treated?

Ulcerative proctitis refers to disease limited to the rectum—not extending above 12–15 cm from the anal verge. Disease in this location is most amenable to topical therapy delivered as suppositories, foam, or enemas. Two drugs are established as effective topical therapy for proctitis: hydrocortisone and 5-aminosalicylic acid (5-ASA). Budesonide, a potent topical steroid metabolized almost 100% in one pass through the liver, will soon join these drugs on the American market. The preparation best tolerated by the irritable rectum is hydrocortisone foam (Cortifoam). The standard dose is 100 mg nightly, retained overnight. The 100 mg hydrocortisone enema (Cortenema) is equally effective if it can be retained. 5-ASA enemas and suppositories (Rowasa) are reserved for steroid-resistant proctitis because of their excessive expense and occasional paradoxical exacerbation of disease. Oral 5-aminosalicylate (sulfasalazine, mesalamine, olsalazine) or intermittent rectal 5-ASA should be continued indefinitely to maintain remission.

Recurrent exacerbations of ulcerative proctitis and occasional cases resistant to topical therapy may require systemic therapy with oral prednisone, 40–60 mg daily, to achieve remission. Every effort should be made to treat proctitis locally and without resort to prednisone. Biddle and colleagues have reported that prolonged use of nightly Rowasa enema eventually (after as long as 34 weeks) brings 80% of patients with resistant proctitis into remission.

8. What is the best way to squelch a flare of ulcerative colitis?

Start with 5-aminosalicylate. As long as the patient is not severely ill and has not had 5-ASA drugs previously or has responded well to them in the past, a 5-ASA drug should be the first line of therapy. The initial flare-up of UC, if it is mild to moderate in severity, responds to this therapy with complete remission in at least 50% of cases. Addition of oral prednisone brings the remission rate to near 90%. Subsequent attacks are usually less responsive to both 5-ASA drugs and steroids. Sulfasalazine, 3–5 gm daily in divided doses, should be introduced gradually over 3–5 days to minimize nausea. For sulfallergic patients or those who cannot take sulfasalazine for other reasons, either olsalazine (up to 4 gm/day) or mesalamine (up to 4.8 gm/day) can be used.

9. When is prednisone used as therapy for ulcerative colitis?

Absence of noticeable improvement in 1–2 weeks or prior poor response to 5-ASA makes prednisone the choice, starting at 40–60 mg daily. This high dose should be continued until improvement reaches a plateau or remission is complete. A 5-ASA drug should be started in the meantime, if not already being given, and the prednisone dose tapered by 5 mg/wk for patients who have responded rapidly. Slow responders and patients whose response is not complete may require a slower withdrawal of prednisone over weeks or months. The 5-ASA drug should be continued in therapeutic doses as prednisone is tapered.

Patients with moderate to severely active disease should receive oral prednisone, as described, or be hospitalized for parenteral steroid therapy, depending on their clinical status. Diarrhea of >10 stools daily, abdominal tenderness, distention, fever, tachycardia, anemia, and leukocytosis indicate severe disease and the need for hospitalization. Patients with recent steroid exposure should receive intravenous hydrocortisone (300–400 mg/day) or methylprednisolone (40–60 mg/day). There is some suggestion that administration by continuous infusion is superior to divided dosing. Patients who have not recently (in the past month) received steroids are best treated with intravenous ACTH (80–120 U/day), again as a continuous infusion. If the patient is hungry and there is no evidence of colonic distention, a low-residue diet may be helpful in providing the short-chain fatty acids the colon prefers as metabolic fuel.

10. What if the patient's disease worsens despite medical therapy?

Failure to improve after 5–7 days, clinical deterioration on twice-daily examinations, worsening laboratory values, or increasing colonic dilatation on daily plain abdominal films should prompt serious consideration of **urgent colectomy.** Development of a "lumpy-bumpy" appearance of the gas shadow on the abdominal plain film indicates ulcer penetration into the muscularis propria and imminent perforation (*see* figure on next page). Patients with severe or fulminant colitis should be followed jointly by surgical and medical physicians. Persistence with high-dose intravenous steroids beyond 10 days confers no additional benefit and carries increased risk. Cyclosporine "rescue" of such patients from colectomy is still an experimental procedure to be attempted only when the expertise to manage this therapy is at hand.

If the severely ill patient responds with cessation of bleeding, abdominal pain, and diarrhea and has return of appetite and improvement of laboratory values, a 5-ASA drug should be started and oral prednisone, 60 mg/day, substituted for the intravenous steroid. A one-day overlap of oral and intravenous steroid may avoid deterioration at the switch. Prednisone dose may then be tapered at weekly intervals in an asymptotic fashion (60 mg, 40, 30, 25, 20, 17.5, 15, 12.5, 10, 7.5, 5, 2.5, 0).

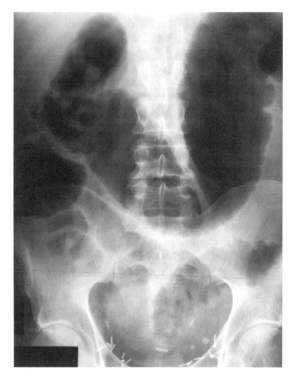

Plain abdominal radiograph demonstrating dilatation of the transverse colon with the "lumpy-bumpy" appearance of the gas shadow, evident particularly at the margins.

11. How can recurrent flares of ulcerative colitis be prevented?

Numerous prospective controlled trials document the efficacy of 5-ASA drugs in maintaining remission in UC. Sulfasalazine at a dose of 2 gm/day was shown to be prophylactically effective even after a full year had passed since the patients' last exacerbation. Olsalazine (1–3 gm/d) and mesalamine (Asacol, 0.8–4.8 gm/d), or Pentasa, 1.5–4 gm/d) have been shown to decrease the frequency of recurrent attacks of UC. Patients who are not sulfallergic and who are tolerant may prefer sulfasalazine because it is much less expensive than its newer congeners. A recent prospective, controlled withdrawal trial demonstrated that long-term use of azathioprine is effective in preventing attacks of colitis in patients who achieved remission by use of azathioprine and prednisone together.

12. What should cause me to hospitalize my patient with ulcerative colitis?

Severe colitis (*see* question 3) requires hospitalization and parenteral steroid therapy or surgery. Impressive abdominal tenderness, in a patient whose abdomen is ordinarily nontender, is cause for great concern that the disease may have become transmural. Somewhat milder disease in a patient who has an appetite, normal vital signs, and no abdominal tenderness or leukocytosis may be safely treated at home with daily follow-up.

13. When should colectomy be considered?

In acute colitis, absence of objective improvement after 5–7 days of high-dose parenteral steroids should prompt serious consideration of colectomy. Deterioration in such circumstances can be subtle; it is important for the treating physician not to be fooled with minor positive changes when the overall course is downhill. Colonic perforation increases the mortality risk of colectomy at least fourfold to over 40%. When daily abdominal films show progressive dilation of the transverse and proximal colon, and especially when the "lumpy-bumpy" appearance of deep, penetrating ulceration appears (see figure on p. 288), it is time for colectomy. Diarrhea may actually decrease in these circumstances as the colon dilates. Less commonly, severe and unremitting hemorrhage prompts colectomy, often requiring total colectomy, including the rectum.

Patients with steroid-dependent or steroid-resistant disease of 8–10 years' duration, consequently at increased risk of colon cancer, are often well advised to have a colectomy. Almost without exception, such patients realize after surgery how much healthier they are, rid of both colon and steroids.

14. Are immunosuppressant drugs ever indicated in ulcerative colitis, given that the disease is cured by colectomy?

The immunosuppressant drugs **azathioprine** and **6-mercaptopurine** have been used much more widely in treatment of Crohn's disease than in ulcerative colitis. Recently, enthusiastic anecdotal reports of their use in UC have appeared, and a controlled trial has shown that azathioprine is effective in maintaining remission achieved on that drug. Steroid-resistant or steroid-dependent UC confined to the rectosigmoid is the most frequent setting in which azathioprine is useful. Anecdotal series suggest that its use conveys a 70–80% chance of significant steroid reduction or discontinuance. Azathioprine and 6-mercaptopurine characteristically take 1–4 months to manifest a beneficial effect, so they have no role in treatment of severe or fulminant colitis. Concern about the oncogenic potential of these drugs has abated with their widespread use in autoimmune disease without an apparent increase in malignancies.

Cyclosporine has recently been introduced as a means to "rescue" patients with severe colitis from imminent colectomy. Its use in this setting requires careful monitoring of blood levels of the drug and expert medical and surgical supervision of the patient's progress.

15. How good is the pouch pull-through operation as an alternative to ileostomy following total colectomy?

Total colectomy with pouch-anal anastomosis has emerged as the operation of choice for young persons with fulminant or medically refractory UC. Operative mortality is <1% in most series and 0.015% in the Mayo Clinic series. Among its complications, the incidence of pouchitis (symptomatic inflammation of the pouch) continues to rise as patients are followed for longer postoperative periods, reaching 50% or more in recent reports. However, persistent, treatment-refractory pouchitis occurs in <10% of patients. Reversion to abdominal ileostomy is required in <3% of patients.

Complications of Pouch Pull-through Operation

COMPLICATION	INCIDENCE
Intestinal obstruction	
After pouch formation	13%
After ileostomy closure	9%
Pelvic sepsis	5%
Wound infection	3%
Anastomotic leakage	2%
Anastomotic stricture	5%
Pouchitis	31%

From Pemberton JH, Kelly KA, Beart RW Jr, et al: Ileal pouch–anal anastomosis for chronic ulcerative colitis: Long-term results. Ann Surg 206:504–513, 1987, with permission.

The functional result is generally excellent. Stool frequency at 1 year averages 6/day in persons 50 years or less. Daytime spotting occurred in 33% of women and 14% of men; nighttime spotting occured in 56% of women and 44% of men. Over 85% of patients are satisfied or very satisfied with the outcome of surgery, and almost none would choose to return to an abdominal ileostomy.

Patients over 50 years of age who desire rapid return to good health and normal activity, and for whom body image is less important, may still choose the relatively uncomplicated and highly satisfactory Brooke ileostomy. A Brooke ileostomy is certainly the proper choice for patients with significant comorbidities.

16. What is the risk of colon cancer in ulcerative colitis?

Published estimates of the risk of colon cancer in colitis vary wildly from no increased risk to a >50% risk at 20 years of disease. Risk clearly varies both with duration of disease and extent of colonic involvement. Patients whose disease never extended proximal to the splenic flexure are at less risk than those with extensive or pancolitis. Some series suggest that the development of cancer is simply delayed about 10 years in left-sided disease as compared with pancolitis.

The most accurate estimates of risk come from population-based studies, exclusively European. A very credible population-based study from Copenhagen (99.9% follow-up; median observation time, 11.7 years) reported a 3.1% cumulative colon cancer risk at 25 years of disease, no different than that in the population from which these patients came. It should be noted that the cumulative colectomy rate in this cohort was 32.4% at 25 years.

17. Is there any way of reducing the risk of colon cancer short of total colectomy?

Although considerable skepticism prevails in some quarters, most American gastroenterologists believe that prospective surveillance colonoscopy with multiple biopsies is effective in reducing the risk of incurable colon cancer in patients with ulcerative colitis. A well-designed and carefully conducted prospective study at the Lahey Clinic found that when either low-grade or high-grade dysplasia was present on *initial* colonoscopy, subsequent follow-up revealed a high incidence of cancer (7 of 18 patients), leading to the recommendation that colectomy be seriously considered upon such a finding. Low-grade or high-grade dysplasia found on surveillance colonoscopies *subsequent to the first examination* was not associated with cancer on subsequent follow-up, although only 6 of 213 patients fell into this group. Finally, among the 175 patients whose initial colonoscopy yielded no dysplasia, 2 developed cancer, but both had dropped out of the surveillance program prior to discovery of cancer. This experience leads to several important conclusions:

1. Colonoscopic surveillance does not absolutely prevent development of cancer.
2. To be effective, surveillance must be pursued faithfully by patient and physician, and the finding of dysplasia acted upon.
3. Colonoscopic surveillance is arduous and expensive.
4. Expert pathologic consultation is required before any action is taken on the finding of dysplasia.

18. How worried should my patient be about the extraintestinal manifestations of ulcerative colitis?

The minor extraintestinal manifestations (aphthous stomatitis, peripheral arthralgias, erythema nodosum) are common (20–50%), tend to accompany flares of colitis, and are controlled by control of the colonic disease. Major extraintestinal manifestations include sacroileitis, ankylosing spondylitis, eye disease (episcleritis and uveitis), pyoderma gangrenosum, and sclerosing cholangitis.

Sacroiliitis detectable by plain film occurs in about 10% of patients and may be asymptomatic or symptomatic, with progression to spondylitis in 1–2%. Spondylitis' prevalence in patients with inflammatory bowel disease is 3–5% and highly correlated with the presence of the HLA-B27 lymphocyte antigen. Sacroiliitis and spondylitis run a symptomatic course unrelated to activity of colitis.

Eye involvement and **pyoderma gangrenosum** are uncommon, occurring in about 2% of patients. Uveitis causes eye pain, photophobia, and blurred vision and requires prompt intervention to prevent scarring and visual impairment. Episcleritis is more benign and is usually well controlled with topical steroids. Pyoderma gangrenosum, occuring in 1–2% of patients, is generally unrelated to clinical activity of colitis and resistant to therapy.

Sclerosing cholangitis is similarly unrelated in severity to the extent and severity of colitis, often progressing to liver failure in patients with minimal colitis or even appearing after colectomy. It occurs in about 5% of patients with UC and can affect any portion of the biliary tree, from interlobular ducts to common bile duct. Currently, it is the second most frequent reason for orthotopic liver transplantation in the United States, as there is no other effective medical or surgical treatment.

19. How important is diet in the management of ulcerative colitis?

Patients with pancolitis often suffer from malnutrition, manifest as underweight, hypoalbuminemia, and anemia. Significant loss of serum protein and hemoglobin from the inflamed colon occurs in active UC. Anorexia, abdominal pain, and diarrhea discourage oral intake. However, in contrast to Crohn's disease, where both parenteral and enteral formula nutrition have been shown to induce remission, controlled trials in UC have failed to show any ameliorating effect of total parenteral nutrition or elemental diet on the disease process. Nevertheless, adequate nutrition is very important, especially in growing chidren, in whom it has been shown that provision of the excess calories necessary to support growth does indeed result in restoration of near-normal growth rates despite continued presence of disease. Nightly enteral formula feedings via self-inserted nasogastric tube have proven very effective for this purpose.

Patients often ask, "What can I eat that will help heal my colon?" Unfortunately, apart from avoidance of milk and lactose-containing milk products for patients with lactase deficiency, no generally applicable dietary recommendations exist. Common sense suggests that diarrheogenic drugs (caffeine, alcohol, red pepper) and laxative fruits (prunes, fresh cherries, peaches) be avoided. Constipated patients with active proctitis may actually benefit from added bulk in the form of psyllium or bran.

20. What role does "stress" play in causing or exacerbating ulcerative colitis?

Another frequent question from patients is, "What is it about my life that makes me have this awful disease?" Despite decades of study, no certain correlation of disease activity with either a personality type, personal history, or stressful life events has been proven. Prospective studies have failed to find any excess of definable mental illness in patients with UC compared with patients comparably ill with nonintestinal disease. Most patients with UC, and most doctors caring for them, believe that flareups of colitis often occur at times of psychosocial stress. However, it is not helpful for patients to believe that they are somehow responsible for bringing this distressing disease upon themselves. In-depth psychiatric exploration of patients' emotional makeup is more often harmful than helpful; supportive, sympathetic, and realistic counseling by the patient's physician is far preferable, except in cases of overt psychiatric illness.

BIBLIOGRAPHY

1. Adler DJ, Korelitz BI: The therapeutic efficacy of 6-mercaptopurine in refractory ulcerative colitis. Am J Gastroenterol 85:717–722, 1990.
2. Biddle WL, Miner PB Jr: Long-term use of mesalamine enemas to induce remission in ulcerative colitis. Gastroenterology 99:113–118, 1990.
3. Buckell NA, Williams GT, Bartram CI, Lennard-Jones JE: Depth of ulceration in acute colitis: Correlation of outcome and clinical and radiologic features. Gastroenterology 79:19–25, 1980.
4. Connell WR, Kamm MA, Dickson M, et al: Long-term neoplasia risk after azathioprine treatment in inflammatory bowel disease. Lancet 343:1249–1252, 1994.
5. Hawthorne AB, Logan RF, Hawkey CJ, et al: Randomised controlled trial of azathioprine withdrawal in ulcerative colitis. BMJ 305:20–22, 1992.

6. Langholz E, Munkholm P, Davidsen M, Binder V: Colorectal cancer risk and mortality in patients with ulcerative colitis. Gastroenterology 103:1444–1451, 1992.
7. Langholz E, Munkholm P, Davidsen M, Binder V: Course of ulcerative colitis: Analysis of changes in disease activity over years. Gastroenterology 107:3–11, 1994.
8. Lichtiger S, Present DH, Kornbluth A, et al: Cyclosporine in severe ulcerative colitis refractory to steroid therapy. N Engl J Med 330:1841–1845, 1994.
9. Lobo AJ, Foster PN, Burke DA, et al: The role of azathioprine in the management of ulcerative colitis. Dis Colon Rectum 33:374–377, 1990.
10. Lynch DAF, Lobo AJ, Sobala GM, et al: Failure of colonoscopic surveillance in ulcerative colitis. Gut 34:1075–1080, 1993.
11. Meyers S, Sachar DB, Goldberg JD, Janowitz HD: Corticotropin versus hydrocortisone in the intravenous treatment of ulcerative colitis: A prospective, randomized, double-blind clinical trial. Gastroenterology 85:351–357, 1983.
12. North CS, Clouse RE, Spitznagel EL, et al: The relation of ulcerative colitis to psychiatric factors: A review of findings and methods. Am J Psychiatry 147:974–981, 1990.
13. Nugent FW, Haggit RC, Gilpin PA: Cancer surveillance in ulcerative colitis. Gastroenterology 100:1241–1248, 1991.
14. O'Donoghue DP, Dawson AM, Powell-Tuck J, et al: Double-blind withdrawal trial of azathioprine as maintenance treatment for Crohn's disease. Lancet 2:955–957, 1978.
15. Pemberton JH, Kelly KA, Beart RW Jr, et al: Ileal pouch–anal anastomosis for chronic ulcerative colitis: Long-term results. Ann Surg 206:504–513, 1987.
16. Pullan RD, Rhodes J, Ganesh S, et al: Transdermal nicotine for active ulcerative colitis. N Engl J Med 330:811–815, 1994.
17. Yang H, McElree C, Roth M-P, et al: Familial empiric risks for imflammatory bowel disease: Differences between Jews and non-Jews. Gut 34:517–524, 1993.

42. SMALL BOWEL TUMORS

Steven W. Hammond, M.D. and Peter R. McNally, D.O.

1. How common are small bowel tumors?

Small intestinal neoplasms are relatively rare, which is surprising given that the small bowel is 6 meters long and accounts for 75% of the length of the entire GI tract and 90% of its mucosal surface area. Only 1–2% of all GI tract tumors occur in the small bowel. Of the small bowel tumors found at autopsy, 75% are benign, whereas 75% of the symptomatic tumors found at surgery are malignant.

Despite the major advances in surgery and diagnostic imaging in the last 40 years there has been little improvement in the survival of patients with primary malignancies of the small bowel. The only chance for cure of these malignancies is early resection, and unfortunately most patients already have metastases at the time of surgery. These tumors are difficult to diagnose largely because of their typically vague clinical presentations. The delay in diagnosis is due in large part to clinical errors in test selection and interpretation, as opposed to a delay between symptom onset and contact with a physician.

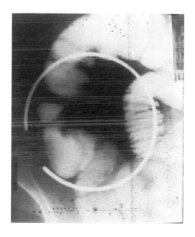

Barium radiograph demonstrating a 1-cm polypoid lesion in the ileum, later found to be a carcinoid tumor.

2. What are the most common malignant tumors of the small bowel?

Most Common Malignant Small Intestinal Tumors and Their Anatomic Distribution

TUMOR	PREVALENCE (PER MILLION POPULATION)	USUAL ANATOMIC LOCATION
Carcinoma	3.7	Duodenum
Carcinoid	2.9	Ileum
Lymphoma	1.6	Ileum
Sarcoma	1.2	Even distribution

3. Do any conditions carry an increased risk for small bowel adenocarcinoma?

Yes. In **adenomatous polyposis coli** (APC), which includes familial polyposis coli and Gardner's syndrome, there is a markedly increased risk of duodenal carcinoma arising from adenomas, primarily in the periampullary region. The risk of developing adenocarcinoma in this condition is 1/1700 person-years. Current recommendations are for periodic surveillance endoscopy of the

UGI tract with both an end-viewing and side-viewing instrument, beginning at the time of diagnosis; biopsies should be done of any ampullary lesions or duodenal polyps found. Endoscopic retrograde cholangiopancreatography (ERCP) should be considered when the ampulla appears abnormal and the alkaline phosphatase level is elevated. Additionally, an index small bowel enteroscopy should be considered when APC is first diagnosed.

Peutz-Jeghers syndrome (mucocutaneous pigmentation and GI polyposis) is an autosomal dominant disease with variable and incomplete penetrance. Patients with this condition have an increased risk for cancer at a number of GI and nonintestinal organs, including the small bowel (duodenum, jejunum, and ileum). Carcinoma appears to arise from foci of adenomatous epithelium within the Peutz-Jeghers polyps, which are unique hamartomas of glandular epithelium supported by branching bands of smooth muscle. The lifetime risk of small bowel adenocarcinoma has been estimated to be 2.4% in patients with this syndrome. Because the small-bowel polyps are relatively inaccessible and the neoplastic potential is unpredictable, surveillance programs remain problematic.

Patients with **Crohn's disease** have a 100-fold greater risk of adenocarcinoma of the ileum compared to age and sex-matched controls. Small bowel carcinomas occur at the site of longstanding disease after a mean of 18 years and occur at an earlier age than patients without Crohn's disease. Because of the risk of carcinoma arising in areas of long-standing disease, it is generally recommended that strictures refractory to medical therapy and bypassed segments of bowel be surgically resected.

In **celiac disease** (gluten-sensitive enteropathy), there is an increased risk of small intestinal malignancies. Most of these are lymphomas, but there is also a significant risk of small bowel adenocarcinoma, which is 80 times higher than that of the general population. Strict adherence to a gluten-free diet appears to reduce the incidence of malignancies in these patients.

4. What is the prevalence of small bowel polyps in asymptomatic patients with familial adenomatous polyposis coli?

In familial APC, adenomatous polyps of the duodenum are very common and present in up to 90% of patients in some series. The polyps are present primarily in the second portion of the duodenum, with clustering in the periampullary region. In a study of Japanese patients with APC, 50% of asymptomatic patients were found to have adenomas of the duodenal papilla. Endoscopically, the papilla had a granular or nodular appearance in most patients; however, 14% of normal-appearing papillae contained adenomatous tissue. A subsequent study in a white American population found a similar 50% prevalence of adenomas of the papilla, with 22% of the adenomas occurring in normal-appearing papillae.

5. What are the two types of small bowel lymphoma, and how do they differ?

The two types of primary lymphoma of the small bowel are lymphoma of immunoproliferative small intestinal disease (IPSID), also known as the Mediterranean type, and non-IPSID, or Western, lymphoma.

Non-IPSID lymphoma is more common in western cultures and is typically a localized ileal tumor with no geographic or socioeconomic pattern of distribution. It arises in the lymphoid tissues of the submucosa, and as it expands, it invades and ulcerates the mucosa and may invade into the serosa. As it invades locally, the lymphoma frequently spreads to regional lymph nodes and, later, to the spleen and more distant sites. Patients typically present with abdominal pain and obstructive symptoms. The vast majority of these tumors are of B-lymphocyte origin, but those arising in patients with celiac disease are of T-cell origin. There is a bimodal age distribution with a peak in children under 10 years and another in the fifth and sixth decades of life.

The **IPSID lymphomas,** also referred to as Mediterranean or Middle Eastern lymphomas, are quite different from non-IPSID lymphomas. Most cases have been reported in countries in the Middle East and North Africa, with a few cases described in other parts of Africa, the Indian subcontinent, Far East, Central America, and Europe. The disease affects persons of low socioeconomic status with poor hygiene and a high incidence of enteric bacterial and parasitic infections in childhood. The peak incidence is in the second and third decades. IPSID usually affects long segments of the proximal small bowel, including the duodenum and proximal jejunum. It is thought that the repeated, intense antigenic stimulation of plasma cells and lymphocytes in the small bowel mucosa leads to eventual emergence of a malignant clone of immunocytes. No specific dietary agent or pathogen has been clearly implicated in the pathogenesis of IPSID.

6. Describe the small bowel pathology seen in IPSID.

In the early stage of the disease, or "prelymphomatous phase," the mucosa of long segments of the proximal small bowel demonstrate a diffuse infiltration by plasma cells and small lymphocytes. The mucosa appears thickened and granular with a thick edematous bowel wall. Initially, the lining epithelial cells are columnar and the brush border is intact, but as the infiltrative process increases, the enterocytes become flattened and small ulcerations are seen. With further progression, tumor nodules appear comprising predominantly immature plasma cells and lymphocytes. The nodules invade the muscularis mucosa and eventually the entire bowel wall. In late-stage disease, there is thickening of the affected bowel, which may be patchy or diffuse, with variable stricturing, dilatation, and gross tumor masses. Mesenteric lymph node changes are seen in parallel with those in the bowel. In advanced cases, tumor may spread to adjacent organs, but spread to spleen, liver, or extra-abdominal lymph nodes is rare. In 20–90% of patients with IPSID, a heavy alpha chain protein can be demonstrated in the serum, though in 50% of these cases, routine serum electrophoresis is insufficiently sensitive to demonstrate the protein.

7. Do patients with IPSID present with any unique symptoms?

Most patients present with chronic abdominal pain and diarrhea, which may be intermittent initially. As the disease progresses, the initially watery diarrhea may give way to frank steatorrhea. Clubbing of the fingers and toes has been observed in one-half to three quarters of patients, and in the later stages of disease, about one-half of patients have fever.

8. How is IPSID treated?

Remission in patients with IPSID has been reported to be induced by treatment with tetracycline, corticosteroids, cyclophosphamide, or a combination of these in early disease. In more advanced disease, abdominal radiation and combination chemotherapy with cyclophosphamide, vincristine, and prednisone with or without doxorubicin has been effective. Remissions may last months to years; however, the prognosis remains poor, with an overall 5-year survival of 22.7% in one large series of 97 patients.

9. Are there risk factors for small bowel lymphoma?

The etiology of non-IPSID lymphoma is, for the most part, unknown. Patients with congenital or acquired immunodeficiency states, including AIDS, organ transplant patients, patients treated with cancer chemotherapy, as well as those with Wiskott-Aldrich syndrome and X-linked immunodeficiency with elevated IgM are at increased risk of developing lymphomas at all sites. Those with prior exposure to ionizing radiation and patients with collagen-vascular disease are also at an increased risk for lymphoma.

There have been a few patients with Crohn's disease reported to develop small bowel lymphoma, but the significance is unclear. There have been no reported cases of patients with ulcerative colitis developing lymphoma in the GI tract outside the colon.

Nodular lymphoid hyperplasia (NLH) of the intestine has been associated with the development of small bowel lymphoma. NLH occurs with primary immunoglobulin deficiency but has also been reported in the absence of hypogammaglobulinemia in underdeveloped countries, probably as a variant of IPSID.

Celiac disease is associated with an increased incidence of small bowel lymphoma. The lymphomas are characteristic T-cell neoplasms which usually arise in the jejunum. About half the malignancies in celiac disease are lymphomas, and lymphoma should be suspected in any patient with celiac disease who fails to improve or deteriorates despite strict adherence to a gluten-free diet.

10. Describe the common presenting symptoms of carcinoid tumors of the small bowel.

The most common presentation of carcinoid tumors of the small bowel is episodic abdominal pain consistent with intermittent bowel obstruction. In a series of 183 consecutive patients with small bowel carcinoids, the duration of symptoms averaged 2 years before the diagnosis was made and extended to as long as 20 years. Because of the deep location and small size of the tumors, intussusception is relatively uncommon and occurs in <3% of patients eventually diagnosed with small bowel carcinoid. The tumor stimulates a fibroblastic reaction in the mesentary as it extends beyond the bowel wall, which causes the mesenteric border of the bowel to buckle and "kink" the intestine. This kinking results in a partial obstruction that can be difficult to demonstrate on small bowel barium x-rays. If the tumor spreads to the mesenteric and celiac lymph nodes, there may be vascular encasement and a peculiar regional vascular thickening that can lead to ischemia and bowel infarction. Even spread to the liver, resulting in large hepatic masses, may cause very few symptoms.

11. What causes the systemic symptoms of carcinoid tumors?

The systemic symptoms of carcinoid tumors are known as the **carcinoid syndrome.** The occurrence of the syndrome is related to the presence of tumor bulk in an area whose blood supply drains into the systemic circulation, implying distant metastasis from a small bowel primary carcinoid. In patients with liver metastasis, the syndrome is common. It is important to note that a large tumor bulk is required for the syndrome. Flushing, triggered by emotional stress, food, alcohol, exertion, or sexual intercourse, is the hallmark of the condition. Other symptoms include diarrhea, asthma, pellagra, and, in late stages, the development of carcinoid heart disease. Carcinoid asthma attacks are uncommon, and pellagra is generally seen only in terminal stages of the disease with associated cachexia. Diarrhea, while common in patients with carcinoid syndrome, may well be related to mechanical factors, such as partial small bowel obstruction or prior bowel resection, as opposed to the carcinoid syndrome itself.

The chemical mediators of carcinoid syndrome are not completely understood. Initially, the large amounts of serotonin produced and released by the tumor were thought to be responsible for the syndrome. Serotonin is metabolized to 5-hydroxyindole acetic acid (5-HIAA), which is readily measured in the urine. Although there is a clear relationship between the urinary 5-HIAA levels and presence of the syndrome, some patients have relatively low 5-HIAA levels with severe flushing, and others have very high 5-HIAA levels with no flushing at all. Other postulated mechanisms include tumor release of kallikrein with induction of bradykinin excess, as well as a role for prostaglandins, gastrin, and histamine. None of these mediators is especially well supported.

12. How does one evaluate a patient with possible carcinoid syndrome?

If a patient presents with symptoms suggesting carcinoid syndrome (flushing, diarrhea, asthma, etc.), a 24-hour urine collection for 5-HIAA is probably the best test. Seventy-five percent of patients with functioning carcinoids excrete >80 mmol/dl. Excessive intake of certain foods, including bananas, pineapples, tomatoes, avocados, walnuts, pecans, and butternuts, can occasionally produce false-positive results. Also, the use of guaifenesin or acetaminophen can produce false-positive results, while levodopa and aspirin may produce false-negative results. Some patients with carcinoid tumors may have classic symptoms of carcinoid syndrome but have a normal urinary 5-HIAA level. In these cases, plasma and platelet serotonin levels should be measured and will demonstrate an elevation.

Imaging studies, such as ultrasonography or computed tomography (CT), should be obtained to evaluate for hepatic metastases, and a directed liver biopsy can then be used to establish a histologic diagnosis. Carcinoid tumors not seen on other imaging modalities may be detected on scans using ^{131}I-labeled MIBG, which accumulates in neuroendocrine cells. The recent development of scintigraphy using radiolabeled somatostatin analogues, which are taken up avidly by a variety of neuroendocrine tumors, provides another tool for assessing for metastatic carcinoid. About 89% of carcinoid tumors can be imaged using ^{111}In-pentetreotide scintigraphy.

13. How are patients with carcinoid tumors managed medically?

Medical management is directed toward controlling symptoms and reducing tumor bulk, although the disease is indolent and some patients with widespread disease can live comfortably for years. Symptoms that are more than a minor annoyance have been managed with a variety of drugs in the past—most with disappointing results—including clonidine, phenoxybenzamine, propranolol, phentolamine, fenfluramine, alpha-methyldopa, and methyldopa. **Cyproheptadine** has been used with some success in relieving the diarrhea, but it seldom reduces flushing and does not decrease urinary 5-HIAA excretion. The dose is 4–8 mg three times daily.

Therapy with **octreotide**, a somatostatin analogue, usually stops flushing within minutes and diarrhea within hours. Serum serotonin levels and 5-HIAA levels also are decreased rapidly. Almost 90% of patients treated with octreotide have >50% reduction in flushing, and urinary 5-HIAA levels decrease by >50% in two-thirds of patients. In an occasional patient, there may even be true tumor regression. Unfortunately, the response to somatostatin analogues is not lasting, with most patients relapsing in just over 1 year. The mechanism of this escape is unknown. An appropriate starting dose for octreotide is 150 µg three times a day, with the dose increased if control is only partial. The side effects are minimal, but at high doses, steatorrhea can be a problem. Chronic octreotide therapy leads to cholelithiasis due to biliary stasis in about a third of patients. Because of its cost and the development of drug resistance, octreotide therapy should be reserved for patients with disabling symptoms and severe impairment in quality of life.

Chemotherapy for carcinoid syndrome is reserved for patients with significant disability and symptoms from the disease or those with poor prognostic signs, including impaired liver function, carcinoid heart disease, or very high 5-HIAA levels. The response rate to any regimen is low and usually very transient with often severe toxicity. Various single-drug and combination regimens have been used in small numbers of patients, including cyclophosphamide, streptozotocin, and 5-fluorouracil, with response rates ranging from 23–40%.

Immunotherapy employing interferon alpha has shown some promise, with a reduction in 5-HIAA levels, relief of symptoms, and tumor regression in some patients. However, the beneficial effects are very transient, and any therapeutic benefit seems outweighed by the high frequency of toxic reactions.

In some patients with extensive hepatic metastases, **hepatic artery occlusion** has been used, with an objective regression rate of 65% and a comparable reduction in 5-HIAA levels and symptoms of flushing and diarrhea. Again, the response was short-lived, lasting a median of only 6.4 months in one study. A combination of hepatic artery occlusion and combination chemotherapy appeared to provide a greater reponse rate (85%) and duration of response (median, 18 months) than either modality alone.

14. What is "carcinoid crisis"?

The situation known as carcinoid crisis is characterized by an intense generalized flush lasting hours or days, CNS abnormalities ranging from lightheadedness to coma, and cardiovascular abnormalities including arrhythmias and hypertension or hypotension. The condition is typically precipitated by physical stress, such as the induction of anesthesia or chemotherapy. Octreotide therapy can be life-saving.

15. How are carcinoid tumors managed surgically?

Carcinoid tumors of the small bowel are seldom recognized until they cause symptoms such as pain or obstruction. They are seldom amenable to endoscopic removal at this point and are usually treated surgically. Cleansing of the bowel is not as important prior to small bowel surgery as it is with colon lesions and should be avoided in patients with obstruction. The treatment of choice is segmental resection of the small bowel, though if the tumor is in the proximal duodenum or extends into the pancreas, a pancreaticoduodenectomy or Whipple procedure may be required. Regional lymph nodes should be resected with the primary lesion. Ileal lesions may require a right hemicolectomy, and if the lesion is in the ileum, care should be taken to preserve as much of the ileum as possible to prevent postoperative diarrhea or vitamin B12 deficiency. If the lesion is unresectable, a bypass procedure should be performed to reestablish continuity of the gut lumen and thus allow oral feeding. The mass should be debulked as much as possible. Pre- and postoperative decompression generally requires only a nasogastric tube, and long intestinal tubes are rarely necessary.

16. What are the characteristic endoscopic ultrasound findings of carcinoid tumor?

Subepithelial mass lesions or nodules found on endoscopy or GI x-rays may be difficult to diagnose precisely. Upper GI endoscopic ultrasonography (EUS) may be very useful in determining whether a lesion is a tumor within the wall of the intestine, a vascular structure, or an extrinsic compression caused by an adjacent organ or mass. If the lesion is found to arise from the gut wall, the sonographic layer of origin and echotexture of the lesion may help infer a diagnosis.

Essentially, the technique involves endoscopically placing a high-frequency transducer in the GI lumen and scanning the area of interest. Studies of the wall of the GI tract with EUS using frequencies from 7.5–12 MHz consistently demonstrate five sonographic layers. The interpretation of these layers remains a matter of some debate, but for practical purposes, the inner three layers correspond to the mucosa and submucosa, including the muscularis mucosa, the fourth hypoechoic layer corresponds to the muscularis propria, and the fifth or outermost layer is the serosa.

Carcinoid tumors arise from one or more of the three innermost sonographic layers of the wall (generally the second layer), unlike leiomyoma or leiomyosarcoma, which arise from the fourth hypoechoic layer. Typically, carcinoid tumors are hypoechoic or of intermediate echogenicity, and they are homogeneous with a smooth, sharply defined border (see figure below). Currently, it is impossible to determine that a lesion is a carcinoid tumor from EUS findings alone.

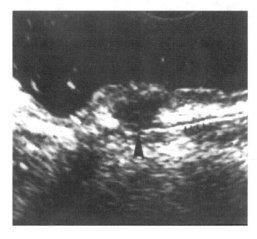

Endoscopic ultrasound of a carcinoid tumor. Note the well-demarcated, hypoechoic tumor (*large arrow*) and the adjacent muscularis propria (*small arrows*).

17. Describe the characteristics of small bowel sarcomas.

Sarcomas are malignancies that arise from cells of mesodermal origin. Leiomyosarcomas are the most common type of sarcoma involving the small bowel. They occur most commonly in the ileum but can be seen anywhere in the small intestine. Typically, leiomyosarcomas present in the fifth to seventh decade of life, with a slight male predominance. Presenting symptoms generally include abdominal pain, nausea, vomiting, and weight loss, but about 9% present with intestinal perforation. Because the tumors are often very bulky, the mass can shift and precipitate a volvulus. Angiosarcomas may acutely hemorrhage due to the tumor's vascularity. More than half of patients with leiomyosarcoma have a palpable abdominal or pelvic mass on physical examination. CT scan often demonstrates a large mass with central necrosis. Lymph node metastases are uncommon, and the tumor spreads most often by direct extension or by hematogenous spread to the liver and lungs.

Treatment is primarily surgical, and 5-year survival rates range from 20–50%. In unresectable or metastatic disease, combination chemotherapy and radiation have been used. The partial response rate to combination chemotherapy is about 50%.

18. Which tumors most commonly metastasize to the small bowel?

Malignant melanoma is the most common tumor metastatic to the small bowel, occurring in 35.6–58% of patients studied at autopsy but in only 8% before death. Melanoma metastatic to the small bowel usually occurs as multiple lesions but may present as diffuse infiltration, a single intraluminal mass, or as bowel implants. The lesions may lead to intussusception, obstruction, or bleeding. In one-third of patients, no primary lesion can be identified, and in many others, the primary tumor had been resected years before.

Other malignancies that metastasize by hematogenous spread are less common but include lung and breast carcinoma. Treatment with corticosteroids for breast cancer seems to predispose to GI metastases. Tumors of the cervix, ovaries, colon, and kidneys may involve the small bowel by direct extension. Renal cell carcinoma is the most common malignancy metastatic to the jejunum.

BIBLIOGRAPHY

1. Alexander JR, Andrews JM, Buchi KN, et al: High prevalence of adenomatous polyps of the duodenal papilla in familial adenomatous polyposis. Dig Dis Sci 34:167–170, 1989.
2. Al-Mondhiry H: Primary lymphomas of the small intestine: East-West contrast. Am J Hematol 22:89–105, 1986.
3. Brophy C, Cahow CE: Primary small bowel maligant tumors. Unrecognized until emergent laparotomy. Am Surg 55:408–412, 1989.
4. Davin Z, Mocitel CG, McIlrath DC: The malignant carcinoid syndrome. Surg Gynecol Obstet 137:637–644, 1973.
5. Domizio P, Talbot IC, Spigelman AD, et al: Upper gastrointestinal pathology in familial adenomatous polyposis: Results from a prospective study of 102 patients, J Clin Pathol 43:738 743, 1990.
6. Iida M, Itoh H, Ohsato K, Watanabe H: Endoscopic features of the duodenal papilla in familial polyposis of the colon. Gastrointest Endosc 27:6, 1981.
7. Iida M, Yao T, Itoh H, et al: Natural history of duodenal lesions in Japanese patients with familial adenomatosis coli (Gardner's syndrome). Gastroenterology 96:1301 1306, 1989.
8. Khojasteh A, Haghshenass M, Haghighi P: Immunoproliferative small intestinal disease: A "third-world lesion." N Engl J Med 308:1401–1405, 1983.
9. Kurtz RC, Sternberg SS, Miller HH, DeCosse JJ: Upper gastrointestinal neoplasia in familial polyposis. Dig Dis Sci 32:459–465, 1987.
10. Laws HL, Han SY, Aldrette JS: Malignant tumors of small bowel. South Med J 77:1087–1090, 1984.
11. Lightdale CJ, Hornsby-Lewis L: Tumors of the small intestine. In Haubrich WS, Schaffner F, Berk JE (eds): Bockus Gastroenterology, 5th ed. Philadelphia, W.B. Saunders, 1995, pp 1274–1290.
12. Luk GD: Cancer surveillance strategies. In Sleisenger MH, Fordtran JS, Scharschmidt BE, Feldman M (eds): Gastrointestinal Disease: Pathophysiology, Diagnosis, Management, 5th ed. Philadelphia, W.B. Saunders, 1993, pp 115–126.
13. Maglinte DDT, O'Connor K, Bessette J, et al: The role of the physician in the late diagnosis of primary malignant tumors of the small intestine. Am J Gastroenterol 86:304–308, 1991.
14. Martin RG: Malignant tumors of the small intestine. Surg Clin North Am 66:779–785, 1986.
15. Matsumoto T, Iida M, Suekane H, et al: Endoscopic ultrasonography in rectal carcinoid tumors: Contribution to selection of therapy. Gastrointest Endosc 37:539–542, 1991.
16. Moertel CG: An odyssey in the land of small tumors. J Clin Oncol 5:1503–1522, 1987.
17. Moertel CG, Sauer WG, Dockerty MB, et al: Life history of the carcinoid tumor of the small intestine. Cancer 14:901–912, 1961.
18. Sarre RG, Frost AG, Jagelman DG, et al: Gastric and duodenal polyps in familial adenomatous polyposis: A prospective study of the nature and prevalence of upper gastrointestinal polyps. Gut 28:306–314, 1987.
19. Spigelman AD, Talbot IC, Williams CB, et al: Upper gastrointestinal cancer in patients with familial adenomatous polyposis. Lancet 2:783–785, 1989.
20. Tio TL, Tytgat GNJ: Endoscopic ultrasonography of normal and pathologic upper gastrointestinal wall structure: Comparison of studies in vivo and in vitro with histology. Scand J Gastroenterol 21(suppl 123):27–33, 1986.
21. Yasuda K, Nakajima M, Yoshida S, et al: The diagnosis of submucosal tumors of the stomach by endoscopic ultrasonography. Gastrointest Endosc 35:10–15, 1989.
22. Zollinger RM, Sternfield WC, Schreiber H: Primary neoplasms of the small intestine. Am J Surg 151:654–658, 1986.

43. EOSINOPHILIC GASTROENTERITIS

Amy M. Tsuchida, M.D.

1. What is eosinophilic gastroenteritis?

Eosinophilic gastroenteritis is an uncommon disease characterized by eosinophilic infiltration in the GI tract, resulting in GI symptoms. The clinical features vary depending on the location as well as which gut wall layer is infiltrated with eosinophils. Parasitic or extraintestinal disease is usually absent.

2. Describe clinical and x-ray features of the three principal patterns of eosinophilic infiltration.

Primary mucosal: Symptoms include nausea, vomiting, diarrhea, crampy periumbilical abdominal pain, watery diarrhea, and weight loss. Mucosal ulcerations may cause fecal occult blood loss and iron-deficiency anemia. Extensive small bowel involvement may result in malabsorption. Barium studies show mucosal edema, nodular polypoid intraluminal masses, and a "saw-toothed" mucosal pattern with diffuse thickening or effacement of the valvulae conniventes.

Primary submucosal/muscularis: This variant presents with complete or incomplete bowel obstruction. Gastric antrum involvement is most common with patients presenting with outlet obstruction. Barium x-rays may demonstrate focal irregular narrowing of the distal antrum or small bowel. Isolated eosinophilic infiltration of the muscularis layer of the esophagus may present with symptoms, manometric findings, and x-ray studies suggestive of achalasia.

Serosal involvement: Serosal involvement presents with eosinophilic ascites and may be seen in conjunction with mucosal and/or muscularis involvement. Eosinophilic pleural effusions have also been reported in patients with predominantly serosal eosinophilic gastroenteritis. Thickened small bowel and colonic serosal infiltrates of eosinophils may be seen on laparotomy.

3. In what other diseases can eosinophilic infiltration of the GI tract be seen?

In chronic inflammation, peptic ulcer disease, Hodgkin's lymphoma, Crohn's disease, carcinoma, and parasitic infection, the magnitude of the eosinophilic infiltrate is less, and histiocytes and plasma cells are often seen in the other chronic inflammatory diseases. Polyarteritis nodosa can present with abdominal pains, peripheral eosinophilia, and nodular masses in the stomach or small bowel on x-rays, but the eosinophilic infiltrates are localized in the perivascular tissue. Allergic gastroenterophathy, usually described in children, is often classified as a variant of eosinophilic gastroenteritis; these children have a history of atopy and food allergy, and symptoms regress as the children get older. Hypereosinophilic syndrome is a multisystem disorder in which eosinophilic infiltrates can be found in a variety of organs. Eosinophilic granulomas, which are localized intramural collections of mature eosinophils, have been reported in the stomach, particularly the gastric antrum.

4. Which parasites should be considered in patients with abdominal symptoms and massive eosinophilic infiltration of the gut?

Trichinella	*Ascaris*
Strongyloides	Hookworm
Toxocara	*Trichara*
Capillaria	Other nematodes

Isospora belli (in immunocompromised hosts).

5. What are Charcot-Leyden crystals?

They are remnants of extruded eosinophil crystals found in the stools of patients with diseases having mucosal infiltration of eosinophils.

6. How reliable is a diagnosis of eosinophilic gastroenteritis established by endoscopic biopsy?

In approximately 10% of patients, mucosal biopsies are nondiagnostic, either because of sampling error or sparing of the mucosa. A minimum of eight specimens is recommended, as the disease may have a patchy distribution. Diagnostic infiltrate is not well defined in most studies, but recently, >20 eosinophils/high-power field, either diffusely or multifocally, within the lamina propria has become the standard. Full-thickness surgical biopsy specimens may be required for diagnosis in those patients with nondiagnostic mucosal biopsies, to exclude tumor or inflammatory bowel disease.

7. What causes eosinophilic gastroenteritis?

It's unknown. Up to 50% of patients have a history of atopic disorders. In some instances, local nonallergic inflammatory responses may be produced to a particular food or parasite.

8. How is eosinophilic gastroenteritis treated?

If certain foods obviously cause symptoms, a trial elimination diet is indicated, but in most individuals, a specific food will not be isolated. A short 7- to 10-day course of oral corticosteroids, with 20 to 40 mg of prednisone daily, will usually produce a clinical remission. Periodic courses of steroids may be necessary for recrudescence of symptoms, with some patients ultimately requiring low-dose corticosteroids to remain in remission. Sodium cromolyn has also been efficacious in some patients. Surgery may be required for complications, such as bowel perforation, pyloric or intestinal obstruction, or refractory disease.

BIBLIOGRAPHY

1. Blackshaw AJ, Levison DA: Eosinophilic infiltrates of the gastrointestinal tract. J Clin Pathol 39:1–7, 1986.
2. Cello JP: Eosinophilic gastroenteritis—A complex disease entity. Am J Med 67:1097–1104, 1979.
3. Lee CM, Changchien CS, Chen PC, et al: Eosinophilic gastroenteritis: 10 years experience. Am J Gastroenterol 88:70–74, 1993.
4. Talley NJ, Shorter RG, Phillips SF, et al: Eosinophilic gastroenteritis. A clinicopathological study of patients with disease of the mucosa, muscle layer, and subserosal tissues. Gut 31:54–58, 1990.

44. BACTERIAL OVERGROWTH

Allan Parker, D.O.

1. What is the mechanism of bacterial colonization of the normal human GI tract?

In utero and at birth, the gut is sterile. Coliform bacteria can be found in the human gut a few hours after birth and propagate from mouth to anus. *Bacteroides* species do not colonize the gut until about 10 days of age. By 1 month of age, the gut flora are essentially the same as in an adult. All bacteria are introduced from the environment via the oral route.

2. What is the normal bacterial density in different areas of the GI tract?

Stomach	<1,000 per ml
Jejunum	<10,000 per ml
Ileum	<100,000 per ml
Colon	<1 trillion per ml

The jejunum is sterile in 30% of normal persons. Lactobacilli and enterococci predominate in the small bowel, whereas *Bacteroides* constitutes the bulk of colonic organisms.

3. How many types of organisms are found in the GI tract?

Up to 400 different species have been noted, excluding the mouth. Most are anaerobes and difficult to culture. Only 0.01% of the bacterial mass in the colon is made up of organisms commonly cultured, such as *Escherichia coli*.

4. What factors are responsible for the variable bacterial populations and densities throughout the gut?

1. Gastric acid kills most swallowed organisms.
2. Rapid motility keeps small bowel bacterial counts low.
3. Mucous secretion may increase clearing by trapping and propelling bacteria.
4. pH and oxygen tension differences support different organisms.
5. Dietary nutrients have little effect.
6. The ileocecal valve is very important in preventing ileal colonization.
7. Slow colonic transit promotes a large population of organisms.

5. What conditions can lead to small bowel bacterial overgrowth?

Conditions Resulting in Bacterial Overgrowth of the Small Bowel

Reduced or absent gastric acid production
    Ulcer surgery
    Omeprazole or high-dose H_2 blockers
    Atrophic gastritis
Stagnation and reduced transit
    Small bowel diverticuli
    Surgical blind loops
    Obstruction (strictures, adhesions, etc.)
    Motility disorders (diabetes, scleroderma, etc.)
    Fistulas between the colon and small bowel (including ileocecal valve resection)

6. Describe the clinical consequences of bacterial overgrowth.

Minor bacterial overgrowth is usually not associated with clinical problems, but severe overgrowth may cause steatorrhea, anemia, bloating, and cramping. Weight loss may be significant in 30% of patients. Very severe overgrowth may result in malabsorption and deficiency syndromes of fat-soluble vitamins and B12, including neuropathy, anemia, osteomalacia, coagulopathy, night blindness, tetany, and diarrhea.

7. Bacterial overgrowth results in malabsorption of minerals and vitamins. Which vitamin is produced by gut bacteria?
Folic acid (vitamin B12) may be produced, but it is not absorbed to any significant degree.

8. What factors lead to hypoproteinemia in severe bacterial overgrowth?
Damaged intestinal epithelium may fail to absorb amino acids. Breakdown and utilization of luminal protein by bacteria may make it unavailable for host utilization. Protein-losing enteropathy may result from mucosal injury.

9. Is the D-xylose absorption test abnormal in bacterial overgrowth?
Yes. A combination of malabsorption secondary to mucosal injury and bacterial metabolism of the xylose in the bowel lumen results in an abnormal result.

10. Diarrhea, which may include watery or foul-smelling steatorrhea, is a common feature of severe bacterial overgrowth. What factors contribute to this diarrhea?
Deconjugation of bile salts by bacteria may lead to bile salt diarrhea. Fat malabsorption with passage of hydroxylated fatty acids, which are osmotic and irritant, contributes to stool volume. Organic acids produced by bacteria increase stool osmolality and fluid, producing an osmotic diarrhea.

11. When should the diagnosis of bacterial overgrowth be considered?
Bacterial overgrowth of the small bowel should be considered in patients presenting with malabsorption, diarrhea, steatorrhea, unexplained weight loss, or anemia (especially macrocytic). The diagnosis is supported by a history of gastric surgery, achlorhydria, Crohn's disease, fistulas, scleroderma or other motility disturbances, surgical pouches or bypasses, small bowel diverticuli, or small bowel radiographs suggestive of malabsorption.

12. Is small bowel biopsy helpful in diagnosing bacterial overgrowth?
It may be helpful but is not diagnostic. An inflammatory infiltrate with lymphocytes and plasma cells is common. Blunting of villi may also be seen. These findings are nonspecific and may be confused with celiac sprue, tropical sprue, and other injuries to the small bowel mucosa.

13. How is the diagnosis of small bowel overgrowth established?
The only means of proving a diagnosis of small bowel bacterial overgrowth is by proper collection and culture of jejunal contents. A bacterial count of $> 10^5$ organisms/ml confirms the diagnosis. This test requires careful intubation of the small bowel to avoid oral contaminants. Usually multiple organisms are cultured. Because of the difficulty in performing this study, it is rarely done except in research settings.

14. Tests have been devised to diagnose bacterial overgrowth by measuring blood levels of compound metabolites resulting from bacterial action, but these are of minimal value. Why?
These tests measure *para*-aminobenzoic acid, indican, phenols, some drugs, and deconjugated bile acids. They are helpful in documenting malabsorption but do not differentiate small bowel bacterial overgrowth from all other causes of malabsorption. Bile acid levels are only helpful if the bacteria that deconjugate bile are present in high numbers. Thus, although the idea sounds good and the tests are relatively simple, their utility in clinical practice is low.

15. Another method used in diagnosing small bowel bacterial overgrowth is breath analysis. What element is common to and critical to all breath tests?
All breath analysis tests are based on bacterial degradation of the substrate in the small bowel lumen and subsequent absorption and excretion of products in the expired air, where it is analyzed. All of the substrates are metabolized normally in the colon. Therefore, documenting *early* me-

tabolism and subsequent *early* breath level elevations are critical to diagnosing small bowel bacterial overgrowth.

16. List three conditions necessary for accurate diagnosis of small bowel overgrowth by breath testing.

1. Normal gastric emptying—Delayed gastric emptying may lead to false-negative results.
2. Normal small bowel transit time—Short transit time may lead to false-negative test results.
3. Absence of enterocolonic fistulas—A fistula from the small bowel to colon allows substrate to reach the colon early and results in false-positive findings.

17 What is a potential problem with the ^{14}C-cholyglycine breath test?

^{14}C-cholyglycine breath testing for bacterial overgrowth depends on the bacterial deconjugation of cholyglycine and eventual metabolism and appearance of $^{14}CO_2$ in the breath. Conditions that result in malabsorption of bile salts may give false-positive results. Examples are Crohn's disease, ileal resection, radiation enteritis, and small bowel lymphoma. The test also has a very high (30%) false-negative rate in patients with proven small bowel bacterial overgrowth.

18. Why is the ^{14}C-xylose breath test superior to the others?

^{14}C-xylose has been adapted for breath testing in the diagnosis of small bowel bacterial overgrowth and is based on the bacterial metabolism of xylose and appearance of $^{14}CO_2$ in the breath. Its sensitivity and specificity are about 90%, with no false-negative studies in one series of patients with culture-proven bacterial overgrowth. Xylose is absorbed proximally in the small bowel such that almost none reaches the colon with its bacterial population. Gram-negative aerobes, which are always part of bacterial overgrowth, readily metabolize xylose.

19. All breath hydrogen is a result of bowel bacterial activity. What are some problems with the hydrogen breath test?

Breath hydrogen testing for small bowel bacterial overgrowth is based on the fact that human tissues do not produce any hydrogen, yet hydrogen produced by small bowel bacteria is readily absorbed from the bowel lumen and appears in the breath. Problems limiting use of this test are as follows:

1. The test is timed to avoid substrate metabolism in the colon and is subject to the variability of GI motility.
2. Large carbohydrate meals the night before the test may result in elevated baseline breath hydrogen levels and false-positive tests.
3. Cigarette smoking, exertion, and hyperventilation must be avoided during testing.
4. The small bowel (early) peak must be clearly distinguishable from the colonic (late) hydrogen peak. This is frequently a problem.
5. The breath hydrogen test has a sensitivity of only 65% and a specificity of 45%.

20. How should breath tests currently be used for diagnosing bacterial overgrowth?

* The breath hydrogen is simple and safe but inaccurate. It involves no radiation and can easily be performed in the clinic.
* The ^{14}C-xylose test is the test of choice. It involves only minimal radiation doses and is accurate.
* Intubation and quantitative culture remains the gold standard but is rarely performed.

21. Successful treatment of small bowel bacterial overgrowth depends on reducing the small bowel bacterial level. What actions may achieve this goal?

1. Eliminate stasis
    Remove diverticulae
    Promotility agents
    Take down blind loops
    Eliminate strictures
2. Remove source of contamination (close fistulas)
3. Antibiotics

22. What antibiotics are commonly used for bacterial overgrowth control?
Augmentin, cephalexin, metronidazole, and tetracycline
Penicillin, ampicillin, gentamicin, and neomycin are ineffective.

23. How long should patients with bacterial overgrowth be treated with antibiotics?
Treatment should last for 7–10 days. A single course may give relief of symptoms for several months. Sometimes, rotating courses of antibiotics is necessary to maintain control of the bacterial population.

24. Is there anything new in the treatment of bacterial overgrowth?
Octreotide recently has been shown to stimulate small bowel motor activity with elimination of bacterial overgrowth. Initial results have been even better than those with antibiotics. Further studies are required, but its utility is limited by the absence of an oral preparation.

BIBLIOGRAPHY

1. Banwell JG, Kistler LA, Giannella RA, et al: Small intestinal bacterial overgrowth syndrome. Gastroenterology 80:834–835, 1981.
2. Bardhan PK, Gyr K, Beglinger C, et al: Diagnosis of bacterial overgrowth after culturing proximal small bowel aspirate obtained during routine upper gastrointestinal endoscopy. Scand J Gastroenterol 27:253–256, 1992.
3. Hamilton JD, Dyer N, Dawson AM: Assessment and significance of bacterial overgrowth in the small bowel. Q J Med 39:265–285, 1970.
4. Kahn IJ Jeffries GH, Sleisenger MH: Malabsorption in intestinal scleroderma: Correction by antibiotics. N Engl J Med 274:1339–1342, 1966.
5. Kerlin P, Wong L: Breath hydrogen testing in bacterial overgrowth of the small intestine. Gastroenterology 95:982–988, 1988.
6. Khin-Maung U, Tin-Aye, Ku-Tin-Myint, et al: In vitro hydrogen production by enteric bacteria cultures from children with small bowel bacterial overgrowth. J Pediatr Gastroenterol Nutr 14.192–197, 1992.
7. Khin-Maung U, Bolin TD, Duncombe VM, et al. Epidemiology of small bowel bacterial overgrowth and rice carbohydrate malabsorption in Burmese (Myanmar) village children. Am J Trop Med Hyg 47.298–304, 1992.
8. Sleisenger MH, Fordtran JS (eds): Gastrointestinal Disease. Philadelphia, W.B. Saunders, 1993.
9. Valdovinos MA, Camilleri M, Thomforde GM, Frie C: Reduced accuracy of ^{14}C-D-xylose breath test for detecting bacterial overgrowth in gastrointestinal motility disorders. Scand J Gastroenterol 28:963–968, 1993.
10. Yamada T, Alpers DH, Owyang C, et al (eds): Textbook of Gastroenterology, 2nd ed. Philadelphia, J.B. Lippincott, 1995.

45. SHORT BOWEL SYNDROME

Philip E. Tanner, MD

1. What is short bowel syndrome?

Short bowel syndrome is a malabsorption disorder that occurs after small bowel resection. The clinical consequences of removing portions of the small intestine are extremely variable and depend on a number of factors, such as the extent of resected bowel and consequent loss of absorptive surface area; the site of resection (jejunum, ileum, colon, or a combination); the presence or absence of the ileocecal valve; the underlying disease process and the potential recurrence of this disease; and the adaptive capacity of the remaining intestine.

2. What are the clinical manifestations of short bowel syndrome?

Although several factors play a role in the clinical features of short bowel syndrome, diarrhea almost invariably occurs. **Early** after surgery, dehydration and marked electrolyte deficiencies from fecal losses are common. An **intermediate phase** consists of malabsorption of virtually all nutrients, including protein and particularly fat and carbohydrates, and produces significant weight loss. A **late phase** manifested by persistent diarrhea but stabilization of body weight may occur, but this is dependent on an adaptive absorption process in the remaining intestine. If this adaptation is not adequate, these patients may require long-term parenteral nutrition supplements to maintain a reasonable body weight.

3. What is the prognosis?

Several thousand patients currently survive with short bowel syndrome. Advances in infection control, intensive care monitoring, surgical technique, and nutritional support have reduced the morbidity and mortality rates of this disease. Approximately 70% of patients who develop short bowel syndrome survive and are discharged from the hospital. Most of these patients are alive 1 year later.

4. Name the causes of short bowel syndrome in children.

     Intestinal atresia
     Gastroschisis
     Midgut volvulus
     Aganglionosis
     Necrotizing enterocolitis

The first four are congenital anomalies and account for about two-thirds of the pediatric cases of short bowel syndrome.

5. Name the causes of short bowel syndrome in adults.

     Crohn's disease with multiple small intestine resections
     Mesenteric ischemia
     Radiation enteritis
     Volvulus
     Trauma
     Jejunoileal bypass

Crohn's disease and mesenteric ischemia account for about 75% of the cases. Jejunoileal bypass was a common surgical procedure to treat morbid obesity in the 1970s and early 1980s. Although not a cause of short bowel syndrome per se, jejunoileal bypass may present as a clinically indistinguishable entity.

6. How does loss of digestive and absorptive processes contribute to the malabsorption seen in short bowel syndrome?

Nutrient absorption is a complex process involving many factors. The villi are taller and the crypts are deeper in the jejunum than in the ileum. The absorptive capacity is severalfold higher in the proximal than in the distal small intestine. The terminal ileum is essential for absorption of vitamin B_{12} and bile acid reabsorption. Gastric hypersecretion has been documented to occur within 24 hours after short bowel resections. Normal nutrient digestion and absorption depends on several interrelated processes, such as gradual emptying of the stomach, release of cholecystokinin and secretin from the proximal small bowel, and secretion of bile and pancreatic enzymes. After small bowel resection(s), gastric emptying is faster and small intestine transit time is quicker, resulting in less time and surface area for absorption to occur.

7. Is there a critical length of small intestine required to maintain positive water and nutrient balance? Does It matter which portion of small intestine remains intact?

The normal small intestine varies from 12 ft (366 cm) to 22 ft (671 cm) in length in autopsy studies. Most digestion and absorption of nutrients occurs in the first 100 cm of jejunum. Furthermore, at least 100 cm of jejunum is required for a positive water, sodium, and potassium balance. Vitamin B_{12} and bile acids are absorbed in the ileum, and any ileal resection may result in some malabsorption of these nutrients. Resections of <100 cm of ileum have been associated with moderate B_{12} and bile acid malabsorption, whereas resections of >100 cm have been associated with severe malabsorption and steatorrhea.

If more than 180 cm of small intestine remains, total parenteral nutrition (TPN) is not usually required. If 60–180 cm remains (with or without the colon), TPN usually is required for at least 1–12 months while "adaptation" occurs. If <60 cm of the small intestine (regardless of colon) remains, patients usually require long-term TPN to maintain adequate nutritional status and body weight.

8. Name the three types of surgical resections typically encountered in short bowel syndrome.

1. Limited jejunoileal resection with preservation of the ileocecal valve
2. Extensive ileal resection and right hemicolectomy
3. Extensive short bowel resection and total colectomy

9. Describe the management of patients with limited jejunoileal resection and preservation of the ileocecal valve.

Patients with short resections (<100 cm removed) are usually the least symptomatic. Diarrhea without steatorrhea is the typical finding. These patients are best assessed by quantitative stool collections for fecal fat, volume/weight, electrolytes, and osmolality. Vitamin B_{12} malabsorption should also be assessed.

10. How are patients with extensive ileal resection and a right hemicolectomy managed?

Often these patients suffer from Crohn's disease and have undergone several resections of ileal strictures. In addition to bile acid and vitamin B_{12} malabsorption because of less surface area, the absence of an ileocecal valve may result in bacterial contamination of the small intestine with colonic anaerobic flora. These bacteria can utilize vitamin B_{12} and deconjugate bile acids, worsening the problem of fat malabsorption.

The optimal **diet** composition for these patients has been extensively debated. A low-fat, high-carbohydrate diet with medium-chain triglycerides does not appear to offer any significant advantage. Increased caloric intake corresponding to two to three times the basal energy expenditure of the patient may be required to maintain nutritional balance. Also, avoidance of lactose, which may worsen diarrhea, is recommended.

Antidiarrheal agents, such as loperamide, diphenoxylate HCl, and codeine, may be helpful in reducing diarrhea. Bacterial overgrowth can occur in these patients, and if it is suspected, a trial of **antibiotics** is warranted.

11. Describe the management of patients with extensive small bowel resection and total colectomy.

These patients suffer from severe short bowel syndrome and often have a short segment of jejunum and a jejunostomy. The length of jejunum is critical in determining the prognosis. Lengths <60 cm (in some studies, 100 cm) cannot sustain adequate nutrient absorption, and long-term parenteral alimentation (TPN) is required. Stomal losses of water and electrolytes can be improved with H_2 blockers and/or somatostatin, but usually a positive balance is not obtained. In addition to protein, fat, and carbohydrate parenteral supplementation, vitamins, minerals, and essential micronutrients should be added to the TPN solution, and serum levels monitored for deficiencies.

12. How does bile acid malabsorption occur in patients with short bowel syndrome? What are the adverse effects of bile acid malabsorption?

Bile acids are necessary for the absorption of fats in the ileum. If the absorptive capacity of the ileum is diminished because of inflammatory bowel disease or resection, malabsorption of bile acids and fats occurs. The incidence of gallstones in short bowel syndrome is increased two- to threefold. Previously, it was generally assumed that interruption of the enterohepatic circulation of bile and depletion of bile salts resulted in hepatic synthesis of bile supersaturated with cholesterol, which in turn resulted in the increased formation of cholesterol gallstones (seen in up to one-third of patients with short bowel syndrome). Although reasonable, this explanation does not explain a similar percentage of patients with radiopaque (calcium-containing) gallstones.

13. How does D-lactic acidosis occur in patients with short bowel syndrome?

An encephalopathy characterized by confusion, ataxia, and slurred speech, unassociated with liver disease, was first reported by DeWind and Payne in patients who had undergone jejunoileal bypass for morbid obesity. As mentioned, this surgery and short bowel syndrome have similar clinical and pathophysiologic features, and this encephalopathy has been subsequently described in several patients with short bowel syndrome. Dahlquist et al. reported a temporal relationship between elevations of D-lactate in the urine and blood, overfeeding with carbohydrates in patients with altered small bowel absorption, an increased anion gap acidosis, and the development of this encephalopathy. D-Lactate can be a normal metabolite of the glycolytic pathway in some bacteria. D-Lactic acidosis is well described in ruminants overfed with grain—the so-called grain engorgement syndrome—and a variety of organisms have been implicated. Whether this fermentation of carbohydrates occurs in the colon or the bypassed small intestine has not been established yet.

14. Are any surgical procedures useful for treating short bowel syndrome?

Surgical Treatment of Short Bowel Syndrome

Techniques to slow transit time and increase absorption
    Construction of intestine valves
    "Antiperistaltic" zones created by reversing segments of small intestine
    Creating "recirculation" loops of small intestine
    Colonic interposition
    Intestinal pacing
Techniques for preserving intestinal length
    Tapering enteroplasty for dilated segments
    Stricturoplasty rather than resection
    Serosal patches

Surgical strategies to slow intestinal transit time, increase absorption, and preserve the intestinal remnant have been investigated. Although successes with different techniques to slow transit time have been reported, the outcomes are very unpredictable, and they may result in obstruction, volvulus, or intussusception. Surgical procedures should be considered only in patients who continue to have severe symptoms despite maximal dietary and pharmacologic therapy and who have waited a sufficient time for intestinal adaptation to occur. Techniques aimed at preserving intestinal length are less controversial and more successful.

15. How does intestinal adaptation occur?

Morphologic and functional adaptive changes in the residual small intestine have been studied extensively in animals, but few similar studies in humans have been performed. After resection of the proximal and mid-intestine in rats, an increase in the circumference, thickness, and height of villi in the residual ileum has been observed. This effect, however, has not been proven in humans. Several studies in humans have shown gradual improvement in the absorption of fat, nitrogen, bile acids, vitamin B_{12}, calcium, and carbohydrates (especially glucose) with time. This appears to be due to an increase in the number of absorption cells (hyperplasia), rather than to an increased capacity of individual cells. Even less is known about the adaptive response of the colon.

Although several possible mechanisms have been proposed for stimulating adaptation (exposure of the residual bowel to dietary nutrients, stimulation by biliary and pancreatic secretions, trophic effects of hormones, stimulation by polyamines, neural factors, and increased blood flow to the residual bowel), the mechanism with considerable scientific support is "exposure of the bowel to dietary nutrients." It has been shown repeatedly that adaptation does not occur in patients receiving TPN, and in fact, hypoplasia occurs.

16. What factors determine the prognosis for patients with short bowel syndrome?

1. Length of resected intestine
2. Portion of intestine resected (jejunum, ileum, colon)
3. Presence or absence of ileocecal valve
4. Underlying disease and risk of recurrence
5. Presence of complications (cholelithiasis, D-lactic acidosis, dehydration, hyponatremia, hypokalemia, bacterial overgrowth, calcium oxalate nephrolithiasis, low body weight, dilated residual small intestine)
6. Adaptive capacity of the remaining small intestine
7. Need for long-term parenteral nutrition and the risks inherent to TPN

BIBLIOGRAPHY

1. Booth IW: Enteral nutrition as primary therapy in short bowel syndrome. Gut 35(suppl 1):S69–S72, 1994.
2. Brasitus TA, Sitrin MD. Short bowel syndrome. In Yamada T, Alpers DH, Owyang C, et al (eds): Textbook of Gastroenterology, 2nd ed. Philadelphia, J.B. Lippincott, 1995.
3. Cullen JJ, Kelly KA: The future of intestinal pacing. Gastroenterol Clin North Am 23(2):391–402, 1994.
4. Dahlquist NR, Perrault J, Callaway CW, Jones JD: D-Lactic acidosis and encephalopathy after jejunoileostomy: Response to overfeeding and to fasting in humans. Mayo Clin Proc 59:141–145, 1984.
5. de Bruin RW, Heineman E, Marquet RL: Short bowel transplantation: An overview. Transpl Int 7:47–61, 1994.
6. Levy E, Frileux P, Sandrucci S, et al: Continuous enteral nutrition during the early adaptive stage of the short bowel syndrome. Br J Surg 75:549–553, 1988.
7. Messing B, Pigot F, Rongier M, et al: Intestinal absorption of free oral hyperalimentation in the very short bowel syndrome. Gastroenterology 100:1502–1508, 1991.
8. Remington M, Malagelada JR, Zinsmeister A, Fleming CR: Abnormalities in gastrointestinal motor activity in patients with short bowels: Effect of a synthetic opiate. Gastroenterology 85:629–636, 1983.
9. Shanghogue LK, Molenaar JC: Short bowel syndrome: Metabolic and surgical management. Br J Surg 81:486–499, 1994.
10. Thompson JS: Management of the short bowel syndrome. Gastroenterol Clin North Am 23(2):403–420, 1994.
11. Thompson JS, Rikkers LF: Surgical alternatives for the short bowel syndrome. Am J Gastroenterol 82:97–106, 1987.
12. Woolf GM, Miller C, Kiurian R, Jeejeebhoy KN: Nutritional absorption in short bowel syndrome—Evaluation of fluid, calorie and divalent cation requirements. Dig Dis Sci 32:8–15, 1987.
13. Westergaard H, Spady DK: Short bowel syndrome. In Sleisenger MH, Fordtran JS (eds): Gastrointestinal Disease, 5th ed. Philadelphia, W.B. Saunders, 1993.
14. Williamson RCN, Chir M: Intestinal adaptation: Pt 1. Structural, functional and cytokinetic changes. N Engl J Med 298:1393–1402, 1978.
15. Williamson RCN, Chir M: Intestinal adaptation: Pt 2. Mechanisms of control. N Engl J Med 298:1444–1450.

VI. Colon Disorders

46. COLON CANCER AND COLON POLYPS

Spencer S. Root, M.D., and Shailesh C. Kadakia, M.D.

COLON CANCER

1. How common is colon cancer?

Colorectal cancer is a major cause of morbidity in western society and in countries that have adopted a high-risk (low-fiber, high-animal fat, high-protein) western diet. It is the third most common cancer in the United States, ranking just below breast and lung cancers. Since 1950, the incidence of colorectal cancer has been increasing in whites; the mortality rates having remained stable in white males, while increasing in white females. In nonwhites, both the incidence and mortality have substantially increased. A recent epidemiologic survey has suggested that African-Americans have a substantially increased risk of dying from colorectal cancer, warranting a more intense screening regimen in this population. It is estimated that 6% of the American population will eventually develop colon cancer.

Worldwide, colon cancer is the second most common cancer in males and ranks number three among females. The risk of colon cancer rises rapidly in those migrating from a low-risk (high-fiber, low-fat diet) area to a high-risk area. Likewise colorectal cancer risk can decrease with migration from a high-risk to a low-risk area.

2. What are some of the causative or predisposing factors thought to be associated with colon cancer?

Multiple dietary and environmental factors have been proposed in the development of colon cancer. Several studies suggest that diets high in fat may lead to colon cancer, especially in the left colon (descending and sigmoid). Studies have also linked low dietary fiber, secondary bile acids, cholecystecomy, charbroiled meats, and diets low in calcium and selenium to colon cancer. Vitamins E and C and foods rich in beta-carotenes have been proposed as chemopreventive agents in colon cancers, but the evidence to suggest a true cause-and-effect relationship to colon cancer is circumstantial and controversial. Other factors linked to the development of colorectal cancer are increasing age (90% of colon cancers occur in those ≥50 years old), personal history of colonic adenoma, and prior history of colon cancer.

3. Is colon cancer a genetic disorder?

The role of genetics in colon cancer is most strikingly obvious in the colonic polyposis syndromes. Genetic predisposition to colon cancer is supported by the threefold increase in colon cancer seen in the first-degree relatives of an index case. In sporadic cases of colon cancer in which no family history exists, an acquired point mutation on chromosome 5q21 has been identified and has been called the MCC gene (mutated in colorectal cancer). C-*myc* and *ras* oncogenes have been associated with colorectal cancer. C-*myc* levels are elevated in most colon cancers. *Ras* point mutations have been found to be an early event in transformation from premalignant adenomas to colon cancers.

4. In what other diseases is there an increased risk of developing colon cancer?

Persons with ulcerative and Crohn's colitis are at an increased risk for developing colon cancer. In *ulcerative colitis*, the increase in risk seems to be related to both the duration and extent of disease. The increased risk of colon cancer begins with a disease duration of 7 years and rises about 10% per decade, reaching about 30% at 25 years. The risk is also greater for those with total colonic involvement than for those with disease limited to the left colon (splenic flexure to rectum). Those with ulcerative proctitis alone have only a slightly increased risk of colon cancer when compared to healthy controls.

In patients with colonic *Crohn's disease,* the risk of colon cancer has been reported to be anywhere from 4–20 times that of the general population. Many of the cancers are mucinous adenocarcinomas. Usually, the cancer arises in a strictured segment of colon or in an area that had been previously bypassed at surgery.

Barrett's esophagus, prior cholecystectomy, and subtotal gastrectomy have also been associated with colon cancer development. No controlled trials have been performed to confirm these associations, and their relationship to colorectal cancer remains controversial.

5. Are there different histologic types of colon cancer?

The vast majority (95%) of colon cancers are adenocarcinomas. In "signet-ring cell" carcinomas, a variant of adenocarcinoma, mucin displaces the nucleus to one side, leaving a large vacuolated space. In a small number of adenocarcinomas, large lakes of mucin are found to contain scattered groups of tumor cells and are known as mucinous or colloid carcinomas. This latter group of tumors is associated with cancers that occur in younger patients, those with hereditary nonpolyposis tumors, and colon cancers occurring in ulcerative colitis. Scirrhous carcinomas of the colon are rare and are characterized by marked desmoplasia and fibrous tissue surrounding sparse glands.

The remaining 5% of colon cancers induce tumors that arise in the anorectum (squamous cell and tumors arising in transitional-zone cells) as well as primary lymphomas and carcinoid tumors.

6. What is the role of carcinoembryonic antigen in colon cancer?

Carcinoembryonic antigen (CEA) is a glycoprotein that is associated with cancer but not specific for neoplasia. Much controversy exists in the literature regarding the use of CEA in the diagnosis and management of colon cancer. Perhaps the best use of CEA in colon cancer is made when both pre- and post-operative levels are obtained. Studies have shown a correlation between high preoperative CEA levels and early tumor recurrence in patients with Duke's B and C stage disease. The CEA levels are usually not of any prognostic value except in stage C disease with four or more lymph nodes involved. Often, the CEA is used postoperatively to monitor recurrence but has a low predictive value in asymptomatic patients. The sensitivity for detecting Duke's A and B lesions is 36%. In Duke's C and D colon cancer, it is 74% and 83%, respectively, when using a cutoff value of 2.5 mg/ml. Because of the combined low sensitivity and specificity, it is inappropriate to use CEA as a mass screening tool.

7. How is colon cancer staged?

Traditionally, colon cancer has been staged with the classification originally developed by Cuthbert Dukes in 1929. The original system was based on the natural history of rectal cancers and has since been modified numerous times to include prognostic information regarding both the colonic and rectal cancers. The most commonly used modification of the Duke's staging classification is that of Turnbull and colleagues from 1967.

Duke's Turnbull Classification of Colorectal Cancer

STAGE	FINDING
A	Limited to mucosa
B	Tumor extension into pericolic fat
C	Regional nodal metastases
D	Distant metastases

The TNM (tumor-node-metastasis) classification for colon and rectal cancers was developed to bring these cancers into line with the classification systems for other solid organ tumors. In the

TNM system, Duke's A colon cancer corresponds to stage I, Duke's B corresponds to stage II, Duke's C to stage III, and Duke's D to stage IV.

TNM Classification of Colorectal Cancer

Stage 0	
Carcinoma in situ	Tis N0 M0
Stage I	
Tumor invades submucosa	T1 N0 M0
Tumor invades muscularis propria	T2 N0 M0
Stage II	
Tumor invades through muscularis propria into serosa or pericolonic, perirectal tissues	T3 N0 M0
Tumor perforates or directly invades other organs	T4 N0 M0
Stage III	
Any perforation with nodal metastases	
N1—1 to 3 nodes	Any T N1 M0
N2—4 or more nodes	Any T N2 M0
N3—Any nodal involvement along any named vascular trunk	Any T N3 M0
Stage IV	
Any invasion of bowel wall with or without lymph node metastasis but with evidence of distant metastasis	Any T Any N M1

8. What is the prognosis with the different stages and histologic subtypes of tumor?

The prognosis of colon cancer in those who undergo potentially curative resection correlates well with the Duke's stage. In stage C disease, the prognosis is greatly influenced by the number of cancerous lymph nodes found at surgery. Four or more nodes decreases the 5-year survival to 25%, whereas three or fewer nodes imparts a 55% 5-year survival rate. Tumor histology also plays a role in patient outcome. The more undifferentiated a tumor is, the worse the prognosis. Mucinous and scirrhous cancers are thought to be more aggressive than well-differentiated adenocarcinomas. Signet-ring cell cancers are usually found at an advanced stage and have a uniformly poor prognosis.

9. Can colon cancer be prevented? Does screening play an important role?

As with all community-based health problems, colon cancer prevention consists of both primary and secondary prevention. In primary prevention, the goal is to identify those at risk and to develop a strategy to reduce that risk. In secondary prevention, the goal is to identify disease at an early stage before it can seriously affect the health of the patient. Although much has been written regarding dietary factors in colon cancer, no hard and fast relationships exist. What is currently considered to be a healthy diet, high in fiber and low in fat, may decrease a person's risk for developing colon cancer.

A family history of colon cancer in at least one first-degree relative or a history of one of the colonic polyposis syndromes places one at increased risk for colon cancer and warrants early screening of these individuals.

The recommendations and techniques for mass screening for colon cancer remain controversial. The availability of screening varies from country to country. In the United States, the American Cancer Society recommends a yearly rectal examination in all persons over 40 years of age. Those over 50 should have stool examined for blood by testing three spontaneously evacuated stools with guaiac-impregnated cards. These individuals should also undergo flexible sigmoidoscopy every 3–5 years. Although the most cost-effective approach remains to be identified, screening for colorectal cancer has been shown to decrease mortality by detecting cancers at earlier stages as well as by allowing the removal of future cancers in the form of colonic adenomas.

10. How is colon cancer treated?

Unless the colon cancer is fortuitously resected at the time of polypectomy, the treatment of choice is surgical resection. The goal of the surgeon is to remove the affected bowel with wide (at least 5 cm) margins and also to remove the blood and lymphatic supply. Adjuvant chemotherapy with 5-fluorouracil and levamisole has been shown recently to be effective in decreasing recurrence and prolonging disease-free survival in patients with Duke's stage C disease. Chemotherapy for advanced disease (stage D) does not seem to offer any benefit to the patient regarding prolongation of life or disease-free intervals, and the resultant toxicity of therapy may lessen the remaining quality of life.

COLON POLYPS

11. What are colon polyps?

A mucosal protuberance into the lumen of the colon is defined as a colon polyp. The word *polyp* has its roots in ancient Greek, derived from *polypus,* which means many footed. This descriptive term is appropriate, as most polyps have many lobes. Histologically, colon polyps can be classified as neoplastic and nonneoplastic. The neoplastic group includes adenocarcinoma (cancer) and adenomas (dysplastic lesions that are not frank cancers).

The prevalence of adenomas is associated with increased age. Recent studies have shown that in healthy persons between age 50–82, there is a 23–41% prevalence rate of colorectal adenomas. Race and sex do not appear to be independent risk factors for adenoma formation. In those with a family history of colon cancer, up to 60% have been found to have adenomas on colonscopy. Family history of adenomatous polyps alone does not influence the prevalence of adenomas. Dietary factors such as a low-fiber diet, large quantities of red meat, cigarette smoking, and diets high in saturated fats have been associated with colon adenomas and colon cancer.

12. Are colorectal polyps precursors to colon cancer?

The predominant theory for many years was that adenomatous polyps left alone long enough would become colon cancers. Recently, the National Polyp Study has shown a definite relationship between adenomas and carcinomas and has given solid footing to the adenoma-to-carcinoma sequence. The few natural history studies that have been performed suggest that it takes at least 5 years, and more often 10 years, for a histologically proven adenomatous polyp to develop into colon cancer. Hyperplastic colorectal polyps impart no risk to the patient of eventual colon cancer.

13. What is the role of endoscopy in the treatment of colorectal polyps?

In Europe and the United States, colonic adenomas are found at autopsy in about 40% of persons over age 60. Individuals with one adenoma found at colonoscopy have a 40–50% chance of having synchronous adenomas. These patients are also at risk for developing adenomas in the future (20–30%). Air-contrast barium enema with flexible sigmoidoscopy and colonoscopy are the primary diagnostic tools used to locate polyps. Colonoscopy is the most sensitive and only therapeutic method available for the nonsurgical removal of colon polyps. According to data from the National Polyp Study, removal of all colonic adenomas reduces the future incidence of colon cancer. After the index colonoscopy has identified a colonic adenoma, follow-up must be individualized based on the difficulty of the procedure, incomplete examination, and a large number as well as on the histology of adenomas found at the time of the procedure. The accompanying table outlines the most recent management recommendations.

Recommendations for Colorectal Cancer Surveillance for the Average-Risk Patient

1. Age 40—Yearly digital rectal exam and fecal occult blood screen
2. Age 50—Sigmoidoscopic exam every 3–5 years in addition to 1
3. If 1 or 2 positive, then colonoscopy should be performed to rule out colonic disease. If colonoscopy is negative, then upper GI evaluation is appropriate.

14. What familial risk factors are associated with colonic polyps?

Because the adenoma-to-carcinoma sequence of polyp to cancer has been well established, it would make sense that familial risk factors that give rise to colorectal cancer play a role in polyp formation as well. Some hereditary forms of colon cancer have been identified other than the polyposis syndromes.

Hereditary nonpolyposis colorectal carcinoma (HNPCC) is characteristic of familial aggregation of colon cancers that behave in mendelian fashion. HNPCC can be further divided into the Lynch syndromes, which are composed of two types. Type I patients tend to have tumors in the proximal colon, are diagnosed at a younger age, and have a higher frequency of metachronous and synchronous lesions. These patients only have colonic neoplasms. In type II, the colorectal cancers are associated with an increased frequency of extracolonic neoplasms, mainly breast, gastric, and gynecologic tumors.

15. How should a malignant polyp be managed?

The initial management of a colorectal polyp depends on its size and whether it is pedunculated (on a stalk) or sessile (flat, not on a stalk). Polyps >2 cm have a markedly increased risk of containing cancer. Pedunculated polyps up to 4 cm can usually be managed by endoscopic removal. Large flat adenomas may require surgical excision.

Following endoscopic polypectomy, further management is dictated by the histologic findings. Patients with hyperplastic polyps can return to the average-risk screening group. Those with adenomas require individualized follow-up that should include colonscopy every 3–5 years. In the case of a malignant polyp where the polyp stalk is free of cancer, the patient should receive regularly scheduled follow-up that includes colonoscopy at 6 and 12 months, followed by colonoscopy each year for 2 years, and then colonoscopy at 3-year intervals.

BIBLIOGRAPHY

1. Doll R: Urban and rural factors in the etiology of colon cancer. Int J Cancer 47:803, 1991.
2. Dukes CE: The classification of cancer of the rectum. J Pathol 35:323, 1932.
3. Fuchs CS, et al: A prospective study of family history and the risk of colorectal cancer. N Engl J Med 331:25, 1994.
4. Kadakla SC: Colonic polyps: A review. Journal of the U.S. Army Medical Department. PB 8-94-1/2, 1994.
5. Metzler SJ, Ahnen DJ: Proto-oncogene abnormalities in colon cancers and adenomalous polyps. Gastroenterology 92:1174, 1987.
6. Nugent FW, et al: Cancer surveillance in ulcerative colitis. Gastroenterology 100:1241, 1991.
7. Ranshoff D, Lange C: Screening for colorectal cancer. N Engl J Med 325:37, 1991.
8. Sleisenger MH, Fordtran JS (eds): Gastrointestinal Disease, 5th ed. Philadelphia, W.B. Saunders, 1993.
9. Toribara NW, Sleisenger MH. Screening for colorectal cancer. N Engl J Med 332:861–867, 1995.
10. Weber CA, et al: Routine colonoscopy in the management of colorectal cancer. Am J Surg 152:87, 1986.
11. Winawer SJ, et al: Colorectal cancer screening. J Natl Cancer Inst 83:243, 1991.
12. Winawer SJ, et al: Prevention of colorectal cancer by colonoscopic polypectomy: The National Polyp Study Workgroup. N Engl J Med 329:1977–1981, 1993.

47. ACUTE AND CHRONIC MEGACOLON

Michael F. Lyons, II, M.D.

1. What is Ogilvie's syndrome?

Ogilvie's syndrome is acute nontoxic megacolon. This entity was first described in 1948, in two patients with metastatic cancer who developed massive dilatation of the cecum and right colon without evidence of more distal colonic obstruction or inflammation. Since that time, numerous other clinical situations have been described and attributed to this syndrome. An alternative term in the literature for Ogilvie's syndrome is **acute colonic pseudo-obstruction.** A distinction must be made between toxic and nontoxic megacolon, however. No infection or inflammation is seen with the latter, unless the colon becomes dilated to the point of inducing ischemic changes in the colonic wall. If this occurs, the patient may show signs more consistent with a toxic megacolon.

2. What is the clinical presentation of Ogilvie's syndrome?

The typical presentation for Ogilvie's syndrome is a postoperative patient who develops a distended abdomen. The patient is on, or recently weaned from, a ventilator. Although there tends to be minimal pain early, some associated nausea and vomiting occur in two-thirds of patients. Individuals typically do not have bowel movements unless in the form of diarrhea. Interestingly, one-half of patients continue to pass flatus. As the syndrome progresses, over 80% of individuals develop a mild, steady pain related to the distention. Bowel sounds are universally present and are often high pitched and quite active during the early phase of the condition. Patients often have a low-grade fever and left-shifted leukocytosis. Although the condition can normalize at any point, patients can proceed to a silent, rigid abdomen, perforation, sepsis, and death. Perforation rates are under 10%, but deaths occur in 15–30%. Of note, patients rarely die of their perforation; rather, death is related to multiorgan system failure.

3. What are the contributing factors of Ogilvie's syndrome?

The cause of Ogilvie's syndrome is not known. Numerous contributing factors have been attributed to its development. However, these factors, in and of themselves, do not cause Ogilvie's syndrome in the vast majority of patients, which suggests that factors other than those described must also be important. In the patients described by Ogilvie, there was **tumor invasion** of the celiac plexus, leading to interruption of the sympathetic innervation of the colon. This was presumed to cause loss of peristalsis and dilatation of the right colon. Most patients with acute nontoxic megacolon do not have intra-abdominal malignancy. Rather, most patients are in the immediate postoperative state, they often have multiorgan system disease, they are often on numerous medications that significantly alter bowel function, and many suffer multiple metabolic derangements that may be contributory.

Factors Associated with the Onset of Acute Nontoxic Megacolon (Ogilvie's Syndrome)

Recent surgery	Chronic obstructive lung disease
Recent general anesthesia	Underlying neurologic disorders
Medications	Diabetes
Congestive heart failure	Uremia
Underlying severe infections	Hip fracture
Electrolyte abnormalities	

4. List some of the medications associated with the development of Ogilvie's syndrome.

Medications Associated with Development of Acute Nontoxic Megacolon

TYPE OF MEDICATIONS	EXAMPLES
Nonsteroidal analgesics	Fenoprofen, naproxen, sulindac
Opiate analgesics	Meperidine, propoxyphene, morphine
Antidepressants	Amitriptyline, protriptyline
Antipsychotics	Thioridazine, chlorpromazine, clozapine
Antiseizure drugs	Phenobarbital, phenytoin
Antacid agents	Sucralfate, aluminum/calcium antacids
Calcium antagonists	Nifedipine, verapamil, felodipine
Cationic agents	Iron/calcium supplements, barium sulfate, bismuth salts
Antiparkinson agents	Procyclidine, benztropine
Ganglionic blockers	Trimethaphan
MAO inhibitors	Sertraline, bupropion, phenelzine
Other agents	General anesthesia, heavy metals (intoxication)

MAO = monoamine oxidase.

5. Does cecal diameter predict perforation in Ogilvie's syndrome?
No. Cecal perforation correlates poorly with cecal diameter. The cecum routinely dilates to 9 or 10 cm in normal individuals undergoing air-contrast barium enema studies. Reported series of perforation in patients with obstructed colons reveal a mean cecal diameter of 11 cm. In patients with Ogilvie's syndrome, cecums have perforated with diameters of <12 cm, and others have had an uncomplicated recovery with a cecal diameter up to 25 cm. One series showed an increase in cecal perforations with cecums above 14 cm in diameter in the setting of postoperative Ogilvie's syndrome. The rate and duration of cecal dilatation are important factors that suggest increased risk of perforation.

6. What is the treatment of acute nontoxic megacolon?
Because a patient with acute nontoxic megacolon is at risk for cecal perforation, aggressive measures must be implemented to prevent this catastrophe. All medications that could contribute to this situation should be discontinued immediately. The patient should have a nasogastric tube with suction placed and should be rotated in bed to assist in mobilizing colonic gas (or ambulated if possible). Measures to correct metabolic, electrolyte, fluid, and oxygenation abnormalities should be implemented.

Serial abdominal radiographs should be obtained every 8–12 hours to assess progression of cecal dilatation. If there is any suggestion of obstruction from more distal colonic lesions, such as volvulus, intussusception, mass, or diverticular disease, further evaluation with a carefully performed water-soluble contrast enema or colonoscopy is warranted. Colonoscopy can be used to decompress the colon immediately. Enemas (other than small-volume tapwater), oral laxatives, lactulose or other osmotic agents, metoclopramide, naloxone, and cholinergic agents (e.g., urecholine, neostigmine) have not been helpful and, in some cases, have been deleterious. If the patient has been on antibiotics for several days prior to the onset of symptoms, strong consideration should be made for pseudomembranous colitis. This diagnosis can be easily overlooked in patients in the intensive care setting who do not present with the typical blood-tinged diarrhea and left-lower-quadrant pain.

If these measures do not lead to clinical resolution of the megacolon or if progression of cecal dilatation is apparent, the patient should undergo colonic decompression endoscopically. Alternatively, radiologists also have decompressed the colon by fluoroscopically passing a wire-guided catheter. Surgical cecostomy should be considered if colonic distention continues or recurs despite endoscopic decompression. Direct percutaneous cecal decompression, a combined technique with radiology and colonoscopy, has also been successful.

7. What causes acute toxic megacolon?
Acute megacolon is a serious complication of **ulcerative colitis** or **Crohn's colitis** and can be life-threatening. The diagnosis of inflammatory bowel disease is almost never in question, as toxic

megacolon tends to be a late manifestation of advanced inflammatory bowel disease. Another cause of this entity is **pseudomembranous colitis.** This presentation is usually seen in a patient in the intensive care unit who has been on antibiotics for several days. The patient is often on a ventilator or in a coma and is unable to relate intestinal symptoms. **Typhlitis** can also be associated with acute toxic megacolon. Other reported causes of acute toxic megacolon are rare but include amebic colitis, cytomegalovirus colitis, typhoid fever, and bacillary dysentery. Finally, colonic ischemia can also present with megacolon and can be catastrophic if not recognized.

8. What is typhlitis?

Typhlitis is a necrotizing process involving the cecum in the setting of neutropenia. Although it was originally described in the setting of children undergoing chemotherapy for leukemia, additional cases have been described in adults undergoing chemotherapy for malignancy, immunosuppressive therapy for organ transplantation, drug induced neutropenia (not associated with malignancy), aplastic anemia, and cyclic neutropenia. Typhlitis may involve the terminal ileum, right colon, and appendix. This necrotizing process can be devastating. Following mucosal denudement (from unclear mechanisms), there is a bacterial invasion with ensuing necrosis, colonic dilatation, and perforation. Death rates are high (averaging 40–50% in series) and are typically due to the perforation.

9. How can one distinguish toxic from nontoxic acute megacolon?

The clinical situation is the best predictor of the various causes of toxic and nontoxic acute megacolon. Vigilant attention to history, medications, metabolism, and oxygenation status are key to establishing a diagnosis. Stool analysis positive for blood, leukocytes, and *Clostridium difficile* toxin are seen with various causes of acute toxic megacolon. If the patient has an associated neutropenia or leukemia, typhlitis must be considered. An abdominal radiograph will distinguish right colon and cecum from pancolonic dilatation. Acute toxic megacolon usually involves the entire colon in ulcerative colitis. Thumbprinting seen on the colonic radiograph can suggest ischemia. Likewise, loss of colonic haustral markings is typical of ulcerative colitis. Ulcerations on the colonic wall can be seen with cytomegalovirus, Crohn's disease, amebiasis, and bacillary infections.

10. What is the clinical presentation for acute toxic megacolon related to inflammatory bowel disease?

Toxic megacolon is the most severe and potentially life-threatening complication of ulcerative colitis. In the era prior to aggressive diagnostic colonoscopy and medical therapy for ulcerative coli-tis, toxic megacolon was not infrequently the initial presentation in patients. With a better understanding of diagnosis and treatment, it is now typically identified during the progression of chronic disease.

Patients usually present with a recent change in their bowel pattern related to their ulcerative colitis. Whereas some may have increased bleeding, the frequency of bowel movements may actually decrease in others. The patients complain of increased abdominal pain, bloating, and distention of the abdomen. They usually have a fever. Depending on the patient's stage of toxicity, there may be signs of hypotension, hypovolemia, and electrolyte abnormalities due to third-spacing of fluids and even mental status changes. There also will be tachycardia, left-shifted leukocytosis, and anemia. Patients have a low serum albumin. An abdominal radiograph will demonstrate a dilated colon, usually involving the entire colon, although in Crohn's disease and some cases of ulcerative colitis, segmental dilatation has been reported. The isolated cecal dilatation of acute nontoxic megacolon is almost never seen with acute toxic megacolon of inflammatory bowel disease. Colonic perforation, septic shock, and death are not rare complications, and in the setting of a very low serum albumin of <1.9 gm/dl, the mortality following perforation approaches 90%.

11. Describe the treatment of acute toxic megacolon associated with inflammatory bowel disease.

As can be seen from the preceding question, patients usually require a certain amount of resuscitation, including correction of fluid and electrolyte status. Blood transfusions may be required at the outset. The patient should be hospitalized and placed at bowel rest, initially including naso-gastric suction. Colonic decompression may be required, but this should be done with patient positioning rather than colonoscopic decompression. Intravenous steroids and antibiotics should be initiated. Central line placement followed by the implementation of parenteral nutrition is required if the patient does not respond rapidly to these measures. Narcotic analgesics and anticholinergic medications should be avoided. It should be remembered that steroids may mask a complication, so very close monitoring of the patient's physical examination, daily laboratory values, and serial abdominal radiographs is vital to assess the need for early surgery.

The timing for surgical intervention is controversial, as data demonstrate that perforation is associated with a very high mortality of up to 50%, and up to 90% if profound hypoalbuminemia is also present. Although there is not total agreement for the timing of surgical intervention, patients should be operated on immediately for colonic perforation, signs of peritonitis, signs of endotoxic shock, rapid clinical deterioration despite aggressive medical therapy, and massively dilated colon (as with acute nontoxic megacolon), especially in the setting of profound hypoalbuminemia (<1.9 gm/dl). If the patient is stabilized with medical management, then elective surgery can be considered, because most patients will relapse within the next several weeks to months. Timing of elective surgery should be between 1 and 4 weeks after medical stabilization, as surgical mortality rates are lowest during this time interval. There are no good clinical discriminators to predict relapse of the megacolon.

12. How is chronic megacolon best classified?

There are congenital and acquired forms of chronic megacolon. The **congenital forms** usually present in the neonatal period (Hirschsprung's disease). This familial disorder is caused by an aganglionosis of the rectum, beginning at the dentate line of the anus and extending variable lengths more cephalad. The length of colonic involvement dictates the clinical presentation: longer segmental disease leads to presentation shortly after birth, whereas very short segmental disease may present as late as adulthood. This had led to further classification of Hirschsprung's disease into **short segment** and **ultra-short segment.** Other variants involving more colon have also been described.

If patients who have a chronic nontoxic megacolon do not have one of the various forms of congenital megacolon, then it is presumed that the patient has an **acquired form.** Numerous causes have been ascribed to the development of chronic acquired megacolon. In some forms, such as idiopathic intestinal pseudo-obstruction, there appears to be a familial clustering with some patients, although it is unclear whether the disease is genetically or environmentally acquired.

Causes of Chronic Acquired Megacolon

Idiopathic (most common)
Amyloidosis
Parkinson's disease
Myopathic idiopathic intestinal pseudo-obstruction
Neuropathic idiopathic intestinal pseudo-obstruction
Muscular dystrophy
Chagas disease
Scleroderma
Diabetes
Psychogenic constipation
Porphyria
Pheochromocytoma
Hypothyroidism
Hypokalemia

13. Does a barium study of the colon help to sort out the various causes of acute and chronic megacolon?

Yes. The following algorithm outlines the classic findings of the various forms of acute and chronic megacolon that may assist in evaluating a patient with a dilated colon. The history usually helps to distinguish acute from chronic megacolon. Once history has been considered, the barium radiograph may be useful in developing a differential diagnosis of the megacolon. One must remember that various types of mechanical obstruction can cause a dilated colon, including volvulus, intussusception, mass, stricture, inflammatory bowel disease, ischemia, and diverticulitis.

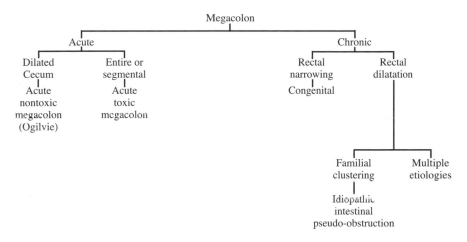

Algorithm for distinguishing nonobstructing types of megacolon.

BIBLIOGRAPHY

1. Barnes PRH, Lennard-Jones JE, Hawley PR, Todd IP: Hirschsprung's disease and idiopathic megacolon in adults and adolescents. Gut 27:534, 1986.
2. Faulk DL, Anuras S, Christensen J: Chronic intestinal pseudo-obstruction. Gastroenterology 74:922, 1978.
3. Fausel CS, Goff JS: Nonoperative management of acute idiopathic colonic pseudo-obstruction (Ogilvie's syndrome). West J Med 143:50, 1985.
4. Greenstein AJ, Sachar DB, Gibas A, et al: Outcome of toxic dilatation in ulcerative and Crohn's colitis. J Clin Gastroenterol 7:137, 1985.
5. Jalan KN, Sircus W, Card WI, et al: An experience of ulcerative colitis: I. Toxic dilation of 55 cases. Gastroenterology 57:68, 1969.
6. Nixon HH: Hirschsprung's disease: Progress in management and diagnostics. World J Surg 9:189, 1985.
7. Preston DM, Lennard-Jones JE, Thomas BM: Towards a radiologic definition of idiopathic megacolon. Gastrointest Radiol 10:167, 1985.
8. Schuffler MD, Rohrmann CA, Chaffee RG, et al: Chronic intestinal pseudo-obstruction: A report of 27 cases and review of the literature. Medicine 60:173, 1981.
9. Vanek VW, Al-Salti M: Acute pseudo-obstruction of the colon (Ogilvie's syndrome): An analysis of 400 cases. Dis Colon Rectum 29:203, 1986.

48. CONSTIPATION AND FECAL INCONTINENCE

R. Matthew Reveille, M.D.

CONSTIPATION

1. How is constipation defined?

The usual frequency of bowel elimination in western society ranges from 3 times per day to 3 times per week. Ninety-five percent of healthy individuals fall within this range of bowel habits. Constipation is defined as stools occurring <3 times per week (decreased frequency), straining at stool >25% of the time, elimination of hard pellet-like stool (scybala), or sense of incomplete evacuation after elimination. Symptoms persisting for >6 weeks continuously constitute chronic constipation.

2. How prevalent is constipation in western society?

Several population-based studies have used a questionnaire format to determine the prevalence of constipation. The average is 2%, but this rate increases after age 65, approaching 10% in patients over age 70. The prevalence of constipation has not changed appreciably in the last three decades. Constipation is more prevalent in individuals of lower socioeconomic status and black race. This symptom is one of the most common complaints encountered in adult medicine, approaching 10% in some practice settings. Economically, consumption of laxatives to relieve constipation symptoms cost over $350 million annually in the United States alone.

3. Describe the normal sequence of physiologic events that result in successful bowel evacuation.

The urge to defecate is triggered by activation of stretch mechanoreceptors in the rectal wall during distention by a fecal bolus propelled from the sigmoid reservoir. Responding to such an urge, an individual seeks a seated or squatting position. Simultaneous closure of the glottis and contraction of abdominal wall musculature (Valsalva maneuver) increase intra-abdominal pressure. Segmental contractions of the colon are inhibited, and feces is propelled toward the rectum. At the same time, pelvic floor musculature relaxes, the pelvic floor descends, and the puborectalis relaxes toward the sacrum, thereby opening the anorectal angle. Filling of the rectum prompts a

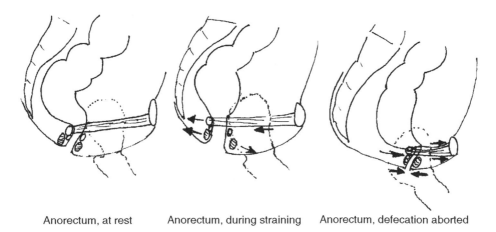

Anorectum, at rest   Anorectum, during straining   Anorectum, defecation aborted

Anorectal function during defecation. Arrows point in the direction of muscle relaxation and contraction during stages of defecation. During defecation, the anorectal angle opens and creates a funnel-type configuration to facilitate rectal emptying.

reflex inhibition of internal anal sphincter tone, and reflex and voluntary relaxation of the external anal sphincter permit expulsion of feces. Following evacuation, anal sphincter tone is restored, and contraction of the puborectalis and pelvic floor muscles restores the anorectal angle.

If the urge to defecate is deemed by the individual to be untimely or inconvenient, voluntary contraction of the puborectalis and external anal sphincters closes the anal canal tightly and sharpens the anorectal angle to pinch off the anal canal from the rectum. The rectum then has time to dilate and accommodate the fecal mass, thereby decreasing rectal wall tension and dissipating the urge to eliminate (see figure below). Such voluntary suppression of the defecatory urge may reflexively inhibit the propulsive movements of the sigmoid colon and restore the segmental, reservoir activity of this region within a few minutes of aborting defecation.

4. Outline the classification scheme for constipation disorders.

The simplest way to classify disorders causing constipation is to group them into intestinal and extraintestinal categories.

Intestinal Causes of Constipation

Organic obstruction of the colon	**Abnormalities of muscle function**
Extraluminal	Irritable bowel syndrome
Tumors	Diverticular disease
Chronic volvulus	Systemic sclerosis
Hernias	Dermatomyositis
Rectal prolapse	Myotonic dystrophy
Luminal	Segmental dilatation of the colon
Tumors	**Rectal disorders**
Strictures	Rectocele
Diverticulitis	Intussusception
Chronic amebiasis	**Anal disorders**
Lymphogranuloma venereum	Anal stenosis
Syphilis	Anal fissure
Tuberculosis	Anismus
Ischemic colitis	Puborectalis syndrome/levator syndrome
Endometriosis	Mucosal prolapse
Corrosive enemas	Anterior ectopic anus
Prior surgery	**Psychogenic constipation**
Radiation injury	(could be considered extraintestinal)
	Functional constipation
	Inadequate fiber intake
	Inadequate water intake
	Reduced physical activity/immobility

Extraintestinal Causes of Constipation

Neurogenic Etiology	
Peripheral nervous system	
Aganglionosis (Hirschsprung's disease)	**Central nervous system**
Hypo/hyper-ganglionosis	Medulla and cord
Ganglioneuromatosis	Cauda equina tumor
Primary	Meningocele
Von Recklinghausen's disease	Shy-Drager syndrome
Multiple endocrine neoplasia, type 2b	Tabes dorsalis
Autonomic neuropathy	Multiple sclerosis
Paraneoplastic	Brainstem trauma
Idiopathic pseudo-obstruction	Brain
Diabetic	Parkinson's disease
Chagas disease	Tumors
	Cerebrovascular accidents
	Alzheimer's disease
	Metabolic/endocrine etiology
	Drug-induced etiology
	Psychogenic/factitious etiology

5. In evaluating a patient's complaint of constipation, a careful medication history is important. List the classes of medications known to cause constipation.

Drugs Inducing Constipation

Opiates	Antihistamines
Anticholinergics/antispasmodics	Nonsteroidal anti-inflammatory drugs
Antidepressants	Diuretics
Anticonvulsants	Antacids (calcium and aluminum salts)
Antihypertensives (esp calcium channel blockers)	Iron, bismuth compounds
Antiparkinson agents	Laxatives (chronic use)

6. What metabolic disorders can give rise to constipation?

A variety of metabolic disorders can cause constipation. As part of the workup for chronic constipation, one should consider screening for and correcting the following where warranted:

Hypokalemia	Uremia
Hypercalcemia (any cause)	Porphyria
Hypo/hypermagnesemia	Pregnancy
Hypothyroidism	Diabetes mellitus (esp long-standing)
Pheochromocytoma	Glucagonoma

7. Is constipation a sign of serious gastrointestinal disease?

Most constipation is due to insufficient dietary intake of fiber and water or decreased caloric intake and therefore is functional and not serious. Acute constipation often occurs as a result of a sudden decrease in physical activity or immobility (e.g., during travel, hospitalization for surgery or other acute illness) and responds to fiber and water supplementation, judicious and temporary use of laxatives, and an increase in physical activity.

Constipation not responding to simple measures warrants further evaluation. The threshold for pursuing additional diagnostic testing depends on the history and circumstances surrounding the constipation complaint (i.e., rectal bleeding, weight loss, anemia) and the patient's age (colonic diseases increase with advancing age).

Specific and potentially serious colonic diseases should be considered (see question 4). Hirschsprung's disease (congenital aganglionosis) must be excluded if no structural cause for chronic constipation is found. Irritable bowel syndrome often has constipation as one of its principal features and is a diagnosis of exclusion after anatomic causes have been ruled out.

For all of these considerations, the minimum diagnostic evaluation should include a barium enema and flexible sigmoidoscopy. Colonoscopy may be indicated in certain circumstances, and surgical intervention may be warranted. In the occasional patient, a reasonable workup fails to disclose the cause of a significant and disabling constipation, and the problem is therefore termed **chronic idiopathic constipation.** Intractable idiopathic constipation accounts for no more than 1% of all patients with constipation.

8. What are the subtypes of chronic idiopathic (intractable) constipation?

Recent advances in the investigation of bowel function have divided chronic idiopathic constipation into three subtypes. **Colonic inertia** refers to a global prolongation in the time it takes to pass feces from cecum to rectum (transit time), presumably from diffuse neuromuscular dysfunction of the colon resulting in infrequent bowel elimination. This entity occurs almost exclusively in women and is of a **painless** variety.

Hindgut dysfunction is localized to a dysfunctional rectosigmoid segment. There appears to be a greater degree of antiperistalsis in this area in affected patients and increased electromyographic activity (increased nonperistaltic contractions) as compared with normal, nonconstipated individuals. Most patients with this subtype of constipation are, again, young women who complain of **painful** constipation.

Outlet obstruction (obstructed defecation) comprises a variety of anatomic and functional aberrations that produce symptoms of excessive straining at stool and sense of incomplete evacuation. Again, this type of chronic constipation occurs mostly in women.

9. What causes outlet-type constipation?

Four major categories of anorectal dysfunction which impair rectal emptying should be considered:

1. **Failure of rectal propulsion** is seen in idiopathic megarectum, radiation proctopathy, systemic sclerosis, and neuromuscular disease. Physiologic changes include impaired rectal sensation such that a larger volume of rectal contents is required to create a defecatory urge.

2. **Failure of internal anal sphincter relaxation** is seen in short-segment Hirschsprung's disease, where there is a loss of myenteric ganglia.

3. **Dysfunction of the puborectalis and/or external anal sphincter** has been termed anismus, dyschezia, spastic pelvis floor syndrome, or paradoxical puborectalis contraction. In essence, in response to straining, either there is failure of voluntary sphincter and pelvic floor muscle relaxation or a paradoxical contraction occurs during excessive straining, which prematurely closes off the anal outlet and aborts rectal evacuation, giving the individual a sense of incomplete evacuation. In most cases, this appears to be a learned phenomenon and responds to bowel retraining with biofeedback.

4. **Misdirection of propulsion** is seen in the setting of a rectocele, where intra-abdominal pressure is transmitted anteriorly against a weak rectal wall, causing pouching of the rectum and direction of feces into the pouch rather than through the anal canal. Partial or complete prolapse of the rectal wall or intussusception of the rectum upon itself results in partial evacuation of feces in the distal rectum, with entrapment of the remaining fecal bolus above the area of collapse, again resulting in incomplete evacuation. Bulking agents, bowel training with timed elimination, and sometimes surgery are often corrective.

10. What diagnostic tests are useful in characterizing the nature and subtype of chronic intractable constipation?

Two main categories of physiologic tests are used in the evaluation and management of chronic constipation. **Assessment of global and regional colonic transit** is done by a marker transit study. Simply, a patient ingests 20 radiopaque markers, and an abdominal x-ray is taken on day 5. At least 80% of the ingested markers should no longer be evident on the x-ray (i.e., they have been evacuated) if transit functions are normal. Persistent and scattered markers throughout the colon suggest a diffuse "colonic inertia" process. An abnormal number of markers localized to the rectosigmoid suggests hindgut dysfunction. Accumulation of markers in the rectum suggests outlet problems. Scintigraphic assessment of colonic transit correlates closely with radiopaque marker results but is not widely available.

Assessment of anorectal functions is accomplished by manometry with electromyography (EMG), balloon expulsion techniques, and defecation proctography. Manometry utilizes a pressure-recording catheter placed across the anal sphincter. Anorectal sensory thresholds and internal anal sphincter relaxation in response to balloon distention of the rectum can be determined with this method. Using concurrent surface electrode or needle EMG techniques with manometry, puborectalis/external anal sphincter dysfunction (failure of relaxation, paradoxical contraction) can be identified and can often be corrected with biofeedback and relaxation techniques. Defecography involves instillation of a barium-oatmeal paste into the rectum. The patient is then seated on a radiolucent commode and instructed to evacuate the rectal contents. This test assesses the completeness of rectal evacuation and demonstrates anatomic abnormalities, such as rectocele, mucosal prolapse, intussusception, and paradoxical pelvic floor motions. In selected circumstances, additional and highly specialized tests, such as pudendal nerve conduction studies and ultrasonography, may be employed.

11. Describe the various categories of laxatives with respect to their mechanism(s) of action.

Bulk-forming laxatives include a variety of vegetable fibers (psyllium), polysaccharides (polycarbophil), and cellulose derivatives. These agents are taken with 8 oz of fluid. In the gut, they swell to form emollient gels, which facilitate passage of intestinal matter and stimulate peristalsis. Onset of laxation is usually within 12–24 hours. The principal side effects of bulk laxatives are flatulence and bloating, a consequence of colonic bacterial fermentation of these substrates. They are contraindicated in patients with intestinal obstruction of any cause.

Emollient laxatives are anionic surfactants that lower fecal surface tension and facilitate mixture of aqueous and fatty substances to soften the stool. They also increase mucosal cyclic AMP in the small intestine and thus stimulate small bowel fluid and electrolyte secretion. These agents are not appreciably absorbed, but because they alter small bowel permeability, they can enhance the absorption of other medications. As a class of laxatives, they are of mild potency.

Osmotic laxatives are typically nondigestible disaccharides (lactulose, sorbitol). These disaccharides are hydrolyzed in the small intestine to organic acids, which lower luminal pH and provide osmotically active particles to stimulate intestinal fluid secretion and motility. They appear to be well tolerated, even in the elderly, unless the patient is lactase deficient. Side effects include bloating, flatulence, and diarrhea.

Saline laxatives contain relatively nonabsorbable cation/anion mixtures of sulfates, phosphates or citrates. Their onset of action is between 0.5 and 3 hours after oral ingestion. This group of agents exerts osmotic action on the small bowel and, through stimulation of cholecystokinin release, stimulate intestinal motility. The principal side effects are volume depletion and the potential for magnesium or phosphate toxicity. They are contraindicated in patients with renal insufficiency.

Lubricant laxatives, such as mineral oil, coat, penetrate, and soften feces and inhibit colonic water absorption. These are seldom used because of their potential for side effects, such as fat-soluble vitamin deficiency (A, D, E, K), lipoid pneumonia, and impaired drug absorption (e.g., warfarin).

Stimulant laxatives comprise a heterogeneous group of compounds, including castor oil, the anthraquinones, and diphenylmethanes. Anthraquinone laxatives include cascara, senna, and aloe. These drugs are hydrolyzed by colonic bacteria to active metabolites, which produce fluid and electrolyte accumulation in the colon and distal ileum. The diphenylmethanes include phenolphthalein and bisacodyl. These agents work by directly stimulating the myenteric plexus of the colon and by inhibiting water and glucose reuptake, which leads to increased luminal fluid accumulation. Onset of stimulants is usually 6–12 hours after oral intake and 15–60 minutes after rectal administration. Side effects include rashes, GI upset, melanosis coli, and, possibly, degeneration of the myenteric plexus with chronic use. Chronic use of this group of laxatives is responsible for the "cathartic colon."

FECAL INCONTINENCE

12. Fecal incontinence is a natural consequence of growing old. True or false?
False. There is no evidence that loss of bowel control is related to the aging process. A common misconception is that this disorder is a disease of the elderly, when in fact nearly one-half of all patients with fecal incontinence are middle-aged (ages 45–60). Nonetheless, fecal incontinence is the second most common reason for institutionalization of the elderly, after dementia. In ambulatory populations, this disorder causes significant psychological and physical disability and has medical and social implications. It contributes to social isolation, depression, loss of sexuality, and divorce.

13. What is the prevalence of fecal incontinence in the United States?
Nearly 3 million persons are estimated to have some degree of fecal incontinence. As many as 40% have combined urinary and fecal incontinence (double incontinence). Currently, over $400 million is spent annually in adult hygiene undergarments to manage incontinence problems.

14. Name the three main anatomic components of the continence mechanism and describe their innervation.
The pelvic floor is made up of the **levator ani complex,** which is innervated by the fourth sacral nerve root on its pelvic surface and the perineal branches of the pudendal nerve (S2–4) on its perineal surface. The **puborectalis** is innervated by S3–4 via the interior rectal nerve. The **anal**

sphincters comprise the internal anal sphincter, which is a continuation of the circular smooth muscle coat of the rectum, and the external and sphincter, which is actually made up of three skeletal muscle rings (deep, superficial, and subcutaneous). The internal anal sphincter is under autonomic control of the pelvic parasympathetics. The external anal sphincter is innervated on the perineal surface by branches of the pudenal nerves (S2–4).

15. What eight factors are responsible for maintaining bowel control?

1. Anal sphincter mechanism
2. Anorectal angle
3. Anorectal sensation
4. Rectal compliance

5. Rectosigmoid motility and evacuability
6. Colonic transmit
7. Stool volume and consistency
8. Awareness and motivation

16. Discuss the role of the anal sphincter mechanism in maintaining bowel control.

The anal sphincter has a mean pressure of 90 mm Hg, with a normal range of 50–120 mm Hg. It is greater in males than in females, and although it declines some with age, this decrease is not usually enough to cause incontinence without other factors. Anal sphincter tone is continuous throughout day and during sleep and is electrically silent during defecation. Recall that the internal anal sphincter is a continuation of the colonic circular smooth muscle and is therefore under

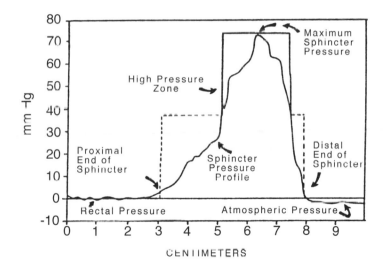

Anal sphincter pressure profile as assessed by manometry. Normal parameters for anorectal sphincter function are also given. (Adapted from Coller JA: Clinical application of anorectal manometry. Gastroenterol Clin North Am 16:17–33, 1987.)

Normal Parameters for Anorectal Sphincter Function

1. Mean maximal resting sphincter pressure—50–120 mm Hg
2. Anal sphincter length—4–6 cm
3. Minimal asymmetry in normals
4. RAIR threshold—begins at 10 ml, complete at 60 ml
5. Sensory threshold—5–10 ml (15 ml is acceptable in age >60)
6. Defecation urge threshold—80–100 ml
7. Painful urge threshold—120–250 ml
8. Squeeze pressure—double the resting pressure, >100 mm Hg, sustain for 40–60 sec
9. Post-squeeze overshoot—absent in normals
10. Pseudodefecation—appropriate relaxation of all sphincter components with rectal volume distention

autonomic and GI peptidergic control, and *not* under conscious control; its tone is responsible for 70–85% of resting sphincter tone. The external anal sphincter is skeletal muscle with a predominance of type I fibers which is under tonic contraction; it contributes most of the additional tone of the resting sphincter. The hemorrhoidal cushions contribute as much as 5% of the resting sphincter tone. In response to coughing, Valsalva maneuvers aside from defecation, and rectal distention, there is *automatic* contraction of the external anal sphincter and puborectalis to augment sphincter pressures to prevent leakage. A typical resting pressure profile of the anal sphincter is shown in the figure below.

17. How does sensory delay affect bowel control?

Anorectal sensation facilitates awareness of enteric contents being presented to the proximal anal canal ("sampling reflex"). The normal threshold for sensation is 5–10 ml of rectal volume, with a 15-ml threshold probably being normal for patients over age 60. Higher-than-normal thresholds for sensation of rectal filling imply neurologic injury. A delay between the time the internal anal sphincter reflexively relaxes (upon rectal distention) and an individual perceives rectal distention at the conscious level is termed **sensory delay** and is an important finding. Normally, there is almost instantaneous perception and therefore no sensory delay. Discovery of a sensory delay during manometric testing is indicative of neurologic injury, and this abnormality may account for up to 10% of incontinence complaints.

18. What is the normal urge threshold?

The rectum is very elastic and distends passively upon filling from above in order to keep intrarectal pressure lower than that of the anal canal. The threshold for normal urge to eliminate is 80–100 ml of rectal volume. Lower-than-normal urge suggests decreased rectal compliance or enhanced sensitivity (e.g., as in irritable bowel syndrome). Higher-than-expected urge threshold suggests increased compliance or a sensory neuropathy (e.g., multiple sclerosis). Dynamic and static rectal compliance can be measured, but the information is of limited clinical value at present.

19. Classify the etiologies of fecal incontinence according to how they affect the anatomical and functional components of the continence mechanism.

Classification of Etiologies of Fecal Incontinence

Abnormal anal sphincter or pelvic floor mechanism
Anatomic sphincter defect
  Traumatic
    Obstetric injury
      3rd or 4th degree tear
      Episiotomy wound complications
      Forceps injury
      Occult sphincter disruption
    Anorectal surgery
      Anal fissure/fistula surgery
      Hemorrhoidectomy
      Sphincterotomy
      Dilatation or stretching injury
      Foreign-body penetrating injury/laceration
  Neoplastic
  Inflammatory*
Pelvic floor denervation
  Primary ("idiopathic" neurogenic incontinence)
    Pudendal neuropathy*
    Chronic straining at stool
    Descending perineum syndrome
    Vaginal deliveries
  Secondary
    Injuries to spinal cord/cauda equina/pelvic floor nerves*

(Continued on next page)

   Diabetic neuropathy*
   Radiation-induced pelvic neuropathy*
   Other toxic/metabolic neuropathies*
  Congenital abnormalities
   Spina bifida
   Myelomeningocele
   Imperforate anus
  Miscellaneous
   Rectal prolapse (procidentia)
Inadequate anorectal sensation
  Neurologic conditions
   Dementia
   Cerebrovascular accidents
   Tabes dorsalis
   Multiple sclerosis
   Nervous system injuries
    Brain
    Spinal cord/cauda equina
   Neoplasms
    Brain
    Spinal cord/cauda equina
   Sensory neuropathies
    Diabetes*
   Radiation-induced neuropathy*
   Other toxic/metabolic neuropathies*
  Overflow incontinence
   Fecal impaction
   Encopresis
   Psychotropic drugs
   Antimotility drugs
Inadequate reservoir capacity or altered compliance
  Inflammatory bowel disease*
  Diverticular disease
  Absent rectal reservoir
   Sphincter-saving operations
    Low anterior resection
    Coloanal anastomosis
    Ileorectal anastomosis
    Ileoanal reservoir
  Rectal ischemia
  Rectal neoplasms
  Extrinsic rectal compression
  Collagen vascular disease
   Scleroderma
   Dermatomyositis
   Amyloidosis
  Radiation proctitis*
  Irritable bowel syndrome*
Altered stool consistency/diarrhea states
  Irritable bowel syndrome*
  Inflammatory bowel disease*
  Infectious diarrhea
  Laxative abuse
  Malabsorption syndromes (incl. short-bowel syndrome)
  Radiation enterocolitis

*Multiple mechanisms for incontinence in these disorders.

20. What important physical findings should one look for when evaluating a patient with fecal incontinence?

A careful and detailed anorectal assessment using inspection and the digital rectal exam can provide substantial information as to the nature of fecal incontinence. Inspection of the anal skin may reveal mucous or fecal soilage and **dermatitis.** The dermatitis is caused by skin irritation from bile acids in feces and implies incontinence of small amounts of liquids due to low resting tone or impaired sensation. Stroking the anal skin lightly should be perceived precisely as to location by a patient. A reflex contraction of the anal sphincters, the **anal wink,** should be present. Its absence suggests neurologic injury, often at the level of the spinal cord, particularly the sacral nerve roots.

On digital examination, the **resting tone** of the anal sphincter can be assessed, although it has been shown that digital assessment of anal sphincter tone by inexperienced examiners correlates poorly with manometric findings. The **length of the anal canal** can also be determined by the digital exam. A length of <2.5 cm is clear evidence of loss of muscle mass, from either previous trauma or surgery or due to atrophy from denervation. The **squeeze pressure** is assessed by having the patient contract the puborectalis and external anal sphincter. With contraction, the puborectalis can be felt moving anteriorly and craniad against the examining finger (toward the symphysis pubis). The external anal sphincter contracts circumferentially to "pinch off" the examining finger. Digital assessment can also detect **asymmetry** and defects in the continuity of the anal ring (local scarring, disruption, "keyhole" deformity), both in the resting state and during the squeeze maneuver. With **pseudodefecation,** the puborectalis should relax toward the coccyx. Paradoxical contraction or failure of relaxation should raise the suspicion of obstructed defecation or neurologic injury.

21. What diagnostic tests should be considered in evaluating a patient with fecal incontinence?

Following a detailed history and anorectal examination to determine the cause and mechanism(s) of a patient's fecal incontinence problem, most individuals should have a *flexible sigmoidoscopy*. This permits examination of the rectosigmoid to rule out tumors, strictures, inflammatory conditions (e.g., proctitis) and diverticular disease, for which specific treatments exist.

The next step is to institute a trial of a bulking agent to increase stool volume, absorb excess fecal water and mucus (to minimize residue for seepage), and promote complete rectal evacuation. Addition of loperamide enhances internal anal sphincter function to a modest degree and slows sigmoid emptying which, in turn, enhances colonic absorption of water from the stool, thereby aiding in firming the stool. Doses of 2–16 mg/day in divided doses can be used safely over extended periods in the management of fecal incontinence.

22. If fecal incontinence persists, which specialized tests can be ordered?

The gold standard for evaluation of refractory fecal incontinence is **anorectal manometry.** The test employs a pressure-recording catheter with a stimulating balloon(s) on its distal aspect to assess various aspects of anal sphincter function. After a single manometric examination, 10% of patients re-learn some aspects of their sphincter function (sensation, proper squeezing technique) and become continent once again.

In selected cases where the cause of the fecal incontinence cannot be determined precisely from the history, physical examination, and anorectal manometric studies, or when corrective surgery is contemplated, assessment of pudendal nerve function may be useful. The **pudendal nerve terminal motor latency** (PNTML) test determines the conduction velocity of the pudendal nerve, from its origin near the ischial spine in the pelvis to the anal sphincter, and the time required for a muscle response. The exam uses a specialized stimulating electrode affixed to a gloved examining finger which is connected to an electromyography (EMG) device. The origin of each pudendal nerve is palpated near the sciatic notch and ischial spine, an electrical stimulus is applied, and the electrical response is recorded by the EMG apparatus. A series of five stimuli per nerve are obtained and averaged, and a characteristic waveform is obtained. The time from the initial stimulus to the onset of the muscle response is termed the *latency*. The normal value for pudendal nerve latency is generally accepted as ≤2.1 msec.

Needle EMG is occasionally used to provide additional information about the degree of denervation or recovery of the external anal sphincter and puborectalis following injury. Detailed EMG mapping of the anal sphincter can identify portions of the sphincter amenable to surgical repair. **Anal endosonography** is a new technique that uses an ultrasound probe to identify areas

Algorithm for Evaluation and Treatment of Fecal Incontinence

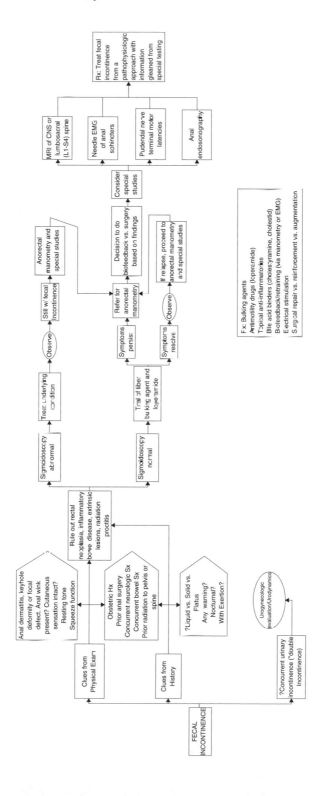

of sphincter disruption or extensive scarring following anal sphincter trauma, which should be considered for surgical repair.

23. What is the role of biofeedback in the treatment of fecal incontinence?

Biofeedback refers to techniques used to regain conscious and voluntary control over visceral functions (e.g., heart rate). With fecal incontinence, this term is a misnomer and should be abandoned in favor of **neuromuscular retraining.** In a patient who does not have a surgically correctable anatomic defect in the anal ring and who does not respond to stool bulking and antimotility drugs, retraining should be considered.

Retraining has been shown to aid in altering colonic function (restoring sigmoid capacity and reservoir functions), improving anal sensation (providing better warning signals), abolishing spontaneous relaxation of the internal anal sphincter (reducing spontaneous seepage and soilage), improving the strength and stamina of the external anal sphincter and puborectalis, and restoring automatic contraction of the voluntary sphincters during rectal filling. Patients with fecal incontinence from spinal cord or CNS diseases do not respond well to retraining. For most patients with the more common causes of fecal incontinence, 80–90% can achieve meaningful improvement in bowel control, and 60–70% can regain complete continence.

24. Outline the approach to diagnosis and treatment of the patient with fecal incontinence.
See algorithm on previous page.

BIBLIOGRAPHY

1. Arhan P, Devroede G, Jehannin B, et al: Segmental colonic transit time. Dis Colon Rectum 24:625–629, 1981.
2. Badiali D, Habib FI, Corazziari E, et al: Manometric and defaecographic patterns of straining. J Gastrointest Motil 3:171, 1991.
3. Bartolo DCC, Kamm MA, Kuijpers H, et al: Working party report: Defecation disorders. Am J Gastroenterol S154–S159, 1994.
4. Bassotti G, Chiarioni B, Vantini I, et al: Anorectal manometric abnormalities and colonic propulsive impairment in patients with severe chronic idiopathic constipation. Dig Dis Sci 39:1558–1564, 1994.
5. Bleijenberg G, Kuijpers HC: Treatment of spastic pelvic floor syndrome with biofeedback. Dis Colon Rectum 30:101–111, 1987.
6. Buser WD, Miner PB: Delayed rectal sensation with fecal incontinence: Successful treatment using anorectal manometry. Gastroenterology 91:1186, 1986.
7. Camilleri M, Thompson WG, Fleshman JW, Pemberton JH: Clinical management of intractable constipation. Ann Intern Med 121:520–528, 1994.
8. Deen K, Kumar D, Williams JG: The prevalence of anal sphincter defects in faecal incontinence: A prospective endosonic study. Gut 34:685–688, 1993.
9. DeLancey JOL: Childbirth, continence, and the pelvic floor. N Engl J Med 329:1956, 1993.
10. Duthie GS, Bartolo DCC: Anismus: The cause of constipation? Results of investigation and treatment. World J Surg 16:881–835, 1992.
11. Enck P: Biofeedback training in disordered defecation: A critical review. Dig Dis Sci 38:1953, 1993.
12. Jacobs PPM, et al: Obstetric fetcal incontinence: Role of pelvic floor denervation and results of delayed sphincter repair. Dis Colon Rectum 33:494, 1990.
13. Jones PN, Lubowski DZ, Swash M: Is paradoxical contraction of puborectalis muscle of functional importance? Dis Colon Rectum 30:667–670, 1987.
14. Jorge JMN, Wexner SD: Etiology and management of fecal incontinence. Dis Colon Rectum 36:77, 1993.
15. Kamm MA, Lennard-Jones JE: Constipation: Pathophysiology. In Henry MM, Swash M (eds): Coloproctology and the Pelvic Floor. Oxford, Butterworth-Heinemann, 1992, pp 411–412.
16. MacLeod JH: Management of anal incontinence by biofeedback. Gastroenterology 93:291, 1987.
17. Metcalf AM, Phillips SF, Zinsmeister AR, et al: Simplified assessment of segmental colonic transit. Gastroenterology 92:40–47, 1987.
18. Miller R, et al: Prospective study of conservative and operative treatment for fecal incontinence. Br J Surg 75:101, 1988.
19. Miner PB: Fecal incontinence. In Bayless TM (ed): Current Therapy in Gastroenterology and Liver Disease, 3rd ed. Philadelphia, B.C. Decker, 1990, pp 363–369.
20. Oliver GC: Clinical examination. In Smith LE (ed): Practical Guide to Anorectal Testing. New York, Igaku-Shoin, 1990, pp 11–15.

21. Orrom WJ, et al: Comparison of anterior sphincteroplasty and postanal repair in the treatment of idiopathic fecal incontinence. Dis Colon Rectum 34:305, 1991.

22. Pearl RK: Anatomy of the pelvic floor, rectum and anal canal. In Smith LE (ed): Practical Guide to Anorectal Testing. New York, Igaku-Shoin, 1990, pp 1–10.

23. Pemberton JH: Anorectal and pelvic floor disorders: Putting physiology into practice. J Gastroenterol Hepatol 1:127, 1990.

24. Pemberton JH, Rath DM, Ilstrup DM: Evaluation and surgical treatment of severe chronic constipation. Ann Surg 214:403–411, 1991.

25. Pescatori M, Pavesio R, Anastasio G, Daini S: Transanal electrostimulation for fecal incontinence: Clinical, psychologic, and manometric prospective study. Dis Colon Rectum 34:540–545, 1991.

26. Preston DM, Lennard Jones JE: Anismus in chronic constipation. Dig Dis Sci 30:413–418, 1985.

27. Speakman CTM: Abnormalities of innervation of internal and sphincter in fecal incontinence. Dig Dis Sci 38:1991, 1993.

28. Sultan AH, Kamm MA, Hudson CN: Pudendal nerve damage during labour: Prospective study before and after childbirth. Br J Obstet Gynaecol 101:22–28, 1994.

29. Sultan AH, et al: Anal sphincter disruption during vaginal delivery. N Engl J Med 329:1905–1911, 1993.

30. Sun WM, Donnelly TC, Read NW: Utility of combined test of anorectal manometry, electromyography, and sensation in determining the mechanism of 'idiopathic' faecal incontinence. Gut 33:807–813, 1992.

31. Wald A: Colonic and anorectal motility testing in clinical practice. Am J Gastroenterol 89:2109–2115, 1994.

32. Wald A: Disorders of defecation and fecal continence. Cleve Clin J Med 56:491, 1989.

33. Wald A, Caruana BJ, Friemanis MG, et al: Contributions of evacuation proctography and anorectal manometry to evaluation of adults with constipation and defecatory difficulty. Dig Dis Sci 35: 481–487, 1990.

34. Wald A: Disorders of anorectal motility. Pract Gastroenterol 17:28, 1993.

35. Wexner SD, Cheape JD, Jorge JM, et al: Prospective assessment of biofeedback for the treatment of paradoxical puborectalis contraction. Dis Colon Rectum 35:145–150, 1992.

36. Whitehead WE, Devroede G, Habib FI, et al: Functional disorders of the anorectum. Gastroenterol Int 5:92–108, 1992.

49. DIVERTICULITIS

Stephen R. Freeman, M.D.

1. How common is diverticular disease, and how frequent are complications?
One-third of the western population has diverticulosis by age 50, and two-thirds by age 80. Most remain asymptomatic, with complications of bleeding or diverticulitis occurring in 10–20%.

2. How do diverticula develop?
Though not known for certain, the presence of diverticula has been correlated with a decrease in dietary fiber; other related factors are aging and increased intraluminal pressure. Decreased fiber in the colonic lumen leads to a decreased stool volume, which results in more colonic segmentation during peristaltic activity in propelling contents aborally. Segmentation generates greater intraluminal pressures. The increased intraluminal pressure may predispose to diverticula formation. Each diverticulum is a result of herniation of mucosa through the muscular colonic wall at points of weakness, which correspond to sites of penetrating arteries.

3. Where are diverticula located?
In western society, 85% of diverticula are located in the **sigmoid colon.** The sigmoid colon is smaller in luminal diameter, and therefore, wall tension during segmentation and intraluminal pressures are greater and probably responsible for diverticula formation. Additionally, the use of western-style toilets results in increased intraluminal pressures compared to defecation performed in the knee-chest position common in third world countries, where the incidence of diverticulosis is much less. Interestingly, because diverticula are site-specific to the right colon in Asians, other factors must also be important, such as genetics and environmental factors. As western-style diets begin to permeate the nonwestern cultures, the incidence of diverticulosis increases, as does the incidence of their left-sided location.

4. What are the common signs and symptoms of diverticulitis?
The most common symptoms are the abrupt onset of abdominal pain and an alteration in bowel pattern. Early acute diverticulitis is characterized by circumscribed abdominal pain and tenderness. The usual location of the pain is the left lower quadrant, but because diverticula, and hence diverticulitis, can develop at any site, inflammation may mimic other conditions. Transverse colon diverticulitis may mimic peptic ulcer disease, for instance, and right colon diverticulitis may mimic acute appendicitis. Signs of inflammation, such as fever and elevated white blood count, help distinguish diverticulitis from the spasm of irritable bowel syndrome.

As the disease progresses in severity, localized abscess and phlegmonous reaction may occur. In addition to pain and tenderness, a mass may develop. Systemic signs of infection become more pronounced, i.e., fever and leukocytosis.

In the elderly and in patients on corticosteroids, the abdominal exam and usual signs are unreliable. Therefore, a high index of suspicion and use of imaging studies, such as CT scan, are important in avoiding a significant delay in diagnosis.

Obstipation has long been taught as a symptom of diverticulitis, but, in fact, diarrhea is not uncommon. Rectal bleeding is not a symptom of diverticulitis. Other causes, such as hemorrhoids, neoplasm, colitis, arteriovenous malformations, or arterial bleeding from diverticulosis, should be considered if bleeding is the problem.

5. Outline the approach to the evaluation and diagnosis of acute diverticulitis, including physical examination and diagnostic procedures.
- **CLINICAL**
  History and physical examination
  Usually >60 years old

LLQ localized tenderness and unremitting abdominal pain
Fever
Leukocytosis
- **DIFFERENTIAL DIAGNOSIS**
  Elderly
Ischemia	Obstruction
Carcinoma	Penetrating ulcer
Volvulus	Nephrolithiasis/urosepsis

  Middle-Aged and Young
Appendicitis	Penetrating ulcer
Salpingitis	Urosepsis
Inflammatory bowel disease	
- **QUALIFIERS**
  Extremes of age (more virulent)
  Oriental ancestry (right-sided symptoms)
  Corticosteroids
  Immunosupression
  Chronic renal failure (abdominal examination insensitive)
- **EVALUATIONS**
  Plain x-rays: Good initial first step. May show ileus, obstruction, mass effect, ischemia, perforation.
  Contrast enema: For mild to moderate cases of diverticulitis when the diagnosis is in doubt, water-soluble contrast exam is safe and helpful; otherwise, delay the exam for 6–8 weeks.
  Endoscopy: Acute diverticulitis is a relative contraindication to endoscopy; must exclude perforation first. Examine only when the diagnosis is in doubt (rectal bleeding, anemia) to exclude ischemic bowel, Crohn's disease, carcinoma, etc.
  CT scan: Very helpful in staging the degree of complications and evaluating for other diseases. Should be considered in all cases of diverticulitis with a palpable mass or clinical toxicity, failure of medical therapy, orthopedic complications, and corticosteroid use. The **test of choice** to evaluate acute diverticulitis in most centers.
  Ultrasound: Can be a safe and helpful noninvasive test to evaluate acute diverticulitis. Over 20% of exams are suboptimal due to intestinal gas; very operator-dependent.

Adapted from Freeman SR, McNally PR: Diverticulitis. Med Clin North Am 77:1152, 1993.

6. What complications of diverticulitis can occur?

Fistula, abscess, obstruction, and peritonitis from perforation are the common complications of diverticulitis.

7. Between what organs may fistulous communications develop?

Bowel, urinary bladder, skin, pelvic floor, and vagina are the areas involved in fistulous disease of diverticulitis. The most common is **colovesicular fistula** (colon to urinary bladder) and is seen almost exclusively in men and in women after hysterectomy. Pneumaturia is a pathognomonic sign of this fistula. Another clue to its presence is recurrent urinary tract infections, especially involving multiple organisms. Demonstration of the fistulous connection is difficult usually. Reflux of contrast through the fistula via contrast enema or cystogram confirms the diagnosis, but such reflux is seen in a minority of patients. Colovesicular fistula represents a strong indication for surgical correction.

Colovaginal fistulae occur almost exclusively in women with prior hysterectomies. A differential diagnosis includes Crohn's disease, previous pelvic irradiation, gynecologic surgery, and pelvic abscess from any cause. Diagnosis is suspected in the proper setting (recent diverticulitis) because of the presence of vaginal symptoms: vaginal discharge, severe vaginitis, flatus vaginalis, and feculant discharge (pathognomonic). Identification of the fistula can be difficult. Barium enema, oral charcoal, vaginography, and combined vaginoscopy and colonoscopy are various means of attempting to localize the fistula. Treatment for colovaginal fistula is a surgical resection of the diseased section of bowel.

8. How is a diverticular stricture differentiated from strictures of other causes?
The signs of a stricture indicating diverticulitis as a cause are the presence of diverticula in the region of the colonic stricture, the suggestion of an extraluminal mass contributing to the stricture, and the suggestion of an intramural or extraluminal extravasation of contrast.

The length of the stricture is helpful, with diverticular strictures usually being longer than malignant strictures. Whereas a **malignant stricture** is usually <3 cm in length and is associated with abrupt shoulders at either end, the **diverticular stricture** is longer, 3–6 cm in length, with smoother contours. Very long strictures, 6–10 cm in length, are more likely to be due to **Crohn's disease** or **ischemia.**

Sometimes, the location of the stricture is helpful in distinguishing its cause. For example, the splenic flexure is an uncommon site for diverticulitis but a common site for ischemia.

9. Extraintestinal complications are known to be associated with inflammatory bowel disease. Are there any extraintestinal complications associated with diverticulitis?
Interestingly, arthritis and pyoderma gangrenosum have been reported in three patients by Klein and coworkers. Resection of the involved colon was effective in eliminating these problems in all patients. All were incorrectly diagnosed as having inflammatory bowel disease originally.

The orthopedic complication of leg pain, possibly associated with thigh abscess or leg emphysema, due to retroperitoneal perforation from diverticulitis has been reported. The 70% mortality associated with this complication is probably due to delayed diagnosis and inadequate treatment. Treatment must include fecal diversion and wide surgical debridement, as well as broad-spectrum antibiotics.

There is an association between diverticulosis and renal disease. Patients who are post-renal transplant, on chronic hemodialysis or peritoneal dialysis, or who have polycystic kidney disease are much more susceptible to life-threatening complications of diverticulitis. Immunosuppression is part of the reason for this. In patients being considered for renal transplantation or continuous ambulatory peritoneal dialysis (CAPD), surgical resection of the involved colon perhaps should be done beforehand, if there has been symptomatic diverticulitis previously.

10. Are any drugs known to exacerbate diverticulitis?
Corticosteroids in high dose have been associated with the development of acute diverticulitis. Whether there is actually a cause-and-effect relationship is debatable, but inhibition of epithelial cell renewal has been hypothesized. Clearly, high-dose steroids may mask the usual signs and symptoms of diverticulitis, leading to a delay in diagnosis.

Nonsteroidal anti-inflammatory drugs also have been associated with more severe diverticulitis. Again, the masking of early signs and symptoms has been hypothesized as the likely reason for this association.

11. What diagnostic tools are available to the clinician to diagnose diverticulitis, and what is the role of each?
Besides clinical and laboratory evaluation, imaging studies play an important role in diagnosis of diverticulitis. Contrast enema, abdominal CT scan, ultrasonography, and endoscopy are all modalities with some role.

Contrast enema might aggravate the disease and prove more harmful than helpful, but several studies have confirmed that this study can be performed safely and prove useful. Because extravasation of barium might worsen peritonitis, water-soluble contrast is favored by many.

Computed tomography (CT) has emerged as the test of choice in the diagnostic evaluation of complicated diverticulitis. It offers the advantage of providing extraluminal information and aids in identifying patients with nondiverticular causes of their symptoms, such as ischemic colitis, mesenteric thrombosis, tubo-ovarian abscess, and pancreatitis. CT criteria used in the diagnosis of acute diverticulitis are localized colonic wall thickening (>5 mm) and inflammation of pericolonic fat or the presence of pericolic abscess.

Abdominal and pelvic **ultrasonography,** in the hands of experienced radiologists, is also a helpful test, with a sensitivity and specificity of 84% and 80%, respectively. Findings by ultrasound are similar to those of CT scan. Wall thickening, inflammation of pericolic fat, intramural and extraintestinal masses, and, occasionally, intramural fistula are supportive findings in the diagnosis of diverticulitis.

Endoscopy is generally felt to be contraindicated in acute diverticulitis due to the fear that scope manipulation and air insufflation might worsen diverticular perforation and subsequent abscess or peritonitis. However, in cases in which the diagnosis is unclear and the differential includes obstructing carcinoma, ischemia, inflammatory bowel disease, and infectious colitis, endoscopy can be very helpful. When performed, the examination should be done very carefully by an experienced endoscopist, with minimal air insufflation and no "slide-by" maneuvers of tight angulations. Findings suggestive of diverticulitis include peridiverticular erythema, edema, and pus.

12. How is mild diverticulitis defined and treated?

Mild diverticulitis is considered if a patient has appropriately localized abdominal pain, usually in the left lower quadrant; fever and/or leukocytosis is usually present. The patient is nontoxic and is able to take food and fluids orally without vomiting. Qualifying factors to consider include age, underlying medical conditions, and concurrent medications. Diverticulitis tends to be more

A Guide to Antimicrobial Therapy in Acute Diverticulitis

MODIFYING CIRCUMSTANCES	ETIOLOGY	FIRST CHOICE	ALTERNATIVE	COMMENT
Mild, nonperforating, with no high-risk factors	Aerobes	TMP/SMX+	Ciprofloxacin or cephalexin	Outpatient, oral
	Escherichia coli *Klebsiella* sp.	Metronidazole	for TMP/SMX Clindamycin for metronidazole	
	Streptococus *Proteus* sp. *Enterobacter* sp. Anaerobes *Bacteroides fragilis* *Peptostreptococcus* *Peptococcus* *Clostridium*			
Moderately ill, possible local abscess, ± high-risk factors	Same including *Pseudomonas aeruginosa*	Ampicillin + Aminoglycoside + Metronidazole	Ciprofloxacin + metronidazole	Inpatient, IV + CT (catheter drainage of abscess)
		Imipenem/cilastatin Ampicillin/ sulbactam Celoxitin Ticarcillin/ clavulanate		Consider surgery
Severely ill, toxic, peritonitis	Same including *Pseudomonas aeruginosa*	Same	Same	Inpatient, IV + CT Consider early surgery

From Freeman SR, McNally PR: Diverticulitis. Med Clin North Am 77:1161, 1993; with permission.

virulent in the young (<40 years) and very old. Immunocompromised patients, such as post-transplant or with chronic renal failure or diabetes mellitus, are also at high risk for more virulent disease, which might be more serious than it first appears. Also, patients with right-sided diverticulitis tend to do less well. Mild disease is defined by a lack of factors placing the patient at higher risk.

Treatment of mild disease is generally done on an outpatient basis. Diet is commonly modified to one of clear liquids, more by convention than proof of efficacy. Antibiotic choice is commonly oral trimethoprim/sulfamethoxazole (TMP/SMX) plus metronidazole. Ciprofloxacin or cephalexin may be substituted for TMP/SMX, and clindamycin for metronidazole. Coverage is aimed at aerobic gram-negative organisms, and usually anaerobic coverage is also added.

13. What antibiotic regimen is appropriate for moderately severe disease, and how is treatment otherwise different?

Antibiotics are usually given intravenously, most often on an inpatient basis. Many combinations are appropriate. Classically and historically, ampicillin, an aminoglycoside, and metronidazole are used. Other choices might be imipenem/cilastatin, ampicillin/sulbactam, cefoxitin, or ticarcillin/clavulanate. Ciprofloxacin plus metronidazole is available as a second choice. One goal of coverage for more severe disease is to cover *Pseudomonas aeruginosa*.

An additional management issue in moderately severe disease, which usually includes the possibility of abscess, is imaging. CT scan or ultrasound is often done, and if localized abscess is found, drainage by percutaneous catheter considered. Surgery for abscess drainage and definitive resection are also a consideration.

14. How is the management of the severely ill patient different?

The severely ill patient is usually toxic with signs of peritonitis. The main difference in treatment from those patients with less serious disease is the threshold for surgery. In the toxic patient, an imaging study, such as CT scan, might be helpful in directing treatment, but early operation is often prudent and the action most likely to result in a favorable outcome.

15. What operations are available in the management of diverticulitis?

Surgical management involves resection of the diseased segment of colon. The surgery may involve abscess drainage and fecal diversion. Surgery, with those measures, may be done in one, two, or three stages (see figure on p. 337).

16. What are the indications for surgery for diverticulitis?

Surgery is indicated for complications of diverticulitis, such as sepsis, fistula formation, and obstruction. Patients with recurrent episodes of diverticulitis are candidates for surgery, as are those who fail medical therapy or who deteriorate during original treatment. Occasionally, patients with a colonic stricture that cannot be shown convincingly not to be cancer are candidates for resection. The threshold for surgery is modified by the presence of higher risk factors: extremes of age, patients on steroids or who are immunocompromised, and patients with right-sided diverticulitis.

17. What are the preferred operations for diverticulitis?

The ideal and preferred situation for a patient requiring surgery for diverticulitis is to have a **single operation**, at which time the diseased bowel is resected and the remaining colon is anastomosed to maintain normal continuity. Examples of clinical scenarios where this operation can be done would be surgery for chronic obstruction, intractable pain, or recurrent episodes of diverticulitis, that are medically responsive. In these cases, surgery is elective, allowing a thorough bowel preparation prior to surgery.

Not uncommonly, a **two-stage procedure** is needed in cases in which a bowel preparation cannot be done beforehand. This approach is usually for medically unresponsive disease. A diverting colostomy is created as the diseased bowel segment is removed. Either a mucous fistula is created with the distal colonic segment, or it is oversewn and placed back in the abdomen (Hartmann's pouch). Later (3–6 months), a second operation is performed to reestablish bowel continuity.

In severely ill patients, a **three-stage procedure** is used. The initial operation is simply

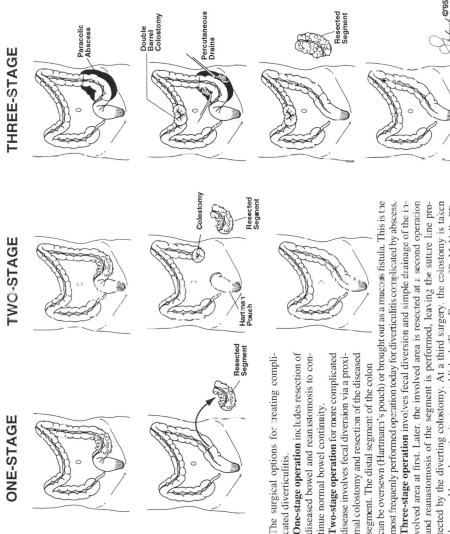

The surgical options for treating complicated diverticulitis.

One-stage operation includes resection of diseased bowel and reanastomosis to continue normal bowel continuity.

Two-stage operation for more complicated disease involves fecal diversion via a proximal colostomy and resection of the diseased segment. The distal segment of the colon can be oversewn (Hartmann's pouch) or brought out as a mucous fistula. This is the most frequently performed operation today for diverticulitis complicated by abscess. **Three-stage operation** involves fecal diversion and simple drainage of the involved area at first. Later, the involved area is resected at a second operation and reanastomosis of the segment is performed, leaving the suture line protected by the diverting colostomy. At a third surgery, the colostomy is taken down and bowel continuity is reestablished. (From Freeman JR, McNally PR: Diverticulitis. Med Clin North Am 77:1149–1167, 1993, with permission.)

drainage of the pericolonic abscess and creation of a diverting colostomy. A second operation in 2–8 weeks is done to resect the diseased bowel, with reanastomosis of the bowel and maintenance of the colostomy to protect the anastomosis. A third surgery is performed in 2–4 weeks to take down the colostomy and restore bowel continuity.

The three-stage approach was the standard operative management for much of the 20th century. Large reviews in the past 20 years have pointed out the considerably reduced mortality and morbidity associated with the two-stage approach. The mortality for the two-stage procedure is 1–12%, whereas that for the three-stage approach is 12–32%. The two-stage approach is now the procedure of choice for perforated diverticulitis.

BIBLIOGRAPHY

1. Almy, TP, Howell DA: Medical progress; Diverticular disease of the colon. N Engl J Med 302:324–331, 1980.
2. Freeman SR, McNally PR: Diverticulitis. Med Clin North Am 77:1149–1167, 1993.
3. Greenall MJ, Levine AW, Nolan DT: Complications of diverticular disease: A review of the barium enema findings. Gastrointest Radiol 8:353–358, 1983.
4. Klein S, Mayer L, Present DH, et al: Extraintestinal manifestations in patients with diverticulitis. Ann Intern Med 108:700–702, 1988.
5. Mendeloff AI: Dietary fiber and gastrointestinal disease. Med Clin North Am 62:165–171, 1978.
6. Mendeloff AI: Thoughts on the epidemiology of divertivcular disease. Clin Gastroenterol 15:855–877, 1986.
7. Painter NS, Burkitt DP: Diverticular disease on the colon: A deficiency disease of western civilization. BMJ 2:450–454, 1971.
8. Reve RV, Nahrwold DL: Diverticular disease. Curr Prob Surg 26:136, 1989.
9. Roberts PL: Current management of diverticulitis. Adv Surg 27:189–208, 1994.
10. Smith TR, Cho KC, Morehouse HT, et al: Comparison of computed tomography and contrast enema evaluation of diverticulitis. Dis Colon Rectum 33:1–6, 1990.
11. Woods RJ, Lavery IC, Fazio VW, et al: Internal fistulas in diverticular disease. Dis Colon Rectum 31: 591–596, 1988.

50. DISEASES OF THE APPENDIX

Theodore R. Schrock, M.D.

1. Is any age group free from the possibility of developing acute appendicitis?
No. All ages are affected, but the peak incidence of acute appendicitis is between 15 and 19 years. From 7–12% of people in western countries develop this condition at some time during their lives. Appendicitis is 1.3–1.6 times more common in males than in females. More important than any of these statistics, however, is recognition that every patient with acute abdominal pain, regardless of age, may have appendicitis.

2. What is meant by simple, gangrenous, and perforated appendicitis?
These terms are a sort of staging system. **Simple** appendicitis is an inflamed appendix that is viable and intact. **Gangrenous** appendicitis has focal or extensive necrosis of the wall, and microscopic perforation is often present. **Perforated** appendicitis implies a grossly disrupted appendix. The risk of postappendectomy wound infection is lowest in simple appendicitis; gangrenous and perforated appendicitis have a similar and much higher risk of this complication.

3. How does acute appendicitis usually develop?
Obstruction of the lumen by fecaliths, viscid fecal masses, calculi, tumors, parasites, or foreign bodies is the primary event in most patients, and bacterial infection is secondary. When the lumen is obstructed, mucosal secretion of fluid continues until the intraluminal pressure reaches 85 cm H_2O; at this point, intraluminal pressure exceeds venous pressure, and the appendiceal mucosa becomes ischemic. Mucosal ulceration permits bacterial invasion of the wall, which leads to thrombosis of small vessels and further ischemia.

Primary infection by viruses, parasites, or bacteria is the probable cause of appendicitis in a few people. Some cases are unexplained.

4. What is the first symptom of classic acute appendicitis?
Pain is the first symptom in nearly every case. This is so universally true that if some other symptom comes first in acute abdominal illness, one should suspect a different diagnosis. The initial pain is visceral—vague or colicky—and is referred from the appendix to other sites. It is localized in the epigastrium or periumbilical area or generalized in the abdomen. Rarely, initial pain is in the right lower quadrant at the onset.

The initial pain typically reaches peak intensity in about 4 hours and then subsides, only to reappear in the right lower quandrant as a progressively severe ache that is worsened by movement. This second type of pain is due to inflammation of periappendiceal tissues and is therefore somatic. The **shift of pain** from initial visceral discomfort in the mid or upper abdomen to a steady pain in the right lower quadrant is an important diagnostic clue when it is present.

Anorexia, nausea, and/or vomiting occur after the onset of pain in 95% of patients. Low-grade fever is present also.

5. Define direct tenderness. Rebound tenderness. Referred tenderness.
Remember that pain is a symptom, and tenderness is a sign. Symptoms are noted by the patient, and signs are elicited by the examiner.

Direct tenderness is pain at the site of pressure. **Rebound** tenderness is pain on sudden release of pressure. **Referred** tenderness is pain at one site while another is palpated.

Before touching the abdomen of a patient with acute abdominal pain, ask the patient to cough and then point to the painful spot with one finger. Usually, a patient with appendicitis can localize the pain to one circumscribed area, and in other conditions, the pain on coughing is diffuse. When the examiner knows the site of pain, systematic one-finger palpation of the abdomen can be carried out, avoiding the point of maximal tenderness until the last, and then applying only gentle pressure.

Rebound tenderness can be misleading if an exaggerated release motion startles the patient. Further, it is cruel and unnecessary to elicit rebound tenderness in most patients. Cough tenderness is essentially the same sign, but it is gentler because the patient controls its severity. Do not accumulate redundant information at the expense of patient discomfort.

In appendicitis, gentle pressure in the left lower quadrant may elicit tenderness over the inflamed appendix in the right lower quadrant—this is referred tenderness. Rebound referred tenderness, as the term implies, is rebound tenderness in one site while palpation pressure is released in another.

A secret: Most patients with acute appendicitis and other "surgical" causes of abdominal pain keep their eyes warily open during abdominal palpation, but most patients with nonspecific abdominal pain keep their eyes closed.

6. How does the position of the appendix affect symptoms and signs of appendicitis?

The appendix is fixed in position in about half of people, and in the other half, it presumably is free to move in response to posture and, perhaps, cecal distention. An inflamed retrocecal or retroileal appendix is shielded from the anterior abdominal wall by the overlying bowel and mesentery so abdominal pain and tenderness may be minimal. The classic shift of pain to the right lower quadrant may not occur. Tenderness is detectable by one-finger palpation lateral to the edge of the rectus abdominis muscle.

In pelvic appendicitis, pain settles quickly in the lower abdomen, sometimes on the left rather than the right. There may be a prominent urge to urinate and defecate. Tenderness may not be apparent on abdominal examination, but it is present on pelvic examination.

Bizarre clinical pictures occur when the cecum is located in the right upper quadrant or on the left side of the abdomen in a patient with malrotation. An exceptionally long appendix can extend into other parts of the abdomen.

7. How is appendicitis different in young children? Elderly people? Pregnancy?

Appendicitis in **infants** and **children** is a diagnostic problem because the patient is unable to describe the symptoms, and one must rely on a parent for the history. Sometimes abdominal pain is unrecognized in infants, and the parent reports lethargy, irritability, and disinterest in feedings. Examination also may be difficult; sedation may be required to perform abdominal and rectal examination.

Symptoms are vague in **elderly people,** the patient often delays, and the physician fails to consider the possibility of appendicitis. The inflammatory response in the elderly may be blunted, so pain is less severe, temperature may be normal, and tenderness may be mild.

In **pregnancy,** symptoms and signs may be attributed to an obstetric problem, but a careful history reveals the same sequence of symptoms as in other patients. The gravid uterus displaces the cecum and attached appendix cephalad and laterally, so tenderness may be subcostal in late pregnancy. Localized tenderness is found at some site, however.

8. Is a normal white cell count a reliable indication that a patient does not have acute appendicitis?

Elevated white cell counts (WBC) are sensitive, but nonspecific, indicators of acute appendicitis. Between 80% and 90% of patients with appendicitis have a WBC >10,000 cells µl, and there is often a "left shift" in the differential cell count, with an elevated percentage of neutrophils. Overall, 96% of patients with acute appendicitis have one or both abnormalities. Therefore, an entirely normal WBC and differential does not exclude appendicitis, but only 4% of patients with appendicitis fall into this category.

9. Which x-rays must be obtained to diagnose acute appendicitis?

None! The sequence of initial visceral pain, anorexia/nausea/vomiting, RLQ inflammatory pain, low-grade fever, localized tenderness in the RLQ, and leukocytosis are diagnostic in all but a few cases. In extreme age groups and other atypical patients, radiographs and other imaging studies can be helpful.

10. When should one suspect that the appendix has perforated?
The appendix can perforate at any time after about 12 hours from the onset of pain, and it becomes increasingly likely after 24 hours. High fever (>38.5°C), toxic appearance, diffuse abdominal tenderness, palpable mass, and a very high WBC (>20,000μl) are suggestive of perforation. Perforation may lead to localized infection (abscess) or spreading or generalized peritonitis, so symptoms and signs vary accordingly.

11. Discuss the most common GI conditions in the differential diagnosis of acute appendicitis.
Good luck with this one, because every condition that can cause acute abdominal pain could be considered. Indeed, according to an old adage, appendicitis should never be lower than second in the differential diagnosis of any acute abdominal problem.

The most common GI condition of concern is **gastroenteritis** and **mesenteric lymphadenitis**. These are really the same problem, i.e., inflammation of the small intestine and/or lymph nodes by viral, bacterial, or protozoal infection. Nausea and vomiting usually precede abdominal pain in these conditions, but in appendicitis, *pain is first!* Also, pain and tenderness are less well localized in gastroenteritis, diarrhea may occur, fever can be higher, and systemic symptoms such as headache, myalgias, or photophobia may be noted. Other GI diseases may be confused with appendicitis too, but many of them also require surgical treatment.

12. What gynecologic conditions are in the differential diagnosis?
Gynecologic diseases that are particularly troublesome in the differential include acute salpingitis and mittelschmerz. **Acute salpingitis** typically begins in the lower abdomen; there is no shift of pain as in appendicitis. Vomiting is infrequent, fever is high (often >38°C), and tenderness is poorly localized. The clinical picture, then, is a young woman with high fever and diffuse lower abdominal pain and tenderness who does not appear ill enough to have perforated appendicitis. Cervical tenderness may be present.

Mittelschmerz is pain caused by bleeding into the pelvic peritoneal cavity at the time of rupture of an ovarian follicle during ovulation. The onset of pain is usually sudden, it is lower abdominal, and it occurs in the middle of the menstrual cycle. Nausea and vomiting are absent, fever and leukocytosis are mild, and symptoms gradually improve without treatment in most cases. Sometimes, however, pain does not subside promptly, and localized tenderness in the right lower quadrant raises the question of appendicitis.

13. Does anyone die of acute appendicitis these days?
Yes—not as frequently as in the past, but still too often to be acceptable. The prognosis of acute appendicitis depends on the state of the disease. The prognosis of simple appendicitis is excellent; some large series have no deaths, and the mortality rate is up to 0.3% in others. However, the outcome of perforated appendicitis is worse. The overall mortality is 1% or less, but in the elderly, deaths may occur in up to 15%.

Remember, the mortality of appendicitis is the mortality of delay. Always consider appendicitis in the differential diagnosis of a patient with acute abdominal pain, and do not delay in making the diagnosis or enlisting the help of someone who can.

Morbidity and Mortality of Appendicitis

	MORBIDITY	MORTALITY
Simple	10%	0.3%
Perforated	15–60%	1.0%

14. Is there such a thing as recurrent appendicitis? Chronic appendicitis?
The answer to the first question is a definite yes. It is not unusual for a patient with appendicitis to relate a history of previous similar episodes that resolved spontaneously. Appendicitis also can

recur if appendectomy is incomplete or if a patient has an appendiceal abscess drained but the appendix is not removed.

Chronic appendicitis is more problematic, but it probably is an authentic entity. There are isolated case reports of patients who underwent successful appendectomy for chronic abdominal pain, and children with cystic fibrosis can have chronic appendicitis due to mucous engorgement of the lumen. However, one should be cautious in diagnosing chronic appendicitis in otherwise healthy people. It is reported that 1 of every 10 school-aged children complains of episodic or persistent abdominal pain, and finding the rare case of chronic appendicitis among them must be very difficult.

15. What would you recommend if the pathologist finds a carcinoid tumor in the appendiceal specimen from a patient with acute appendicitis?

Appendiceal carcinoid tumors may obstruct the lumen and cause acute appendicitis, so this scenario is not far-fetched. Usually, the surgeon will recognize the presence of a carcinoid if it is large, but small ones, including those that are coincidental, may not be appreciated at operation.

The management decision is based on size and location of the carcinoid tumor in the appendix and the general health of the patient. If the tumor is small (<1 cm) and/or situated in the mid or distal appendix so there is a good margin of tissue between the tumor and the transection line, nothing further need be done. Larger carcinoids and those at the base of the appendix are best treated by reoperation to resect the distal ileum, cecum and ascending colon, and associated mesocolon with its lymph nodes. Certainly, the age and general condition of the patient must be weighed as well.

CONTROVERSY

16. Is laparoscopic appendectomy preferred over open appendectomy?

Laparoscopic appendectomy is widely available, safe, and effective, but whether it is preferable to open appendectomy in routine cases is a matter of opinon. There is no doubt that laparoscopy has value in the diagnosis of appendicitis in certain instances, and if the appendix is inflamed, it can be removed laparoscopically most of the time. Laparoscopy is the only diagnostic procedure, other than laparotomy, that permits direct inspection of the appendix — all of the other tests are indirect. Thoroughness of abdominal exploration is greater with laparoscopy than with standard operation, and this is an advantage. Laparoscopy is an operation, however; it is performed under general anesthesia, and it is "invasive," albeit minimally. It is most useful in young women with possible gynecologic causes of acute abdominal pain and in others with atypical symptoms and signs that leave the diagnosis in doubt. As experience has increased, relative contraindications to diagnostic laparoscopy, such as previous abdominal operation, have become less important.

Prospective comparisons of laparoscopic versus open appendectomy have not resolved the issue thus far. The laparoscopic approach has not proved to be as hugely advantageous for appendectomy as it is for cholecystectomy. The incision is small and hospitalization is short with either method. Laparoscopic appendectomy has the disadvantage of higher expense because the tools are costly, but it probably has the advantage of shorter disability before patients can return to full activity.

At the moment, the choice is mainly a matter of the surgeon's — and the patient's — preference. If the diagnosis is in doubt, especially if the odds favor a condition other than appendicitis, it often makes sense to begin the operation with diagnostic laparoscopy and conclude it laparscopically if appendicitis is found.

BIBLIOGRAPHY

1. Andersson R, Hugander A, Thulin A, et al: Indications for operation in suspected appendicitis and incidence of perforation. BMJ 308:107–110, 1994.
2. Blair NP, Bugis SP, Turner LJ, MacLeod MM: Review of the pathologic diagnoses of 2,216 appendectomy specimens. Am J Surg 165:618–620, 1993.

3. Bonanni F, Reed Jr, Hartzell G, et al: Laparoscopic versus conventional appendectomy. J Am Coll Surg 179:273–278, 1994.

4. Ford RD, Passinault WJ, Morse ME: Diagnostic ultrasound for susptected appendicitis: Does the added cost produce a better outcome? Am Surg 60:895–896, 1994.

5. Franz MG, Norman J, Fabri PJ: Increased morbidity of appendicitis with advancing age. Am Surg 61: 40–44, 1995.

6. Frazee RC, Roberts JW, Symmonds RE, et al: A prospective randomized trial comparing open versus laparoscopic appendectomy. Ann Surg 219:725–728, 1994.

7. Guidry SP, Poole GV: The anatomy of appendicitis. Am Surg 60:68–71, 1994.

8. Halvorsen AC, Brandt B, Andreasen JJ: Acute appendicitis in pregnancy: Complications and subsequent management. Eur J Surg 158:603–606, 1992.

9. Mattei P, Sola JE, Yeo CJ: Chronic and recurrent appendicitis are uncommon entities often misdiagnosed. J Am Coll Surg 178:385–389, 1994.

10. Olsen JB, Myren CJ, Haahr PE: Randomized study of the value of laparoscopy before appendectomy. Br J Surg 80:922–923, 1993.

11. Ramirez JM, Deus J: Practical score to aid decision making in doubtful cases of appendicitis. Br J Surg 81:680–683, 1994.

12. Wade DS, Marrow SE, Balsara ZN, et al: Accuracy of ultrasound in the diagnosis of acute appendicitis compared with the surgeon's clinical impression. Arch Surg 128:1039–1044, 1993.

13. Zaninotto G, Rossi M, Anselmino M, Constantini M: Laparoscopic versus conventional surgery for suspected appendicitis in women. Surg Endosc 9:337–340, 1995.

51. COLITIS: RADIATION, MICROSCOPIC, COLLAGENOUS, AND PSEUDOMEMBRANOUS

John S. Goff, M.D.

1. What symptoms suggest that a patient may have an inflammatory colitis?

Typically, patients present with complaints of diarrhea that may be noticeably bloody and is associated with abdominal pain or cramping. Patients may have tenesmus (urgency without passage of much volume), which is very suggestive of rectal inflammation. The diarrhea often wakens them at night, and they may admit to incontinence if queried.

2. What conditions should be considered in the differential diagnosis of a suspected inflammatory colitis?

Differential Diagnosis of Suspected Colitis

BLOODY DIARRHEA OR DISCHARGE	DIARRHEA
Ulcerative colitis	Collagenous colitis
Acute self-limited colitis	Microscopic colitis
Allergic proctitis	Laxative/diuretic use
Pseudomembranous colitis	Pseudomembranous colitis
Invasive pathogens	Noninvasive pathogens
Crohn's disease	Crohn's disease
Drugs	Drugs
Diversion colitis	Irritable bowel syndrome
Solitary rectal ulcer	Hormone excess
Radiation enteritis	Food allergy
Hemolytic uremic syndrome	Malabsorption
Ischemic colitis	Colitis cystica profunda
Caustic colitis	Fecal impaction
Endometriosis	Pneumatosis

There are many possible causes for colitis-like symptoms. Not all patients with colitis-like symptoms have a true inflammatory colitis, which makes examination of the rectosigmoid mucosa very important in the initial evaluation. Historic information from the patient is often critical in making an initial determination of the cause. Useful information includes travel history, exposure to other ill individuals or animals, drug use (particularly antibiotics), dietary history, family history of inflammatory bowel disease, previous GI problems or surgeries, fever or chills, and any associated symptoms in other organ systems (arthritis, skin disorders, eye diseases). Drugs that have been associated with an inflammatory colitis include gold, chemotherapeutic agents, sulfasalazine, flucytosine, methyldopa, and nonsteroidal anti-inflammatory drugs. Vasopressin, ergot derivatives, digoxin, and estrogens/progestins have been associated with ischemic colitis. Patients have been known to use various caustic agents as enemas, either purposely or inadvertently.

3. How does sigmoidoscopy help in the evaluation of a patient with suspected colitis?

Examination of the rectosigmoid can provide useful information on the cause of the patient's symptoms. The most basic information obtained helps differentiate between conditions that cause mucosal disruption or changes from those that have no mucosal changes or only microscopic changes. Biopsies obtained from normal and abnormal mucosa may provide distinguishing information, though many forms of colitis can appear identical grossly and histologically. The final diagnosis may depend on identifying a specific organism, toxin, allergen, or drug; finding other GI lesions; or noting the response to certain medications.

Not all inflammatory bowel lesions involve the rectum. Many patients have significant lesions proximal to the rectosigmoid. Identifying these lesions requires a barium enema or colonoscopy. Colonoscopy is more likely to identify subtle lesions in the proximal colon or terminal ileum than a barium enema. Thus, a patient having a normal sigmoidoscopy but with blood or excessive white blood cells (WBCs) in the stool needs to be considered for a colonoscopy, especially if stool cultures and examinations for parasites are negative.

4. What initial tests should be performed on a patient's stool when one suspects a colitis?
Stool must be examined in the laboratory for occult blood, relative number of WBCs, bacteria, and parasites. Stool should also be tested for *Clostridium* toxin if the patient has been on antibiotics. Laboratories routinely look and culture for limited organisms in the stool, so specific cultures or tests should be requested if unusual organism are suspected (e.g., *Yersinia* cultures or special stains for *Cryptosporidium*). These tests can be very useful, but results may be negative because of inhomogeneity of stool specimens. In the past it was recommended that three separate stool specimens be submitted for parasite examination, but the increase in yield beyond the first specimen may be so small as to make such a recommendation cost-ineffective.

RADIATION ENTEROCOLITIS

5. Describe the acute effect of therapeutic irradiation on the GI tract.
Therapeutic radiation—usually for prostate, bladder, gynecologic, or rectal cancers—results in a dose-dependant acute injury to any bowel that is within the treatment port. This injury develops shortly after the onset of the radiotherapy, leaving the bowel mucosa edematous, erythematous, or dusky and friable. Histologically, there is an acute inflammatory cell infiltrate, and often there are crypt abscesses composed of eosinophils. The patients have typical colitis symptoms of diarrhea, tenesmus, abdominal cramping, and, sometimes, blood in the stools.

6. What is the course of acute therapeutic radiation injury to the bowel, and how does one treat it?
The acute injury induced by the radiation will totally resolve, both grossly and histologically, without specific therapy. The injury may improve despite continued irradiation but, if severe, may require discontinuation of treatment at least temporarily. Medical management consists of symptomatic therapy with antidiarrheal agents and anticholinergic drugs. Anti-inflammatory agents are rarely required to treat an acute radiation colitis.

7. Does therapeutic irradiation produce any delayed effects on the GI tract beyond the acute period?
Anywhere from 6 months to 30 years after irradiation, with a mean of about 2 years, patients may develop symptoms from previous irradiation. The incidence is generally reported at 2–10% but up to 20% has been reported. Because therapeutic irradiation is usually aimed at low pelvic structures most symptoms occur in the rectosigmoid colon, but injury can occur in the small bowel and produce problems related to inflammation or stricturing of the intestine. Patients complain of hematochezia, diarrhea or constipation (or both), and rectal or abdominal pain. The most serious problems are severe bleeding, significant stricturing, and fistula forming between bowel loops and other organs, such as the vagina.

8. Are there any factors that predispose to developing these problems after radiotherapy?

Hypertension	Thin physique
Diabetes mellitus	Prior abdominal or pelvic surgery
Pelvic inflammatory disease	Concomitant chemotherapy

The amount of radiation exposure and the presence of bile and pancreatic secretions within the small bowel may increase the likelihood of injury. Interestingly, having acute radiation injury does not seem to correlate with the development of chronic radiation injury.

9. What is the pathophysiology of the delayed radiation injury syndrome?
The delayed injury seems to be due to a vasculitis with endarteritis developing. All layers of the bowel wall are affected, including the serosa. Vessel walls are hyalinized, and there may be venous or arteriolar thrombosis. This thrombosis results in relative ischemia or tissue hypoxia, which is manifested by serosal thickening, muscularis propria fibrosis and mucosal thickening, and mucosal atrophy or ulceration. Telangiectatic vessels are commonly found. Malnutrition can result if a substantial portion of the small bowel, especially the terminal ileum, is damaged. Patients will have an abnormal small bowel motility (fed) pattern and decreased intensity of the migrating motor complexes. Severe cases may present as pseudo-obstruction.

10. How is delayed radiation injury diagnosed?
The appropriate clinical setting (history of radiation treatment) with exclusion of other causes is the usual means of making a diagnosis. Barium studies help by showing lack of haustra, mucosal effacement, narrowing, ulcerations, and fistula in involved segments of bowel. The endoscopic appearance is usually characterized by some combination of ulcerations, inflammatory change, atrophic mucosa, luminal narrowing, or telangiectasia. Biopsies of the mucosa taken at endoscopy may be suggestive of radiation injury but are rarely diagnostic, because the superficial mucosal changes are nonspecific.

11. How is delayed radiation injury to the bowel treated?
Initial therapy is symptomatic, with bulk agents and anticholinergic drugs depending on the primary symptoms. Attention to nutritional deficiencies may be necessary depending on the location and extent of bowel damage. Improvement in the inflammatory changes in the mucosa has been reported after use of 5-aminosalicylic acid (5-ASA) compounds, such as sulfasalazine, but improvement is more likely to develop after use of systemic or topical steroids. If patients have partial obstruction, poor motility, or interbowel fistulae, they may need to be treated for bacterial overgrowth.

Bleeding telangiectasias that do not respond to medical therapy can be treated by extensive ablative therapy using endoscopically applied energy from a Nd-YAG laser. Although this may be time-consuming therapy, it will decrease the number of transfusions required by the patient. Surgery for major complications can be undertaken, but the difficulty level is high, because radiation injury is often accompanied by extensive intraabdominal adhesions. Anastomoses are prone to leaking if they are created with injured bowel. Consequently, one common approach to these problems is to perform bypass or diversion surgery rather than direct corrective interventions.

MICROSCOPIC/COLLAGENOUS COLITIS

12. Under what circumstances should a diagnosis of microscopic or collagenous colitis be considered?
The typical patient with microscopic or collagenous colitis is a middle-aged to elderly woman with a history of large-volume, watery diarrhea that is intermittent, often nocturnal, and possibly incontinent. The patient may experience weight loss, though malabsorption has not been documented in these patients. There is no osmotic gap measurable in the stool. The patient may have an elevated sedimentation rate, and an increased incidence of arthritis, diabetes mellitus, and thyroiditis is seen in these patients. Symptoms may be present for years before a diagnosis is made. The female predominance may be more marked in the group with collagenous colitis.

13. How does one diagnose microscopic or collagenous colitis?
These patients have normal-appearing small and large bowels on both radiography and endoscopy, and biopsies are necessary to identify the disorder. The typical finding is a lymphocytic infiltrate in the mucosa of the colon, but the characteristic feature that is not usually seen in either ulcerative colitis or acute self-limited colitis is intraepithelial lymphocytes. This infiltrate is associated with flattening or loss of the surface epithelial cells. In addition, distorted or inflamed crypts, as is seen in ulcerative colitis, are not present, but this finding also is not seen in acute self-limited colitis. There

is no goblet cell depletion, and eosinophils may be part of the inflammatory infiltrate. Collagenous colitis is distinguished by a >15-μm band of subepithelial collagen (see figure below).

The microscopic findings in these two conditions are very similar except for the collagen band. In fact, it has been proposed that they are two ends of the spectrum of the same condition, because cases have been reported in which the collagen component seems to come or go while the inflammatory component remains unchanged. This condition often has a patchy distribution involving any portion of the colon or terminal ileum. Thus, a diagnosis is not absolutely excluded until a full colonoscopy with multiple random biopsies is performed.

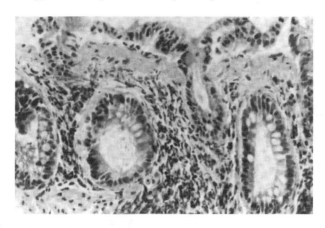

Photomicrograph showing the typical subepithelial collagen band, epithelial injury and detachment, and lymphocytic infiltrate of the mucosa in a patient with collagenous colitis.

14. Why do these patients have diarrhea?

Careful steady-state perfusion studies have shown that these patients have impaired water and electrolyte absorption in the colon, which is presumably the reason the patients complain of large-volume watery diarrhea.

15. What causes microscopic and collagenous colitis?

Bacterial cytotoxins and nonsteroidal anti-inflammatory drugs have been proposed as causes of the microscopic or collagenous colitis, but the evidence of this association is not very convincing. An autoimmune mechanism may be involved, given the association with other autoimmune disorders.

16. How is microscopic or collagenous colitis treated?

The natural history of these conditions is not known. Therapeutic responses to many agents (octreotide, clonidine, sulfasalazine, metronidazole, loperamide, steroids, and quinacrine) have been reported in individual or a few cases, but there have been no controlled trials of therapy. Initial treatment should be with a 5-aminosalicylic (5-ASA) compound that delivers the drug to the involved part of the colon or small bowel. If this approach is ineffective, adding or switching to systemic steroid therapy is often helpful. Because of the often diffuse and patchy distribution of these conditions, there is usually no reason to attempt topical therapy with enemas. It has been suggested that microscopic colitis responds better than collagenous colitis, but both disorders can be difficult to bring under control, and relapse after successful therapy is common.

PSEUDOMEMBRANOUS COLITIS

17. What is pseudomembranous colitis (PMC)?

PMC is one of several presentations of antibiotic-associated diarrhea that is caused by *Clostridium difficile* toxin. About 20% of patients with diarrhea after antibiotic use have *C. difficile* isolated in their stool, but if they have associated colitis, the positivity rate is closer to 75%. If they have widespread pseudomembranes in their colon, then the positivity rate for *C. difficile* approaches 100%. The characteristic pseudomembranes of PMC are due to the effect of endotoxin A, produced by the infecting strain of *C. difficile*, on the colonic mucosa.

18. What is a pseudomembrane?

The hallmark of PMC is the presence of yellow plaques on the colonic mucosa that range in size from a few millimeters to confluent plaques covering many centimeters (see figure below). These plaques represent collections of fibrin, mucus, and inflammatory cells and are called pseudomembranes.

Microscopically, an inflammatory exudate is seen spewing from the epithelial glands (see figure below). Usually, the intervening mucosa is normal, but it may be inflamed. The lesions typically start

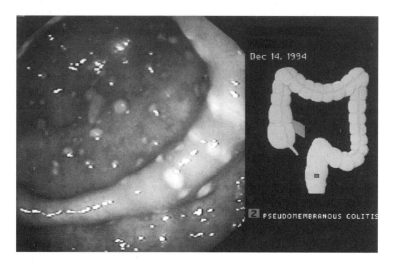

Endoscopic view of typical pseudomembranes in the rectum of a patient with antibiotic-associated diarrhea caused by *C. difficile*.

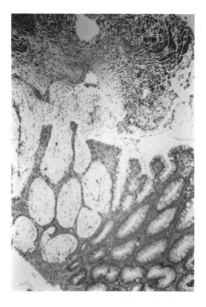

Photomicrograph of a pseudomembrane in a patient with pseudomembranous colitis. Note how the exudate spews from the epithelial glands; adjacent glands appear completely normal.

in the rectum and are thus easily identified at sigmoidoscopy. However, up to 10% of patients with PMC have the typical pseudomembranes found proximal to the reach of a flexible sigmoidoscope.

19. How is PMC diagnosed?

The presence of toxin-producing *Clostridium difficile* can be detected in the stool by assaying for the presence of cytotoxin B or detecting endotoxin A with antibodies. Cytotoxin B will damage and disrupt cells in culture, but this effect can be blocked by specific antibodies to cytotoxin B. Stool ultrafiltrate can be placed in a tissue culture, and if the cells are damaged, one can suspect *C. difficile* as the cause. Repeating the test with specific antibodies against cytotoxin B in the culture media blocks the effect and thus confirms the diagnosis. This technique is quite specific and sensitive, but costly and time-consuming (at least 48 hours to a proven diagnosis). A quicker, though less accurate, method for detecting *C. difficile* is the latex-agglutination test to detect endotoxin A, which is the pathogenic endotoxin produced by *C. difficile*. Stool can be cultured for *C. difficile*, but this organism is difficult to culture and all strains are not endotoxin-producing.

20. How and why do patients acquire PMC?

Patients usually acquire *Clostridium difficile* in the hospital from personnel and contaminated surfaces, but some patients are carriers of this organism. When the patient's usual GI flora is altered by the use of antibiotics with broad-spectrum activity against enteric organisms, *C. difficile* can proliferate and damage the colonic mucosa via its endotoxins. Prevention of spread in the hospital is best accomplished by using gloves and gowns, careful washing between patients, and sterilizing any objects (such as thermometers and endoscopes) placed in a patient's rectum. PMC also has been described after the use of chemotherapeutic agents with no exposure to antibiotics.

21. Which antibiotics are associated with the development of PMC?

Antibiotics Associated with the Development of PMC

HIGH FREQUENCY	MODERATE FREQUENCY	LOW FREQUENCY
Ampicillin	Sulfonamides	Aminoglycosides
Amoxicillin	Erythromycin	Metronidazole
Clindamycin	Tetracyclines	Vancomycin
Cephalosporins	Chloramphenicol	Rifampin
	Trimethoprim	Bacitracin
	Quinolones	

22. Describe the usual clinical presentation of a patient with PMC.

Patients with antibiotic-associated diarrhea and colitis not caused by *Clostridium difficile* are much less sick than those with typical PMC. PMC patients have moderate to severe diarrhea, often with gross blood, abdominal cramping, malaise, and low-grade fevers. The abdomen is often tender, especially when palpated over the colon. In advanced cases of PMC, a fulminant, life-threatening colitis can develop. These patients have severe pain, rapid heart rates, fever, and lethargy. Their colons become quite dilatated and are at risk of perforation (toxic megacolon). Thickened bowel wall may be detected by the appearance of "thumbprinting" on abdominal radiographs. Leukocytosis is common in PMC. Older patients can be difficult to diagnose by clinical features alone, because they may not manifest fever or leukocytosis and their pain can be minimal, at least initially. PMC can develop anywhere from a few days to 4 weeks after use of an antibiotic.

23. What is unique about neonates and *Clostridium difficile*?

The carriage rate for *C. difficile* among neonates can run as high as 80%, with many of these neonates harboring toxigenic strains. The neonates seem to be resistant to the development of PMC because they lack the necessary colonocyte receptors for the toxins to bind to and subsequently produce their damaging effects. The receptors become present after about 1 year of life.

24. How is PMC treated?

Mild cases of diarrhea associated with *Clostridium difficile* can be managed expectantly after stopping the offending antibiotic. True PMC should be managed by stopping the initiating antibiotic, if at all possible, and then starting metronidazole, 250 mg four times daily, orally or intravenously if the patient cannot take oral medications. Alternatively, one can use vancomycin, 125 mg four times daily orally (intravenous is not effective). Higher doses of vancomycin have been advocated, but this agent is very expensive and the lowest effective dose seems to be 125 mg. Cholestyramine, 4 gm three times daily, or colestipol, 5 gm three times daily, may be useful as single therapy in mild cases or as an adjuvant in resistant or recurrent cases of PMC. These drugs are felt to work by binding the endotoxin before it can bind to an enterocyte. Bacitracin, 25,000 U four times daily, is a bit less effective and has a higher relapse rate. Rifampin, 300 mg twice daily, may be useful in recurrent cases. Treatment with *Lactobacillus* or *Saccharomyces boulardii* has been suggested as useful adjuncts to antibiotic therapy, particularly in recurrent cases of PMC.

BIBLIOGRAPHY

1. Alam MJ: Chronic refractory diarrhoea: A manifestation of endocrine disorders. Dig Dis 12:46–61, 1994.
2. Bo-Linn GW, Vendrell DD, Lee E, Fordtran JS: An evaluation of the significance of microscopic colitis in patients with chronic diarrhea. J Clin Invest 75:1559–1569, 1985.
3. Fortson WC, Tadesco FJ: Drug-induced colitis: A review. Am J Gastroenterol 79:878–883, 1984.
4. Haddad GK, Grodsinsky C, Allen H: The spectrum of radiation enteritis: Surgical considerations. Dis Colon Rectum 26:590–594, 1983.
5. Husebye E, Hauer-Jensen M, Kjorstad K, Skar V: Severe late radiation enteropathy is characterized by impaired motility of proximal small intestine. Dig Dis Sci 39:2341–2349, 1994.
6. Kamthan AG, Bruckner HW, Hirschman SZ, Agus SG: *Clostridium difficile* diarrhea induced by cancer chemotherapy. Arch Intern Med 152:1715–1717, 1992.
7. Kelly CP, Pothoulakis C, LaMont JT: *Clostridium difficile* colitis. N Engl J Med 330:257–262, 1994.
8. Kingham JGC: Microscopic colitis. Gut 32:234–235, 1991.
9. Kongham JC, Levison DA, Ball JA, Dawson AM: Microscopic colitis—a cause of chronic watery diarrhea. BMJ 285:1601–1604, 1982.
10. Lewis FW, Warren GH, Goff JS: Collagenous colitis with involvement of the terminal ileum. Dig Dis Sci 36:1161–1163, 1991.
11. McFarland LV, Surawicz CM, Stamm WE: Risk factors for *Clostridium difficile* carriage and *C. difficile*-associated diarrhea in a cohort of hospitalized patients. J Infect Dis 162:678–683, 1990.
12. Mulholland MW, Levitt SH, Song CW, et al: The role of luminal contents in radiation enteritis. Cancer 54:2396–2402, 1984.
13. Russell JC, Welch JP: Operative management of radiation injuries of the intestinal tract. Am J Surg 137: 433–441, 1979.
14. Surawicz CM, McFarland LV, Elmer G, Chinn J: Treatment of recurrent *Clostridium difficile* colitis with vancomycin and *Saccharomyces boulardii*. Am J Gastroenterol 84:1285–1288, 1989.
15. Yoonessi M, Romney S, Dayem H: Gastrointestinal tract complications following radiotherapy of uterine cervical cancer: Past and present. J Surg Oncol 18:135–142, 1981.

VII. General Symptoms and Conditions

52. UPPER GASTROINTESTINAL TRACT HEMORRHAGE

John Schaefer, M.D.

1. What immediate historical information is important in patients with acute upper GI (UGI) hemorrhage?

A brief directed history should document the presence or absence of hematemesis, melena, blood per rectum, peptic symptoms, and use of nonsteroidal anti-inflammatory drugs. It is also important to know about past ulcer history, previous bleeds, dizziness or syncope, alcohol consumption, and current medications. Further details can be obtained after initial resuscitation procedures are underway.

2. What should be noted on initial physical examination?

An assessment of hemodynamic status takes first priority. A rapid evaluation of blood volume status is made by measuring the blood pressure and pulse and checking for postural changes. The patient is surveyed for signs of associated illnesses, especially liver, heart, or lung diseases, or a bleeding diathesis betrayed by petechiae, purpura, or hematoma. A rectal exam is mandatory.

In selected patients with no apparent clinical clue as to the cause of hemorrhage, look carefully for the tell-tale lesions of hereditary hemorrhagic telangiectasia or pseudoxanthoma elastica. It will "make your day" if you are first to recognize these rare causes of intestinal bleeding.

3. What can be learned from the rectal exam?

The color of the material obtained on rectal examination should be recorded: usually brown, black, or red. It takes <50 ml of UGI bleeding to make the stool positive for occult blood. A melenic stool virtually always indicates a bleeding source proximal to the ligament of Treitz and can be seen with as little as 200 ml of blood loss. A melenic stool may be seen rarely from a right-sided colon lesion if there is prolonged fecal transit time, 72 hours or more, as may be seen in bedridden nursing home patients. Red blood per rectum (hematochezia) means either a mid or lower intestinal tract hemorrhage or a massive UGI bleed. The latter patients usually show hemodynamic instability and a transient rise in the blood urea nitrogen level. Clinical studies show that stool may remain positive for occult blood for 7–14 days after a single large instillation of blood into the stomach.

4. What else needs to be done right away?

Adequate intravenous access should be guaranteed by placement of at least one large-bore intravenous line and initial resuscitation begun with intravenous crystalloid solution, normal saline, or Ringer's lactate. A large-bore nasogastric tube should be placed for gastric lavage. Older patients need an electrocardiogram.

5. What laboratory tests are urgently obtained?

Complete blood count
Prothrombin time

Partial thromboplastin time
Platelet count
Serum electrolytes
Liver function tests
Blood type and crossmatching
The clinical assessment may dictate additional tests.

6. Of what value is the nasogastric (NG) tube in a patient with UGI hemorrhage?

The NG tube is of no proven therapeutic benefit. A grossly bloody return, however, confirms the presence of UGI hemorrhage. Keep in mind that perhaps 10% of patients with bleeding from a duodenal ulcer may not show blood on gastric aspiration. Others with no recent fresh bleeding may have rapidly emptied old blood from the stomach. HemOccult testing of gastric contents is of little or no clinical value.

For most patients, once the stomach has been cleared of retained blood, repeat gastric lavage is the most reliable online indicator for the presence or absence of ongoing hemorrhage. A gastric tube of adequate size, 24 French or larger, is required for adequate removal of blood clots. A clean stomach is required for the best possible endoscopic examination. Gastric irrigation with the newer large-bore, 34 French, closed lavage system is particularly efficient in evacuating the gastric contents. Contamination of personnel and surroundings with blood is also minimized. Irrigation with tap water at room temperature is recommended.

7. How can the amount of acute blood loss be estimated?

500 ml—Up to 500 ml of blood may be lost without discernible clinical findings.

1000 ml—Blood loss exceeding 1000 ml usually causes postural changes in blood pressure and pulse (supine-to-upright drop in systolic blood pressure of at least 10–20 mm Hg and a rise in the pulse rate of 20/min or more).

2000 ml—Acute hemorrhage exceeding 2000 ml often presents with clinical shock. Patients appear pale, diaphoretic, and restless with supine blood pressure of 90 mm Hg or less.

8. Are hematocrit levels useful in acute hemorrhage?

During acute hemorrhage, there is an interplay of multiple factors influencing the hematocrit level. Interpretation is difficult but not useless. Very early in hemorrhage, the hematocrit remains at baseline levels. Subsequent levels fall in response to the quantity of blood lost, the amount, type, and rate of administered intravenous fluids, and the body's efforts to reestablish intravascular volume by shifting interstitial fluid into the vascular space. The most rapid drop in hematocrit is caused by blood volume expansion from intravenous fluids. When bleeding stops and intravenous fluids are curtailed or stopped, there is often a slow continuation of compensatory hemodilution. The consequent downward drift of the hematocrit and the prolonged stool positivity for occult blood may give rise to a misinterpretation of mild recurrent bleeding or continued oozing from the lesion.

When the patient is first seen and before any resuscitative fluids are given, the hematocrit level can be interpreted in light of the presumed starting level and the estimated time of onset of bleeding, allowing one to approximate the percent fall of the final hematocrit. After an episode of hemorrhage without intravenous fluids, the hematocrit drops approximately 25% of its total fall within 2 hours, 50% by 8 hours, and takes up to 72 hours to reach the final value.

9. Is a flow chart necessary?

Yes! A flow chart allows the attending physicians and consultants to appraise rapidly a patient's hospital course. It should clearly identify time of admission, initial and timed subsequent vital signs, serial hematocrit values, type and amount of intravenous fluids, urine volume, frequency and description of stools, and findings on frequent gastric irrigations.

10. Where and by whom are patients with UGI bleeding best managed?

Patients with moderate or severe hemorrhage are best evaluated on an intensive care unit by combined medical and surgical consultants. Patients judged to have mild hemorrhage can be admitted to a general care ward. Findings that identify patients with mild bleeding include age <65 years, stable vital signs, no evidence of chronic liver disease or other significant coexisting disease, and nasogastric aspirate that clears of retained blood rapidly and shows no evidence of fresh blood. These low-risk patients do not share the same degree of diagnostic urgency as those with evidence of more severe hemorrhage.

11. What are the most common causes of UGI hemorrhage?

The frequency of the various causes of UGI hemorrhage depends on the population surveyed. Overall, peptic ulcer, duodenal or gastric, remains the most common cause. In recent years, hospitalization for peptic ulcer disease has been substantially reduced, but the frequency of patients admitted with bleeding ulcers remains unchanged. Undoubtedly, hemorrhage from gastropathy induced by nonsteroidal anti-inflammatory drugs (NSAIDs), especially in patients over 60 years of age, contributes to this finding. Other common causes of UGI hemorrhage are erosive gastritis, esophageal varices, and Mallory-Weiss tears. These latter causes are seen more often in hospitals serving a population with a high prevalence of alcoholism. Acute bleeding from esophagitis, neoplastic tumors, and vascular abnormalities is uncommon and often mild.

12. Why is endoscopy the favored diagnostic procedure in UGI hemorrhage?

Early endoscopy is by far the most sensitive and specific way to identify the cause of bleeding. The clinical diagnosis is accurate in only about one-half of cases. Radiographic examination cannot detect most mucosal lesions and is unreliable in patients with previous gastric surgery. Because their management is radically different, patients with liver disease require an accurate assessment of variceal versus other sources of hemorrhage. Rarely, a patient may bleed so massively as to require immediate surgery. Endoscopy in the operating room after endotracheal intubation may be useful to the surgeon, particularly in excluding an esophageal site of hemorrhage.

13. Of what value is angiography?

Upper GI endoscopy has virtually eliminated angiography for diagnosing the cause of UGI hemorrhage. In patients with prohibitively high surgical risk and hemorrhage uncontrolled by other measures, the angiographer may extend one last therapeutic attempt. If a bleeding vessel can be identified, hemorrhage may be stopped on occasion by selective intra-arterial infusion of vasopressin or thromboembolization with various substances.

14. What is the expected clinical course of patients having UGI bleeding?

More than 80% of patients have spontaneous cessation of hemorrhage and, thus, require only supportive care. Most hemorrhage already has stopped or stops within a few hours of admission, and almost all that stop spontaneously do so within the first 12 hours. Often such patients with nonvariceal causes of hemorrhage can be discharged after 2 or 3 days.

An additional group of patients with persistent or recurrent active hemorrhage respond to therapeutic endoscopic procedures with heater probe or bipolar electrocoagulation of the bleeding site. Less than 10% of patients require emergency surgery to control bleeding. Patients with bleeding from esophageal varices are exceptions, in that a greater proportion require endoscopic variceal banding, sclerosis, or balloon tamponade for control of hemorrhage.

15. Which patients require blood transfusions?

Patients presenting with overt clinical shock, tachycardia, and recumbent systolic blood pressure <90 mm Hg require blood transfusions. Transfusions should be given in patients with active bleeding if the hematocrit can be predicted to fall below 30%. Hematocrit values maintained near this level provide for adequate tissue oxygenation and a buffer against continued or recurrent hemorrhage.

16. What findings predict potential mortality?

The overall mortality varies from 8–10% in most recorded series of UGI bleeding. The mortality rate may be reduced in future studies with the increaed use of therapeutic endoscopic intervention, especially in surgically high-risk patients. The major factors associated with high mortality risk include serious concomitant illness, age >65 years, presentation in clinical shock, and intractable hemorrhage after hospitalization. These latter patients show persistent hemodynamic instability and often copious red blood on both nasogastric lavage and per rectum. Such patients have massive hemorrhage, and their mortality approaches 30%. Patients with variceal hemorrhage also have a mortality rate of 30–40%. An advanced stage of liver failure is the major risk factor for variceal hemorrhage and for high mortality.

17. Who is at risk for rebleeding from a peptic ulcer?
If clinically significant rebleeding occurs after initial control, it usually occurs within the first 3 days after admission. The endoscopic appearance of the ulcer allows an estimation of the rebleeding potential:

Ulcer with clear whitish base	<5% chance of rebleeding
Flat pigmented spot within crater	~10%
Adherent blood clot that cannot be irrigated off the ulcer base	20%
Raised fibrinous clot over site of eroded artery (visible vessel)	40%

In a stabilized patient, if active arterial bleeding is present on endoscopy, there is almost an 80% chance for continued or recurrent bleeding if endoscopic hemostasis is not performed. Each of the markers for potential rebleeding approximately doubles the preceding rate and, thus, forms a convenient means for estimating the risk.

18. Which patients with a peptic ulcer benefit from an endoscopic therapeutic procedure?
No therapeutic maneuver is advocated for peptic ulcers having a clean base or a flat pigmented spot. Most favor leaving an adherent clot alone, but some argue for remvoal and endoscopic coagulation applied at the site of adherence. Controlled studies show significant benefit from endoscopic treatment of ulcers with a "visible vessel" or active arterial bleeding. The most common form of endoscopic treatment is local injection with epinephrine, 1/10,000 dilution, followed by arterial electrocoagulation with a heater or multipolar probe. About 20% of patients so treated will rebleed. For patients at high risk for surgery, a second attempt for endoscopic control may be warranted. The others require urgent surgery.

19. How is the diagnosis of bleeding from esophageal varices made?
Most patients with esophageal varices never bleed from them. When bleeding occurs, however, it is usually more severe than that from other causes. Patients with alcoholic liver disease admitted with UGI hemorrhage are often bleeding from a cause other than varices (50%). Therefore, early endoscopy is necessary for accurate diagnosis. If a bleeding varix is seen, the cause is unequivocal. A presumptive diagnosis of variceal bleed is made if varices are found and no other potential bleeding lesion is seen within the stomach or duodenum.

Esophageal varices of large size are the most likely to bleed. Stigmata of recent rupture (pigmented spots or venules on the surface of the varices) add to the likelihood of a recent variceal bleed. If varices and a coexisting potential bleeding lesion are found in the stomach or duodenum, the conservative approach is to assume that the varices did not bleed. If hemorrhage recurs after initial control in these patients, repeat endoscopic evaluation is required. Oral beta-blocker therapy has been reporred to reduce to incidence of initial hemorrhage from esophageal varices.

20. What measures are used to stop variceal hemorrhage?
Hemorrhage from esophageal varices is best controlled by endoscopic variceal sclerosis or banding (see figures on next page). Sclerotherapy has about a 20% rate of complications, such as ulceration, stricture formation, dysmotility, or mediastinitis. Endoscopic banding is just as effective and has fewer complications. Both procedures are effective in obliterating esophageal varices and reducing recurrent hemorrhage if repeated on five or more occasions at 1–2-week intervals.

Intravenous vasopressin may be effective in stopping variceal hemorrhage but has not been shown to improve survival. Concomitant use of intravenous nitroglycerin reduces the adverse cardiovascular effects of vasopressin. Reportedly, intravenous somatostatin is equally effective

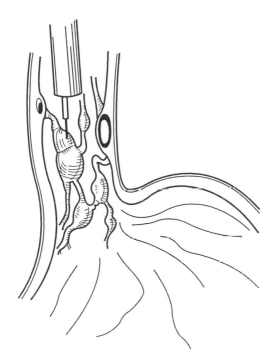

A 22-gauge sclerotherapy needle is shown
during treatment of a distal esophageal varix.

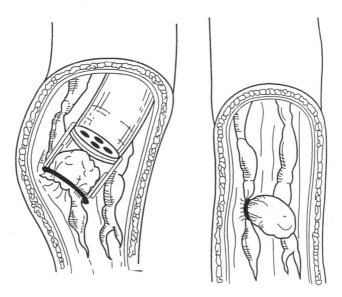

Stiegmann-Goff variceal band ligation device. The varix and esophageal mucosa are suctioned into the banding device (*left*), and an O-ring is deployed over the varix (*right*).

in hemostasis with less hemodynamic side effects. Both vasopressin and somatostatin are secondary measures often used in conjunction with other forms of therapy.

If these procedures fail, the use of balloon tamponade, Sengstaken-Blakemore or Minnesota-Linton tube, can be used (see Figure A below). Properly positioned, these control esophageal variceal bleeding most of the time. Bleeding, however, often recurs with deflation. Because of the high incidence of potential complications, only those physicians with considerable experience in placement should use these tubes.

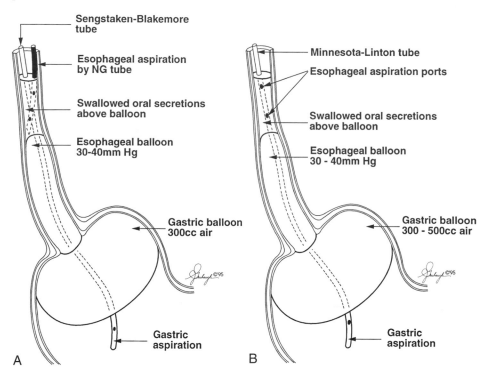

A, Modified Sengstaken-Blakemore tube with nasogastric (NG) tube. B, Minnesota-Linton variceal tamponade device. This device contains an internal esophageal aspiration port, obviating the need for an additional nasogastric tube.

21. What is the TIPS procedure?

This acronym stands for transvenous intrahepatic portosystemic shunt. It is performed by interventional radiologists, usually with only conscious sedation of the patient. Under fluoroscopic guidance, an expandable metallic shunt is placed within the liver parenchyma, bridging between the portal vein and hepatic vein (see figure on next page). The shunt decompresses portal hypertension.

The prime use is for control of recurrent variceal hemorrhage, particularly for patients awaiting hepatic transplantation. It is also valuable for patients who bleed from gastric varices that are not generally amenable to other forms of treatment. Some patients with intractable ascites may benefit. Portosystemic encephalopathy can be troublesome, and long-term use may be compromised by shunt stenosis or thrombosis.

22. Which patients require emergency surgery?

There are no simple rules to define which patients require surgery to stop hemorrhage. The decision usually depnds on the experienced clinical judgment of both medical and surgical attendings. Surgery for patients with ongoing hemorrhage carries a multifold risk of mortality compared to elective surgery in a similar patient population. This is particularly true for patients >60 years of age.

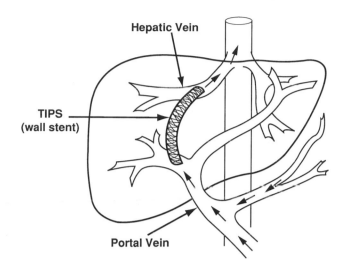

Hepatic Vein

TIPS (wall stent)

Portal Vein

TIPS procedure requires placement of a metallic wall stent between the hepatic and portal veins.

Some general guidelines are useful:

- Almost all patients should have had diagnostic endoscopy and failed at least one attempt at endoscopic hemostasis.
- Surgical candidates include patients failing to stop bleeding after vigorous resuscitation, including blood transfusions, or those with clinically important rebleedng after 12–24 hours of initial control.
- Aside from the urgency of hemorrhage, all patients must otherwise be acceptable surgical candidates. For example, patients with overtly decompensated liver disease, Child's class C, are prohibitive surgical risks.
- Patients >age 60 are likely to have surgery sooner than younger patients.
- Those with a point source of hemorrhage, such as peptic ulcer, are more readily accepted for surgery than patients with diffuse erosive gastritis or variceal hemorrhage.

The most important decision occurs when patients first become potential candidates for emergency surgery. This time is particularly critical for the high-risk patients, and the decision for or against surgery should be decisive. Whatever adverse findings bear upon the surgical risk will persist or become progressively more severe as bleeding continues. Thus, if surgery is to be considered, any further delay compromises the chance for success.

BIBLIOGRAPHY

1. Bordley DR, Mushlin AI, Dolan JG, et al: Early clinical signs identify low-risk patients with acute upper gastrointestinal hemorrhage. JAMA 253:3282–3285, 1985.
2. Cochran TA: Bleeding peptic ulcer: Surgical therapy. Gastroenterol Clin North Am 22:751–778, 1993.
3. Galamabos MR, Galambos JT: How to cope with bleeding esophageal varices. J Crit Illness 5:603–623, 1990.
4. Gier DL, Cooke AR: Upper GI bleeding: A five-step approach to diagnosis and treatment. J Crit Illness 7:1676–1695, 1992.
5. Kandel G: Management of nonvariceal upper GI hemorrhage. Hosp Pract (Jan):121–138, 1990.
6. Kleber G,Sauerbruch T, Ansari H, Paumgartner G: Prediction of variceal hemorrhage in cirrhosis: A prospective follow-up study. Gastroenterology 100:1332–1337, 1991.
7. Laine L: Bleeding peptic ulcer. N Engl J Med 331:717–727, 1994.
8. Laine L: Rolling review: Upper gastrointestinal bleeding. Aliment Pharmacol Ther 7:207–232, 1993.
9. Quinn PG, Issa K, Mullen KD: Techniques for managing acute variceal bleeding. J Crit Illness 9:289–299, 1994.
10. Wara P: Endoscopic prediction of major rebleeding: A prospective study of stigmata of hemorrhage in bleeding ulcer. Gastroenterology 88:1209–1214, 1985.
11. Weisz N, Jensen DM: Improved strategies for managing upper GI bleeding. Contemp Intern Med (Jul/Aug):42–59, 1990.

53. LOWER GASTROINTESTINAL TRACT BLEEDING

Ian M. Gralnek, M.D., and Dennis M. Jensen, M.D.

1. Define lower gastrointestinal bleeding.

Lower GI bleeding is defined generally as bleeding distal to the ligament of Treitz, but in most considerations it is limited to that from the colon. Bleeding between the ligament of Treitz and the ileocecal valve is considered small bowel bleeding. Bleeding from the esophagus, stomach, or duodenum is considered upper GI bleeding.

Lower GI bleeding can be divided further as **gross** bleeding, where red or maroon blood is visible in the stool, versus **occult** bleeding, where blood is not visible and discovered by chemical testing of the stool (i.e., with guaiac-impregnated cards).

2. How common is lower GI bleeding?

In 1991, approximately 0.4% of individuals admitted to nonfederal, short-stay hospitals had a "first-listed" diagnosis of GI hemorrhage without hematemesis or melena. Although the causes of such hemorrhage were unspecified, many presumably were lower GI lesions. In addition, survey studies have shown that 15% of adults report gross red blood on the toilet paper following defecation, and 2–3% of "apparently healthy individuals" notice blood in the toilet or intermixed with stool.

3. What is hematochezia? What is melena?

Hematochezia is the passage of red or maroon-colored blood per rectum. This may be pure blood, blood clots, blood intermixed with or coating formed stool, or bloody diarrhea. Hematochezia is usually a manifestation of bleeding from the lower GI tract, but in approximately 20% of cases, it is seen with brisk upper GI or small bowel bleeding with rapid transit of blood.

Melena is black-colored stool that is shiny, sticky, and foul-smelling. It results from conversion of hemoglobin to hematin by bacteria of the gut. Melena is generally secondary to bleeding from an upper GI tract or small bowel source, yet it can be a manifestation of colonic bleeding, especially a right-sided colon lesion, with slow transit time.

4. Which "normal" conditions might masquerade as hematochezia?

Natural red pigments from beets may cause maroon-appearing stools. Patients who ingest laxatives to induce defecation and simultaneously drink cranberry juice or other red-colored drinks (such as Koolaid, soda pop, or fruit or vegetable juice) may have red or maroon stools. The stool is HemOccult-negative and easily distinguished from blood, even though it may alarm the patient.

5. Describe the different clinical presentations of patients with lower GI bleeding.

Patients with lower GI bleeding usually present with hematochezia. However, a proximal colon lesion may present with melena or a combination of melena and hematochezia. Lower GI bleeding is acute, self-limited, and not hemodynamically significant (no resting tachycardia or postural hypotension) in approximately 85% of patients. These patients can be evaluated electively as outpatients. Fifteen percent of patients have more severe, ongoing, hemodynamically significant (resting tachycardia, postural hypotension) bleeding. These patients require hospital admission to an intensive care unit and urgent evaluation.

6. How important is the history in assessing a patient with lower GI bleeding?

Eliciting a complete history is very important and can help identify a possible etiology of the bleeding. The duration of bleeding should be determined. When did the bleeding start? Was this the first time bleeding had been noticed, or was it a recurrent event? The quality of the bleed should be determined. What color is the blood—red, maroon, or black? Is the blood coating formed stools or intermixed? Are blood clots being passed? If the patient drips or squirts blood after defecation, this usually indicates bleeding internal hemorrhoids. Is there associated abdominal or perianal pain?

Comorbid medical conditions and past medical history should be determined, and prior surgeries may be relevent (i.e., for peptic ulcer disease). A history of surgery for an abdominal aortic aneurysm suggests possible aortoenteric fistula. Medication use, such as anticoagulants, aspirin, or nonsteroidal anti-inflammatory drugs (NSAIDs), needs to be determined because these can cause any GI lesion to bleed.

7. What physical findings are important clues to the diagnosis?
The physical examination should be directed yet complete.

1. Orthostatic vital signs assessing the hemodynamic status of the patient should be performed first.

2. Examination of the lips and mucous membranes for telangiectasias or pigmented macules may indicate Osler-Weber-Rendu disease, Peutz-Jeghers syndrome, or vascular ectasia in the gut.

3. Cardiac auscultation should be performed with attention to a possible murmur of aortic stenosis. Presence of a murmur may be insightful because some reports suggest an association between aortic stenosis and vascular ectasia of the GI tract.

4. Abdominal examination should assess for bowel sounds, tenderness, masses, and surgical scars. In addition, hepatosplenomegaly, ascites, and/or caput medusae may indicate chronic liver disease with portal hypertension, suggesting an esophageal or colonic variceal bleed.

5. Skin examination for cutaneous purpura or petechiae suggest a coagulopathy, and spider angiomata may be another indicator of chronic liver disease.

6. Joint swelling or deformity may indicate an arthritic condition and possible patient use of aspirin or NSAID products.

7. Digital rectal exam to evaluate for prolapsed internal hemorrhoids or masses and stool examination for color and guaiac testing are mandatory.

8. Does anoscopy have a role in the diagnosis of lower GI bleeding?
Anoscopy with a lighted, slotted anoscope is important to determine whether there is active bleeding from internal hemorrhoids. A visualized, nonbleeding hemorrhoid implies bleeding is *unlikely* to be hemorrhoidal in origin. Anoscopy is also helpful to exclude an anal fissure as the source of bleeding.

9. Which laboratory tests are helpful for patient evaluation in lower GI bleeding?
All patients: hemoglobin, hematocrit, platelets, prothrombin time, partial thromboplastin time
Acute severe bleeding: blood type and cross-matching
Chronic GI blood loss: liver function tests, reticulocyte count, serum iron, total iron-binding capacity, ferritin, red blood cell indices (mean cell volume, red blood cell distribution width)

10. When should a nasogastric (NG) tube be used for diagnostic evaluation of suspected lower GI bleeding?
Approximately 15–20% of patients with severe, ongoing hematochezia and anemia have an upper GI source of bleeding. To exclude this source, an NG or orogastric tube should be placed and gastric contents aspirated. An NG aspirate that is clear and nonbloody does not exclude an upper GI tract bleed unless bile is present. A *bilious*, nonbloody aspirate virtually excludes a bleeding site proximal to the ligament of Treitz when a patient has ongoing hematochezia. Guaiac testing of the NG aspirate is of no clinical utility, leads to many false-positive and false-negative results, and should not be performed.

11. What should the initial management strategy be?
The history, physical, and laboratory findings must be assessed to determine the severity of bleeding.

"Severe" lower GI bleeding is defined as persistent or recurrent bleeding that fails to stop spontaneously, with evidence of orthostatic hypotension and/or a decrease in baseline hematocrit of at least 8% after volume resuscitation. These patients should be directly admitted to an intensive care unit (ICU) or monitored bed for volume resuscitation, cardiopulmonary monitoring, further diagnostic evaluation, and treatment. Volume resuscitation should include placing an intravenous line and administering crystalloid fluids (normal saline or lactated Ringer's solution) to correct the estimated volume depletion, packed red blood cells to correct anemia (hematocrit ≤ 30%), and fresh frozen plasma or platelets to correct any coagulopathy or thrombocytopenia. Intravenous access should include at least two peripheral catheter lines, one being at least 16 gauge. A general or GI surgeon should also be consulted at the time of the patient's ICU admission. The importance of these initial resuscitative measures cannot be overemphasized.

Patients without persistent or recurrent bleeding or evidence of hemodynamic instability are defined as having a **"mild" lower GI bleed.** These patients may be electively evaluated as outpatients or as inpatients if the patient is older (> 50 years) and/or has comorbid medical conditions.

12. What causes most lower GI bleeding in ambulatory adults?

Internal hemorrhoids. Hemorrhoidal disease is estimated to occur in 50–80% of the U.S. population. This rate is in sharp contrast to that in developing countries, where the lifetime prevalence is estimated to be < 5%. Hemorrhoidal disease is uncommon in adolescents and children.

13. How do hemorrhoids develop? How does hemorrhoidal bleeding present?

Many theories have been proposed on the pathogenesis of hemorrhoids. Today, it is generally thought that chronic straining at defecation and a low-fiber diet predispose persons to hemorrhoidal disease. Over time, with increased colonic intraluminal pressure, submucosal and connective tissue support weakens and deteriorates with further enlargement of veins. As the anal lining descends, the hemorrhoids are more exposed to pressure from straining and/or direct trauma from stool. This leads to stasis of blood, swelling, erosions, and subsequent bleeding (see figure below).

Bleeding from internal hemorrhoids is usually intermittent, sometimes massive, and often noted by patients at the time of defecation. Bright red blood is generally seen coating the stool or on toilet paper, or it may drip or squirt into the toilet water. Patients may have associated symptoms of anorectal discomfort or pain, pruritus, discharge, or prolapse. Bleeding internal hemorrhoids may simulate or mask other, more serious anorectal pathology, and a more complete endoscopic examination of the colon is required.

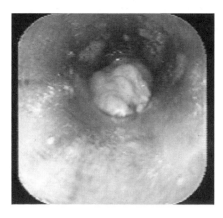

Internal hemorrhoid seen on slotted anoscopy. The patient was a 45-year-old white man with self-limited hematochezia and anemia.

14. What are other common causes of lower GI bleeding?

Diverticulosis, vascular ectasia, and neoplasms.

15. Describe diverticulosis as a cause of lower GI bleeding.

Diverticulosis is an age-acquired condition that is usually asymptomatic and most often diagnosed incidentally by barium enema. The prevalence of diverticular disease of the colon increases with age and is > 50% in individuals over age 60. It is uncommon in persons < 40 years old.

Dietary factors are theorized to play an important role in its pathogenesis. The high prevalence of diverticulosis in western countries is attributed to the consumption of a low-fiber diet, which presumably results in decreased stool bulk, prolonged fecal transit time, increased colonic muscle contractions, and elevated colonic intraluminal pressure, resulting in the formation of diverticuli.

Complications, such as inflammation or bleeding, occur in up to 20% of persons with colonic diverticular disease. Diverticular hemorrhage is reported to occur in 3–5% of persons with colonic diverticulosis. Recurrence of bleeding occurs in up to 25% of patients, and of those with recurrent bleeding, the chance of a second recurrence is 50%. Although diverticula are predominantly a left-sided colonic lesion, diverticula that bleed are most often right-sided in location. Males and females are equally affected.

Patients usually present with acute, massive, painless hematochezia, although some have melena with slow transit from right-colon bleeding. Bleeding is usually self-limited and stops spontaneously or with conservative therapy in 75–95% of patients. Diverticular bleeding is not chronic and does not cause chronic, occult blood loss.

16. Describe the vascular anatomy of bleeding diverticula.

The vasa recta, the intramural branches of the marginal artery supplying the colon, consistently penetrate the colonic wall from the serosa to the submucosa. A vas rectum intimately courses in the serosa over the dome of a diverticulum. Therefore, the vas rectum is separated from the diverticular lumen by only mucosa and a few muscle fibers. Histologic examination of bleeding colonic diverticula shows rupture of the underlying vas rectum, usually at the dome or neck of the diverticulum. The arterial defect is eccentric and faces the lumen of the diverticulum. With time, the arterial wall weakens and ruptures into the diverticulum. Arterial bleeding occurs via this communication.

17. What is vascular ectasia? How does it cause lower GI bleeding?

Vascular ectasia of the colon is a well-recognized, common cause of lower GI bleeding in older patients. These are age-acquired lesions, especially found in individuals > 50 years old, and occur with equal frequency in men and women. Sporadic vascular ectasias are also referred to as **angiodysplasias,** arteriovenous malformations, or angiomas.

Vascular ectasias are predominantly located in the cecum and proximal ascending colon, although they can occur throughout the rest of the colon, small bowel, and stomach. Twenty-five percent of patients have multiple lesions. Endoscopically, these lesions appear flat and bright red and have a fern-like pattern. Washing of the lesion can precipitate bleeding, helping to confirm the diagnosis.

Histologically, vascular ectasias consist of ectatic, distorted, thin-walled veins, venules, and capillaries in the mucosa and/or submucosa. It is theorized they develop secondary to repeated episodes of colonic distention, resulting in increased colonic wall tension. This leads to obstruction of submucosal venous outflow where these vessels penetrate the colonic muscle layers; over time, these submucosal veins, venules, and capillaries dilate and eventually form an arteriovenous communication.

The clinical presentation of patients with bleeding from colonic vascular ectasia is variable. Bleeding is usually subacute and recurrent, although 15% of patients present with acute, massive hemorrhage. Another 10–15% present with occult blood loss and iron-deficiency anemia. Bleeding ceases spontaneously in > 90% of cases.

18. Is there an association between colonic vascular ectasia and other vascular GI disorders?

Sporadic colonic vascular ectasias are clinically and pathologically unrelated to other vascular anomalies, such as hereditary hemorrhagic telangiectasias (Osler-Weber-Rendu disease), congenital arteriovenous malformations, hemangiomas, or radiation telangiectasia, that also can involve the GI tract.

19. What extrasystemic conditions are associated with colonic vascular ectasia?

There is controversy regarding the association of vascular ectasia and aortic stenosis. Several reports describe cessation of GI bleeding after aortic valve replacement, but others have failed to corroborate this. Other conditions associated with colonic vascular ectasia are chronic renal failure, cirrhosis, and collagen vascular disease.

20. How often do colonic neoplasms cause lower GI bleeding?

Colon cancer and colonic polyps more commonly present with occult GI blood loss and iron-deficiency anemia rather than gross hematochezia (see figure below). In adults over age 40 with hematochezia, colon cancer must be excluded as a possible cause of bleeding since early detection improves survival. Unfortunately, colon cancer that presents with hematochezia usually is at an advanced tumor stage. Patients with colon cancer may report an associated change in bowel habits and/or weight loss. Physical examination may reveal a palpable abdominal or rectal mass.

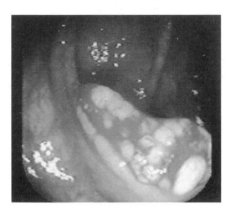

Bleeding sessile polyp (villous adenoma) of the right colon in a 57-year-old Hispanic woman. This polyp was resected endoscopically by piecemeal polypectomy.

21. Describe ischemic colitis as a cause of lower GI bleeding.

Ischemic colitis can be classified into occlusive and nonocclusive types. Most episodes have no identifiable cause. Patients present with acute onset of crampy, LLQ abdominal pain and urge to defecate, subsequently passing bloody diarrhea. Nausea, vomiting, fever, and tachycardia may also be present. Abdominal examination is often unremarkable or reveals only mild to moderate tenderness. Rarely, patients present with peritoneal signs indicative of transmural damage and perforation. "Watershed areas" of the colon, such as the splenic flexure and sigmoid colon, are more commonly involved due to their poor collateral blood flow.

Plain film abdominal radiographs may demonstrate "thumbprinting," caused by submucosal hemorrhage and edema in the colon wall. Flexible sigmoidoscopy or colonoscopy reveals segmental colonic involvement with erythema, ulceration, and/or necrosis.

Treatment consists of supportive care with optimization of hemodynamic status and correction of any underlying medical condition that may have contributed to the ischemic event. If there are peritoneal signs or ongoing hemorrhage, laparotomy with surgical resection of the involved colon is indicated. There is no role for therapeutic endoscopy in the management of these patients, who often have diffuse, segmental colitis.

22. List the less frequent causes of lower GI bleeding in an adult with hematochezia.

There are literally dozens of obscure and rare causes of lower GI bleeding that must be considered in the differential diagnosis.

Radiation-induced proctitis/colitis: This may be an acute or chronic complication of ionizing radiation for treatment of a gynecologic, prostatic, bladder, or rectal malignancy. Acute radiation injury occurs during or shortly after radiation therapy; chronic injury manifests clinically months to years later. Radiation-induced vascular damage causes ischemia, fibrosis, and mucosal ulcerations. Patients may complain of recurrent hematochezia, diarrhea, and tenesmus. Endoscopy reveals multiple, mucosal telangiectasias that are almost always the bleeding sites (see figure below).

Inflammatory bowel disease: Hematochezia occurs more commonly in ulcerative colitis than in Crohn's disease. Endoscopic findings include mucosal erythema, edema, friability, and ulcerations. Infectious causes must be ruled out. There is no role for endoscopic therapy. Medical

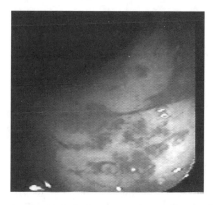

Bleeding radiation telangectasia in a 72-year-old white man with anemia and recurrent hematochezia, occurring 1 year after radiation therapy for prostate cancer. The rectal telangectasias were treated with a heater probe, which controlled the bleeding in three treatment sessions

treatment includes systemic corticosteroids, 5-aminosalicylate products, and, recently, cyclosporine. Surgery is reserved for patients not responding to medical therapy.

Infectious colitis: Bloody diarrhea can occur in colitis secondary to *Shigella, Salmonella, Campylobacter jejuni,* enteroinvasive *Escherichia coli,* enterohemorrhagic *E. coli* serotype 0157:H7, *Clostridium difficile,* or *Entamoeba histolytica* infection. Diagnosis is made by stool culture, ova and parasite examination, and/or flexible sigmoidoscopy with biopsy. In patients with impaired immunity, cytomegalovirus or herpes simplex ulcerations and Kaposi's sarcoma lesions of the colon may cause bloody diarrhea. There is no role for therapeutic endoscopy, and antibiotic treatment is pathogen-specific.

Colonic varices: These portosystemic collaterals develop secondary to portal hypertension, usually in the rectosigmoid area. Hematochezia from colonic varices has been well documented and is usually intermittent, yet severe. Colonoscopy and arteriography are the primary methods for diagnosis. On colonoscopy, the varices appear as bluish, serpiginous columns. Like gastroesophageal varices, bleeding colonic varices respond to protosystemic shunt surgery, segmental colonic and endoscopic sclerotherapy.

Intussusception of the colon: This clinical entity is rare in adults and usually has an underlying malignancy or polyp acting as the lead point for involution. Patients may present with crampy abdominal pain and hematochezia. Barium enema, ultrasonography, and abdominal CT have been used for diagnosis. Surgical resection of the involved bowel is the treatment of choice.

Other "less frequent" causes include the solitary rectal ulcer syndrome (SRUS), portal colopathy, diversion colitis, mesenteric ischemia, aortoenteric fistula, vasculitis, colonic endometriosis, and runner's colitis.

23. What is the most common cause of lower GI bleeding in children?

Meckel's diverticulum is the most common cause of lower GI bleeding in children, although rarely adults also may present with hemorrhage of this source. Meckel's diverticulum is the most common congenital anomaly of the gut, occurring in 1–3% of the population and is caused by failure of the vitelline duct to obliterate completely. It is located on the antimesenteric border of the ileum, within 100 cm of the ileocecal valve. Most Meckel's diverticula remain asymptomatic; however, GI bleeding is the most common complication. Those that bleed almost all contain functioning heterotopic gastric mucosa, which secretes acid that causes ulceration within the diverticulum or the adjacent ileal mucosa, leading to subsequent bleeding. Patients present with painless melena or hematochezia, commonly referred to as "currant jelly" stools.

24. How is the diagnosis of Meckel's diverticulum established?

Diagnosis can be made with a technetium-99m pertechnetate scintiscan (Meckel's scan), which demonstrates the heterotopic gastric mucosa by binding to the parietal cells. This test has a sensitivity of 75–100% in children, but a lower rate in adults. There is a 15% false-positive and 25% false-negative rate. In actively bleeding Meckel's diverticula, arteriography may be diagnostic. In the symptomatic patient, surgical resection of the diverticulum in the treatment of choice. Asymptomatic patients do not require treatment.

25. What are other common causes of lower GI bleeding in adolescents and young adults?
1. Anal fissures related to constipation and rectal pain with bowel movements
2. Inflammatory bowel disease and infectious diarrhea in some families and travelers
3. Internal hemorrhoids in pregnant women (and some young adults)
4. Familial polyposis and juvenile polyps in those with a family history

26. Can radiographic studies be used for diagnosis of severe lower GI bleeding?
Emergency **barium enema** has no role in a patient with severe lower GI bleeding. Barium enemas are rarely diagnostic and never therapeutic in such patients. In a critically ill patient, a technically adequate study is impossible to obtain because of the inability to prep the patient, and barium remaining in the colon precludes emergency colonoscopy or visceral arteriography for several days.

Abdominal CT may be helpful in diagnosing aortoenteric fistula in an individual presenting with severe hematochezia. A prior history of abdominal vascular surgery (i.e., abdominal aortic aneurysm repair) should indicate the need for this diagnostic test. The limitation of CT is that patients are often too ill to be safely transported and monitored in the radiology department during this examination. Most patients with severe hematochezia do not require such diagnostic testing.

27. What is the role of radionuclide scanning for diagnosis of lower GI bleeding?
Two types of radionuclide "bleeding" scans are available: technetium-labeled sulfur colloid (^{99m}Tc sulfur colloid), and technetium-"tagged" autologous red blood cells (^{99m}Tc RBC scan). Each has a threshold rate of bleeding for localization by scanning of 0.05–0.1 ml/min. Sulfur colloid is rapidly cleared, within minutes, from the intravascular space by the reticuloendothelial system. The tagged RBCs have a longer half-life and allow imaging up to 24 hours after intravenous injection. Because of its limitations, sulfur colloid scanning has largely been replaced by tagged RBC scans.

Sequential images of the abdomen, using a gamma camera, are obtained. Images within the first 1–4 hours of radionuclide injection are often the most useful for localizing severe, active bleeding (see figure below). Delayed RBC scans at 12 and 24 hours may detect intermittent GI bleeding. These scans may be useful for localizing colonic sites of actively bleeding diverticuli, vascular ectasia, or tumors, particularly if early scans at 1–4 hours are positive. However, scintigraphy has a significant rate of incorrect localization of GI bleeding, and performing surgery on the basis of a positive RBC scan alone is not recommended. Radiologists usually prefer scintigraphy as the initial diagnostic test and, if it is positive, proceed with visceral arteriography. We recommend initial colonoscopy and, if nondiagnostic, proceed to a tagged RBC scan. In many institutions, scintigraphy has replaced emergency visceral arteriography as an adjunct to colonoscopy because of its higher sensitivity, noninvasive technique, and lower cost.

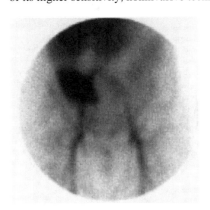

Positive Tc-tagged RBC scan in a patient with recurrent hematochezia. A cecal vascular ectasia was later confirmed by colonoscopy. (Courtesy of Carl Hoh, M.D.)

28. When is visceral arteriography indicated for diagnosis and therapeutic intervention in patients with lower GI bleeding?
Selective visceral arteriography is potentially diagnostic as well as therapeutic. The diagnostic yield varies with patient selection, timing of the procedure, and skill of the angiographer

but ranges from 12–72%. Extravasation of contrast material into the gut lumen may be seen when there is active bleeding at a rate of at least 1–1.5 ml/min (see figure below). Selective arterial catheterization can also be used to diagnose abnormal vessels consistent with tumors or vascular ectasia as well as actively bleeding colonic diverticula.

Therapeutic interventions include vasopressin infusion and embolization techniques using autologous clots, absorbable gelatin (Gelfoam), metal coils, oxidized cellulose, and polyvinyl alcohol particles. Potential complications from visceral arteriography and transcatheter treatment are bowel ischemia and infarction, arterial thrombosis and embolization, hematoma formation, and contrast-induced renal failure.

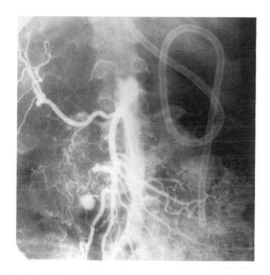

Positive emergency arteriogram in a patient with ongoing hematochezia and multiple diverticuli by colonoscopy. (Courtesy of Antoinette Gomes, M.D.)

29. When is flexible sigmoidoscopy indicated for diagnosis of patients with lower GI bleeding?
Flexible sigmoidoscopy, performed with a 65-cm instrument, can diagnose lesions beyond the view of the anoscope and up to the descending colon. For patients with severe hematochezia who are being evaluated as an emergency, this examination should be done before colonoscopy, because diagnosis of a bleeding source would potentially obviate the need for further endoscopic examination. Preparation is important, with enemas until clearance of stool and blood, although such clearance may not be possible in very ill patients. However, a diagnostic flexible sigmoidoscopy examination may obviate the need for other emergency examinations, whereas a normal examination indicates the need for further studies. Turnaround examination (retroflexion) in the rectum allows for visualization of lesions potentially missed by rigid sigmoidoscopy or anoscopy. In addition, biopsies of involved colonic mucosa or suspicious lesions may be obtained at the time of examination.

30. When is esophagogastroduodenoscopy (EGD) recommended in a patient with the presumptive diagnosis of lower GI bleeding?
Exclusion by EGD of a bleeding lesion proximal to the ligament of Treitz is recommended if the nasogastric aspirate is grossly bloody, a nonbilious nonbloody aspirate returns, the history is suggestive of an upper GI source, or anoscopy and flexible sigmoidoscopy fail to identify a probable rectosigmoid bleeding source. A bile-containing, nonbloody gastric aspirate virtually excludes an upper GI source of bleeding. In our experience, 11% of patients presenting with severe hematochezia had an upper GI source of bleeding diagnosed at EGD. This percentage is consistent with other published data on etiologies of hematochezia. EGD should be performed before oral purge and urgent colonoscopy. Some authorities advocate EGD in all patients presenting with acute, severe hematochezia regardless of nasogastric aspirate results.

Etiologies for 100 Patients with Severe Hematochezia

LESION SITE	NO. OF PATIENTS
Colonic	74 (74%)
Vascular ectasia	30 (41%)
Diverticulosis	17 (23%)
Polyps or cancer	11 (15%)
Focal colitis	9 (12%)
Rectal lesions	4 (5%)
Other	3 (4%)
Upper GI	11 (11%)
Small bowel*	9 (9%)
No site found	6 (6%)

*A diagnosis of presumed small bowel site of bleeding was made when panendoscopy and colonoscopy were negative, but fresh blood or clots (or both) were coming through the ileocecal valve. (Courtesy of CURE Hemostasis Research Group.)

31. What is "urgent" colonoscopy? What is its role in diagnosing lower GI bleeding?

Urgent colonoscopy involves a full colonoscopic examination to the cecum and terminal ileum in a patient with severe hematochezia after the colon has been cleansed of stool and blood. In our experience, these colonoscopies are performed in the ICU with videocolonoscopes and necessary accessories available for diagnosis and treatment. Until recently, urgent colonoscopy in patients with severe hematochezia was thought to be dangerous, often nondiagnostic, and impractical. However, this technique is feasible with adequate prior colonic cleansing. Colonoscopy also allows for biopsies to be obtained and definitive endoscopic hemostasis if clinically indicated.

At colonoscopy, diagnosis of a bleeding site can be made by visualization of active bleeding, a nonbleeding visible vessel, an adherent clot resistant to washing with an endoscopic catheter, or blood in an area around a clean lesion without other lesions in that segment of bowel. In our experience, initial colonoscopy and/or EGD can make a definitive diagnosis in approximately 90% of patients with ongoing hematochezia (see algorithm below).

Recommended Diagnostic Approach to the Patient with Severe Lower GI Bleeding

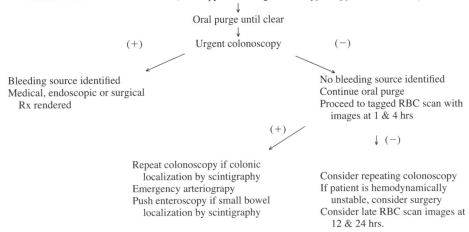

32. Describe colon cleansing as used prior to "urgent" colonoscopic evaluation.

Best results are achieved with an electrolyte-polyethylene glycol (PEG) solution, such as GoLytely, CoLyte, or NuLytely, performed simultaneously with resuscitation measures. The purge solution, administered orally or via nasogastric tube, is given at a rate of 1 liter every 30–45 minutes over 3–5 hours, until the rectal effluent is clear of stool and blood clots. Usually, 5–8 liters is sufficient to achieve this goal. Metoclopramide (10 mg intravenously before and then every 3–4 hours) helps to decrease the nausea and facilitate gastric emptying. The PEG solution should be administered at room temperature so as to maintain patient core body temperature. Once the rectal effluent is clear of stool and blood clots, colonoscopy can be performed safely and effectively.

33. What bleeding colonic lesions are amenable to endoscopic treatment?

Lower GI bleeding secondary to internal hemorrhoids, vascular ectasia, diverticula, colonic tumors or polyps, radiation telangiectasia, colonic varices, and colonic ulcers are all amenable to endoscopic hemostasis techniques.

34. List the main risks of endoscopic hemostasis performed via colonoscopy.

Perforation

Post-coagulation syndrome (abdominal pain, focal rebound tenderness, fever, and leukocytosis without evidence of perforation)

Delayed bleeding

Rectal or colonic stenosis (rarely, due to repeated circumferential coagulation with Nd:YAG laser of radiation telangectasia or villous adenomas)

These risks are minimized if hemostasis procedures are performed by trained endoscopists.

35. When is "emergency" surgery indicated for acute lower GI bleeding?

A general or GI surgeon should be consulted upon admitting the patient to the hospital. Emergency surgery is reserved for those patients who have:

(1) Ongoing bleeding and persistent hypovolemic shock despite resuscitation efforts;

(2) Ongoing bleeding and transfusion requirements > 6 units of packed red blood cells and no diagnosis by emergency colonoscopy, scintigraphy, or arteriography; or

(3) A specific segmental diagnosis made by colonoscopy and/or arteriography, in which surgery is determined to be the best mode of treatment.

Emergency surgery, in the face of ongoing bleeding, has a much greater mortality (> 25%) than elective surgery performed once bleeding has ceased (< 10%). The ability to localize the bleeding site preoperatively allows for segmental resection with decreased patient morbidity and mortality.

BIBLIOGRAPHY

1. Dennison AR, Wherry DC, Morris DL: Hemorrhoids: Nonoperative management. Surg Clin North Am 68:1401, 1988.
2. Freeman ML: The current endoscopic diagnosis and intensive care unit management of severe ulcer and other nonvariceal upper gastrointestinal hemorrhage. Gastrointest Endosc Clin North Am 1:209, 1991.
3. Hosking SW, Johnson AG, Smart HL: Anorectal varices, haemorrhoids, and portal hypertension. Lancet 1:349, 1989.
4. Jensen DM, Machicado GA: Management of severe lower gastrointestinal bleeding. In Barkin JS, O'Phelan CA (eds): Advanced Therapeutic Endoscopy, 2nd ed. New York, Raven Press, 1994, p 201.
5. Jensen DM, Machicado GA: Diagnosis and treatment of severe hematochezia: The role of urgent colonoscopy after purge. Gastroenterology 95:1569, 1988.
6. Meyers MA, Alonso DR, Gray GF: Pathogenesis of bleeding colonic diverticulosis. Gastroenterology 71:577, 1976.
7. Miller LS, Barbarevech C, Friedman LS: Less frequent causes of lower gastrointestinal bleeding. Gastroenterol Clin North Am 23:21, 1994.
8. Randall GM, Jensen DM, Machicado GA: Prospective randomized comparative study of bipolar versus direct current electrocoagulation for treatment of bleeding internal hemorrhoids. Gastrointest Endosc 40:403, 1994.
9. Reinus JF, Brandt LJ: Vascular ectasias and diverticulosis: Common causes of lower intestinal bleeding. Gastroenterol Clin North Am 23:1, 1994.
10. Savides TJ, Jensen DM: Colonoscopic hemostasis for recurrent diverticular hemorrhage associated with a visible vessel: A report of three cases. Gastrointest Endosc 40:70, 1994.
11. Schrock TR: Colonoscopic diagnosis and treatment of lower gastrointestinal bleeding. Surg Clin North Am 69:1309, 1989.
12. Zuckerman DA, Bocchini TP, Birnbaum EH: Massive hemorrhage in the lower gastrointestinal tract in adults: Diagnostic imaging and intervention. AJR 161:703, 1993.

54. OCCULT AND OBSCURE GASTROINTESTINAL BLEEDING

Thomas Kepczyk, MD

1. What is occult gastrointestinal bleeding?

Bleeding that is hidden and not grossly apparent on stool inspection, but is manifested by a positive chemical test for stool blood, iron-deficiency state, or anemia.

2. What is obscure gastrointestinal bleeding?

Recurrent bouts of acute or chronic bleeding that have been evaluated with routine endoscopic or radiologic procedures, with no definitive source identified.

3. What are HemOccult cards?

HemOccult cards, used to detect the presence of occult blood in stool, are made of a guaiac-impregnated paper and used with a developing solution of hydrogen peroxide and denatured alcohol. Hemoglobin in stool has a pseudoperoxidase activity that allows the oxidative conversion of guaiac from colorless to a blue color. HemOccult is the tradename for one such test (made by SmithKline Beecham Diagnostics), but other similar cards are available from other sources with equal sensitivity.

4. What factors can give a false-positive or false-negative result on an occult blood test?

Foods containing pseudoperoxidase can produce a **false-positive** reaction: rare red meat, raw broccoli, turnips, cauliflower, radishes, cantaloupe, and parsnips. Some have advocated rehydrating the cards with water prior to development, but this can result in a higher false-positive rate. **False-negative** results have been attributed to ascorbic acid (vitamin C), improper storage and developing (i.e., delayed testing), degradation of hemoglobin by colonic bacteria, and absence of bleeding at the time of testing. In a recent study oral iron preparations did not result in false-positive HemOccult tests, and therefore a positive test in the setting of iron supplementation should be evaluated.

5. Describe the proper way to test stool for occult blood.

For 3 days prior to the collections, the patient should avoid rare red meat, peroxidase-containing vegetables (*see* Question 4), vitamin C, aspirin, and nonsteroidal anti-inflammatory drugs (NSAIDs). They should collect two samples from three consecutive stools. The slides should be developed within 4–6 days, and for average-risk patients, you should not rehydrate the slides prior to developing, as this results in a higher false-positive rate.

6. How much blood loss is required to give a positive HemOccult test? How much blood loss is required to result in gross bleeding?

Only 2 ml of blood is needed to produce a positive HemOccult test. Melena is apparent when 200 ml of blood is acutely present in the stomach, and melena or hematochezia is apparent if 150 ml of blood are released in the cecum. However, if the bleeding is lower in the colon (i.e., anorectal), then as little as 1–2 ml will be apparent as streaks of blood on the stool.

One exception to this rule is in the setting of hematochezia or maroon stools in a hemodynamically unstable patient: approximately 10% of patients with massive upper GI hemorrhage have a negative nasogastric lavage. Therefore, some have advocated a diagnostic upper GI endoscopy as part of the evaluation in this setting.

7. How effective is occult blood testing in detecting colorectal cancer or colon adenomas in asymptomatic patients?

In large population studies, the positivity rate of HemOccult testing ranges from 2–6%. The predictive value of a positive test (true-positives) for colon cancer is 5%, and for adenomas is 20%.

However, the cancers found using screening HemOccult testing usually are of a lower stage: 65–90% are Duke's stage A or B in the screened group versus 33–55% in a control group. False-negative tests occur in approxiately 40%, probably due to an intermittent bleeding pattern. False-positive results occur in 2%.

8. An asymptomatic patient over age 50 without anemia has a positive HemOccult test. What should the further evaluation be?
In this situation, the goal is to exclude colorectal carcinoma. The most sensitive and specific approach would be to perform a colonoscopy. However, the combination of sigmoidoscopy and air-contrast barium enema probably is equally sensitive in detecting cancer, although this approach may miss small lesions. If the colon examination does not reveal a cancer or significant lesion, then it is acceptable to stop further evaluation, as long as there are not symptoms and no anemia, and repeat the HemOccult testing in 6–12 months. Some have advocated checking a serum ferritin level in addition, as it is inexpensive and may give an early clue to chronic blood loss. If the ferritin is low, then further evaluation is warranted.

9. How common is iron deficiency, and what are some of the physical signs and symptoms of iron-deficiency anemia?
In the United States, an estimated 20 million people are iron deficient, and the global prevalence is estimated at 15%, or 600 million people, making this a common problem. In men and post-menopausal women, GI bleeding is the most common etiology. Symptoms include fatigue and tachycardia due to the anemia. Pica has also been reported, and pagophagia, or ice eating, is not uncommon in iron-deficient women and children. Physical signs include chcilitis (fissuring and scaling of lips), glossitis (erythema and loss of lingual papillae), and koilonychia (nails become brittle, furrowed, or spooned). An associated finding is upper esophageal webs, also known as Plummer-Vinson syndrome or Paterson-Kelly syndrome.

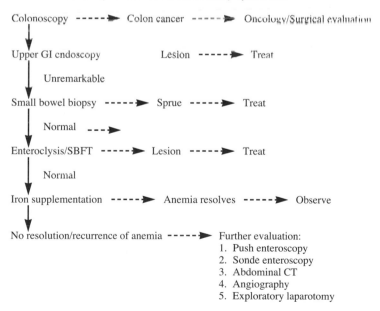

Algorithm for evaluation of iron-deficiency anemia. SBFT = small bowel follow-through.

10. What should the evaluation consist of in an elderly patient with iron-deficiency anemia?

Most physicians agree that a colon examination is indicated, with colonoscopy being the preferred method. If colonoscopy is unremarkable or if any findings suggest an etiology of the blood loss, then upper GI endoscopy needs to be performed. Some studies have supported doing both colonoscopy and upper endoscopy as the initial evaluation. In a recent study, 17% of patients with iron-deficiency anemia had potential upper and lower sources of blood loss. Also, if no suspicious lesions are noted on colonoscopy and upper endoscopy, then a small bowel biopsy is warranted at the time of upper endoscopy, as celiac sprue is found in approximately 5% of patients with occult iron deficiency. Some of these sprue patients will present with iron deficiency as the only manifestation of the celiac disease, i.e., no symptoms of weight loss or diarrhea. Also, if angiodysplasias are suspected, substitution of the usual meperidine (Demerol) analgesia with naloxone may make the lesions more apparent, because meperidine has been reported to cause blanching of the lesions.

11. What lesions are found in the evaluation of iron-deficiency anemia?
The most common lesions found are peptic lesions, such as gastric erosions, esophagitis, and ulcers, which are found in 38%. Neoplastic lesions (cancer and large adenomas) are found in approximately 15%, in the order of frequency of colorectal cancer > primary gastric cancer > esophageal cancer > ampullary cancer.

Etiologies Associated with Iron-Deficiency Anemia

Peptic lesions	Neoplastic lesions
Gastric erosions	Primary GI cancer (any site)
Esophagitis	Metastatic lesions to GI tract
Gastric and duodenal ulcers	Large polyps (any location)
Vasular lesions	Small bowel lesions
Angiodysplasia	Meckel's diverticulum
Hemangioma	Sprue
Gastric vascular ectasia/watermelon stomach	Eosinophilic gastroenteritis
Blue rubber bleb nevus syndrome	Whipple's disease
Inflammatory lesions	Infectious causes
Crohn's disease	Hookworm
Ulcerative colitis	Strongyloidiasis
Miscellaneous etiologies	Ascariasis
Gastric surgery, Billroth II procedure	Tuberculous enterocolitis
Long-distance running (runner's colitis or gastritis)	
Small bowel ulcers due to NSAIDs	
Solitary rectal ulcer syndrome	
Severe hemorrhoidal bleeding	

12. What should be done if the initial evaluation with upper and lower endoscopy is negative in an iron-deficient patient?
If the endoscopic evaluation is negative, then the small bowel should be evaluated. Small bowel follow-through has a 5% yield, and this rate can be increased to 10% with an enteroclysis. If this evaluation is negative, then the patient should be placed on iron supplements and observed for a response. If the patient's hemoglobin normalizes, then continued observation is warranted. However, if the patient's hemoglobin fails to improve or anemia recurs, then special studies are warranted: push enteroscopy, sonde enteroscopy, angiography, abdominal CT, and interoperative endoscopy, depending on the severity of blood loss (*see* Figure 1).

13. How often will the source of recurrent or chronic bleeding remain obscure after standard upper and lower endoscopic or barium evaluation?
In 3–5% of the cases. The lesions typically are located between the second portion of the duodenum and the ileocecal valve. These small bowel sources are difficult to diagnose.

14. Name the most common small bowel lesions found in this setting.
Small bowel angiodysplasias account for 80% of lesions found in several studies, followed by small bowel tumors. Of all patients with angiodysplasias, 10% eventually bleed.

15. Which radiologic techniques can be used in further evaluating recurrent obscure bleeding?

In patients who are relatively stable, numerous options are available. Some advocate **barium small bowel follow-through,** but this test has a yield of only 5%, and that of enteroclysis is only 10%. **Radioisotope bleeding scans** reportedly can isolate 5 ml of intraluminal blood after 1–2 hours and have the advantage of allowing a repeat scan at 24 hours; however, in one series, bleeding scans failed to localize the source in 85%. **Angiography** can detect bleeding at a rate of 0.5 ml/min; this technique will localize bleeding in 50–72% with massive hemorrhage but in only 25–50% with slow or intermittent bleeding, and it is especially poor for small bowel angiodysplasias. **Stress angiography,** or pharmacoangiography, which uses heparin or vasodilators during angiography to induce or continue bleeding, has also been advocated. However, the true yields are unknown, and extreme caution should be used in performing these procedures.

16. What are the endoscopic options in further evaluating recurrent obscure bleeding?

Push enteroscopy, with passage of a colonoscope (160 cm) peroral, generally reaches beyond the ligament of Treitz and has a yield of 38% over standard upper GI endoscopy. If this technique fails to localize a source, then intraoperative endoscopy or enteroscopy is indicated. Newer push enteroscopes (250–300 cm) can reach approximately 100 cm beyond the ligament of Treitz and increase the yield by a further 25–30%. Both the colonoscope and enteroscopes allow treatment of lesions, i.e., coagulation of angiodysplasias.

Another type of enteroscope is **sonde enteroscope,** which is a small-diameter scope passed transnasally and allowed to pass via peristalsis to the distal small bowel (75% of exams reach the ileum or colon). This technique allows a more complete evaluation of the small bowel and has a higher yield, between 29–40%. Its disadvantage is that no treatment can be applied through the scope.

Intraoperative endoscopy presently is the most widely used technique and involves passage of a peroral colonoscope while the surgeon has the abdomen open. The surgeon assists in passage of the scope by "sleaving" the small bowel over the colonoscope. This technique is very successful, with a source identified in 83–100% of cases.

17. So what is a rational approach to evaluate obscure gastrointestinal bleeding?

Massive bleeding: If there is massive bleeding and initial esophagogastroduodenoscopy (EGD) and colonoscopy are negative or unhelpful, then acute angiography is indicated. If this is unhelpful, or if bleeding continues to be severe, then surgery is indicated and intraoperative endoscopy may be used.

Occult or intermittent bleeding: If the initial EGD and colonoscopy are unrevealing, then push enteroscopy is warranted. If this is negative and the patient is <50 years old, exploratory laparotomy is indicated, as in this age group, a Meckel's diverticulum or small bowel tumor is likely. If no lesions are palpated, then intraoperative endoscopy may localize the lesion. If the patient is >50 years old, then sonde enteroscopy, if available, should be considered, or interoperative endoscopy to help localize the site, as angiodysplasia is much more likely in this setting (see algorithm on next page).

18. Some patients with obscure GI bleeding have multiple angiodysplasias throughout the small bowel and colon, and endoscopic or surgical treatment may not be an option. What are other options?

This situation occurs typically in the elderly, renal failure patients, and patients with Osler-Weber-Rendu disease. Medical management has included iron supplementation to keep up with blood loss, and more recently, reports have shown some success using hormonal therapy with estrogen/progesterone. This approach has been most effective in patients with renal failure or Osler-Weber-Rendu disease, where it reportedly stops bleeding in 57% of patients on dialysis. However, other studies have shown no benefit. Recent case reports have shown the use of octreotide, a somatostatin analog, to be promising in preventing rebleeding from angiodysplasias.

Massive Bleeding

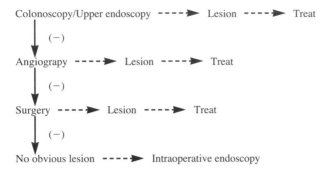

Intermittent Bleeding

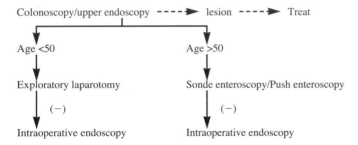

Algorithms for evaluation of obscure GI bleeding.

BIBLIOGRAPHY

1. Ahlquist DA: Approach to the patient with occult gastrointestinal bleeding. In Yamada T (ed): Textbook of Gastroenterology. Philadelphia, J.B. Lippincott, 1991.
2. Berner JS, Mauer K, Lewis BS: Push and sonde enteroscopy for the diagnosis of obscure gastrointestinal bleeding. Am J Gastroenterol 89:2139, 1994.
3. Chong J, Tagle M, Barkin JS, Reiner DK: Small bowel push-type fiberoptic enteroscopy for patients with occult gastrointestinal bleeding or suspected small bowel pathology. Am J Gastroenterol 89:2143, 1994.
4. Coles EF, Starnes ED: Use of HemoQuant assays to assess the effect of oral iron preparations on stool hemoccult tests. Am J Gastroenterol 86:1442, 1991.
5. Foutch PG, Sawyer R, Sanowski RA: Push-enteroscopy for diagnosis of patients with gastrointestinal bleeding of obscure origin. Gastrointest Endosc 36:337, 1990.
6. Keller FS, Rosch J, Barton RE: Pharmacoangiography, a visceral stress test. Pract Gastroenterol 17(10):16C, 1993.
7. Kepczyk T, Kadakia SC: Prospective evaluation of the gastrointestinal tract in patients with iron-deficiency anemia. Dig Dis Sci 40:1283–1289, 1995.
8. Lewis BS: Occult gastrointestinal bleeding. In Clinical Update—American Society for Gastrointestinal Endoscopy. 2(3):1, 1995.
9. Lewis BS, Waye J: Small bowel enteroscopy for obscure GI bleeding. Gastrointest Endosc 37:277, 1991.
10. Lewis BS: Intraoperative techniques in patients with obscure bleeding. Pract Gastroenterol 18(1):28A, 1994.
11. Peterson WL, Laine L: Gastrointestinal bleeding. In Sleisenger MH, Fordtran JS (eds): Gastrointestinal Disease: Pathophysiology, Diagnosis, Management. Philadelphia, W.B. Saunders, 1993.
12. Peterson WL: Obscure gastrointestinal bleeding. Med Clin North Am 72:1169, 1988.
13. Rossini FP, Arrigoni A, Pennazio M: Octeotide in the treatment of bleeding due to angiodysplasia of the small intestine. Am J Gastroenterol 88:1424, 1993.

55. EVALUATION OF ACUTE ABDOMINAL PAIN

James E. Cremins, M.D. and Peter R. McNally, D.O.

1. Provide a useful clinical definiton of an acute abdomen.
This clinical scenario is characterized by severe pain, often of rapid onset, that prevents bodily movement. When patients experience symptoms of pain for more than 6 hours, surgical intervention is usually necessary.

2. What are the four types of stimuli for abdominal pain?
Stretching or tension, inflammation, ischemia, and neoplasms.

3. What are the three categories of abdominal pain?
Visceral, parietal, and referred.

Visceral pain occurs when noxious stimuli affect an abdominal viscus. The pain is usually dull (cramping, gnawing, or burning) and poorly localized to the ventral midline. The pain is poorly localized because the innervation to most viscera is multisegmental. Secondary autonomic effects such as diaphoresis, restlessness, nausea, vomiting, and pallor are common.

Location of Visceral Pain

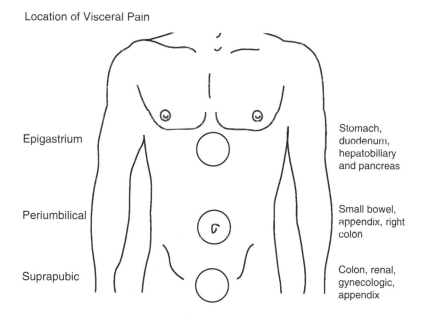

Epigastrium — Stomach, duodenum, hepatobiliary and pancreas

Periumbilical — Small bowel, appendix, right colon

Suprapubic — Colon, renal, gynecologic, appendix

Parietal pain occurs when noxious stimuli irritate the parietal peritoneum. The pain is more intense and more precisely localized to the site of the lesion. Parietal pain is likely to be aggravated by coughing or movement.

Referred pain is experienced in areas remote from the site of injury. The remote site of pain referral is supplied by the same neurosegment as the involved organ, e.g., gallbladder pain may be referred to the right scapula and pancreatic pain may radiate to the mid back.

4. How does the character of the abdominal pain help in the evaluation?

Classification of Pain by the Rate of Development

Explosive and excruciating (instantaneous)	Myocardial infarction Perforated ulcer Ruptured aneurysm Biliary or renal colic (passage of a stone)
Rapid, severe, and constant (over minutes)	Acute pancreatitis Complete bowel obstruction Mesenteric thrombus
Gradual and steady pain (over hours)	Acute cholecystitis Diverticulitis Acute appendicitis
Intermittent and colicky pain (over hours)	Early subacute pancreatitis Mechanical small bowel obstruction

5. What are the important components of the physical examination for the patient with acute abdominal pain?

General status	Is the patient hemodynamically unstable? Does he or she need immediate hemodynamic resuscitation and emergent laparotomy, e.g., ruptured spleen, hepatic tumor, aneurysm, ectopic pregnancy, or mesenteric apoplexy.
Inspection	Visually evaluate for distention, hernias, scars, and hyperperistalsis.
Auscultation	Hyperperistalsis suggests obstruction; absence of peristalsis >3 minutes suggests peritonitis (silent abdomen); bruits suggest presence of an aneurysm.
Percussion	Tympany suggests either intraluminal or free abdominal air.
Palpation	Start the examination away from the area of tenderness and be gentle. Abdominal pain with voluntary coughing suggests peritoneal signs. Deeply palpating the abdomen in this case will only diminish patient trust and cooperation. The enlarged gallbladder will be missed on deep palpation. Inspiratory arrest during light palpation of the right hypochondrium suggests gallbladder pain—Murphy's sign. Localized pain suggests localized peritonitis, e.g., appendicitis, cholecystitis, diverticulitis. The abdominal examination of visceral ischemia/infarction is characteristically disproportionate to the degree of abdominal pain.
Pelvic and rectal exam	These exams should be done in any patient with abdominal pain. A painful rectal examination may be the only sign of pelvic appendicitis, diverticulitis, or tuboovarian pathology. Bimanual examination is critical in order to exclude obstetric or gynecologic cause.
Iliopsoas test	With the patient supine and the legs fully extended, the patient is requested to raise the legs. Pain occurs when the psoas muscle is inflamed, e.g., appendicitis.
Obturator test	This test is performed by flexing the patient's thigh at right angles to the trunk and then rotating the leg externally. Inflammation of the obturator internus muscle will cause pain to be elicited with this test, e.g., tuboovarian abscess or pelvic appendicitis.

6. What laboratory tests should be obtained in the patient with acute abdominal pain?
Although laboratory tests are helpful in confirming that a disease process is evolving, they are frequently not helpful in localizing the cause of the abdominal pain.
- Complete blood count (CBC): elevation of the white blood count suggests inflammation;

however, absence of leukocytosis may be unhelpful early. A low hematocrit with a normal MVC suggests acute blood loss, whereas a low hematocrit with a low MCV suggests iron deficiency from chronic GI blood loss or malabsorption.

- Amylase elevations (> 500 IU) suggest pancreatitis but are not specific. Lipase enzyme elevations are more specific for pancreatic origin.
- Liver enzyme elevations may be suggestive of hepatobiliary causes of pain. Aminotransferase (AST or ALT) elevations suggest hepatocyte injury. Alkaline phosphatase or gamma glutamine transferase (GGT) elevations suggest canalicular or biliary injury. Total bilirubin elevations over 3 mg/dl suggest common bile duct obstruction or associated intrahepatic cholestasis.
- Evidence of pyuria on urinalysis suggests urinary tract infection but also may be seen in nephrolithiasis or even pelvic appendicitis.
- Chemistry analysis can be helpful in the global assessment of patient health, hyperglycemia, acidosis, electrolyte disturbances.
- Pregnancy tests (β-HCG) should be ordered for all premenopausal women.
- Stool examination for occult blood is necessary.
- ECG is performed for all patients with possible myocardial infarction or over 50 years of age.

7. What radiologic test(s) should be ordered to evaluate the patient with acute abdominal pain?
The selection of tests depends on the likelihood of the pretest clinical diagnosis and the ability of the radiologic test to confirm the clinical suspicion.

- Plain x-rays of the abdomen are quick, readily available, and can be done at the bedside. They are reliable in detecting bowel obstruction and viscus perforation. Occasionally they may suggest stone disease (1/3 of gallbladder and 2/3 of renal stones are calcified) or ruptured aortic aneurysm (separation of aortic wall calcium and mass effect). Free intra-abdominal air is best detected with the patient in the left lateral decubitus position for 10 minutes (see chapter 72).
- Ultrasound of the abdomen is quick, noninvasive, and can be performed at the bedside. The disadvantages of ultrasound include variable operator expertise and suboptimal examination in the obese or gaseous abdomen. Ultrasound is excellent for evaluating the gallbladder, bile ducts, liver, kidneys, and appendix (see chapter 74).
- Computerized tomography (CT) of the abdomen provides a detailed view of the anatomy. It is expensive, requires transportation of the patient, and is not always readily available. Oral and intravenous contrast agents are usually required. It provides the best evaluation of the pancreas (see chapter 74).
- HIDA scan is the most accurate test for acute cholecystitis (see chapter 74).

8. Pain referred to the abdomen can be confusing to the clinician. What are some of the extra-abdominal causes of referred abdominal pain?

Thoracic	Pneumonia, pulmonary embolism, pneumothorax, myocardial infarction or ischemia, esophageal spasm, or perforation
Neurogenic	Tabes dorsalis, radicular pain (spinal cord compression from tumor, abscess, compression, or varicella zoster)
Metabolic	Uremia, porphyria, acute adrenal insufficiency
Hematologic	Sickle cell anemia, hemolytic anemia, Henoch-Schonlein purpura
Toxins	Insect bites (scopine bite-induced pancreatitis), lead poisoning

9. What are the common causes of acute abdominal pain in gravid females?
Appendicitis, ovarian cysts complicated by torsion, rupture, and hemorrhage, and gallbladder problems.

10. When the appendix is found to be entirely normal during a laparotomy performed for presumed appendicitis in a gravid woman, should the appendix be removed?
No. Removal of the normal appendix triples the risk of fetal loss.

11. What is the most common cause of acute abdominal pain in the elderly?
Biliary tract disease is responsible for 25% of all cases of acute abdominal pain in the elderly requiring hospitalization. Bowel obstruction and incarcerated hernia are the next most common, followed by appendicitis.

12. What symptom(s) are helpful in evaluating for appendicitis?
It is decidedly uncommon for acute appendicitis to present with nausea, vomiting, or diarrhea *before* abdominal pain. Usually acute appendicitis is heralded by pain and often followed by anorexia, nausea, and sometimes single-episode vomiting. Acute appendicitis should be first on the differential diagnosis list in anyone with acute abdominal pain without a prior history of appendectomy. The diagnosis of typical appendicitis requires only careful history and physical examination. Laboratory tests and radiographic studies are ancillary.

13. What are some atypical forms of appendicitis?
When the appendix is retrocecal or retroileal in location, the inflamed appendix is often shielded from the anterior abdomen. Here the pain is often less pronounced and localizing signs on physical examination uncommon. Symptoms and signs of appendicitis in the elderly are subtle. Pain is often minimal, fever only mild, and leukocytosis unreliable. A high index of suspicion is essential.

14. Describe the ultrasound findings of acute appendicitis.
The appendix appears as a round target with an anechoic lumen, surrounded by a hypoechoic and thickened (>2 mm) appendiceal wall. This finding with reproduction of pain under the transducer has a diagnostic accuracy of 95% and a negative predictive value of 97%.

15. When laparotomy is performed for presumed appendicitis, what is the acceptable false-negative rate. How often is another cause identified in this circumstance?
A false-negative laparotomy of 10–20% is reported. In roughly 30% of these cases some other cause of abdominal pain is identified, such as mesenteric lymphadenitis, Meckel's diverticulum, cecal diverticulitis, pelvic inflammatory disease, ectopic pregnancy, ileitis.

16. What is the single best test to evaluate patients with immunodeficiency syndrome complaining of acute abdominal pain?
Due to the variety of causes of abdominal pain in these patients, it has been argued that CT scan is the single best test.

17. What are the cardinal features of a ruptured tubal pregnancy?
- Amenorrhea—missed period or scant menses
- Abdominal and pelvic pain
- Unilateral, tender adnexal mass
- Signs of blood loss

18. What are the characteristics of acute intestinal obstruction?
- Nausea and vomiting
- Failure to expel flatus
- Prior abdominal surgery or presence of hernia
- Peristaltic pain (colicky pain—every 10 minutes for jejunal obstruction and every 30 mintues for ileal obstruction)

19 What are the characteristics of large bowel obstruction?
- Most patients are over 50 years of age.
- Lower abdominal cramping pain is gradual in onset.
- Abdominal distention is a prominent feature.
- Dilated loops of bowel with haustra distinguish the colon from the small bowel.
- Sigmoidoscopy or single-column barium enema is important.
- Causes include obstructing neoplasm, and cecal or sigmoid volvulus.

20. What are the clinical characteristics of diverticulitis?
- most patients are over 50 years of age
- localized left lower abdominal pain
- palpable mass in the left lower quadrant

21. What are the clinical hallmarks of acute cholecystitis?
- Patients often give a history of prior episodes of milder abdominal pain.
- Abdominal pain usually arises after a meal, especially in the evening after a large meal.
- Pain typically crescendos over 20–30 minutes and then plateaus.
- Pain lasting longer than 1–2 hours is usually accompanied by gallbladder wall inflammation.
- Associated nausea occurs in 90%; vomiting may follow the onset of pain in 50–80% of cases.
- Radiation of the pain to the back is common, to the right scapula in 10%.
- Low-grade fever is common.
- Right hypochondrium tenderness is generally seen. Inspiratory arrest during gentle palpation of the right upper quadrant—Murphy's sign—is suggestive of acute cholecystitis.
- Diagnostic tests include HIDA scan or ultrasound.

22. What is the differential diagnosis of acute cholecystitis?
- Liver: alcoholic hepatitis, liver metastasis, Fitz-Hugh–Curtis syndrome, congestive hepatopathy
- Pancreas: pancreatitis, pseudocyst
- Gastrointestinal tract: peptic ulcer disease with or without perforation, acute appendicitis (retrocecal)
- Kidney: pyelonephritis, renal colic
- Lung: pneumonia, pulmonary embolism, emphysema
- Heart: myocardial infarction, pericarditis
- Pre-eruptive varicella zoster

23. When should a patient undergo surgery for an acute abdomen?
When, in the judgment of the surgeon, a problem will be identifiable or treatable by surgical intervention. There is no substitute for good surgical judgment and intuition.

BIBLIOGRAPHY

1. Brandt CP, Priebe PP, Eckhauser ML: Diagnostic laparoscopy in the intensive care patient: Avoiding the non therapeutic laparotomy. Surg Endosc 7:168–172, 1993.
2. Clement DJ: Evaluation of the acute abdomen with CT: IS image everything? Am J Gastroenterol 88:1282–1283, 1993.
3. Connor TJ, Garcia IS, Ramshaw BJ, et al: Diagnostic laparoscopy for suspected appendicitis. Am Surg 61:187–189, 1995.
4. de Dombal FT: Acute abdominal pain in the elderly. J Clin Gastroenterol 19:331–335, 1994.
5. Epstein FB: Acute abdominal pain in pregnancy. Emerg Med Clin North Am 12:151–165, 1994.
6. Haubrich WS: Abdominal pain. In Haubrich WS, Schaffner, F, Berk JE (eds): Bockus Gastroenterology, 5th ed. Philadelphia, WB Saunders, 1995, pp 11–29.
7. Klein KB: Approach to the patient with abdominal pain. In Yamada T (ed): Textbook of Gastroenterology, 2nd ed. Philadelphia, J.B. Lippincott, 1995, pp 750–771.
8. Kovachev LS: "Cough sign": A reliable test in the diagnosis of intra-abdominal inflmmation. Br J Surg 81:1542, 1994.
9. Mulhohhand MW: Approach to the patient with acute abdomen and fever of abdominal origin. In Yamada T (ed): Textbook of Gastroenterology, 2nd ed. Philadelphia, J.B. Lippincott, 1995, pp 783–796.
10. Ridge JA, Way LW: Abdominal pain. In Sleisenger MH, Fordtran JS (eds): Gastrointestinal Disease: Pathophysiology/Diagnosis/Management, 5th ed. Philadelphia, W.B. Saunders, 1993, pp 150–162.
11. Silen W: Cope's Early Diagnosis of the Abdomen. New York, Oxford University Press. 1979.
12. Taourel P, Baron MP, Pradel J, et al: Acute abdomen of unknown origin: Impact of CT on diagnosis and management. Gastrointest Radiol 1992;17:287–291, 1992.
13. Wyatt SH, Fishman EK: The acute abdomen in individuals with AIDS. Radiol Clin North Am 32:1032–1043, 1994.

56. EVALUATION OF ACUTE DIARRHEA

Kent C. Holtzmuller, M.D.

1. What are the most common causes of acute bloody diarrhea?
Infectious dysentery, inflammatory bowel disease (ulcerative colitis and Crohn's disease), and ischemic colitis.

INFECTIOUS DYSENTERY

2. What is dysentery?
Dysentery is a disease process characterized by diarrhea that contains blood and polymorphonuclear cells. Dysentery results when an organism causes an inflammatory reaction, either by direct invasion of the colonic/ileal epithelium or by producing a toxin that causes cellular death and tissue damage. Symptoms associated with dysentery may include abdominal pain and cramping, tenesmus (painful urgency to evacuate stool), fever, and dehydration.

3. Name the common causes of infectious dysentery in the United States.
Campylobacter and *Salmonella* are the principal causes of dysentery in the United States. *Shigella* and certain strains of *Escherichia coli* are less common. Rarer causes include *Yersinia, Entamoeba, Aeromonas,* and *Plesiomonas.*

4. What is the significance of stool leukocytes?
The presence of fecal polymorphonuclear cells and mononuclear leukocytes aids in distinguishing inflammatory diarrhea from noninflammatory diarrhea. Under normal circumstances, fecal leukocytes are not present in the stool. Fecal leukocytes are usually found in the stool of infectious diarrhea caused by *Campylobacter, Salmonella, Shigella, Yersinia, Clostridium difficile,* enterohemorrhagic and enteroinvasive strains of *Escherichia coli,* and *Aeromonas.* Fecal leukocytes are also seen in ischemic colitis and in the inflammatory bowel conditions ulcerative colitis and Crohn's disease. Diarrhea secondary to a noninflammatory cause does not contain stool leukocytes.

5. How do you evaluate a stool specimen for leukocytes?
The study is best performed on liquid stool or mucus.
1. Place a drop of liquid stool or mucus on a glass microscope slide.
2. Add several drops of methylene blue or Gram stain.
3. Mix the material thoroughly.
4. Place a coverslip over the mixture.
5. Wait several minutes to allow for nuclear staining.
6. Scan the slide under high power to observe for leukocytes and red blood cells (positive if ≥3 leukocytes are present in four or more fields).

6. By what mechanisms do toxigenic organisms produce diarrhea?
The toxins produced by organisms can be classified into two categories, cytotonic and cytotoxic. **Cytotonic toxins** cause a watery diarrhea by activation of intracellular enzymes, which cause net fluid secretion into the intestinal lumen. Examples of cytotonic toxins are toxins produced by *Vibrio cholerae* and enterotoxigenic strains of *E. coli.* **Cytotoxic toxins** cause structural injury to the intestinal mucosa, which, in turn, causes inflammation and resultant diarrhea that contains red and white cells. An example of a cytotoxic toxin is that produced by enterohemorrhagic *E. coli.*

7. Which *Campylobacter* species are implicated as causes of dysentery? How is *Campylobacter* transmitted?
C. jejuni accounts for 98% of isolates reported. The less common isolates are *C. fetus* and *C. fecalis.* Direct contact with fecal matter from infected persons or animals and the ingestion of contaminated food or water have been implicated in the transmission of *Campylobacter.*

8. Describe the clinical and endoscopic features of *Campylobacter* diarrhea.
Incubation, from ingestion of organisms to the onset of symptoms, is 1–7 days. Symptoms include diarrhea (often bloody), abdominal pain, malaise, headache, and fever (sometimes high). With or without antibiotic therapy, most patients recover within 7 days. Relapse may occur. The sigmoidoscopic findings in the rectum and sigmoid colon may be indistinguishable from those of ulcerative colitis or Crohn's disease. A tentative diagnosis of *Campylobacter* infection can be made if Gram stain of the stool shows comma-shaped, gram-negative bacteria.

9. How are *Salmonella* organisms classified?
Salmonella are gram-negative, aerobic and facultative anaerobic bacteria of the Enterobacteriaceae family. There have been 2200 different serotypes identified utilizing O and H antigens. The term *nontyphoidal salmonellosis* is used to denote disease caused by serotypes of *Salmonella,* with the exception of *S. typhi.*

10. List the types of illnesses that can be caused by *Salmonella*.
  1. Acute gastroenteritis: The degree of colonic involvement determines the extent of the dysentery-like symptoms.
  2. Bacteremia with or without GI involvement
  3. Localized infection: Bacteremia can result in localized nonintestinal infections (e.g., bone, joints, meninges).
  4. Typhoidal or enteric fever
  5. Asymptomatic carrier state: Asymptomatic chronic carriers often have cholelithiasis.

11. What is typhoid fever?
Typhoid fever is a clinical syndrome characterized by prolonged high fever, sustained bacteremia, hepatosplenomegaly, and abdominal pain. The illness can be caused by any serotype of *Salmonella* but most commonly occurs with *S. typhi* and less commonly with *S. paratyphi*. Humans are the only known reservoir of *S. typhi,* so transmission is primarily fecal-oral. The illness usually lasts for 3–5 weeks. Up to 90% of patients may experience a "rose spot" rash within the first or second week of illness, typically on the upper anterior trunk. Diarrhea is unusual, although the illness may be complicated by intestinal hemorrhage or perforation secondary to ulceration of Peyer's patches in the small and large intestine. A number of vaccines are successful against typhoid.

12. Describe the characteristics of *Shigella* infection.
Shigella is a gram-negative rod and member of the Enterobacteriaceae. Most (90–95%) *Shigella* infections are caused by four species: *S. sonnei, S. flexneri, S. dysenteriae,* and *S. boydii.* The organism is highly infectious, with transmission by the fecal-oral route. Infection can occur with the ingestion of as few as 10–100 organisms. Intestinal damage occurs primarily from direct invasion of the organism into the colonic epithelium and, to a lesser extent, by the production of an enterotoxin. The *Shigella* toxin is composed of an A sunbunit, which is catalytic, and a B subunit, which is responsible for binding. The endoscopic appearance of shigellosis shows intense involvement of the rectosigmoid with varying levels of proximal colonic involvement. Approximately 15% of *Shigella* cases will have a pancolitis. In children, *Shigella* infection has been associated with the occurrence of seizures.

13. What are the diarrheogenic illnesses caused by *Escherichia coli*?
   E. coli belong to the family Enterobacteriaceae and are facultative anaerobic, gram-negative bacteria. They are common inhabitants of the human GI tract, and most strains do not have virulence factors to cause disease. The four pathogenic strains of *E. coli,* and the syndromes they cause, are listed below:

Enterotoxigenic *E. coli* (ETEC): ETEC accounts for most traveler's diarrhea but is relatively rare in the United States. Fecal-oral transmission through the ingestion of contaminated food or water is the primary means of spread. Disease is produced by the adherence of ETEC to the mucosa, followed by the production of toxins. Invasion of the mucosa does not occur. The usual course of the disease is a self-limited, 3–5-day illness characterized by watery diarrhea and abdominal cramping. Occasionally, a low-grade fever and, rarely, a bloody diarrhea are associated with this illness.

Enteropathogenic *E. coli* (EPEC): This strain also lacks invasive properties, and disease results from its enteroadherent properties. Illness caused by EPEC primarily affects the young ($<$ 2 years of age) and must be considered as a probable cause in outbreaks of diarrhea in hospitalized infants. Profuse watery diarrhea, which can become chronic, is the usual presentation of this disease. As with ETEC, EPEC-caused illnesses rarely result in bloody diarrhea.

Enteroinvasive *E. coli* (EIEC): This strain can invade the intestinal mucosa and usually presents with symptoms of bloody diarrhea, fever, abdominal cramping, tenesmus, and myalgias. EIEC strains are not commonly found in the United States.

Enterohemorrhagic *E. coli* (EHEC): Although a number of serotypes have been identified as the etiology of EHEC, *E. coli* 0157:H7 is the principal serotype. Acquisition of *E. coli* 0157:H7 is primarily from the ingestion of contaminated beef, although outbreaks have also been associated with contaminated water, raw milk, and person-to-person transmission among household members. The patient usually presents with severe abdominal cramps and watery diarrhea, which then progresses to bloody diarrhea. The organism is not invasive but produces disease from a Shiga-like toxin, which is cytotoxic to vascular endothelial cells in vitro. The disease can produce the hemolytic uremic syndrome and thrombotic thrombocytopenia purpura, although fewer than 10% of cases will develop these conditions. The very young and old are the most susceptible for fatal complications.

14. Describe the clinical presentation of infection with *Yersinia enterocolitica.*

The most common presentation of *Y. enterocolitica* infection is diarrhea, abdominal pain, and low-grade fever. Most cases are self-limited and do not require antibiotic therapy. Microscopic examination of the stool usually shows red and white cells. Approximately 25% of the diarrhea cases are grossly bloody. Children and young adults can present with a pseudoappendicular syndrome manifested by symptoms of RLQ abdominal pain and tenderness, fever, and leukocytosis. Findings at surgery show mesenteric lymphadenitis and terminal ileitis. On rare occasions, a patient may progress to a fulminant enterocolitis with possible perforation, peritonitis, and major intestinal hemorrhage. Pharyngitis is common in children with *Y. enterocolitica* infection and is seen in up to 10% of adult cases. Patients with an iron-overload state (hemochromatosis) are susceptible to sepsis from *Yersinia*. Postinfectious manifestations of reactive arthritis erythema nodosum, Reiter's syndrome, thyroiditis, myocarditis, and glomerulonephritis have been reported.

15. Which organisms are associated with seafood-induced dysentery?

Vibrio parahaemolyticus is a member of the Vibrionaceae family and is a halophilic organism (grows only in media containing salt). This organism has been isolated in fish, crustaceans, and shellfish. The resulting diarrhea is commonly watery, but up to 15% of patients present with bloody diarrhea.

Other organisms that cause dysentery and are associated with seafood ingestion are *Plesiomonas shigelloides* (a Vibrionaceae) and *Campylobacter.*

16. What parasites cause bloody diarrhea?

Entamoeba histolytica, Balantidium coli, Dientamoeba fragilis, and *Schistosoma.* Amebiasis, caused by *Entamoeba histolytica,* is the most common cause of parasitic-induced dysentery in the United States. Although parasitic diarrhea is rare in the United States, it is a significant cause of morbidity and mortality worldwide.

17. Who is at risk for amebiasis? What are the potential complications of amebic dysentery?
Individuals at high risk include travelers and immigrants from endemic areas, institutionalized patients, and homosexual men. Complications include toxic megacolon, intestinal perforation, peritonitis, ameboma, and liver abscess.

18. What is an ameboma?
An ameboma is a segmented mass of granulation tissue and inflammatory swelling of the mucosa and submucosa of the colon. This inflammatory process can present as a tender, palpable abdominal mass but is usually located in the cecum or ascending colon. Approximately 0.5–1.5% of patients with amebic colitis will have an ameboma. Barium enema may show an "apple-core" appearance. Diagnosis is confirmed with colonoscopy, and biopsy is necessary to rule out carcinoma or tuberculosis. Amebomas respond to antiamebic therapy, and surgery is generally not required.

19. Are any laboratory studies useful in the diagnosis of amebic dysentery?
An **ova and parasites exam** of a stool specimen may show cysts and trophozoites. Symptomatic disease is produced when the trophozoites invade the colonic mucosa. The **indirect hemagglutination test** to detect antibody titers to *E. histolytica* is the most commonly used serologic test. Approximately 80–90% of patients with amebic dysentery have a positive serology, although a negative serologic study does not rule out the possibility of infection. A positive serologic study in a patient with diarrhea who has a tentative diagnosis of inflammatory bowel disease should raise the possibility that the actual diagnosis is amebiasis.

20. How do you obtain a stool specimen for ova and parasites exam?
Stool examination for patients with suspected protozoan infection should be properly performed to obtain the highest yield possible. A hat-like container is a convenient receptacle in which to collect the stool, as the specimen should be free of contamination from urine and toilet water. Because protozoan trophozoites degenerate rapidly, the specimens should be fresh and processed expeditiously, or they should be preserved using a two-vial preservation technique. One vial contains a buffered formalin mixture, and the other, a polyvinyl alcohol fixative. Because of the uneven shedding of some forms of parasites, it is recommended that a total of three specimens be obtained, each collected every second or third day. A number of substances may interfere with this stool examination, including barium, antibiotics, mineral oil, antacids, bismuth, and enemas.

21 Describe the treatment of amebic dysentery. What are the potential side effects of metronidazole?
Treatment of acute amebic dysentery is metronidazole, 500–750 mg three times daily for 5–10 days. Metronidazole can induce an "Antabuse" effect (abdominal cramps, nausea, emesis, headache, flushing) if alcohol is consumed during therapy, and so alcohol should be avoided during therapy and for 1 day after cessation. Other important drug effects may be the potentiation of the effects of warfarin and lithium. A peripheral neuropathy manifested by numbness or paresthesia in the distal extremities has also been seen with metronidazole. This symptom has been reported to be persistent in patients taking prolonged metronidazole therapy. Other possible symptoms include a metallic taste and GI distress manifested by nausea, flatus, and diarrhea.

22. What causes pseudomembranous colitis (PMC)? What are the risk factors for this disease?
PMC is caused by *Clostridium difficile*, a gram-positive, spore-forming, anaerobic bacillus. The colitis induced by *C. difficile* is mediated by two toxins, enterotoxin A and cytotoxin B. Patients are suceptible to *C. difficile* diarrhea during and after the cessation of antibiotic therapy. The diarrhea typically presents 10 days after initiation of antibiotics but may begin several days following initiation and up to 8 weeks after cessation. Clindamycin, the penicillins, and the cephalosporins are most frequently associated with this syndrome. Less frequently associated are

tetracycline, erythromycin, and metronidazole, and rarely associated are the quinolones, parental aminoglycosides, and vancomycin. Other risk factors for PMC are cancer chemotherapy, immunosuppression, and hospitalization. Improper washing of hands by hospital personnel is a major route of transmission of PMC in hospitals.

23. How do you diagnose pseudomembranous colitis?

A **stool assay for** *C. difficile* **toxin** should be obtained in any patient suspected of having PMC. Culture is available and is very sensitive but not very specific, because up to 20% of hospitalized patients are colonized with *C. difficile*. The endoscopic appearance of the involved colonic mucosa can range from normal to the classic appearance of a **pseudomembrane**—i.e., 1–3-mm, yellow-whitish, plaque-like lesions that are scattered or confluent over the colonic mucosa. The histologic appearance of the pseudomembrane shows a "summit" or "volcano" lesion on the surface of the colonic epithelium, which is composed of inflammatory cells, fibrin, and mucus. However, a lack of pseudomembranes on sigmoidoscopy does not exclude *C. difficile* colitis; 50% of patients present without characteristic pseudomembranes and 10% of patients have mucosal changes confined to the right colon. Isolated pseudomembranes in the right colon have also been reported.

24. What is the treatment of pseudomembranous colitis?

First, stop the incriminated antibiotic. Discontinuation of the antibiotic therapy alone results in complete cessation of symptoms in many patients.

Consider drug therapy in any patient with moderate to severe symptoms. Oral vancomycin, metronidazole, and Bacitracin have all been shown to be effective. Vancomycin is expensive (up to $500 for a 5–10-day course). Intravenous metronidazole can be used in a patient who cannot tolerate oral intake. A symptomatic relapse rate of 15–20% is seen following treatment with all three therapies.

An alternative to antibiotic therapy is the oral anion exchange resin, cholestyramine. The resin allows binding of *C. difficile* toxin while the colonic flora reconstitutes itself. Resin therapy has been advocated for use in mild cases and for treatment of relapses in patients treated with antibiotics.

Fecal enemas have been used experimentally to reestablish bacterial flora. Although interesting from a theoretical standpoint, the value of fecal enemas in clinical practice could be diminished by limited patient acceptance of this therapy.

25. Outline the differential diagnosis of a patient with AIDS who presents with bloody diarrhea.

As with nonimmunosuppressed patients, colitis secondary to the invasive bacteria (*Salmonella, Shigella, Campylobacter,* and *Yersinia*), bacteria which produce cytotoxins (EHEC), and amebiasis must be considered. Infections that can result in a proctitis and bloody diarrhea include rectal gonorrhea, lymphogranuloma venereum (*Chlamydia trachomatis*), primary anorectal syphillis, and herpes simplex. The hallmark of herpes proctitis is severe rectal pain and tenesmus. In addition, a purulent rectal discharge is frequently present, and difficulty with urination, inguinal lymphadenopathy, and perianal ulcerations may also be noted.

Colitis characterized by abdominal pain, diarrhea, hematochezia, and fever is a common manifestation of cytomegalovirus (CMV) infection. Patchy involvement of the colonic mucosa is often seen on colonoscopy in patients with CMV infection, and diagnosis is aided by the identification of cytomegalic inclusion cells. Pseudomembranous colitis must also be in the differential for individuals with AIDS who are taking or have recently completed antibiotic therapy. It should be noted that more than one cause of diarrhea may be present concurrently in this population.

Cryptosporidium, Isospora belli, Microsporidia, Giardia, Mycobacterium avium-intracellulare, and lymphoma, all of which can cause diarrhea in this population, typically affect the small bowel but do not cause a bloody diarrhea. Patients who have inflammatory bowel disease and then acquire AIDS have been reported to show improvement in their inflammatory bowel disease, probably secondary to the immunosuppression from the HIV.

26. List the risk factors and therapy for infectious dysentery.

Infectious Dysentery

ORGANISM	RISK FACTORS/RESERVOIRS	THERAPY
*Campylobacter**	Contaminated food, water, raw milk, infected animals and humans	Erythromycin Ciprofloxacin
*Salmonella** (nontyphoidal)	Food (milk, eggs, poultry, meats), water, infected humans	Ampicillin TMP/SMX
*Shigella**	Food, water, infected humans	Ciprofloxacin TMP/SMX Ampicillin Tetracycline
Escherichia coli (EHEC)	Beef, raw milk, direct contact	Supportive care
*Aeromonas**	Untreated water	TMP/SMX
Plesiomonas	Uncooked shellfish	TMP/SMX
*Yersinia**	Food (milk products, tofu), water	TMP/SMX
Entamoeba histolytica	Travel to endemic areas (food, water, fruit)	Metronidazole
Clostridium difficile	Antibiotic use, chemotherapy	Metronidazole Vancomycin Cholestyramine

*Mild to moderate symptoms do not require antibiotic therapy. TMP/SMX = trimethroprim/sulfamethoxazole.

27. Are antimotility agents contraindicated in patients with dysentery?
Antimotility agents, such as diphenoxylate-atropine (Lomotil) and loperamide (Imodium), have historically been contraindicated in patients with bloody diarrhea. It was felt that reduced colonic motility would promote overgrowth of the pathogens. However, a recent study of patients with bloody diarrhea due to *Shigella* showed that loperamide, when used in conjunction with antibiotic therapy, shortened the duration of the diarrhea. No adverse side effects were seen in these patients or in patients with dysentery caused by other organisms. However, no benefit was seen in the patients with other organisms. Antimotility agents continue to be contraindicated in children with dysentery due to case reports of adverse outcomes.

28. What is Reiter's syndrome? Which enteric infections are associated with its development?
Reiter's syndrome is a triad of arthritis, urethritis and conjunctivitis. *Salmonella, Shigella, Campylobacter jejuni,* and *Yersinia enterocolitica* have been associated with this syndrome. Approximately 80% of patients affected by Reiter's syndrome are HLA-B27 antigen-positive. The male-to-female ratio is 9:1.

INFLAMMATORY BOWEL DISEASE

29. How does one differentiate between an acute infectious dysentery and the acute onset of inflammatory bowel disease as the cause of bloody diarrhea?
The clinical symptoms and endoscopic findings of the colon are often similar in these two diagnoses. When evaluating a patient with bloody diarrhea, the clinician must use historical data, assess the patient's potential risk factors and associated symptoms, and evaluate endoscopic appearance, radiologic findings, and laboratory data to narrow the differential. Many of the infectious dysentery illnesses are self-limited in nature. Dysenteric illnesses that do not spontaneously resolve and are culture-negative should undergo investigation for inflammatory bowel disease.

30. Can a mucosal biopsy obtained on flexible sigmoidoscopy assist in differentiating among acute bacterial dysentery, ulcerative colitis, and Crohn's disease?
Some overlap can be seen on histologic evaluation of mucosal specimens in these three conditions, and biopsy findings are not 100% specific. However, there are distinguishing features

among the three diseases. Acute, self-limited **bacterial infection** shows mucosal edema, neu-
trophilic infiltration of the superficial lamina propria, absence of plasmacytosis of the deep lamina propria, and preservation of the crypt architecture. Histologic findings of **ulcerative colitis** include crypt abscesses (clumps of neutrophils in the crypt lumen), chronic inflammation limited to
the mucosa and submucosa, atrophy, and possibly dysplasia. The presence of granulomas and
granulomatous features is the hallmark of **Crohn's disease.** However, the absence of granulomas
does not exclude Crohn's disease, because up to 50% of patients may not show granulomas on
biopsy. Submucosal inflammation, focal ulceration, and patchy involvement in the biopsy specimen are also suggestive of Crohn's disease.

31. Describe the endoscopic differences between ulcerative colitis and Crohn's disease.

Ulcerative colitis is marked by continuous inflammatory changes of the colonic mucosa,
consisting of granularity with loss of vascular markings, erosions, ulcerations, and pseudopolyps
that begin at the anal verge and extend to variable lengths proximally.

A diagnosis of **Crohn's** disease is favored when there is discontinuous mucosal involvement,
a "cobblestone" appearance of the mucosa, perianal disease, terminal ileal disease (if the exam is
performed to the terminal ileum), and stricturing in the colon. Continuous involvement of the
colonic mucosa alone does not rule out the possibility of Crohn's disease. Approximately 5–15%
of cases will be indeterminate on edoscopic evaluation.

32. Contrast the distinguishing features of ulcerative colitis and Crohn's disease.

Distinguishing Features of Ulcerative Colitis and Crohn's Disease

	CROHN'S DISEASE	ULCERATIVE COLITIS
Symptoms	Pain is more common; bleeding is uncommon	Diarrhea with a bloody-mucoid discharge, cramping
Location	Can affect the GI tract from mouth to anus	Limited to the colon
Pattern of colonic involvement	Skip lesions	Continuous involvement
Histology	Transmural inflammation, granulomas, focal ulceration	Mucosal inflammation, crypt abscesses, crypt distortion
Radiologic	Terminal ileal involvement, deep ulcerations, normal haustra between involved areas, strictures, fistulas	Rectum involved, shortened colon, absence of haustra (lead-pipe sign)
Complications	Obstruction, fistulas, abscesses, kidney stones, gallstones, B12 deficiency	Bleeding, toxic megacolon, colon cancer

33. What is toxic megacolon? What are its risk factors?

Toxic megacolon is a complication of colitis manifested by dilatation of the colon, with associated fever, tachycardia, leukocytosis, anemia, and postural hypotension. The colonic dilatation
occurs following an inflammatory process that involves the entire colonic wall and causes the
colon to lose its ability to contract. Ulcerative colitis patients with severe pancolitis are at highest risk for toxic megacolon, but this process can be seen in any type of severe colitis. Barium enema, colonoscopy, the antimotility agents loperamide and diphenoxylate, anticholinergics, and
opiates have been implicated as precipitating risk factors.

34. What is the treatment of ulcerative colitis?

5-Aminosalicylic (5-ASA) compounds (sulfapyridine, mesalamine, olsalazine) should be the initial therapy for mild or moderate symptoms. Colitis located in the distal colon can be treated with

5-ASA enemas or steroid enemas. Prednisone should be used for moderate symptoms unresponsive to 5-ASA compounds and for severe symptoms. Immunosuppressants (6-mercaptopurine, azathioprine, cyclosporine) can be used for colitis refractory to steroid therapy. Patients with severe refractory colitis, toxic megacolon unresponsive to medical management, exsanguinating hemorrhage, severe refractory extraintestinal manifestations, and dysplasia or cancer on biopsy should be treated with removal of the colon. The surgical alternatives are proctocolectomy with Brooke ileostomy formation or an ileoanal anastomosis (a pouch is formed from the terminal ileum and sewn into the dentate line).

35. Does treatment of ulcerative colitis differ from that of Crohn's disease?

Mild to moderate ileocolonic Crohn's disease should also undergo an initial trial of a 5-ASA compound. Metronidazole is used for patients with perianal disease and is an alternative therapy for patients with ileocolonic disease unresponsive to 5-ASA. Disease unresponsive to metronidazole and severe disease should be treated with prednisone. Steroid-refractory disease can be treated with trials of immunosuppressants. Surgery should be reserved for disease unresponsive to medical management and limited to resection of the disease which necessitated the surgery. Ileoanal anastomoses are not advocated for Crohn's disease because of the possibility of disease recurrence in the ileal pouch.

36. How does sulfasalazine work? What are its potential side effects?

Sulfasalazine is composed of sulfapyridine azo bonded to 5-ASA. The compound enters the colon, where bacteria cleave the azo bond, releasing the two moieties. Although the exact mechanism of action of sulfasalazine is unknown, it is believed that the 5-ASA portion, by interfering with prostaglandin production in the colonic mucosa, is the active component.

Symptoms of nausea, dyspepsia, anorexia, and headache are the most common side effects associated with sulfasalazine use. Additional side effects include sulfa allergic reactions, low-grade hemolysis, folate deficiency, and reduction in sperm count (reversible).

37. How are the other 5-ASA compounds formulated?

Other 5-ASA compounds include olsalazine, a compound in which two 5-ASA molecules are azo-bonded, and mesalamine, a slow-release form of 5-ASA. These two compounds do not have a sulfa component as part of their structure. Absorption of 5-ASA would occur in the upper GI tract if it were not azo-bonded.

38. What extraintestinal manifestations are associated with inflammatory bowel disease?

Extraintestinal Manifestations of Inflammatory Bowel Disease

Rheumatologic	Peripheral large-joint arthritis
	Sacroiliitis
	Ankylosing spondylitis
Dermatologic	Pyoderma gangrenosum
	Erythema nodosum
Ophthalmologic	Episcleritis
	Uveitis
Hepatobiliary	Primary sclerosing cholangitis
	Fatty liver
Hematologic	Iron-deficiency anemia
	Thrombosis
	Vitamin B12 deficiency (Crohn's disease)
	Folate deficiency (sulfasalazine)

ISCHEMIC COLITIS

39. Are there predisposing factors for ischemic colitis?
Most patients with ischemic colitis are middle-aged or elderly and have a history of atherosclerotic heart disease and/or peripheral vascular disease. Medications that have been implicated in colonic ischemia include digitalis, NSAIDs, diuretics, vasopressin, gold compounds, and some cancer chemotherapeutic agents. A common complication of surgical repair of an abdominal aortic aneurysm is colonic ischemia. During surgery, mucosal ischemia occurs from the prolonged low blood flow state to the colonic mucosa or from disruption of blood flow in the inferior mesenteric artery.

40. Name the segment of colon most commonly affected by ischemic disease.
The left colon is the segment most commonly affected (75%). The next most common segments are the transverse colon (15%) and right colon (5%). Although any area of the colon can be affected by ischemia, the rectum is rarely involved due to its rich blood supply.

41. How is the diagnosis of ischemic colitis established?
Clinically, the patient complains of sudden-onset abdominal pain. The degree of bloody diarrhea is variable. An acute abdominal series may show "thumbprinting" of the colonic mucosa.
Flexible sigmoidoscopy is the mainstay of diagnosis. The rectum is usually spared due to its collateral blood flow. Above the rectum, the mucosa becomes friable and edematous, and there may be hemorrhagic areas and ulcerations resembling those of Crohn's disease. Angiography is generally not helpful in the evaluation of ischemic colitis; ischemic colitis is a small-vessel disease (nonocclusive), as opposed to mesenteric midgut ischemia of the small bowel, which involves thrombosis or embolism in the superior mesenteric artery (occlusive). A barium enema is contraindicated in the patient with suspected ischemic colitis, because colonic expansion during a barium enema may produce further ischemia of the colonic mucosa.

42. What is the therapy for ischemic colitis? What are the possible patient outcomes?
Treatment of a patient with ischemic colitis is supportive, involving abdominal exam, complete blood count, and close monitoring of the patient's vital signs. Broad-spectrum antibiotic therapy is recommended.
There are three possible outcomes of ischemic injury:
1. The patient progressively improves and the symptoms resolve over several days to weeks. Most patients have this outcome.
2. The patient proceeds to bowel infarction with the eventual development of peritonitis and possible perforation.
3. The patient improves but develops a stricture in the colon that may or may not be symptomatic.

OTHER ETIOLOGIES

43. What is diversion colitis?
Diversion colitis is an inflammatory process that is seen in the portion of colon from which the fecal stream has been diverted. This is usually seen in a Hartmann's pouch that is formed after a sigmoid resection. The endoscopic and histologic appearance of the mucosa is similar to that of ulcerative colitis. These changes resolve promptly following anastomosis of the bowel and restoration of the fecal stream. Proposed theories as to the cause of this inflammatory reaction include overgrowth of normal bowel flora and a nutritional deficiency of short-chain fatty acids. Short-chain fatty acids are produced by anaerobic bacteria and are used as an energy source by the colonic epithelium cells.

44. Describe the evaluation of a patient with acute bloody diarrhea.

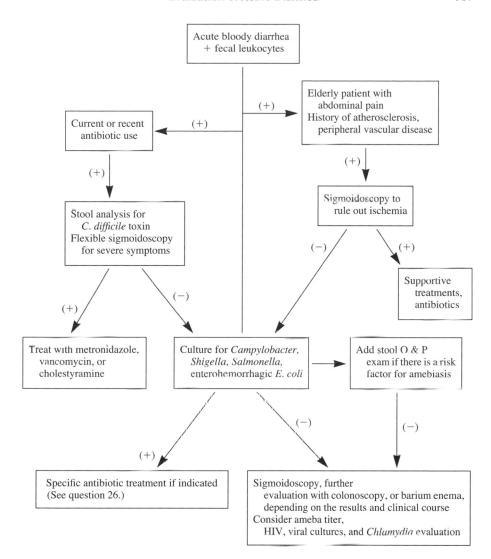

45. List the rare or unusual causes of acute bloody diarrhea.

Bloody diarrhea, like many other illnesses, has many different causes, some of which show up only rarely.

Unusual Causes of Bloody Diarrhea

Vasculitides	Neoplastic
Beçhet's disease	Chemotherapy
Henoch-Schönlein purpura	Graft-versus-host disease (bone marrow
Polyarteritis nodosa	transplantation)
Churg-Strauss disease	Radiation therapy
Wegener's granulomatosis	Hematologic
Cryoglobulinemia	Sickle cell disease
Systemic lupus erythematosus	Iatrogenic
Mechanical	Glutaraldehyde-sterilizing solution (residue
Intestinal intussusception	on equipment)

BIBLIOGRAPHY

1. Cover TL, Aber RC: *Yersinia enterocolitica.* N Engl J Med 321:16–24, 1989.
2. Gorbach SL: Bacterial diarrhoea and its treatment. Lancet 2:1378–1382, 1987.
3. Goldberg MB, Rubin RH: The spectrum of *Salmonella* infection. Inf Dis Clin North Am 2:571–598, 1988.
4. Goodell SE, Quinn TC, Mertichian E, et al: Herpes simplex virus in homosexual men. N Engl J Med 308:868–871, 1983.
5. Griffen PM, Ostroff SM, Tauxe RV, et al: Illnesses associated with *Escherichia coli* 0157:H7 infections. Ann Intern Med 109:705–712, 1988.
6. Farmer RG: Infectious causes of diarrhea in the differential diagnosis of inflammatory bowel disease. Med Clin North Am 74:29–38, 1990.
7. Finch MJ, Riley LW: Campylobacter infections in the United States. Arch Intern Med 144:1610–1612, 1984.
8. Holmberg SD, Schell WL, Fanning GR, et al: Aeromonas intestinal infections in the United States. Ann Intern Med 105:683–689, 1986.
9. Krogstad DJ, Spencer HC, Healy GR: Amebiasis. N Engl J Med 298:262–265, 1978.
10. Murphy GS, Bodhidatta L, Echeverria P, et al: Ciprofloxacin and loperamide in the treatment of bacillary dysentery. Ann Intern Med 118:582–586, 1993.
11. Park SI, Giannella RA: Approach to the adult patient with acute diarrhea. Gastroenterol Clin North Am 22:483–497, 1993.
12. Sawyer MK, Gehlbach SH: Bacterial diseases of the colon. Prim Care 15:125–145, 1988.
13. Smith PD: Infectious diarrheas in patients with AIDS. Gastroenterol Clin North Am 22:535–548, 1993.
14. Stenson WF, MacDermott RP: Inflammatory bowel disease. In Yamada T, Alpers DH, Owyong C, et al (eds): Textbook of Gastroenterology. Philadelphia, J.B. Lippincott, 1991.
15. Yaun SK, Liu FJ: Laboratory diagnosis of gastrointestinal tract and exocrine pancreatic diseases. In Henry JB (ed): Clinical and Diagnosis Management by Laboratory Methods. Philadelphia, W.B. Saunders, 1991, pp 536–549.

57. CHRONIC DIARRHEA

Jorge L. Herrera, M.D.

1. What is the definition of chronic diarrhea?

Diarrhea is defined as abnormal frequency and liquidity of fecal discharges. More precisely, diarrhea is present if daily stool weight exceeds 250 gm and the number of movements are >2/day. Increased stool weight without increased liquidity is not considered diarrhea and most likely represents increased fiber intake.

Most cases of diarrhea are self-limited and resolve within 7–12 days. Diarrhea that persists for >4 weeks is considered chronic. In some cases, it is difficult to assess whether the patient is actually having diarrhea or frequent passage of small amounts of stool. A 24-hr stool collection for volume and weight can be used to resolve the issue. A value of **<200 gm/day** indicates that no true diarrhea exists; in this case, proctitis with tenesmus or fecal incontinence may be considered. Stool weights of 200–350 gm/day are typically found in patients with functional diarrhea, such as irritable bowel syndrome. A stool weight **>800 gm/day** suggests small bowel disease rather than isolated colonic disease.

2. List the four major mechanisms of diarrhea.

Osmotic diarrhea is caused by the presence of poorly absorbable, osmotically active solutes that are either ingested or remain in the bowel as a result of maldigestion or malabsorption

Secretory diarrhea is caused by abnormal secretion or inhibition of absorption by the intestinal epithelium.

Deranged intestinal motility decreases intestinal transit time and reduces the amount of time that intestinal contents are in contact with the mucosa for proper absorption of nutrients, water, and electrolytes.

Inflammatory diarrhea results from exudation of mucus, blood, and protein from sites of inflammation.

3. What important historical features may help in the differential diagnosis of diarrhea?

Medication and dietary history: Many prescription and nonprescription medications can induce diarrhea. Elixirs, in particular, may contain significant amounts of sorbitol. Ingestion of lactose-containing products can cause diarrhea in lactase-deficient patients. Fructose-induced diarrhea may result from excessive ingestion of fruits, fruit juices, or soft drinks. Soft-drink manufacturers have substituted high fructose corn syrup for cane sugar, which may cause fructose-induced diarrhea in patients drinking large quantities of these products. Use of sugar free gum in excess may lead to diarrhea secondary to nonabsorbable sugars. Caffeine-containing beverages, if consumed in excess, may also cause diarrhea.

Travel and occupational history: Recent camping, hiking, or fishing trips, trips to Russia or the Colorado mountains suggest giardiasis. Close contact with small children in diapers, such as in a day care environment, is also a risk factor for giardiasis.

Timing of the diarrhea: Diarrhea that wakes a patient from sleep suggests an organic etiology. Diarrhea that occurs only at night, particularly if associated with incontinence, suggest autonomic neuropathy, such as seen with diabetes. Diarrhea that occurs mainly between breakfast and lunch and tapers off as the day progresses suggests a functional etiology, such as irritable bowel syndrome.

Volume of stool: Large-volume diarrhea suggests small bowel or right colonic dysfunction. Small-volume diarrhea, particularly if associated with urgency, indicates a colonic source of diarrhea.

Location of pain: If the diarrhea is associated with abdominal pain, pain localized in the periumbilical area suggests a small bowel etiology. Pain in the hypogastrium (RLQ or LLQ) or in the sacral region suggests a large bowel etiology.

Blood in stool: Presence of blood in the stool suggests an inflammatory, infectious, or neoplastic etiology and makes less likely the possibility of a functional or factitious cause.

Weight loss: Weight loss suggests malabsorption or an inflammatory or neoplastic etiology.

Dehydration and electrolyte disturbances: The presence of these signs suggests a secretory process, such as endocrine tumors or laxative abuse.

Incontinence: Many patients refer to episodes of incontinence as having "diarrhea". It is important to differentiate incontinence from true diarrhea.

4. **What are the clinical characteristics of osmotic diarrhea?**
   • The diarrhea stops when the patient fasts or stops taking the osmotically active agent.
   • Stool electrolyte analysis reveals an osmotic gap >100 mOsm/kg H_2O.

5. **How are the results of the stool electrolyte analysis interpreted?**
   A fresh, liquid sample of stool is submitted to the laboratory for **sodium** and **potassium** determination. The **stool osmolality** is calculated with the formula 2(Na + K). The normal stool osmolality is 290–300 mOsm/Kg H_2O. The **osmotic gap** is calculated by measuring the difference between the calculated stool osmolality and 300 (the normal stool osmolality). It is not recommended to measure the actual stool osmolality because there is an artifactual increase in the gap caused by fermentation that occurs during transportation and handling of the specimen.

   In patients with secretory diarrhea, the osmotic gap is <50. In patients with osmotic diarrhea, the presence of an unabsorbed osmotic agent causes an osmotic gap >100.

   The intestinal epithelium is incapable of secreting free water. Thus, the colon is incapable of producing a hyposmolar stool. A stool osmolality calculated at <270 mOsm/kg H_2O suggests that the patient has added water or urine to the stool specimen.

6. **List the potential causes of osmotic diarrhea.**
   • Carbohydrate malabsorption from lactase deficiency
   • Intestinal mucosal disease such as celiac sprue or tropical sprue
   • Excessive intake of poorly absorbed carbohydrates, such as lactulose, sorbitol, or fructose
   • Magnesium-induced diarrhea from laxatives, antacids, or oral magnesium supplements
   • Laxatives containing poorly absorbable anions

7. **What are the clinical characteristics of secretory diarrhea?**
   1. The diarrhea persists after a 48–72-hour fast (although the volume may be reduced due to the lack of oral itake).
   2. The stool osmolar gap is <50 mOsm/kg H_2O
   3. Secretory diarrhea secondary to laxative ingestion may stop during fasting if the patient does not take the laxative during this period.

8. **List the potential causes of secretory diarrhea.**
   Bacterial or viral infections
   Neuroendocrine tumors (VIPoma, gastrinoma, other pancreatic islet-cell tumors, bronchogenic carcinoma, carcinoid)
   Bile acid malabsorption
   Stimulant laxative use (bisacodyl, cascara, docusate sodium, senna)
   Microscopic colitis
   Collagenous colitis
   Hyperthyroidism
   Medullary carcinoma of the thyroid
   Collagen vascular diseases (systemic lupus erythematosus, mixed connective tissue disease, scleroderma)

9. **Describe the clinical characteristics of diarrhea due to deranged motility.**
   - Alternating diarrhea and constipation
   - Mucus in the stool, with no blood
   - Bloating
   - Onset of abdominal pain with the onset of diarrhea, and relief of the pain with defecation
   - Worsening of the diarrhea during periods of stress
   - Nocturnal diarrhea in patients with long-standing diabetes

10. **What are some conditions associated with diarrhea due to deranged motility?**

Irritable bowel syndrome	Hyperthyroidism
Postvagotomy and postgastrectomy diarrhea	Malignant carcinoid syndrome
Diabetic neuropathy	Scleroderma
Post-ileal resection	

11. **List the clinical characteristics of inflammatory diarrhea.**
    Blood and mucus in the stool, urgency, and fever.

12. **What are some conditions associated with inflammatory diarrhea?**
    - Inflammatory bowel disease (ulcerative colitis, Crohn's disease, Bechet's syndrome)
    - Invasive bacterial disease
    - Intestinal neoplasms

13. **What is the likely differential diagnosis in a patient with chronic nonbloody diarrhea who is not systemically ill?**
    1. Functional diarrhea (irritable bowel syndrome)
    2. Laxative abuse
    3. Lactase deficiency (lactose maldigestion)
    4. Giardiasis
    5. Bile salt induced diarrhea (if recent ileal resection)
    6. Dumping syndrome (if prior vagotomy or antrectomy)
    7. Zollinger-Ellison syndrome (gastrinoma)
    8. Pancreatic insufficiency
    9. Villous adenoma of the rectum causing secretory diarrhea

14. **In a patient with chronic nonbloody diarrhea who is systemically ill?**
    1. Crohn's disease
    2. Diabetic neuropathy
    3. Malabsorption syndrome (celiac sprue, tropical sprue, Whipple's disease)
    4. Hyperthyroidism
    5. Scleroderma with small bowel bacterial overgrowth

15. **List the common causes of chronic bloody diarrhea in a nonsystemically ill patient.**
    Rectal carcinoma, ulcerative proctitis, and diarrhea of other cause associated with bleeding from hemorrhoids or anal fissures.

16. **What are the likely causes of chronic bloody diarrhea in a systemically ill patient?**
    Ulcerative colitis, Crohn's colitis and chronic GI infections (*Plesiomonas, Aeromonas, Campylobacter jejuni*).

17. **What tests should be obtained in the stool of patients with chronic diarrhea?**
    - Occult blood: Its presence suggests an inflammatory process.
    - Stain for white blood cells: Their presence suggests an inflammatory or infectious process.
    - Parasites: Amebic trophozoites, giardia cysts, or parasitic ova may be diagnostic.
    - Sudan stain for fat: The presence of an abnormal amount of fat suggests a malabsorption process or the use of oil-containing laxatives.

- Stool electrolytes: An increased osmotic gap may indicate the presence of a nonabsorable agent.
- Culture may detect the presence of organisms causing a chronic infection.
- Stool pH: A low pH may indicate carbohydrate malabsorption.
- Alkalinization of the stool: A positive test indicates the presence of phenolphthalein-containing laxatives.

18. What additional tests are useful in the evaluation of patients with chronic diarrhea?

Tests Useful in the Evaluation of Chronic Diarrhea

Routine blood tests	Suspected endocrine etiology
Complete blood count	Serum cortisol
Chemistry profile	Serum gastrin
Sedimentation rate	Serum vasoactive intestinal peptide (VIP)
Triiodothyronine (T_3)	Serum calcitonin
Stool tests	Serum somatostatin
Occult blood	Urine 5-HIAA, VMA, and metanephrines
Stain for white blood cells	Pancreatic ultrasound or CT scanning
Cultures	Suspected malabsorption
Ova and parasites	72-hr stool collection for fat
Sudan stain for fat globules	B12 and folate levels
Stool electrolytes	Serum carotene
Stool pH	D-Xylose absorption test
Alkalinization of stool	Small intestinal biopsy
Endoscopic evaluation	Breath hydrogen test for lactose
Flexible sigmoidoscopy with mucosal biopsies	malapsorption
Colonoscopy with biopsies	Quantitative immunoglobulins
Upper endoscopy with small bowel biopsies	Suspected bacterial overgrowth
	Serum B12, folate levels
	Small bowel aspirate and culture
	Fasting breath hydrogen level
	Lactulose or glucose breath tests

All patients should have a complete blood count, chemistry profile, erythrocyte sedimentation rate, and T_3 measurement. In more difficult cases, or if the history points to a specific diagnosis, additional tests to consider include amebic serologies, serum cortisol, serum gastrin, VIP level, and calcitonin. Serum peptide levels should only be measured when the index of suspicion for a neuroendocrine tumor is high. Indiscriminate use of fasting plasma peptide concentration determinations in patients with chronic diarrhea is discouraged, because elevated levels usually represent an epiphenomenon and are not the cause of the diarrhea.

To evaluate for possible malabsorption, a 72-hour stool collection for fat may reveal significant steatorrhea. Vitamin B12 levels may be low in patients with bacterial overgrowth or after ileal resection. Quantitative immunoglobulin may uncover preexisting common variable hypogammaglobulinemia or selective IgA deficiency, which can be associated with intestinal villus atrophy or chronic infection with *Giardia lamblia*.

Urine collection for 5-hydroxyindoleacetic acid (5-HIAA), vanillylmandelic acid (VMA), and metanephrines may help in the diagnosis of carcinoid syndrome or pheochromocytoma. Urine for laxative screen may reveal laxative abuse.

A string test allows for sampling of duodenal contents and may be diagnostic for giardiasis or strongyloides infection.

A lactose breath hydrogen test can be used to diagnose lactose maldigestion. Lactose maldigestion is caused by a deficiency in the brush border enzyme lactase, which is needed to break down lactose into galactose and glucose for proper absorption. The most sensitive and specific test for diagnosing lactose maldigestion is the lactose breath hydrogen test. After a baseline breath hydrogen level is measured in a fasting patient, an oral dose of lactose is administered.

Breath samples are collected hourly for 4 hours, and the amount of hydrogen in the exhaled breath is measured. If lactose maldigestion is present, nonabsorbed lactose will be digested by intestinal bacteria and hydrogen will be produced. A rise in exhaled hydrogen of >20 ppm over baseline indicates lactose maldigestion.

Bacterial overgrowth can be diagnosed by performing small bowel aspiration and quantitative cultures of jejunal aspirates. Several breath tests are also available to diagnose bacterial overgrowth. These include the lactulose or glucose breath H_2 tests, the ^{14}C-D-xylose test, and the ^{14}C-glycocholate breath test. A fasting breath hydrogen concentration >42 ppm is also considered a reliable indicator of bacterial overgrowth.

19. What is the role of endoscopic studies in the evaluation of chronic diarrhea?

Colonoscopy or flexible sigmoidoscopy allows for inspection of the mucosa to detect changes consistent with inflammatory process, such as friability or ulceration. The appearance of the mucosa may be diagnostic. Patients who abuse anthracene cathartics, such as cascara, senna, aloe, or rhubarb, develop a brown to black pigment in the colonic mucosa. This condition, known as melanosis coli, can be easily detected on endoscopic examination of the colon. Even in patients with normal-looking colonic mucosa, random biopsies may reveal the presence of microscopic or collagenous colitis.

Upper GI endoscopy is indicated in patients with suspected malabsorption. Small intestinal biopsies may confirm the diagnosis of celiac or tropical sprue, Whipple's disease, intestinal lymphoma, or Crohn's disease of the upper GI tract. Multiple ulcerations may indicate the presence of the Zollinger-Ellison syndrome. Duodenal aspirates and biopsies may diagnose infections, such as giardiasis or strongyloidiasis.

20. What is the role of radiologic studies in the evaluation of chronic diarrhea?

Small bowel series can detect changes suggestive of malabsorption. These include flocculation of the contrast material in the intestinal lumen, dilatation of the jejunum and ileum, and thickening of the jejunal folds. The presence of small bowel diverticulosis may predispose to small bowel bacterial overgrowth. Tumors or strictures of the small bowel may cause intestinal hypersecretion leading to diarrhea.

Barium enema may be helpful in patients who have not undergone colonoscopy. A barium enema may reveal changes suggestive of inflammatory bowel disease, a mass lesion of the colon, or a villous adenoma causing secretory diarrhea.

21. What are the most common etiologies found in patients with chronic diarrhea and negative initial evaluation?

Laxative abuse, iatrogenic diarrhea (diet, medications, prior surgery, or prior radiation), fecal incontinence, microscopic or collagenous colitis, and carbohydrate malabsorption.

22. List the laxatives that can be detected in stool or urine.

Phenolphthalein-containing laxatives can be identified by alkalinizing stool water. If phenolphthalein is present, a red color will be seen. Anthraquinone laxatives can be found by a chemical test on urine or by chromatography in stool water. Chromatography of stool water can also detect bisacodyl and emetine. Magnesium, sulfate, and phosphate can be detected in stool water by atomic absorption spectrophotometry.

23. What is the definition of chronic diarrhea of obscure origin?

In general a patient is categorized as having chronic diarrhea of obscure origin when, after extensive evaluation, a clear etiology is not found. Patients with chronic diarrhea of obscure origin should meet the following criteria:
1. Loose or frequent stools
2. Chronicity (>4 weeks)

3. Negative stool microbiologic studies
4. Negative GI x-rays, sonogram, CT scan, endoscopic, and colonoscopic evalution, including colonic and small bowel biopsies
5. No evidence of endocrine disease (diabetes, adrenal insufficiency, thyroid disease)
6. No evidence of diarrheogenic tumors (carcinoid syndrome, pheochromocytoma, gastrinoma, medullary carcinoma of the thyroid, VIPoma, glucagonoma, somatostatinoma, etc.)
7. No evidence of systemic immunodeficiency (AIDS, immunoglobulin deficiency)
8. Poor or incomplete response to nonspecific antidiarrheal therapy

24. How is chronic diarrhea treated?

If an etiology is found, treatment should be directed to the underlying etiology. In cases of chronic diarrhea of obscure origin, treatment is problematic. Nonspecific antidiarrheal agents should be used to alleviate symptoms. Caution is advised on prescribing dephenoxylate for long-term use, because dependency may occur with long-term use of high doses. Loperamide is a safe choice for long-term control of diarrhea, although high doses may be required. The use of fiber supplements adds bulk to the stool and decreases the liquidity.

For patients with large-volume diarrhea, particularly those prone to dehydration or electrolyte imbalance, who do not respond to antidiarrheal agents, codeine or tincture of opium may be tried, although both can be habit-forming. Other agents that have been reported to decrease diarrhea in anecdotal reports include clonidine, aspirin, indomethacin, and phenothiazines. Octreotide is a somatostatin analog and, as such, is a potent inhibitor of intestinal secretion. It has been shown to be effective in controlling symptoms associated with endocrine tumors, such as carcinoid syndrome or VIPoma. Its use in the treatment of diarrhea of other causes is not approved, but anecdotal evidence suggests that it may help in cases of diarrhea secondary to dumping syndrome and in AIDS patients with diarrhea of unknown cause.

In many patients with sporadic idiopathic chronic diarrhea, the symptoms may resolve spontaneously without specific therapy after a mean of 15 months. Reassurance and supportive care are important aspects in the care of these patients.

BIBLIOGRAPHY

1. Afzalpurkar RG, Schiller LR, Little KH, et al: The self-limited nature of chronic idiopathic diarrhea. N Engl J Med 327:1849–1852, 1992.
2. Ammon HV: Diarrhea and constipation—Part I. Diarrhea. In WS Haubrich, F Schaffner, JE Berk (eds): Bockus Gastroenterology, 5th ed. Philadelphia, W.B. Saunders, 1995, pp 87–99.
3. Bertomeu A, Ros E, Barragan V, et al: Chronic diarrhea with normal stool and colonic examinations: Organic or functional? J Clin Gastroenterol 13:531–536, 1991.
4. Fine KD, Krejs GJ, Fordtran JS: Diarrhea. In Sleisenger MH, Fordtran JS (eds): Gastrointestinal Disease: Pathophysiology, Diagnosis and Management, 5th ed. Philadelphia, W.B. Saunders, 1993, pp 1043–1072.
5. Fine KD, Santa Ana CA, Fordtran JS: Diagnosis of magnesium-induced diarrhea. N Engl J Med 324:1012–1017, 1991.
6. Goldfinger S, Phillips S, Rogers A: Diarrhea: A Practical Guide to Diagnosis and Management. New York, Projects in Health, Inc., 1976, pp 1–101.
7. Kacere RD, Srivatsa SS, Tremaine WJ, et al: Chronic diarrhea due to surreptitious use of bisacodyl: Case reports and methods for detection. Mayo Clin Proc 68:355–357, 1993.
8. Moriarty KJ, Silk DBA: Laxative abuse. Dig Dis 6:15–29, 1988.
9. Schiller LR: Chronic diarrhea of obscure origin. In Current Topics in Gastroenterology: Diarrheal Diseases. New York, Elsevier, 1991, pp 219–238.
10. Schiller LR, Rivera LM, Santangelo WC, et al: Diagnostic value of fasting plasma peptide concentrations in patients with chronic diarrhea. Dig Dis Sci 39:2216–2222, 1994.
11. Topazian M, Binder HJ: Factitious diarrhea detected by measurement of stool osmolality. N Engl J Med 330:1418–1419, 1994.

58. AIDS AND THE GI TRACT

Wheaton J. Williams, M.D., and Donald R. Skillman, M.D.

1. What is bacillary peliosis hepatis (BPH)?

BPH is a manifestation of infection with *Bartonella* species (formerly *Rochalimaea*) and is an uncommon complication of advanced HIV infection. Clinical features include fever, weight loss, abdominal pain or fullness, and GI symptoms such as nausea, vomiting, or diarrhea. Cutaneous bacillary angiomatosis (reddish vascular papules) may be present. Physical examination and imaging studies may reveal hepatomegaly, splenomegaly, and abdominal or retroperitoneal lymphadenopathy. Laboratory evaluation demonstrates marked elevations of gamma-glutamyltransferase and alkaline phosphatase and only mild elevations of aminotransferase levels. Histopathologic examination reveals multiple cystic blood-filled spaces with surrounding fibromyxoid stroma. Warthin-Starry staining shows clumps of bacilli within the fibromyxoid areas. *Bartonella henselae* has been isolated from blood and tissue samples of patients with BPH. Erythromycin is the drug of choice for treating BPH, although doxycycline appears to be a good alternative. A prolonged course of therapy, usually 4–6 weeks, is needed to prevent relapse.

2. What are the major causes of biliary tract disease in AIDS?

Patients with advanced HIV infection may develop signs and symptoms of biliary tract disease, such as fever, RUQ abdominal pain, and elevation of alkaline phosphatase. Many of these patients have bile duct abnormalities referred to as **HIV-associated cholangiopathy.** The ductular changes include combined papillary stenosis and sclerosing cholangitis, as well as isolated papillary stenosis, sclerosing cholangitis, or long extrahepatic bile duct strictures. Infection of the biliary tract with cytomegalovirus (CMV), cryptosporidia, or microsporidia has been associated with this disorder. Most patients with HIV-associated cholangiopathy have evidence of ductular abnormalities on ultrasound or CT scans, but a negative scan does not exclude the diagnosis. Patients with papillary stenosis often have improvement in pain following endoscopic sphincterotomy. Balloon dilatation or stent placement may be beneficial for patients with bile duct obstructions.

Acute acalculous cholecystitis is another cause of biliary tract disease in HIV-infected patients. Most cases are attributed to CMV infection, but *Cryptosporidium* and *Isospora belli* have also been implicated. Cholecystectomy is indicated for these patients.

3. Name the most common cause of pancreatitis in HIV-infected patients.

Pancreatitis should be considered in the differential diagnosis of acute abdominal pain in HIV-infected patients. Most cases of pancreatitis are drug-induced in this population, with the most common offending agents being pentamidine and didanosine (ddI). Pancreatitis is associated with the administration of **pentamidine** by both the intravenous and inhaled routes and usually occurs >7 days after initiating therapy. The use of pentamidine may also result in impaired glucose metabolism. Hypoglycemia, defined as a blood glucose <60 mg/dl, may occur in up to 50% of HIV-infected patients receiving intravenous pentamidine and is associated with elevated serum levels of pentamidine, renal insufficiency, and prolonged therapy. Hypoglycemia appears to result from inappropriate insulin release. Hyperglycemia can also occur during pentamidine therapy and seems to be due to B islet cell destruction.

About 5% of patients taking **didanosine** (ddI) develop pancreatitis, which in rare instances can have a fulminant course resulting in death. Risk factors for ddI-related pancreatitis include a prior history of pancreatitis, advanced HIV infection, and CD4 count <50/mm³. Pancreatitis can also complicate treatment with **zalcitabine** (ddC), but this occurs in <1% of patients receiving ddC. Alcohol consumption may increase the likelihood of drug-induced pancreatitis.

Possible **infectious causes** of pancreatitis in patients with HIV infection include CMV, herpes simplex virus (HSV), *Mycobacterium tuberculosis, M. avium* complex, and *Cryptococcus neoformans.*

4. Describe the effect that coinfection with HIV has on the clinical course of hepatitis B infection.

HIV and hepatitis B virus (HBV) share similar routes of transmission and occur in similar risk groups, so coinfection with these two viruses is common. Up to 90% of patients with AIDS have serologic evidence of past or present infection with HBV. HIV-infected patients who acquire HBV infection are three to eight times more likely to become chronic carriers of HBV than HIV-seronegative patients. About 10% of AIDS patients are chronic HBV carriers.

HIV infection does not appear to significantly alter the clinical course of acute HBV infection, although there is a trend for patients with HIV to have more prolonged symptoms and ALT elevations associated with acute HBV infection. HIV-infected patients who develop chronic HBV infection are more likely to have lower median ALT levels in the 36 months after infection onset. In addition, patients with HIV and chronic HBV infection have less severe histologic evidence of inflammation but have higher levels of serum HBV DNA polymerase. Interferon-α appears to be less effective in the management of chronic HBV in HIV-positive patients.

Cell-mediated immunity is believed to be critical for both clearance of HBV infection and pathogenesis of the HBV-associated hepatocellular damage. The impaired cell-mediated immunity associated with HIV-infection is the most likely cause of the increased risk of HBV carriage and the reduced risk of HBV-related liver damage observed in patients with HIV infection.

5. How effective is hepatitis B immunization in HIV-infected patients?

The rationale for providing immunization against HBV infection for HIV seropositive patients without evidence of HBV infection includes the following:

- HIV and HBV share similar routes of transmission.
- HIV-infected patients are more likely to become chronic HBV carriers.
- HIV-infected patients are potentially more infectious since they are more likely to demonstrate HBV viremia.

HIV-infected patients have an impaired immune response to both plasma-derived and recombinant hepatitis B vaccines, with only 22–56% of patients demonstrating protective levels of hepatitis B surface antibody following immunization. In contrast, >90% of HIV-seronegative patients develop protective antibody after vaccination against hepatitis B. The relationship between vaccine response and immunologic parameters, such as CD4 cell count or delayed-type hypersensitivity, is not well-established, but the information available suggests that vaccine response is improved in patients with CD4 cell counts >500. HIV-infected patients who develop a protective antibody response appear to be protected against the development of the HBV carrier state. HIV-infected patients who are nonresponders after completing the three-dose hepatitis B vaccine series, and those who have received two or less doses of vaccine, have rates of HBV infection comparable to unvaccinated patients.

The optimal dose and schedule of hepatitis B vaccine for HIV-infected patients has not been determined. It is recommended that the hepatitis B surface antibody response be measured after vaccination, and nonresponders should be revaccinated with one to three additional doses.

6. Describe the prevalence of hepatitis C infection in patients infected with HIV and the effect of coinfection on the natural history of hepatitis C infection.

The overall prevalence of hepatitis C virus (HCV) infection, as determined by recombinant immunoblot assay (RIBA), is about 10% in HIV-positive patients attending U.S. military clinics or a university clinic. In contrast, the prevalence of HCV infection in healthy blood donors in the United States is <1%. The risk of HCV infection is significantly increased in certain subpopulations of HIV-infected patients, such as intravenous drug users, hemophiliacs, and recipients of multiple blood transfusions.

The effect of coinfection with HIV on the natural history of HCV infection is not well-established. Because liver disease in HCV infection appears to be due to cytopathic effects of the virus rather than immune-mediated damage, immunosuppression from HIV infection could promote increased viral replication and increased liver damage. A study of a cohort of hemophiliacs suggested that liver failure occurred more frequently in coinfected patients than in those with HCV infection alone. The efficacy of interferon-α for the treatment of chronic HCV infection in coinfected patients is not yet clear.

7. What are the major causes of bowel perforation in AIDS patients?

Bowel perforation needs to be considered in the differential diagnosis of acute abdominal pain in AIDS patients. The most common etiology of bowel perforation is probably CMV infection involving either the distal small bowel or colon. Infections with *Histoplasma capsulatum* and *Clostridium difficile* have also been associated with bowel perforation. Noninfectious conditions associated with perforation include lymphoma and Kaposi's sarcoma.

8. Name the major causes of gastrointestinal bleeding in AIDS patients.

GI hemorrhage is an uncommon condition in HIV-infected patients but can represent a diagnostic dilemma. Bleeding is often due to disorders not unique to AIDS, such as duodenal ulcers, gastric ulcers, Mallory-Weiss tears, varices, ulcerative colitis, bacterial colitis, proctitis, and hemorrhoids.

Several conditions associated with HIV infection can result in GI hemorrhage. Kaposi's sarcoma can occur throughout the GI tract, and large bulky lesions can occasionally bleed spontaneously. Non-Hodgkin's lymphoma occurs with increased frequency in AIDS patients and can involve both the upper and lower GI tract. GI lymphomas, especially gastric lymphomas, may cause significant bleeding. Aphthous ulcerations of the colon can cause rectal bleeding.

CMV infection of the esophagus, stomach, small intestine, and colon can potentially result in bleeding. HSV and candida esophagitis are rarely associated with hemorrhage. Enteric pathogens such as *Campylobacter*, *Shigella*, *Salmonella*, and *Entamoeba histolytica* can cause colitis and lower GI bleeding. Finally, HSV and *Chlamydia trachomatis* can cause proctitis and rectal bleeding.

9. Discuss the diagnosis and management of aphthous ulcerations of the GI tract in patients with AIDS.

Aphthous ulcerations involving the mouth and oropharynx or the GI tract can cause significant morbidity in AIDS patients. These ulcerations can present during acute HIV infection or after the onset of AIDS. Aphthous ulcers in HIV-positive patients tend to be larger and more persistent than those occurring in HIV-seronegative patients. Clinical manifestations include pain and dysphagia with esophageal ulcers and rectal bleeding with colonic ulcers. Biopsies and cultures of these ulcers must be obtained to rule out ulceration due to CMV or HSV.

If aphthous ulcers are limited to the mouth and oropharynx, topical corticosteroids may be effective. Other potentially effective therapies for oral aphthous ulcers include oral prednisone, thalidomide, H_2 blockers, and sucralfate. Aphthous ulcers involving the esphagus or colon should be treated with oral prednisone, starting at 40 mg/day and tapering over 2–3 weeks.

10. What are the gastrointestinal manifestations of disseminated *Mycobacterium avium* complex (MAC) infection?

MAC causes disseminated disease in about 40% of HIV-infected patients in the United States but usually occurs only when the CD4 cell count is $<100/mm^3$. The GI tract appears to be a common portal of entry for MAC, following ingestion from environmental sources.

Many of the clinical manifestations of disseminated MAC are referable to the GI tract. Common symptoms include fever, night sweats, weight loss, anorexia, nausea, diarrhea, and abdominal pain. Findings on physical examination and/or imaging studies include cachexia, hepatomegaly, splenomegaly, and abdominal or retroperitoneal lymphadenopathy. Laboratory abnormalities include severe anemia and an elevated serum alkaline phosphatase. The diagnosis of disseminated

MAC is established by the isolation of MAC from a normally sterile site, such as blood, bone marrow, lymph node, or liver. Isolation of MAC in a stool specimen does not confirm the diagnosis of disseminated infection.

MAC infection can involve the bowel, most commonly the duodenum, and may produce white mucosal nodules noted at endoscopy. Histopathologic features include poorly formed granulomas and, occasionally, an appearance similar to Whipple's disease (focal collection of macrophages with foamy cytoplasm).

11. What is the currently recommended treatment for disseminated MAC?

A multidrug regimen is recommended for the treatment of disseminated MAC because of the potential for the emergence of resistant isolates following monotherapy. Unfortunately, the optimal treatment regimen has not been established. Currently, use of at least two drugs is recommended. The regimen should include either clarithromycin or azithromycin, in combination with one to three of the following agents: ethambutol, rifampin, rifabutin, ciprofloxacin, clofazimine, or amikacin.

Rifabutin, 300 mg by mouth daily, is recommended for prophylaxis against disseminated MAC for HIV-infected patients with a CD4 cell count <100/mm³. Before initiating prophylaxis, it is important to rule out active disease due to MAC or *M. tuberculosis*. Consider obtaining a PPD, chest x-ray, and mycobacterial blood culture before initiating MAC prophylaxis.

12. What is the difference between thrush and oral hairy leukoplakia?

Oral candidiasis can take several forms, the most common being **pseudomembranous candidiasis,** or thrush. Thrush presents as removable white plaques on any oral mucosal surface. Plaques can be 1–2 mm in size or large and extensive. They can be wiped off, yielding an erythematous or bleeding mucosal surface.

The **erythematous** form of oral candidiasis presents as smooth red patches on the hard or soft palate, buccal mucosa, or dorsal surface of the tongue. Occasionally *Candida* causes **hyperkeratosis** or **leukoplakia.** This can be on the tongue, buccal mucosa, and hard palate and is difficult to distinguish from hairy leukoplakia except by smears, histopathology, and response to therapy. **Angular cheilitis** due to *Candida* produces erythema, cracks and fissures at the corners of the mouth. Oral candidiasis is a prognostic indicator for HIV progression and the development of AIDS.

Diagnosis involves KOH or lactophenol cotton blue preparation of a smear. Culture can identify the species of *Candida* involved, which is important as some species do not respond to azole antifungal agents. Biopsy is helpful to diagnose candidal leukoplakia.

Hairy leukoplakia (HL) has been described on the buccal mucosa, soft palate, and floor of the mouth but is usually seen on the lateral margins of the tongue. It produces white thickening of the mucosa with vertical folds or corrugations. Lesions can be a few millimeters in size or cover the entire dorsal surface of the tongue. In addition to candidal leukoplakia, the differential diagnosis includes smoker's leukoplakia, epithelial dysplasia or oral cancer, white sponge nevus, and the plaque form of lichen planus. Epstein-Barr virus has been identified in biopsy specimens.

13. What is the work-up for diarrhea in HIV-infected patients?

Immunodeficiency predisposes the GI tract to infection with a wide spectrum of viral, fungal, bacterial, and protozoan pathogens. A thorough evaluation will yield a specific diagnosis in up to 85% of cases.

A geographic **travel history** can help direct the work-up. For example, 18% of HIV-infected persons with diarrhea in Australia have rotavirus, but this etiology is rare in the U.S. If necessary, as many as three **stool specimens** should be cultured for enteric pathogens, screened for ova and parasites (including acid-fast smears for *Cryptosporidium* and *Isospora belli*), and assayed for *Clostridium difficile* toxin. If this is nondiagnostic, or if therapy for identified pathogens is ineffective, then proceed with **esophagogastroduodenoscopy** and/or **colonoscopy** to visualize the mucosa, obtain luminal fluid, and acquire biopsy specimens. Colonoscopy may be reserved for patients with clinical signs suggestive of colitis.

Duodenal biopsy specimens should be cultured for CMV and mycobacteria. **Colonic biopsy** specimens should be cultured for CMV, adenovirus, mycobacteria, and HSV. Formaldehyde-fixed biopsy specimens should be stained with hematoxylin-eosin (to identify histologic changes, protozoa, and viral inclusion cells), Grocott methenamine silver or Giemsa (for fungi), and Fite for mycobacteria). Examine duodenal fluid for parasites.

If still without a diagnosis, proceed with **electron microscopic examination** of glutaraldehyde-fixed duodenal biopsies (to identify *Microsporidium*) or colonic biopsies (to identify adenovirus). At least 15% of HIV-infected patients with diarrhea will have a negative evaluation and are felt to have AIDS-associated enteropathy.

14. What are the primary features of Herpes simplex virus proctitis?

HSV proctitis is the most common cause of nongonoccal proctitis in sexually active homosexual men. Its distinctive clinical presentation distinguishes it from other infectious causes of acute proctitis, but the diagnosis should be confirmed by culture. It is associated with fever, inguinal adenopathy, anorectal pain, tenesmus, constipation, rectal discharge, and hematochezia. Severe anorectal pain is a universal finding and is usually greater than with other forms of proctitis. Only rectal lymphogranuloma venereum infection also produces so much pain.

Neurologic symptoms in the distribution of the sacral roots may be present. Difficulty in initiating micturition, posterior thigh pain or paresthesias of the buttocks or perineal region, and impotence were reported by 52% of 23 men with HSV proctitis, compared to <1% of 63 heterosexual men and 1.6% of 123 women with primary HSV-2 genital infections in a study by Goodell et al.

Perianal or anal lesions on anoscopy, vesicular or pustular rectal lesions, and diffuse ulceration of the distal rectum on sigmoidoscopy are each associated with HSV proctitis. Rectal mucosal abnormalities 10 cm above the anal verge are unusual, in contrast to those due to pathogens such as *Chlamydia trachomatis, Campylobacter jejuni, Clostridium difficile,* and *Entamoeba histolytica,* which also involve the sigmoid mucosa.

15. An HIV-infected Spanish man presents with fever, hepatosplenomegaly, hyperglobulinemia, and pancytopenia. What is the diagnosis, and how can you prove it?

He probably has visceral leishmaniasis (kala-azar). This disease is endemic in Spain and other Mediterranean areas. Over 150 cases of kala-azar and HIV coinfection have been reported, most of them from Spain. It is estimated that 50% of kala-azar cases in adults are associated with HIV and that 1–3% of AIDS patients in southwest Europe acquire visceral leishmaniasis. In HIV-infected persons, kala-azar usually presents in this classic acute fashion.

Diagnosis requires a bone marrow aspirate with culture on Novy-MacNeal-Nicolle (NNN) media or identification of the organism in tissue. Parasites can usually be demonstrated in the marrow and sometimes on biopsy of the liver or skin lesions. In Kenya, a splenic aspirate may be the diagnostic method most commonly employed.

In most cases associated with HIV infection (93%), no antileishmanial antibodies are found at presentation, during relapses, or during the chronic course of disease. This is in contrast to findings in immunocompetent individuals or non–HIV-infected immunocompromised persons, in whom significant antibody levels are usually found. Most patients intitially respond to pentavalent antimony treatment, but relapses are very common, and some success has been achieved by adding interferon-γ to the treatment regimen.

16. What are the clinical features of cryptosporidiosis?

In normal hosts, *Cryptosporidium* causes a self-limiting, noninflammatory diarrhea. In AIDS patients, this intracellular protozoan can cause a chronic severe diarrhea and cholangitis. It infects and reproduces in epithelial cells lining the GI and respiratory tracts of most vertebrates. Twenty species have been named, with *C. parvum* responsible for clinical disease in humans. Infection follows person-to-person, animal-to-person, or waterborne transmission. The life cycle is completed in a single host, with autoinfectious cycles following ingestion of a few oocysts, leading to severe disease and persistent infections in immunodeficient persons.

Diarrhea, with or without crampy abdominal pain, may be intermittent or scant, or it may be continuous, watery, and exceedingly voluminous (12–17 l/day). There is considerable variation between patients, and the disease may wax and wane or be relentlessly persistent in a given individual. Stool may contain mucus but rarely blood or leukocytes. Constitutional symptoms include low-grade fevers, malaise, anorexia, nausea, and vomiting. Eosinophilia has been reported, but there are no characteristic laboratory features. Radiography is nonspecific, showing prominent mucosal folds, air-fluid levels, distended loops of bowel, and disordered motility.

17. How do you establish the diagnosis of cryptosporidiosis?
Diagnosis requires identification of organisms in small bowel biopsy specimens or oocysts in the stool, bowel aspirates, bile, or respiratory secretions. Most labs use at least two methods to find oocysts: a concentration method and a staining technique for permanent record. Multiple specimens may be required, and the lab should be informed to specifically seek cryptosporidia. Modified acid-fast staining is the most popular diagnostic stain, although other stains such as malachite green and fluorescent stains (e.g., acridine orange, auramine-carbol-fuchsin) will also demonstrate the organism.

The gallbladder may be affected in as many as 10% of AIDS patients with cryptosporidiosis. Presenting features are acalculous cholecystitis or sclerosing cholangitis, fever, RUQ pain, nausea, and vomiting. Diarrhea may or may not be present. Sonography reveals an enlarged gallbladder with a thickened wall, dilated biliary ducts, and, sometimes, a stenotic distal common bile duct. Diagnosis is made by histologic examination following cholecystectomy, ampullary biopsy, or identification of oocysts in bile. Prognosis is poor. There is no reliable palliative or curative treatment for cryptosporidiosis, although some success has been achieved with paromomycin.

18. Describe the clinical features of infection by *Isospora belli*.
I. belli is a host-specific coccidian protozoan. The sexual and asexual phases of the life cycle occur within the human small intestinal epithelium. Immature, unsporulated (thus noninfectious) oocysts are released in the feces. After a few days, sporulation occurs, yielding a mature oocyst. Transmission is believed to be via fecally contaminated food and water.

Infection with *I. belli* is an uncommon cause of chronic diarrhea in AIDS patients in the United States. *I. belli* infection is most common in AIDS patients from developing tropical countries.

In normal hosts, *I. belli* produces a nonspecific watery diarrheal illness with malaise, anorexia, abdominal cramps, and occasionally fever. Blood or leukocytes are not present in the stool. Chronic, persistent diarrhea is rare in immunocompetent hosts. In AIDS patients, the diarrhea is protracted and profuse, similar to cryptosporidiosis. Weight loss, abdominal cramping, and fever are typical. In contrast to other protozoal diseases, with *I. belli* infection, peripheral blood eosinophilia and stool Charcot-Leyden crystals may be present.

The infection is diagnosed via oocyst identification in the stool using an acid-fast stain. *I. belli* oocysts are readily distinguished from those of *Cryptosporidium* or *Cyclospora* by their size and shape. Oocysts may be shed intermittently, so several stool specimens may be needed to make the diagnosis. Treatment with trimethoprim-sulfamethoxazole (TMP-SMX) usually leads to a prompt response, but relapse is common with AIDS. Consequently, lifelong therapy is usually necessary with a low dose of TMP-SMX. Alternative drug choices include pyrimethamine, with or without sulfadiazine.

19. What are the unique clinical features of salmonellosis in HIV infection?
The clinical course of salmonellosis infection in persons with asymptomatic HIV infection, or even in those with AIDS-related complex (ARC), is similar to that of infection in immunocompetent hosts. However, in persons with full-blown AIDS, the infection has been associated with acute enterocolitis, fulminant diarrhea, and rectal ulcerations. Overwhelming diarrhea and/or recurrent or refractory bacteremia can lead to death, even if appropriate treatment is instituted. Bacteremia can develop during the course of antibiotics.

Recurrent *Salmonella* bacteremia is an AIDS-defining illness. *Salmonella* bacteremia was more common before the widespread use of zidovudine (AZT), but this drug has activity against *Salmonella* in vitro and within macrophages infected with the organism.

20. What are the gastrointestinal features of the acute retroviral syndrome?

The acute retroviral syndrome associated with acquisition of HIV is probably both underreported and overdiagnosed. It is seen in 53–93% of cases. Asymptomatic seroconversion does occur, but a high index of clinical suspicion and prior experience with primary HIV infection greatly increase the recognition rate. The time from exposure to the onset of clinical illness is typically 2–4 weeks, although longer times have been reported.

Onset is acute and lasts 1–2 weeks. Many persons require hospitalization. Most clinical manifestations are self-limited and do not recur after resolution. The main features reflect the lymphocytic and neurologic tropism of the virus. Typical symptoms are fever, lethargy and malaise, myalgias, lymphadenopathy, and a maculopapular rash. Mucocutaneous ulceration is a distinctive sign. Ulcers can be present on the buccal mucosa, gingiva, palate, esophagus, anus, or penis. They are round to oval, with sharply demarcated borders, and the surrounding mucosa is normal. Electron microscopy has shown viral particles in the lesions consistent with HIV.

Other GI features include a sore throat, pharyngeal edema, anorexia, nausea, vomiting, and diarrhea. Oral and esophageal candidiasis is sometimes seen, associated with significant reduction in CD4$^+$ T-cell number. Elevated alkaline phosphatase and AST have been noted, infrequently associated with clinical hepatitis.

21. How do you evaluate symptoms of esophagitis in a person with AIDS?

Start with a physical examination. If oropharyngeal candidiasis is found, then esophageal candidiasis is strongly suggested. A trial of antifungal therapy (fluconazole) is probably warranted before pursuing other diagnostic tests. If symptoms resolve with therapy, then the diagnosis is established empirically. In the absence of oral thrush or with failure to respond to presumptive antifungal therapy, proceed with an upper GI contrast radiography study or esophagogastroduodenoscopy (EGD). On upper GI, *Candida* esophagitis has a cobblestone appearance with diffuse ulcerations and plaques. CMV typically causes single or multiple large shallow ulcerations, whereas HSV usually causes multiple deep ulcerations.

Endoscopy is preferred over radiologic studies for patients with dysphagia or odynophagia. Friable cheesy plaques (easily removed with forceps) are consistent with candidiasis. Diffuse erythematous ulcerations are commonly seen with viral infections. More than one pathogen can be found, so lesions should be biopsied and cultured for fungi and viruses. Biopsies should be done to seek viral inclusion bodies and/or invasive fungi.

Esophageal Kaposi's sarcoma, lymphoma, aphthous ulcers, reflux esophagitis, carcinoma, achalasia, and peptic ulcer disease may also be discovered in HIV-infected patients.

22. What is the most common cause of viral diarrhea in AIDS patients, and what are the primary features of the illness?

Cytomegalovirus (CMV) causes a painful colitis in late-stage HIV-infected persons. Symptoms include small-volume diarrhea, cramping and bloating, pain, fever, and, often, tenesmus. Colonic perforation may result from severe CMV colitis. CMV has even been reported to cause appendicitis in HIV-infected patients. Treatment with ganciclovir or foscarnet is usually effective, with improvement in clinical symptoms seen within 1 week of starting therapy. Because these drugs have significant toxicities, a specific diagnosis should be established by histologic exam before initiating therapy. Culture of CMV from secretions or excretions alone is not sufficient evidence that CMV is causing disease, nor is the clinical presentation of CMV colitis sufficiently specific to establish CMV as the diagnosis. The clinical scenario should be correlated with histologic and culture findings before concluding that CMV infection is present which requires specific antiviral treatment.

Other viruses associated with diarrhea in AIDS patients include astrovirus, adenovirus, calcivirus, and picobirnavirus.

BIBLIOGRAPHY

 1. Alvar J, Gutierrez-Solar B, Molina R, et al: Prevalence of *Leishmania* infection among AIDS patients. Lancet 339:1427, 1992.
 2. Bach MC, Howell DA, Valenti AJ, et al: Aphthous ulceration of the gastrointestinal tract in patients with the acquired immunodeficiency syndrome (AIDS). Ann Intern Med 112:465, 1990.
 3. Bonacini M: Pancreatic involvement in human immunodeficiency virus infection. J Clin Gastroenterol 13:58, 1991.
 4. CDC: Recommendations of the Advisory Committee on Immunization Practices (ACIP): Use of vaccines and immune globulins for persons with altered immunocompetence. MMWR 42(RR-4):1, 1993.
 5. CDC: Recommendations on prophylaxis and therapy for disseminated *Mycobacterium avium* complex for adults and adolescents infected with human immunodeficiency virus. MMWR 42(RR-9):17, 1993.
 6. Cello JP, Wilcox CM: Evaluation and treatment of gastrointestinal tract hemorrhage in patients with AIDS. Gastroenterol Clin North Am 17:639, 1988.
 7. Cello JP: Human immunodeficiency virus-associated biliary tract disease. Semin Liver Dis 12:213, 1992.
 8. Eyster ME, Diamondstone LS, Lien J, et al: Natural history of hepatitis C virus infection in multitransfused hemophiliacs: Effect of coinfection with human immunodeficiency virus. J Acquir Immune Defic Syndr 6:602, 1993.
 9. Friedman SL: Gastrointestinal manifestations of acquired immunodeficiency syndrome. In Sleisenger MH, Fordtran JS (eds): Gastrointestinal Disease, 5th ed. Philadelphia, W.B. Saunders, 1993, pp 239–258.
10. Goodell SE, Quinn TC, Mkrtician E, et al: Herpes simplex proctitis in homosexual men. N Engl J Med 308:868, 1983.
11. Hadler SC, Judson FN, O'Malley PM, et al: Outcome of hepatitis B virus infection in homosexual men and its relation to prior human immunodeficiency virus infection. J Infect Dis 163:454, 1991.
12. Horsburgh CR Jr: *Mycobacterium avium* complex infection in the acquired immunodeficiency syndrome. N Engl J Med 324:1332, 1991.
13. Mandell GL, Bennett JE, Dolin R (eds): Principles and Practice of Infectious Diseases, 4th ed. New York, Churchill Livingstone, 1995.
14. Perkocha LA, Geaghan SM, Yen TSB, et al: Clinical and pathological features of bacillary peliosis hepatis in association with human immunodeficiency virus infection. N Engl J Med 323:1581, 1990.
15. Sande MA, Volberding PA (eds): The Medical Management of AIDS, 4th ed. Philadelphia, W.B. Saunders, 1995.
16. Smith PD, Quinn TC, Strober W, et al: Gastrointestinal infections in AIDS. Ann Intern Med 116:63, 1992.

59. INTESTINAL ISCHEMIA

Eugene D. Jacobson, M.D.

1. What are the anatomical differences between the splanchnic circulation, the mesenteric circulation, and the small intestinal and colonic circulations?

The **splanchnic** circulation consists of the blood vessels (arteries and veins) that deliver blood to and from the splanchnic viscera—i.e., the digestive organs of the abdomen (stomach, small intestine, colon, liver, gallbladder, and pancreas) and the spleen. Its major inflow vessels include the celiac, superior mesenteric, and inferior mesenteric arteries; its major outflow vessels are the portal and hepatic veins.

The **mesenteric** circulation is composed of the vessels that course through the mesentery, conveying blood to and from the small and large bowel—i.e., the superior and inferior mesenteric arteries and veins. Nearly all of the blood supply to the small intestine is provided by superior mesenteric arterial branches. This artery also distributes blood to the proximal half of the colon. The inferior mesenteric arterial branches supply blood to the distal colon (*see* Figure 1).

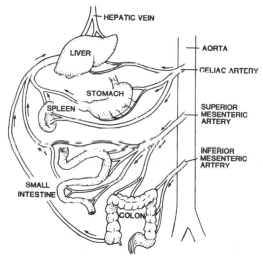

Figure 1. Major splanchnic organs and blood vessels.

2. Name the three main types of blood vessels in the intestinal microcirculation. What are their major functions?

When blood vessel diameters are <0.1 mm, the vessels cannot be seen by the unaided eye. The microcirculation consists of such small vessels. The three main vessel types in the intestinal microcirculation are arterioles, capillaries, and venules (*see* Figure 2). All microscopic vessels serve as conduits for flowing blood. They also contain blood and especially the formed elements of blood within the vascular compartment. These vessels are lined by endothelial cells that have immunologic functions.

The unique circulatory property of **arterioles** is to resist the free flow of blood; therefore, arterioles are the primary site in the overall circulation for the dissipation of the energy driving blood through the tissues. Accordingly, mean blood pressure in a visible artery may be 100 mm Hg but will have declined to 35 mm Hg by the terminal portion of the arteriole.

The unique function of **capillaries** is to permit the exchange of materials between cells in the

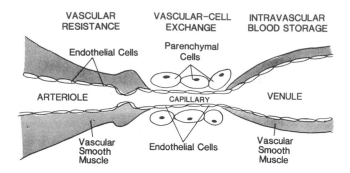

Figure 2. Intestinal microcirculation: vessel types and functions.

gut wall and blood flowing through the organ. Substances moving from blood to cells include oxygen, water, nutrients, electrolytes, and hormones. The most important items diffusing from cells into the blood include CO_2, water, metabolites, electrolytes, hormones, and heat.

The major function of intestinal **venules** is short-term storage of blood, which will be mobilized and directed to the heart in response to exercise or the consumption of a meal.

3. How important is the splanchnic circulation in mobilizing blood to support physical exercise?

Although the splanchnic organs contain only 33% of the resting blood volume, their venous vessels contain the body's major reservoir of readily mobilized blood. The spleen, liver, and intestines are capable of releasing 70% of the blood mobilized from the entire body to the heart during exercise.

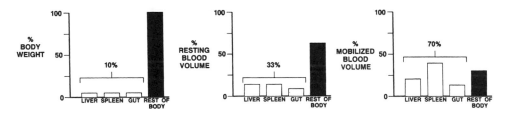

Figure 3. Comparison of percentages of body weight, resting blood volume, and mobilized blood of splanchnic organs versus rest of body.

4. What factors in the body regulate blood flow to the gut?

Normal levels of intestinal blood flow are maintained by a balance between factors that increase blood flow (vasodilators) and those that decrease blood flow (vasoconstrictors). These factors include autonomic neurotransmitters (neurocrines), circulating hormones (endocrines), tissue substances (paracrines), and intravascular physical forces. These vasoactive influences operate in the context of general cardiovascular system factors which maintain normal blood flow to each organ of the body (*see* Figure 4).

5. What general cardiovascular factors contribute to normal intestinal blood flow?

The general cardiovascular factors upon which intestinal blood flow depends are hemodynamic forces and their interactions (i.e., arterial blood pressure, cardiac output, and blood volume). For bowel blood flow to be normal, these general cardiovascular factors must be normal (*see* Figure 5). For example, if a previously healthy young man suffers serious leg trauma with massive

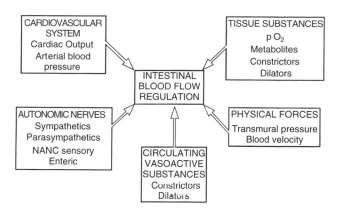

Figure 4. Factors that regulate normal gut blood flow.

femoral arterial hemorrhage, blood volume will be reduced, thereby diminishing venous return to the heart. The result will be a decrease in both cardiac output and arterial blood pressure, which will compromise blood flow to the gut. In addition, there will be peripheral vasoconstriction which will further diminish blood flow to the gut. The mesenteric circulation is quite sensitive to general cardiovascular dysfunction. Thus, the trauma of open-heart surgery may reduce arterial blood pressure and cardiac output by <25% but will be associated with a 50% or greater reduction in GI blood flow.

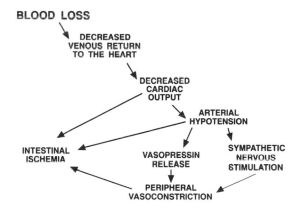

Figure 5. Hemorrhage prompts intestinal low flow in several ways.

6. How do neurocrines control blood flow to the bowel?

The autonomic nerves are organized into four components in the gut, each with its array of neurocrine substances which are released at nerve termini. Many of the neurocrines bind to vascular smooth muscle cell receptors and constrict or dilate arterioles. Autonomic nerves also alter actions of venous and cardiac smooth muscle, thereby changing general cardiovascular factors upon which gut blood flow depends. For example, the sympathetic nerves constrict veins and mobilize blood flow back to the heart, thereby increasing cardiac output and arterial blood pressure. Conversely, parasympathetic nerves reduce heart rate and cardiac output. Furthermore, neurocrine substances can vasoconstrict or vasodilate intestinal arterioles, thereby respectively decreasing or increasing bowel blood flow.

The four components of the autonomic nervous system that project nerve fibers to mesenteric arterioles are:
(1) extrinsic sympathetic nerves which release mainly constrictor neurocrines;
(2) extrinsic parasympathetic nerves;
(3) extrinsic nonadrenergic, noncholinergic (NANC) sensory nerves; and
(4) the intrinsic enteric nervous system.

The latter three autonomic nervous components release predominately dilator neurocrines. The major constrictor neurocrines are norepinephrine and ATP. The major dilator neurocrines are neuropeptides (vasoactive intestinal peptide [VIP], calcitonin gene-related peptide [CGRP], substance P), nitric oxide, and acetylcholine.

Types of Autonomic Nerves that Innervate Intestinal Blood Vessels

AUTONOMIC NERVE TYPE	EXTRINSIC OR INTRINSIC	MAJOR NEUROTRANSMITTERS	VASOACTIVE EFFECT ON INTESTINAL CIRCULATION
Sympathetic	Extrinsic	Norepinephrine	Constriction
		ATP	Constriction
Parasympathetic	Extrinsic	Acetylcholine	Dilation
		VIP	Dilation
NANC sensory	Extrinsic	CGRP	Dilation
		Substance P	Dilation
		Nitric oxide	Dilation
Enteric	Intrinsic	Norepinephrine	Constriction
		Acetylcholine	Dilation
		VIP	Dilation
		Nitric Oxide	Dilation

7. What endocrines regulate gut blood flow?

Endocrines include substances that are synthesized by endocrine gland cells and then are released into the blood. These circulating substances eventually diffuse out of the capillaries and bind to receptors on the surface of target cells, such as vascular smooth muscle, visceral muscle, and secretory cells. Endocrines, such as vasopressin from the posterior pituitary gland, angiotensin II from the juxtaglomerular apparatus (JGA), and norepinephrine from the adrenal medulla, contract intestinal vascular smooth muscle and reduce bowel blood flow. Other endocrines, such as gastrin, cholecystokinin (CCK), and secretin, stimulate overall digestive system functions, including GI motility, exocrine secretion by the stomach, pancreas, and liver, and absorption of nutrients and electrolytes in the small intestine and colon. The heightened cellular activity associated with these augmented digestive system functions increases blood flow to support the enhanced metabolism.

Endocrines that Influence Intestinal Blood Flow

ENDOCRINE SUBSTANCE	TISSUE SOURCE	VASOACTIVE EFFECT IN THE GUT	EVENT STIMULATING ENDOCRINE RELEASE
Norepinephrine	Adrenal medulla Peripheral sympathetics	Direct constriction	Heavy exercise
Angiotensin II	Renal JGA	Direct constriction	Heart failure
Vasopressin	Posterior pituitary	Direct constriction	Oligemia
GI hormones: gastrin, CCK, secretin	GI mucosa	Indirect dilation via increased metabolism	Eating a meal

8. Which paracrines influence intestinal blood flow?

Paracrine substances are released by different cells in the tissue and diffuse through the interstitial space before reaching receptors on the surface of their target cells. Many of the paracrines are vasoactive substances that bind to vascular smooth muscle cell receptors. Two widely distributed cell types generate most of these vasoactive paracrines. **Endothelial cells,** which line all blood vessels, are one of the most common cells of the body. In the gut arteriolar wall, endothelial cells lie adjacent to vascular smooth muscle cells. Endothelial cells synthesize and release vasoconstrictor paracrines, such as endothelins, interleukins, platelet-activating factor (PAF), thromboxanes, and leukotrienes; these cells also elaborate vasodilator paracrines, such as nitric oxide, prostacyclin, and bradykinin. The other cells that produce vasoactive paracrines are the **immunocytes,** such as mast cells and leukocytes. These cells generate vasoconstrictor paracrines such as active oxidants, PAF, and leukotrienes, and vasodilator paracrines such as histamine, prostacyclin, and bradykinin. Some of these vasoactive substances play a physiologic role in regulating bowel blood flow, some are involved in the inflammatory response, and some play roles in both physiologic and pathophysiologic intestinal circulatory states.

Paracrines that Influence Intestinal Blood Flow

PARACRINE SUBSTANCE	CELL SOURCE	VASOACTIVE EFFECT IN THE GUT	EVENTS STIMULATING PARACRINE RELEASE
Nitric oxide	Endothelial	Dilation	Dilator mediators
Prostacyclin	Endothelial	Dilation	Increased metabolism
Bradykinin	Endothelial	Dilation	Inflammatory response
Endothelin-1	Endothelial	Constriction	Intestinal ischemia
PAF	Endothelial	Constriction	Intestinal ischemia
Interleukins	Endothelial	Constriction	Intestinal ischemia
Active oxidants	Neutrophil, mast	Constriction	Intestinal ischemia
Histamine	Mast	Dilation	NANC sensory nerves
Leukotrienes	Mast	Constriction	Intestinal ischemia

9. What are intravascular physical forces, and how do they regulate mesenteric blood flow?

Two physical forces influence blood flow in an intestinal arteriole: transmural pressure and the velocity of streaming blood. **Transmural pressure** is the difference in pressure between the inside of the blood vessel and the outside. When this pressure is raised, the vascular smooth muscle wall contracts to offset the stretch imposed by the rising transmural pressure. The result is usually a decrease in blood flow.

A change in the **velocity of streaming blood** is sensed by the endothelial lining of arteriolar walls as a change in shear stress. Acceleration of this velocity increases endothelial surface shear stress and stimulates release of endothelium-derived relaxing factors, such as nitric oxide. The result is usually an increase in blood flow.

10. What is intestinal ischemia? What are the major mechanisms involved in ischemic injury to the gut?

Intestinal ischemia is a low blood flow state in the gut with at least a 50% reduction from normal blood flow values. If ischemia is protracted, severe structural and functional damage to the bowel wall and especially to the mucosa result.

Intestinal ischemia encompasses many disorders of the small intestine or colon, with a variety of underlying etiologies and pathophysiologic mechanisms. In most of these conditions, the ischemia is life-threatening, is difficult to diagnose and treat successfully, and is likely to end with the death of the patient. The major pathophysiologic mechanisms involved in intestinal ischemia include loss of epithelial integrity, neutrophil chemotaxis and adherence to endothelial cells, formation of active oxidants, release of other cytotoxic chemicals, depletion of intracellular chemical energy stores, and suppression of natural defense mechanisms.

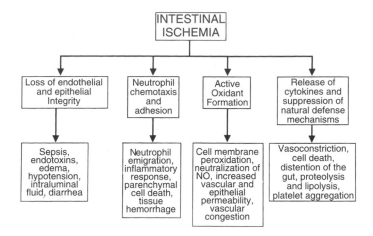

Figure 6. Major pathophysiologic events: intestinal ischemia. (NO = nitric oxide.)

11. Where does cell death start in intestinal ischemia?

The gut cells most vulnerable to ischemic hypoxia are the enterocytes that cover the distal half of the small intestinal villi (*see* Figure 7). The susceptibility to hypoxic injury is due to several factors:

(1) These cells are the major absorptive units in the entire gut for the active transport of sodium, calcium, iron, galactose, glucose, and amino acids and, therefore, are metabolically the most active cells of the mucosa.

(2) The distal half of the villi contains the highest concentration of xanthine dehydrogenase in the gut and is, therefore, the site with the highest concentration of active oxidants during intestinal ischemia.

(3) The villus microcirculation operates as a countercurrent exchanger for oxygen during the ischemic states, which causes especially low tissue pO_2 values at the villus tips.

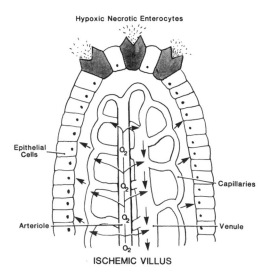

Figure 7. Blood flow and ischemic cell death in a small intestinal villus.

12. Describe the consequences of hypoxic necrosis in the small intestinal villi.

The first sites of necrosis in the ischemic bowel wall examined histologically by the pathologist are the tips of the villi. As intestinal ischemia progresses, the enterocytes lining the distal villus are lifted away from their underlying lamina propria by the growing tissue edema. Then they are sloughed into the intestinal lumen, thereby exposing the uncovered tissue to luminal contents. Two consequences of this loss of epithelial integrity are the **absorption of toxic luminal contents** and the **loss of vital tissue materials** into the lumen. The gut lumen contains many noxious agents that now have access to the circulation, such as pathogenic bacteria and their exotoxins and endotoxins, digestive enzymes such as proteases and lipases, tissue breakdown products from sloughed epithelial cells, lysosomal cathepsins and hydrolases, and electrolytes. The translocation of bacteria and these other noxious luminal materials into the mucosal tissue and the vascular compartment leads to progressive necrosis of the gut wall and septic shock. Simultaneously, vital materials are leached out of the exposed mucosal tissue into the lumen, such as structural macromolecules (hyaluronic acid, phospholipids, glycoproteins, intracellular enzymes) and ions, which leads to a massive osmotic fluid shift into the lumen, decomposition of the tissue, and advancing cellular necrosis.

13. What happens to neutrophils in intestinal ischemia?

Leukocytosis is a common finding in patients with intestinal ischemia. Much of the leukocytosis is caused by the chemical attraction (chemotaxis) of neutrophils in the body to the ischemic gut, where these leukocytes adhere to endothelial cells and then migrate out of the blood into the ischemic tissue.

Normally, neutrophils flow in or near the axial stream of a blood vessel. In response to ischemia, however, neutrophils marginate to the endothelial lining of the vessel. The margination is mediated by macromolecules, called **selectins**, located on the surfaces of both the neutrophils and endothelial cells. Selectins cause neutrophil behavior inside the vessel to change from cells flowing in the streaming blood to cells rolling along the endothelial lining. Then, another class of macromolecules, called **integrins**, is elaborated by the involved cells and causes firm binding of neutrophils to the endothelium. Next, the endothelial cells contract, thereby opening spaces between endothelial cells to allow neutrophils to penetrate and emigrate out of the vascular compartment into the perivascular interstitium. The result is an accumulation of massive numbers of neutrophils in the mucosa of the ischemic bowel. These translocated leukocytes become the major component of acute inflammatory cells observed microscopically in intestinal ischemia.

Neutrophils are equipped with cytotoxic mechanisms that can be used against pathogenic bacteria to kill those infectious agents. Neutrophils can generate such noxious agents as active oxidants and H^+, which can be injected into nearby cells. In the ischemic inflamed gut mucosa, neutrophils turn these antibacterial systems against parenchymal cells of the gut that have already been damaged by ischemic hypoxia. The end result is a killing field in which neutrophils contribute to the massive necrosis characteristic of intestinal ischemia.

14. What are active oxidants?

Active oxidants are metabolites in which the outer ring of the molecule contains an unpaired electron. Some of the common active oxidants include the oxygen free radical (O_2), hydrogen peroxide, and the hydroxyl radical (OH*). When present in larger than normal quantities, active oxidants are cytotoxic because they peroxidize the lipid component and oxidize –SH groups on proteins in cell membranes, thereby making the membranes leaky to water, macromolecules, and ions. The flooding of the cytosol with water and Ca^{2+}, for example, prompts intracellular swelling and cessation of vital cytosolic chemical reactions, leading to cell death.

In the intestinal mucosa subjected to ischemia, three adverse events occur related to tissue energetics and formation of cytotoxic active oxidants.

1. Ischemic hypoxia reduces production of ATP, on which all cells depend for normal metabolism and ion transport.
2. Hypoxia causes conversion of the small intestinal enzyme, xanthine dehydrogenase, into an isoform, xanthine oxidase.
3. Hypoxia imposes anaerobic metabolic conditions on mucosal tissue, which causes catabolism of AMP into adenosine, inosine, and hypoxanthine.

As ischemic mucosa is reperfused with blood containing a bit more oxygen, xanthine oxidase catabolizes hypoxanthine into xanthine and then into uric acid, with the production of excess quantities of active oxidants at each step of these last two metabolic conversions.

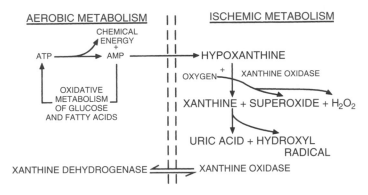

Figure 8. Intestinal ischemia reduces ATP production, converts xanthine dehydrogenase into xanthine oxidase, and generates active oxidants.

15. Describe the other pathophysiologic processes and cytotoxic agents involved in intestinal ischemia.

There are numerous naturally occurring agents in the gut wall that are not particularly harmful to nearby cells, as long as these agents are present in minute concentrations. In intestinal ischemia, however, many of these substances are overproduced, and they become lethal to nearby cells in their elevated concentrations. These endogenous injurious chemicals interfere with a range of important intestinal functions, including:

(1) Endothelial impermeability to macromolecules (i.e., vascular leakage of macromolecules, water, and electrolytes occurs, causing edema and oligemia);

(2) Epithelial impermeability to macromolecules (its loss leads to a decline in intestinal absorptive capacity and intraluminal fluid accumulation);

(3) Translocation of both leukocytes and erythrocytes from blood to the interstitial space;

(4) Intravascular aggregation of leukocytes and platelets;

(5) Local circulatory failure characterized by ischemic hypoxia and venous congestion;

(6) Loss of normal visceral smooth muscle tone and propulsive ability, leading to paralysis and distention of the gut wall;

(7) Cytotoxicity starting with the most superficial epithelial cells and advancing inexorably into the deeper gut wall;

(8) Release of proteolytic and lipolytic enzymes which digest cellular plasma membranes; and

(9) Aggregation of platelets and deposition of fibrin in mucosal microcirculatory blood vessels.

The changing chemical environment of the intestine includes declining availability of oxygen and other blood-borne nutrients, an increase in toxic active oxidants, tissue acidosis, and excess quantities of such naturally occurring paracrine substances as histamine, serotonin, bradykinin, nitric oxide, leukotrienes, thromboxanes, interleukins, endothelins, PAF, complement, and thrombin.

16. Which naturally occurring defense systems of the gut are suppressed in intestinal ischemia?

Endogenous defense systems in the bowel include secretion into the lumen of mucus which adheres to the epithelium, epithelial impermeability to luminal contents, a viable mucosal blood flow, vascular impermeability to macromolecules, active mucosal immunocytes, and responsive epithelial regenerative mechanisms. With intestinal ischemia, each of these protective processes is inhibited as a result of their dependency on oxidative metabolism, which has declined because of intestinal ischemic hypoxia.

In addition, ischemia inhibits several enzyme systems that produce protective agents. Among the more notable enzymes that are inhibited by intestinal ischemia are nitric oxide synthase, cyclooxygenase, and certain proteases. Nitric oxide synthase converts L-arginine into nitric oxide, which maintains normal mucosal blood flow as well as epithelial and vascular impermeability to macromolecules, certain ions, and water. Cyclooxygenase converts arachidonic acid into protective eicosanoids, such as prostacyclin and prostaglandin E_2. These eicosanoids contribute to the maintenance of normal gut blood flow and stimulate secretion of mucus; they are also essential for epithelial regeneration. These eicosanoids stabilize lysosomal membranes, thereby preventing autodigestion of injured cells, and they antagonize platelet aggregation. Certain proteases maintain low levels of autolytic enzymes in healthy cells.

Thus, with ischemic inhibition of defense processes and supressed generation of cytoprotective agents, the gut is in poor position to minimize hypoxic injury or to replace necrotic tissue.

17. What are the major pathophysiologic steps involved in nonocclusive intestinal ischemia?

The time frame of events is usually sufficiently slow in nonocclusive intestinal ischemia to appreciate the pathophysiologic progression. By contrast, in intestinal ischemia caused by a thrombus or embolus of a mesenteric artery, the events are telescoped into an acute abdominal catastrophe with rapid evolution into infarcted bowel, peritonitis, and death of the patient (see Figure 9).

The typical patient with nonocclusive intestinal ischemia is elderly and has coexistent serious cardiovascular disease, most often congestive cardiac failure. With heart failure, cardiac output is reduced, which reduces blood flow to the gut. In addition, there is sympathetic nervous overactivity and release of angiotensin II in heart failure, which further constricts splanchnic blood vessels. Patients with heart failure are often medicated with cardiac glycosides that constrict the mesenteric circulation and also prompt peripheral release of catecholamines. Other drugs used in heart failure patients include diuretics, which produce hypovolemia, and beta-adrenergic blocking agents, which constrict the mesenteric circulation. These general circulatory and pharmacologic conditions impose a persistent low blood flow state in the gut that progresses into symptomatic intestinal ischemia requiring hospitalization of the patient.

Symptoms and signs of intestinal ischemia at this stage may include continuous deep abdominal pain, hypotension, hematochezia, and diarrhea. Positive specific routine laboratory tests for intestinal ischemia are nonexistent, although abdominal films may show evidence for an edematous bowel wall. Mesenteric angiography, if ordered, will demonstrate vascular insufficiency in the involved gut. For the patient to survive at this point in nonocclusive intestinal ischemia, it is essential that an early diagnosis be made and that effective intervention with mesenteric vasodilator therapy be undertaken. If these steps are not made in a timely fashion, the patient will slowly slide into the irreversible phase of intestinal ischemia over several days and die.

As the disorder progresses, ischemic hypoxia destroys the epithelial lining, starting at the villus tips. Simultaneously, ischemic hypoxia causes a massive mucosal inflammatory response with chemotaxis and emigration of neutrophils, generation of active oxidants and a variety of other toxic substances, and suppression of natural defense mechanisms. As mucosal infarction evolves, there is absorption of toxic luminal contents. The superimposition of sepsis in an elderly patient suffering from heart failure and ischemic bowel leads to periotonitis, irreversible shock, and death. Reported mortality rates for patients not diagnosed and treated early in nonocclusive intestinal ischemia are about 90%.

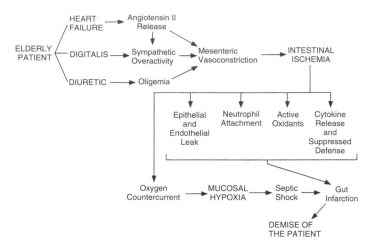

Figure 9. Pathophysiologic progression of nonocclusive intestinal ischemia.

18. List the four types of intestinal ischemic diseases and their underlying pathophysiologic mechanisms.

There are four major classes of intestinal ischemic disease, three of which occur in the small bowel and one in the colon. Most of these entities involve the arteries primarily, but ischemia caused by veno-occlusion is not rare. The mortality rate exceeds 50% in most of these disorders. The table lists the more common entities. Under small intestinal ischemia, the prevalence is more readily ascertained, because most of these patients die from their low flow state, and the diagnosis can be made postmortem. By contrast, many patients with colonic ischemia survive the disorder without a diagnosis having been established.

Classification of Small Bowel Ischemic Disorders

MAJOR PATHOLOGICAL PROCESS	EXAMPLES OF DISEASE ENTITIES
SMA occlusion	SMA thrombosis or embolus
SMA vasospasm	Nonocclusive intestinal ischemia
Miscellaneous mechanisms	
Bacterial translocation	Necrotizing enterocolitis
Mesenteric venous occlusion	Hepatic tumor compression
Connective tissue disorder	Periarteritis

SMA = Small mesenteric artery.

19. Can structural abnormalities be seen in the histopathology of intestinal ischemia?

The major determinant of the abnormal findings in intestinal ischemia is the severity and duration of the low blood flow state, rather than the underlying disease process which caused the ischemia.

With **mild degrees** of ischemia from whatever cause, there may be no histopathologic findings in the bowel, despite the patient's having suffered diarrhea, hematochezia, and abdominal pain. The earliest structural abnormalities would be necrosis of scattered enterocytes at or near the small intestinal villus tips or colonocytes at the luminal surface of the large bowel. Next, edema in the underlying lamina propria lifts the epithelial cells off their mucosal attachments. If the ischemia is resolved at this stage, recovery is complete without structural evidence of the ischemic disease.

With **moderate degrees** of ischemia, there is morphologic evidence of mucosal infarction, which includes extensive epithelial cell necrosis and sloughing of enterocytes or colonocytes into the lumen; engorged venules with extravasation of both leukocytes and erythrocytes into the lamina propria; fibrin deposition in microcirculatory vessels; widespread edema; and increased cellularity with a mix of necrotic parenchymal cells, neutrophils, and erythrocytes in the mucosa.

The inflammatory response to ischemia usually involves the muscularis propria. Resolution of the disease at this stage is often followed by severe fibrosis and bowel strictures and is a common outcome in ischemic colitis.

With **severe degrees** of intestinal ischemia, the infarction involves the full wall thickness, including serosal inflammation and peritonitis. In the case of the large bowel, toxic megacolon may result. At this stage, the gut wall displays extensive coagulation necrosis, and the mucosa gives the appearance of ghost tissue lacking cellular detail (*see* Figure 10). This stage of intestinal ischemia is terminal for the patient, and most victims die despite surgical resection of the involved gut.

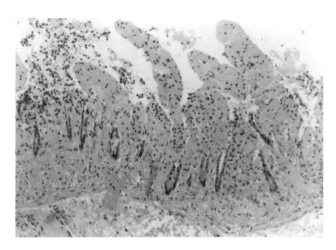

Figure 10. Histopathologic appearance of gut wall mucosa in intestinal ischemia, showing the lack of cellular detail (ghost tissue).

20. Why is the diagnosis of intestinal ischemia usually made too late to save the patient?

1. Intestinal ischemia is regarded as an uncommon and obscure set of illnesses. This viewpoint works against a high level of clinical suspicion. This view is also out of touch with the fact that intestinal ischemia is responsible for as many deaths in the United States as is colon cancer. About 5% of hospital deaths in this country involve intestinal ischemia as the major cause of demise.

2. Intestinal ischemia usually coexists with another life-threatening and more obvious disease, such as heart failure, septic shock, thromboembolic conditions, cardiac arrhythmias, or recovery from major cardiovascular surgery.

3. There is no specific routine laboratory test available for bowel ischemia. Nevertheless, delay in the diagnosis of intestinal ischemia ensures a fatal outcome. The lateness of the diagnosis is evidenced by the fact that most patients in whom the diagnosis is made die from the illness.

21. What clues suggest intestinal ischemia in a patient with abdominal pain?

Although intestinal ischemia can occur at any age starting with neonatal life, the typical patient with a low flow state in the bowel is elderly. Indeed, the acute onset of abdominal pain in an elderly patient who has other serious cardiovascular disease should lead to considering ischemia in the initial differential diagnosis. The pain is often severe and periumbilical but is not associated with either rebound tenderness or guarding on examination. An abrupt onset of pain suggests an embolus, whereas more gradual onset is associated with gut ischemia caused by thrombotic occlusion or nonocclusive intestinal ischemia.

22. Why should hematochezia lead to the suspicion of intestinal ischemia?

The colon may be the site of ischemia, in which case hematochezia reflects large bowel mucosal injury. Ischemic hematochezia may occur with or without diarrhea in younger adults as a catastrophic consequence of pregnancy, as a side effect of birth control medication, with cocaine or

amphetamine use, as a manifestation of a hypercoagulable state with venous thrombosis, with an-
tibiotic-related *Clostridium difficile* infection, or with enteroinvasive *Escherichia coli* infection.
Colonic ischemia can also occur in elderly patients with cardiovascular disease or following aortic bypass surgery.

**23. Given the advances in diagnostic technology, why is it difficult and time-consuming to
prove that a patient has intestinal ischemia?**
  Routine laboratory tests that may be positive in an elderly patient with new-onset abdominal
pain include blood pH, white blood cell count, amylase, and abdominal x-rays. None of these tests
is specific for intestinal ischemia, however.
  More specific diagnostic procedures, such as mesenteric angiography in an elderly patient in
heart failure or colonic endoscopy in an elderly subject with hematochezia, are not undertaken
lightly. These interventions are not screening procedures and are likely to be ordered only after
other common causes of an acute abdomen have been excluded by many other time-consuming
tests and procedures.

24. Outline the major elements of the treatment plan for a patient with intestinal ischemia.
  The first step after diagnosing intestinal ischemia is to resuscitate and stabilize the seriously
ill patient, who may be hypotensive, acidotic, in electrolyte imbalance, or under respiratory distress. Lines are inserted to monitor central venous pressure and pulmonary artery pressure and to
deliver intravenous fluid/electrolyte resuscitation. Inotropic and antiarrhythmic drugs are commonly required, along with broad-spectrum antibiotics following blood and peritoneal cultures.
More specific diagnosis is achieved by angiography and/or colonoscopy.
  In the small intestine, about half of the cases involve an embolus or thrombus in the superior
mesenteric artery, and 25% of cases reflect nonocclusive intestinal ischemia. The mainstay of
treatment for an embolus is rapid surgical exploration with appropriate bowel resection or em-
bolectomy and selected use of a second-look operation 1–2 days later. With mesenteric thrombosis, definitive treatment includes timely reconstructive vascular surgery coupled with protracted intra-arterial infusion of papaverine for vasodilation if the thrombus is in the distal
mesenteric circulation. In patients with nonocclusive intestinal ischemia, intra-arterial papaverine infusion for 24 hours is accepted therapy.

BIBLIOGRAPHY

1. Brandt LJ, Boley SJ: Ischemic and vascular lesions of the bowel. In Sleisenger M, Fordtran J (eds): Gas-
     trointestinal Disease, 5th ed. Philadelphia, W.B. Saunders, 1993, pp 1927–1961.
2. Clavien PA: Diagnosis and management of mesenteric infarction. Br J Surg 77:601–603, 1990.
3. Granger DN: Role of xanthine oxidase and granulocytes in ischemia-reperfusion injury. Am J Physiol
     255:H1269–H1275, 1988.
4. Kvietys PR, Granger DN: The vascular endothelium in gastrointestinal inflammation. In Wallace J (ed):
     Immunopharmacology of the Gastrointestinal Tract, vol 5. New York, Academic Press, 1993, pp 65–
     93.
5. Levine JS: Acute bloody diarrhea. In Levine JS (ed): Decision Making in Gastroenterology, 2nd ed.
     St. Louis, C.V. Mosby, 1992, pp 110–111.
6. Levine JS, Jacobson ED: Intestinal ischemic disorders. Dig Dis 13:3–24, 1995.
7. Moore WM, Hollier LH: Mesenteric artery occlusive disease. Cardiology Clin 9:535–541, 1991.
8. Norris HT: Vascular disorders. In Ming SC, Goldman H (eds): Pathology of the Gastrointestinal Tract.
     Philadelphia, W.B. Saunders, 1992, pp 214–239.
9. Whittle BJR: Nitric oxide in gastrointestinal physiology and pathology. In Johnson LR (ed): Physiology
     of the Gastrointestinal Tract, 3rd ed. New York, Raven Press, 1994, pp 267–294.

60. NUTRITIONAL ASSESSMENT AND THERAPY

Jonathan P. Kushner, M.D., and Sandra E. Smith, R.D., M.S.

1. What is meant by nutritional status?
Nutritional status reflects how well nutrient intake contributes to healthy **body composition** and **function,** affected also by the existing metabolic environment. The four major body composition compartments include water, protein, mineral, and fat. The first three compose the lean body mass (LBM); functional capacity resides in a portion of the LBM called the body-cell mass. The nutritionist focuses his or her greatest efforts on the preservation or restoration of this vital component.

2. What is malnutrition? How do different types of malnutrition impact on function and outcome?
Malnutrition refers to states of over- (e.g., obesity) or undernutrition. **Marasmus** is calorie malnutrition in which there is significant physical wasting of energy stores (adipose tissue and somatic muscle protein) while visceral and serum proteins are preserved. These patients do not demonstrate edema and may have mild immune dysfunction. **Hypoalbuminemic malnutrition** occurs in those with stressed metabolism and is common in hospitalized patients. They may have greater energy stores and body weight but have expanded extracellular and depleted intracellular mass, edema, depressed serum protein levels, and immune dysfunction. A similar state of relative protein deficiency occurs in classic **kwashiokor,** where caloric provision is adequate while quantity and quality of protein is not.

A 40% loss of LBM is generally incompatible with survival. Elegant studies reveal that muscle and immune function may be affected by a loss of 20% body protein; patients with 10–20% loss of body weight may have lost 20% of body protein. The state of hydration and edema must be considered when judging weight parameters.

3. Explain the differences between unstressed starvation and stressed metabolism.
In **unstressed starvation,** the body utilizes fat stores to preserve the functioning tissue. Obligatory glucose-utilizing tissues, such as brain and red blood cells, derive energy from liver glycogen stores and gluconeogenesis. Gluconeogenic precursors include muscle amino acids, particularly alanine. Fortunately, after several days of starvation, the brain adapts to ketones for energy and muscle protein is spared. Daily urinary nitrogen excretion drops from 12–15 gm early to 3–4 gm in the adapted state. Survival for months is possible.

In **stressed metabolism,** hormones and cytokines mobilize lean tissue amino acids for the synthesis of beneficial reactive proteins and glucose. Unlike in unstressed starvation, gluconeogenesis and amino acid mobilization are not easily suppressed by exogenous energy provision, and nitrogen losses remain high. While beneficial to the host early on, lean mass catabolism, when prolonged, has deleterious consequences, including a shortened survival.

4. How do you accomplish a simple nutritional assessment? What additional tools and techniques exist?
Simple bedside assessment may be as valuable in predicting nutrition-associated outcomes as more sophisticated composition and function tests. One popular method, the **Subjective Global Assessment,** incorporates basic questions on weight history, intake, GI symptoms, disease state, functional level, and a physical examination to classify patients as well-nourished, mild to moderately malnourished, or severely malnourished.

Adequate recent intake may improve function before a noticeable change occurs in composition or weight. Low **serum proteins** may indicate hypoalbuminemic malnutrition but are nonspecific nutritional markers. They may decline rapidly under stress or after surgery, yet are relatively preserved in unstressed starvation.

SERUM PROTEIN	NORMAL	HALF-LIFE	PPV	NPV
Albumin	3–5 gm/dl	14–20 d	86	17
Transferrin	200–400 mg/dl	8–9 d	87	27
Prealbumin	10–40 mg/dl	2–3 d	93	56
Retinol-binding protein	3–8 mg/dl	0.5 d	73	19

PPV and NPV = positive and negative predictive values of rising nitrogen balance.
Adapted from Church J, Hill G: Assessing the efficacy of intravenous nutrition in general surgery patients. JPEN 11:135–139, 1987, with permission.

Some laboratory tests for **micronutrients** (red cell folate, vitamin B12, ferritin) are available and may help to interpret total body status. Others (zinc, copper) are less easily obtained and unreliable markers of whole body status. **Urinary creatinine-height index** to estimate muscle mass and **anthropometric measures** of skinfolds and circumferences are less reliable tools. Bedside **bioelectric impedance analysis** discerns fat from fat-free mass but needs further validation. Isotopic body water determination, underwater densitometry, dual x-ray absorptiometry, neutron activation analysis, assays of involuntary muscle function and cellular energetics are research tools.

In summary, a weight history, estimate of recent intake, brief physical exam, consideration of disease stress/medications, and assessments of functional status and wound healing allow for a good estimate of nutritional status. They predict the risk for malnutrition-associated complications as well as or better than available laboratory data. Poor intake for greater than 1–2 weeks or a weight loss of 10% or more warrants closer nutritional assessment and follow-up.

5. What are the components of energy expenditure? How are they affected clinically?

Energy is required for the maintenance of the living state, to do work, for repletion, and for growth in children. Energy is derived largely from macronutrient oxidation of carbohydrate, fat, and protein.

Caloric equivalents

Carbohydrate	4.0 kcal/gm	IV dextrose	3.4 kcal/gm
Protein	4.0 kcal/gm	Fat	9.0 kcal/gm

Energy expenditure

Total energy expenditure (TEE) = Resting energy expenditure (REE) + thermic effect of feeding (TEF) + energy expenditure of activity (EEA)

REE = Basal energy expenditure (BEE) ($\sim$ 20 kcal/kg or obtained from standard regression equation such as Harris-Benedict) modified for disease state/stress (often 25–30 kcal/kg or 1.0–1.5 $\times$ BEE in recent studies) or measured by indirect calorimetry.

TEF = 10% of REE if meals in typical bolus fashion; negligible if continuous feeds.

EEA = Quite variable; 5–30% of BEE in hospitalized patients.

The BEE is determined primarily by the LBM. When energy expenditure is estimated from standard equations, the body weight used for the calculation is critical. Use of an edematous or obese weight will overrepresent the LBM; therefore, a dry weight is estimated in the case of edema, and an adjusted weight is used in significantly obese patients as follows:

0.25 (actual weight − desirable weight) + desirable weight

Desirable weights from the 1983 Metropolitan Life Tables are estimated as 135 lbs for a 5 ft, 3 in male plus 3 lbs per additional inch ($\pm$ 10%), and 119 lbs for a 5 ft, 0 in woman with 3 lbs per additional inch ($\pm$ 10%).

We can directly measure the REE using indirect calorimetry with a metabolic cart. The energy of activity must be estimated and added to the REE. Use of the cart also provides the RQ (respiratory quotient) where RQ = VCO_2/VO_2. An RQ of 0.7 reflects pure fat oxidation; an RQ of 1.0, pure carbohydrate oxidation; and values in between, mixed fuel oxidation. An RQ > 1.0 suggests that lipogenesis from carbohydrate exceeds fat oxidation; i.e., overfeeding. Although use of the metabolic cart has not been demonstrated to improve outcome, bear in mind the significant individual variability of energy expenditure and the limitations of predictive formulas.

6. Describe the types of oral diets commonly prescribed.

The **clear liquid diet** supplies fluid and calories in a form that requires minimal digestion, stimulation, and elimination by the GI tract. It provides about 600 cal, 150 gm carbohydrate, 15 gm protein, 1 gm fat, and inadequate vitamins and minerals. These foods are hyperosmolar; GI symptoms may be minimized by diluting the beverages and eating slower. If clear liquids are needed for > 3 days, a dietitian can assist with supplementation.

The **full liquid diet** is used often in progressing from clear liquids to solid foods. It may also be used in patients with chewing or swallowing problems, gastric stasis, or partial ileus. Typically, this diet provides > 2000 cal, about 340 gm carbohydrate, 70 gm protein, and 85 gm fat. It may be adequate in all nutrients, except fiber, especially if a high-protein supplement is added. Patients with lactose intolerance will need special substitutions, and the significant amounts of fat may not be well tolerated in all patients. A dietitian can help to modify this diet, if indicated. Progression to solid foods should be accomplished with modifications or supplementation, as needed.

One of the most challenging populations to feed well are patients recovering from recent gastric surgery. In addition to the anorexia that is common in sick individuals, these patients may suffer from early satiety, slow recovery of GI function, and delayed gastric emptying or rapid GI transit and dumping syndrome. They are at increased risk for chronic iron, calcium, vitamin D, magnesium, and vitamin B_{12} malabsorption. The typical postgastrectomy diet limits simple sugars, size of meals, and fluids with solids, but encourages fluids and snacks between meals.

7. When should nutritional support be considered?

Situations that warrant potential intervention with nutritional support (forced feeding) include:

1. Protein and calorie deprivation for 7–10 days in a previously well-nourished or mildly malnourished adult
2. Hypermetabolism or hypercatabolism and protein-calorie deprivation for > 4 days
3. Moderate to severe degree of malnutrition at presentation
4. Starved or critically ill children who are not consuming adequate oral intake

8. What types of enteral formulas may be prescribed?

Classification of Adult Enteral Formulas

CATEGORY	EXAMPLES	CHARACTERISTICS	INDICATIONS
Blenderized	Compleat Compleat Mod.	Contains some blenderized whole foods. 1 kcal/ml. 16% of kcal as protein. Expensive. Unpalatable.	Regulation of bowel function. Long-term feeding. Normal digestive and absorptive capacity.
Standard	Isocal (HN) Osmolite (HN) Ensure (HN)	Low residue. 1 kcal/ml. 13–17% of kcal as protein. May have MCT. May or may not be palatable.	General feeding. Fairly normal digestive and absorptive capacity. Low fecal residue.
Fiber supplemented	Ultracal, Jevity Ensure with fiber Profiber	12–14 gm fiber/l. 1 kcal/ml. 14–18% of kcal as protein. Generally unpalatable.	Regulation of bowel function. Long-term feeding. Normal digestive and absorptive capacity.
High protein	Ensure High Protein Promote, Replete Protain XL	1 kcal/ml. 20–25% of kcal as protein. Elevated levels of some vitamins and zinc. Some contain added fiber.	Catabolism. Wound healing. Normal digestive and absorptive capacity.
Concentrated	Ensure Plus (HN) Sustacal Plus, Magnacal, Nutren 2.0	1.5–2.0 kcal/ml. 14–17% of kcal as protein. 69–77% water. Hyperosmolar.	Fluid/volume restriction. Normal digestive and absorptive capacity.
Hydrolyzed protein	Vital HN, Accupep Peptamen, Alitraq Vivonex Plus	Amino acids and/or peptides. Some have added glutamine and/or arginine. Most low in LCT. May have added MCT. Expensive.	Limited digestive capacity and absorptive surface.

Table continues on following page.

Classification of Adult Enteral Formulas (Continued)

CATEGORY	EXAMPLES	CHARACTERISTICS	INDICATIONS
Renal	Suplena, Nepro Travasorb Renal Amin-Aid	Restricted in water, Na, K, P, Mg, and vitamin A. Some have no "nonessential" amino acids, minerals, or vitamins. Expensive.	Supplement or total feeding during renal failure, predialysis or with dialysis. Avoid using only essential amino acids for > 2 wk.
Hepatic	Hepatic-Aid II Travasorb Hepatic	Higher in branched-chain amino acids and reduced in aromatic amino acids and methionine. Expensive.	Hepatic encephalopathy, when standard formulas are not tolerated.
Modular additives	Propac, Promod Polycose Microlipid, MCT	Protein powder Glucose polymers MCT oil; vegetable oil.	To modify the kcal:N ratio of the base formula.

All formulas listed are lactose-free except Compleat.
MCT = medium-chain triglyceride; LCT = long-chain triglyceride.

Specialty formulas exist for respiratory failure, diabetes, trauma/sepsis, and immune dysfunction; however, research demonstrating the superiority of these products over traditional formulas is limited.

9. What precautions should be taken when forced enteral feeding is used? What are the potential complications?

Aspiration: Most feared complication; incidence depends on definition; greatest risk in those with inability to protect airway or with very poor gastric emptying. Elevate head of bed, avoid bolus delivery, monitor residuals, feed post-pyloric or jejunal.

Mechanical complications: Nasopharyngeal/labial irritation, sinusitis, esophageal/laryngeal ulceration, tube displacement, feeding tube obstruction. Use small-bore ($\leq$ 10 F) nasal/oral feeding tubes; tape tube securely; verify tube placement; flush tube (20–30 ml water) before and after administration of medications and feedings; declog with distilled water, solution of papain, or pancreatic enzymes and bicarbonate.

GI complications: (1) Nausea, vomiting, distention, gastric residual ($>$ ~ 150 ml), pneumatosis intestinalis. Position tube distal to ligament of Treitz; use continuous feeding vs bolus; initiate feeding at low rate (20–25 ml/hr) and gradually increase; maintain head of bed $\geq$ 30°; consider prokinetic medications; use isotonic and lower fat formulas; do not feed during hemodynamic instability. (2) Diarrhea (etiology is often multifactorial) and infectious complications. Stool assay for *Clostridium difficile*; modify medications (e.g., dilute hyperosmolar medications); start slow infusion rate and advance gradually; dilute hypertonic formulas; use sterile products and avoid feeding contamination; avoid boluses of cold formula; if needed, supplement with pancreatic enzymes; consider change to a peptide, amino acid, low-fat or fiber-containing formula (esp soluble fiber); administer MCT gradually, if used; attempt to correct severe hypoalbuminemia ($<$ 2.0–2.5 gm/dl).

Metabolic complications: Abnormal fluid, minerals, glucose, triglyceride. Use appropriate formula; advance feeding gradually, monitor lab values, avoid overfeeding; supplement or restrict water.

10. When should an enterostomy replace a nasoenteric tube for enteral access? Which enterostomies are preferable?

When forced enteral feeding will exceed 4–6 weeks duration, an enterostomy may be preferable to a nasal tube for patient comfort and, perhaps, tube stability. In many instances, the percutaneous endoscopic gastrostomy (PEG) has replaced surgically placed gastrostomies. Cost and operative time are reduced. Immediate and longer term morbidities have been equal in controlled trials. Complications (about 5–10%) may include tube displacement, peristomal leaks and infections, GI bleeds, peritonitis, or fasciitis, though major complications are rare. Jejunal feeding may reduce aspiration/reflux risks compared to gastric or duodenal feeds, but the placement of a J-tube through a PEG has proved difficult with frequent failures. Patients at high risk of aspiration or with upper GI tract compromise may best be served by placement of a surgical jejunostomy.

11. Discuss the basic types of parenteral nutrition.

The first major distinction in types of parenteral nutrition is the site of administration. Either peripheral or central veins may be used, and the choice is determined by the osmolality of the solution, the anticipated duration of therapy ($<$ or $>$ 10 days), the condition of the patient's veins, and fluid tolerance.

About 75–85% of the kilocalorie and protein needs of most patients can be met in 2.4–3.0 l/day of **peripheral parenteral nutrition** (PPN), which is lower in dextrose and thus osmolality—i.e., 600–900 mOsm/l. The risk of phlebitis can be decreased with use of heparin or hydrocortisone.

For patients who require large amounts of nutrients, fluid restriction, or long-term parenteral feeding, central venous access is needed for **total** or **central parenteral nutrition** (TPN/CPN). There are shorter-term and longer-term access devices, including peripherally inserted central catheters.

Parenteral solutions can be delivered as total nutrient admixtures, which have the fat added to the TPN solution, or the fat can be given separately via a Y-catheter or peripheral vein. There are advantages and disadvantages to each method.

The adult standard parenteral nutrition multivitamin supplement contains all known vitamins, except vitamin K, which can be added to the formula, if needed. The adult multitrace-5 mineral supplement contains zinc, copper, chromium, selenium, and manganese. Long-term patients can be switched to the multitrace-7 which also contains iodine and molybdenum. The essentiality of some trace minerals was first identified when TPN patients not receiving these minerals presented with clinical and laboratory abnormalities that resolved with supplementation.

TPN does not generally contain iron; it is not compatible in lipid-containing parenteral solutions, and most people, especially men, do not require it during short-term support. Long-term patients, especially children, who cannot obtain sufficient iron enterally, will probably need parenteral iron supplementation. Intravenous iron supplementation has been associated with an increased risk of gram-negative sepsis, hemosiderosis, and allergic reactions, including fatal anaphylaxis.

Research suggests that the normal dosage of vitamin D (5 μg ergocalciferol) added to TPN may be one factor in the development of metabolic bone disease associated with long-term TPN.

12. What are the potential complications of parenteral nutrition?

Potential complications include pneumothorax, thrombosis, embolism, improper tip location, catheter-related sepsis, metabolic abnormalities, GI atrophy, and hepatobiliary abnormalities. As the number of lumens increases (from single to triple), so may the incidence of infection. Precautions include careful and sterile line insertion, adherence to insertion and dressing change protocols, and confirmation of line placement. Nutrient delivery should be gradually increased and the patient monitored (e.g., labs) often. Because patients can easily be given large amounts of kilocalories in TPN, including dextrose, previously starved patients may exhibit "refeeding syndrome" (salt/volume overload, and an acute drop in serum K, P, and possibly Mg). Overfeeding calories, especially dextrose ($>$ 4–6 mg/kg/min in stressed patients), may result in hyperglycemia, increased CO_2 production, and hepatic steatosis. Excess long-chain fat ($>$ 1.5 gm/kg/day or infusion rate $>$ 0.1 gm/kg/hr) may exceed clearance capacity and interfere with the reticuloendothelial system.

13. What are "hidden" sources of calories?

Watch out for significant glucose absorption (30–50%) across peritoneal dialysis or continuous arteriovenous hemodialysis membranes, large amounts of dextrose from other intravenous drips, or lipid calories from propofol, a sedative (1.1 kcal/ml).

14. Why is enteral nutrition preferable to parenteral nutrition?

Nutrients are metabolized (e.g., "first pass") and may be utilized more effectively via the enteral than the parenteral route. Production of secretory IgA is maintained by enteral nutrition and may prevent bacterial adherence to the intestinal mucosa. Enteral nutrition may result in less gut bacterial translocation, macromolecule permeability, sepsis, and multiorgan failure compared to TPN. Most enteral products contain glutamin. Fiber-containing enteral formulas result in the production of short-chain fatty acids that help promote intestinal and colonic growth. Catabolic response may be lessened, and proliferation of gut mucosal cells enhanced with early enteral nutrition after injury or stress. Obviously, there are no venous catheter-related risks and lower costs with enteral feeding. Long-term patients, especially with a short gut, experience more hepatic failure when they are primarily TPN-dependent. Therefore, when the gut works and can be safely used, use it!

15. A 56-year-old white man, who is 5 ft, 6 in tall and weighs 210 lbs, has been on ventilator support for 2 days following surgery. He is sedated and febrile. Calculate his current energy requirements.

For **energy requirements,** we would use 76 kg as an adjusted weight for obesity (*see* Question 5) and estimate a basal energy expenditure (BEE) of 1540 kcal/day. The patient's current postoperative, febrile state may warrant a 20–30% increment above BEE. No thermic effects of feeding are taking place. His activity is minimal while sedated and ventilated, warranting perhaps 5% added to BEE. Thus, his estimated total daily energy expenditure is:

$$1540 \text{ (BEE)} + 385 \text{ (stress)} + 77 \text{ (activity)} = 2000 \text{ kcal}$$

In unstressed patients, provision of at least 125–150 gm of carbohydrate per day (1.2–2.0 mg/kg/min) will spare the gluconeogenic amino acids that would be used for obligatory glucose needs. Above that level, fat and carbohydrate are equivalent energy sources for protein sparing.

16. Calculate his protein requirements.

Most healthy people require no more than 0.8 gm of protein/kg/day to maintain protein (nitrogen) balance. The average hospitalized patient requires 1.0–1.5 gm of protein/kg. A highly stressed patient often requires 1.5–2.0 gm of protein/kg/day. More than 2.0–2.5 gm of protein/kg may exceed the body's capacity for net protein gains.

In our sample patient, the provision of 1.5 gm of protein/kg, 114 gm of protein/day, would be a good place to start, and his nitrogen balance should then be checked periodically. Whereas a nonprotein calorie-to-nitrogen ratio of 150:1 is felt to be optimal for patients with mild to moderate stress levels, a 100:1 ratio may be more appropriate with severe stress. Whether total or nonprotein calories are used to meet the estimated energy requirements, care should be taken to avoid gross overfeeding.

17. What are his fluid requirements? Vitamin and mineral requirements?

For fluid requirements, one simple estimation is 30–35 ml/kg for most adults. Using the adjusted weight of 76 kg, this would be 2280–2660 ml/day for this patient. This estimate may need to be revised based on his postoperative fluid status and sensible and insensible losses.

Vitamin and mineral requirements for hospitalized patients are not known. It is general practice to provide 100–200% of the recommended daily allowances (1989 RDAs) for enterally delivered micronutrients and the American Medical Association-recommended daily levels of vitamins and trace minerals for parenteral administration. Most enteral formulas contain 100% of the RDA for the micronutrients in 1200–2000 calories.

18. Thus, what is your nutritional prescription for this patient?

Assuming the patient had good nutritional status preoperatively, nutritional support would be appropriate in this stressed, postoperative patient by the fourth or fifth postoperative day, or sooner if it is anticipated that he will not be eating by day 4 or 5. His intubated status precludes oral diets. If the gut is functional and there are no absolute contradictions to enteral tube feeding, this should be considered.

Enteral formula (for 2000 kcal, 114 gm protein/day, and no fluid or renal limitations): A high-protein formula (e.g., 1 kcal/ml, 50–60 gm protein/l) should be used, starting at 20–25 ml/hr and advancing to a goal rate of 80–85 ml/hr. If a lower protein formula is used, he may need the addition of a protein module.

Parenteral feeding: If the patients's gut is unusable or fails, PPN might be tried, provided peripheral veins are adequate and short duration use is anticipated. However, it will take 3.0 l/day of PPN to meet 80% of kcal/protein needs. If CPN/TPN is indicated, the following format may be used to order TPN:

Protein grams = gm/kg × kg	e.g., 1.5 × 76 = 114 gm
Dextrose grams = (50–80% nonprotein kcal) / 3.4	e.g., 70% × 2000 / 3.4 = 412 gm
Fat grams = (20–50% nonprotein kcal) / 10	e.g., 30% × 2000 / 10 = 60 gm

Volume: Minimal volume here should be about 2000–2100 ml/day, which is 30 ml/kg in this patient. Order a higher volume if desired.

Minerals: For approximately 2 liters volume or 2000 kcal, average requirements are:

Na 60–180 meq	K 80–120 meq
Cl 60–180 meq	Mg 12–30 meq
Ca 5–15 meq	P 20–30 mmol

A typical order for 2000 ml would be:

30 meq NaCl	70 meq Na acetate
40 meq KCl	10 meq Ca gluconate
16 meq MgSO$_4$	24 mmol KP

Acetate: chloride ratios may be altered if needed (e.g., more acetate, less chloride for a metabolic acidosis). Other electrolytes may be increased or decreased as needed for preexisting electrolyte abnormalities or to provide more salt if greater volume is ordered.

Micronutrients: Standard multivitamin/ multitrace mineral solutions should be ordered.

Medications: Regular insulin may be added at two-thirds of prior doses or sliding scale requirements. Other compatible medications may be added.

19. What monitoring should be done for patients on forced feedings?

Before starting parental nutrition and for the first few days until the patient is stable, the following variables should be monitored closely. These variables should be checked 1–2 times a week along with albumin and prealbumin.

Fluid status	Calcium	Triglycerides
Sodium	Magnesium	Complete blood count
Potassium	Glucose	Prothrombin time
Chloride	Blood urea nitrogen	pH
Bicarbonate	Creatinine	PCO$_2$
Phosphorus	Liver function tests	

20. How is nitrogen balance estimated and utilized?

After a patient has had a stable intake for at least 2 days, a 24-hour urine can be analyzed for urine urea nitrogen (UUN). To calculate nitrogen balance, subtract the grams of the 24-hour UUN (plus about 4 gm for nonurea urine, skin, and fecal nitrogen losses) from the intake of N over 24 hours (grams of dietary protein divided by 6.25). This formula is only grossly accurate if the collection is complete, if glomerular filtration rate is > 50 ml/min, and if the patient does not have large nonurea N losses.

Although negative N-balance is undesirable, bed rest, high-dose corticosteroids, and poorly controlled disease may maintain the patient in negative N-balance despite generous quantities of calories and protein. Optimal efforts may only attenuate some of the losses. If balance remains unsatisfactory, check electrolyte, acid-base and blood glucose control. Increase protein delivery, if tolerated, and confirm energy requirements with a metabolic cart. Consider use of branched-chain amino acids. Initiate enteral feeding when possible. Once the patient's medical condition has stabilized and, if possible, some ambulation resumed, a positive 2–4 gm N-balance may be attainable. The goal of nutritional support is to avoid unnecessary harmful starvation, but at the same time, avoid potentially dangerous overfeeding that is immunosuppressive or benefits inflammatory or infectious processes more than the host.

21. What are the typical findings in deficiency or excess of various micronutrients?

Vitamin and Mineral Deficiencies and Toxicities

MICRONUTRIENT	DEFICIENCY	TOXICITY
Vitamin A	Follicular hyperkeratosis, night blindness, corneal drying, keratomalacia	Dermatitis, xerosis, hair loss, joint pain, hyperostosis, edema, hypercalcemia, hepatomegaly, pseudotumor
Vitamin D	Rickets, osteomalacia, hypophosphatemia, muscle weakness	Fatigue, headache, hypercalcemia, bone decalcification
Vitamin E	Hemolytic anemia, myopathy, ataxia, ophthalmoplegia, retinopathy, areflexia	Rare; possible interference with vitamin K, arachidonic acid metabolism; headache, myopathy
Vitamin K	Bruisability, prolonged prothrombin time	Rapid iv infusion: possible flushing, cardiovascular collapse
Vitamin C	**Scurvy:** poor wound healing, perifollicular hemorrhage, gingivitis, dental defects, anemia, joint pain	Diarrhea, poss hyperoxaluria, uricosuria, interf. with glucose, occult blood tests, dry mouth, dental erosion
Vitamin B1 (thiamine)	**Dry beriberi** (polyneuropathy): anorexia, low temperature **Wet beriberi** (high output CHF): lactic acidosis **Wernicke-Korsakoff:** ataxia, nystagmus, memory loss, confabulation, ophthalmoplegia	Large dose iv: anorexia, ataxia, ileus, headache, irritability
Vitamin B2 (riboflavin)	Seborrheic dermatitis, stomatitis, cheilosis, geographic tongue, burning eyes, anemia	None
Vitamin B3 (niacin)	Anorexia, lethargy, burning sensations, glossitis, headache, stupor, seizures **Pellagra:** diarrhea, pigmented dermatitis, dementia	Hyperglycemia, hyperuricemia, GI symptoms, peptic ulcer, flushing, liver dysfunction
Vitamin B6 (pyridoxine)	Peripheral neuritis, seborrhea, glossitis, stomatitis, anemia, CNS/EEG changes, seizures	Metabolic dependency, sensory neuropathy
Vitamin B12	Glossitis, paresthesias, CNS changes, megaloblastic anemia, depression, diarrhea	None
Folic acid	Glossitis, intestinal mucosal dysfunction, megaloblastic anemia	Antagonize antiepileptic drugs, decrease Zn absorption
Biotin	Scaly dermatitis, hair loss, papillae atrophy, myalgia, paresthesias, hypercholesterolemia	None
Pantothenic acid	Malaise, GI symptoms, cramps, paresthesias	Diarrhea
Calcium	Paresthesias, tetany, seizures, osteopenia, arrhythmia	Hypercalciuria, GI symptoms, lethargy

Table continued on following page.

Vitamin and Mineral Deficiencies and Toxicities (Continued)

MICRONUTRIENT	DEFICIENCY	TOXICITY
Phosphorous	Hemolysis, muscle weakness, ophthalmo-plegia, osteomalacia	Diarrhea
Magnesium	Paresthesias, tetany, seizures, arrhythmia	Diarrhea, muscle weakness, arrhythmia
Iron	Fatigue, dyspnea, glossitis, anemia, koilonychia	Iron overload (hepatic, cardiac), possible oxidation damage
Iodine	Goiter, hypothyroidism	Goiter, hypo/hyperthyroidism
Zinc	Lethargy, anorexia, loss of taste/smell, rash, hypogonadism, poor wound healing, immunosuppression	Impaired copper, iron metabolism, reduced HDL, immunosuppression
Copper	Anemia, neutropenia, lethargy, depigmen-tation, connective tissue weakness	GI symptoms, hepatic damage
Chromium	Glucose intolerance, neuropathy, hyperlipidemia	None
Selenium	Keshan's cardiomyopathy, muscle weakness	GI symptoms
Manganese	Possible weight loss, dermatitis, hair disturbances	Inhalation injury only
Molybdenum	Possible headache, vomiting, CNS changes	Interfere with copper metabolism, possible gout
Fluorine	Increased dental caries	Teeth mottling, possible bone integrity/fluorosis

22. What nutritional problems are encountered in patients with inflammatory bowel disease (IBD)? What are the therapeutic nutrition options?

Causes of malnutrition in IBD include anorexia, active inflammation, steroid use, bleeding, malabsorption, protein-losing enteropathy, surgical loss of bowel, infections, and fistulous losses. Besides protein loss, Crohn's patients may have difficulty with the absorption of fat and fat-soluble vitamins, vitamin B12, magnesium, zinc, and other trace nutrients. Diarrhea may lead to salt, water, and potassium depletion.

Caloric requirements for the noninfected patient with IBD may be 30–50% above BEE. Consider 1.5 gm/kg/day protein, perhaps up to 2 gm/kg in the patient on steroids or with significant losses of gut protein, fistulas, or bleeds.

Mild or quiescent IBD may be treated with a standard oral diet. Fat, lactose, or fiber restrictions may benefit selected patients. Patients with more active disease present the challenge of maintaining or restoring the nutritional state while alleviating the disease. Studies suggest that neither enteral nor parenteral nutrition are superior to medical therapy at inducing remission. Bowel rest removes gut stimulation and potential antigens; whether or not it achieves remission sooner remains unproven. Large-scale randomized trials to compare bowel rest/TPN with enteral use have not been accomplished, but existing data show no difference in short-term remission rates.

A reasonable approach may be to combine medical therapy with enteral usage; an elemental or semi-elemental formula might be tried if food or polymeric formulas are not tolerated. Bowel rest/TPN should be reserved for unresponsive cases or when gut use is contraindicated (obstruction, toxic megacolon, severe ileus, substantial GI bleed, or a high-output fistula).

23. What are the nutritional concerns and therapy for patients with short bowel syndrome?

Loss of bowel surface puts the patient at great risk for dehydration and malnutrition. The small bowel averages 600 cm in length and absorbs about 10 liters of ingested and secreted fluids a day.

An individual may tolerate substantial loss of small bowel, though preservation of < 2 ft with an intact colon and ileocecal valve, or < 5 ft in the absence of the colon and ileocecal valve, may make survival impossible by enteral use alone. In addition, the loss of the distal ileum precludes absorption of bile acids and vitamin B12. Remaining bowel, especially ileum, may adapt its absorptive ability over several years, but this may be hampered by underlying disease.

Therapy in the acute postsurgical phase is aimed at intravenous fluid and electrolyte restoration. Parenteral nutrition may be required while the remaining gut function is assessed and adaptation takes place. Attempts at oral feeding should include frequent, small meals with fluid and fat limitations initially. Osmolar sugars (e.g., sorbitol), lactose, and high-oxalate foods are best avoided. Antimotility drugs and attempts to reduce gastric acid secretion should be used if stool output remains high. Oral rehydration with glucose- and sodium-containing fluids (e.g., sports drinks) may help prevent dehydration. Pancreatic enzymes, bile-acid-binding resins (if bile acids are irritating the colon), and octreotide injections may play a role in selected cases. If oral diets are failing, the use of elemental feedings (via enteral tube) may enhance absorption and nutritional state. Studies looking at gut rehabilitation using growth hormone and glutamine, as well as intestinal or combined intestinal-liver transplantation, are available at selected centers.

24. What is the approach to nutritional support in patients with acute pancreatitis?
Pancreatitis can resemble other cases of stressed metabolism. If the disease process precludes the normal intake of food beyond 4–5 days, consideration should be given to nutrition support. The route of feeding remains controversial, and there are no randomized studies to clarify the issue. Bowel and pancreatic rest have not been shown conclusively to alter the clinical course, and parenteral nutrition added to bowel rest does not accelerate recovery beyond improvement of the nutritional state. Energy expenditure is variable but most likely only 20–30% above basal. The enteral route may be tried if GI dysfunction (e.g., ileus) does not exist. Distal delivery of a low-fat formula, preferably jejunal, should minimize pancreatic stimulation and might be tried if oral clear liquids and low-fat foods are not tolerated. Use PPN or TPN if the enteral approach fails. Experiments suggest that parenteral nutrition, including intravenous fat, elicits little significant pancreatic secretion. All pancreatitis patients should have triglyceride levels checked at the outset and during nutritional therapy to exclude severe hypertriglyceridemia.

25. What are the nutritional considerations in patients with advanced liver disease? What forms of protein should be given?
Because the liver is the "first pass" organ for nutrients delivered via the enteral route, both acute and chronic liver disease pose challenges to the nutritionist.

Protein intolerance is always of concern. Most amino acids, except for the branched-chain group (BCAA—leucine, isoleucine, valine), are metabolized at the liver. Excessive levels of the aromatic amino acids may gain access across the blood-brain barrier (they share a carrier with the BCAAs) and predispose to hepatic encephalopathy in the form of false neurotransmitters. Many patients with chronic liver disease show signs of malnutrition attributable to reduced intake. Also, in fulminant liver failure or post-transplantation state, adequate protein delivery is desired to facilitate regeneration or offset the higher turnover rates.

Thus, there exists the dilemma of adequate protein delivery without precipitating encephalopathy. Although enteral protein may be more encephalopathic than intravenously administered amino acids, the enteral route of feeding should still be used when possible. Current recommendations suggest starting with 0.8–1.0 gm/kg protein in oral diets or enteral formulas, monitoring tolerance. Vegetable protein produces encephalopathy less often than animal-derived protein. If tolerated, advance toward 1.5 g/kg in more catabolic patients. Only if encephalopathy ensues should either protein be restricted or a specialized hepatic formulation (high BCAA/low aromatics and methionine) used. Controlled trials using hepatic formulas have suggested improvement in mental status and outcome of encephalopathic patients. As in other diseases where amino acid delivery must be limited, adequate calories must be provided to minimize endogenous protein breakdown.

26. What are the roles for conditionally essential nutrients, antioxidants, and nutritional immunomodulation?

Glutamine has become the prototypical conditionally essential nutrient. Not needed from exogenous sources in healthy individuals and traditionally omitted from TPN solutions (instability), it remains a primary fuel for intestinal cells and the immune system. In stressed illness, it is redistributed and may be relatively deplete. Evidence of improved outcome has accumulated in several controlled trials where glutamine was provided with TPN.

Arginine, like glutamine, is a nonessential amino acid in healthy people. In larger doses, however, it may stimulate growth hormone secretion, the immune system, and wound healing. **Nucleotides,** present in food but absent from parenteral and traditional enteral preparations, play an important role in the immune response.

Modification of **dietary fat** remains an area of intense interest. The most commonly used polyunsaturates, the ω 6 vegetable oils (corn, safflower, sunflower), may prove deleterious in higher quantities. Although their major component, linoleic acid, is essential to humans at 2–3% of total calories, it serves as the precursor for arachidonic acid and prostaglandins and leukotrienes that, at higher levels, are immunosuppressive and proinflammatory. Fats of the ω-3 variety (linolenic acid or eicosapentenoic and decosahexanoic acid, the "fish oils") competitively inhibit the formation of the arachidonic acid-derived eicosanoids and may improve immune parameters and outcome. Adverse effects of ω-3 fats may be impairment of wound strength, glucose tolerance, and formation of ω-3 lipid oxidation products.

Medium-chain triglycerides are used due to ease of transport and oxidation, with less tendency to immunosuppression and hyperlipidemia. Structured intravenous lipids, using combinations of long, medium, and short-chain fats, are under investigation.

Enteral use of **viscous dietary fiber** may be an important source of nutrition to colonocytes and perhaps other organs. Bacterial fermentation of soluble fiber to short-chain fatty acids can meet 5–10% of daily energy needs.

There is growing recognition of the role that **oxidative damage** plays in aging, critical illness, tumorigenesis, and vascular disease. Nutrients act as both pro-oxidants (metals such as iron and copper) and antioxidants (vitamins A, C, and E, β-carotene, selenium) in a finely balanced system. Epidemiology suggests that those with lower iron stores and higher antioxidant intake and blood levels suffer less from cancer and cardiovascular disease. Thus far, controlled trials using pharmacologic doses of a number of antioxidants have failed to reduce disease occurrence as hoped. Large-scale trials are still underway, but at present, intake of antioxidant-containing *foods* may prove more beneficial than large doses of isolated antioxidants. As in other metabolic manipulations, we must find the right balance between benefit and harm to the host.

27. What guidelines help in deciding whether or not to use nutritional support in a terminal patient?

Recent court rulings and consensus opinions have treated nutritional support as a form of medical therapy, rather than an unquestionable necessity for all patients. Decisions on when to consider nutritional support and in what form should still be based on sound medical and nutrition principles. What is more difficult to determine is how much improvement in quantity or quality of life is gained from adequate nutrition, and how much suffering is or is not incurred from relative starvation. Remember that forced feeding itself can be life-threatening. Each patient should be evaluated as an individual, and the principles of patient autonomy, beneficence, and integrity should be respected.

BIBLIOGRAPHY

1. ASPEN Board of Directors: Guidelines for the use of parenteral and enteral nutrition in adult and pediatric patients. JPEN 17(4 suppl):1SA–52SA, 1993.
2. Church J, Hill G: Assessing the efficacy of intravenous nutrition in general surgery patients. JPEN 11:135–139, 1987.

3. Daly J, Weintraub F, Shou J, et al: Enteral nutrition during multimodality therapy in upper gastrointestinal cancer patients. Ann Surg 221:327–338, 1995.
4. Detsky A, McGlaughlin J, Baker J, et al: What is subjective global assessment of nutritional status? JPEN 11:8–13, 1987.
5. Grimble R: Nutritional antioxidants and the modulation of inflammation: Theory and practice. N Horiz 2(2):175–185, 1994.
6. Hill G: Body composition research: Implications for the practice of clinical nutrition. JPEN 16:197–218, 1992.
7. Hunter D, Jaksic T, Lewis D, et al: Resting energy expenditure in the critically ill: Estimation vs. measurement. Br J Surg 75:875–878, 1988.
8. McClave S, Snider H: Use of indirect calorimetry in clinical nutrition. Nutr Clin Pract 7:207–221, 1992.
9. Moore F, Feliciano D, Andrassy R, et al: Early enteral feeding compared with parenteral reduces postoperative septic complications: Results of meta-analysis. Ann Surg 216:172–183, 1992.
10. Naylor C, O'Rourke K, Detsky A, Baker J: Parenteral nutrition with branched chain amino acids in hepatic encephalopathy: A meta-analysis. Gastroenterology 97:1033–1042, 1989.
11. Pomposelli J, Bistrian B: Is total parenteral nutrition immunosuppressive? N Horiz 2:224–229, 1994.
12. Rombeau J, Caldwell M (eds): Clinical Nutrition: Enteral and Tube Feeding, 2nd ed. Philadelphia, W.B. Saunders, 1990.
13. Rombeau J, Caldwell M (eds):Parenteral Nutrition, 2nd ed. Philadelphia, W.B. Saunders, 1993.
14. Schlictig S, Ayres S: Nutrition Support of the Critically Ill. Chicago, Year Book Medical Publ, 1988.
15. Sitrin M: Nutrition support in inflammatory bowel disease. Nutr Clin Pract 7:53–60, 1992.
16. Solomon S, Kirby D: The refeeding syndrome: A review. JPEN 14:90–97, 1990.
17. VA TPN Cooperative Study Group: Perioperative total parenteral nutrition in surgical patients. N Engl J Med 325:525–532, 1991.
18. Wilmore D: Catabolic illness: Strategies for enhancing recovery. N Engl J Med 325:695–702, 1991.
19. Zaloga G: Physiology and effects of peptide enteral formulas. Nutr Clin Pract 5:231–237, 1990.

61. MALABSORPTION AND MALDIGESTION

John S. Goff, M.D.

1. Compare and contrast sugar (starch), fat, and protein absorption.
Starches are broken down by amylase from the salivary glands and pancreas into glucose molecules and limit dextrins. Disaccharides (sucrose, lactose, etc) and limit dextrins are split into simple sugars by intestinal brush-border disaccharidases and then are absorbed. **Protein** is denatured in the stomach by acid, and its initial breakdown is started by pepsins. Proteolysis is completed in the intestine by pancreatic proteases (e.g., trypsin, chymotrypsin, carboxypeptidase) and intestinal brush-border peptidases. Dietary **fat** is generally in the form of triglycerides, which are broken down by pancreatic lipase in the presence of colipase and bile salts into two free fatty acids and one monoglyceride. These are absorbed and then reassembled in the intestinal cells before being transported in the form of chylomicrons. Lingual and gastric lipase contribute modestly to lipid digestion.

2. Are there any specific sites in the bowel that are devoted to certain absorptive functions?
Yes. Iron tends to be absorbed mostly in the proximal duodenum, whereas vitamin B12 and bile salts are exclusively absorbed in the ileum.

3. What clinical signs and symptoms should raise your suspicions about malabsorption?
The classic symptoms of malabsorption include weight loss and diarrhea, with the patient often seeing oil in the toilet or having trouble clearing the toilet of adherent stools. However, patients may have quite variable degrees of diarrhea, and weight loss is often a later manifestation. More subtle hints are related to vitamin deficiencies that accompany malabsorption or maldigestion: transverse nail ridging, easy bruising or bleeding, follicular hyperkeratosis, night blindness, cheilosis, glossitis, decreased taste or smell, bleeding gums, dementia, peripheral neuropathy, loss of position or vibratory sense, tetany, bone pain, amenorrhea, parotid enlargement, edema, and poor wound healing. Gas and bloating are also common symptoms in patients with various types of malabsorption but are nonspecific symptoms. Similarly, fatigue is not very helpful by itself as a predictor of malabsorption.

4. What biochemical findings are suggestive of malabsorption?
Various findings on routine blood tests that might suggest malabsorption is present to some degree include abnormal mean cell volume, anemia, prolonged prothrombin time, elevated alkaline phosphatase, hypokalemia, hypocalcemia, hypomagnesemia, hypophosphatemia, hypoalbuminemia, hypotriglyceridemia, and hypocholesterolemia. Unfortunately, many of these findings can be caused by other conditions besides malabsorption or are not seen in the early stages of a malabsorption disorder. More specific and potentially more sensitive blood tests include folate, vitamin B12, iron, carotene, immunoglobulin levels, or other specific vitamin levels.

5. Does radiography have a role in a malabsorption evaluation?
Radiography has a limited, but often a helpful, role in detecting or defining some of the potential causes of malabsorption. A simple **abdominal film** may show pancreatic calcification, suggesting chronic pancreatitis or Looser's zones in the pubic and ischial rami consistent with a diagnosis of osteomalacia. **Barium studies** of the upper GI tract may show clumping or flocculation of the barium as a general indication of increased fluid in the small bowel consistent with malabsorption, but this finding is less frequent with newer formulations of barium that do not break up as easily. Though the traditional small bowel follow-through (SBFT) can show abnormal folds which may suggest a source of malabsorption, the small bowel **enteroclysis** or **enema** is much

more likely to detect subtle mucosal abnormalities. Normally, there are two to four folds per inch, and these are no more than 2 mm wide. Small (2–3 mm) nodules in the mucosa suggest either intestinal lymphangiectasia or Whipple's disease. Besides making an assessment of the small bowel fold pattern, a small bowel enema can identify anatomic abnormalities that can result in bacterial overgrowth, such as diverticula, blind loops, and stasis. A small bowel study can also provide valuable information about Crohn's disease. A **CT scan** can be important in identifying thickened loops of small bowel and extension of the process into the mesentery or retroperitoneum.

6. How is small bowel biopsy used in the evaluation of malabsorption?

Currently, the easiest and most reliable way to obtain small bowel mucosal biopsies of good quality is with a therapeutic endoscope and jumbo biopsy forceps. The tissue obtained can be analyzed for brush-border enzyme levels (lactase, sucrase-isomaltase, trehalase) and examined microscopically. The limitations of small bowel biopsy are that not all disorders have a characteristic biopsy appearance and many conditions have a patchy distribution. Conditions with a diffuse lesion and diagostic histologic appearance include Whipple's disease, agammaglobulinemia, and abetalipoproteinemia. Disorders with an abnormal mucosa but a nondiagnostic histologic appearance include celiac disease, tropical sprue, and bacterial overgrowth. Lymphoma, eosinophilic gastroenteritis, mastocytosis, lymphangiectasia, amyloidosis, and Crohn's disease have diagnostic histologic findings but have a patchy distribution that may be missed on biopsy. Small bowel mucosa can have flatted villi from severe protein-calorie malnutrition; this finding could be misinterpreted as the cause of the nutrition problem and will make correction of the problem by enteral feeding more difficult because of malabsorption. Small bowel biopsies are indicated if there are abnormal radiographic findings or test abnormalities consistent with a mucosal disorder.

7. Why do patients with lactase deficiency develop gastrointestinal symptoms?

A lack of lactase in the mucosal brush-border results in no breakdown (hydrolysis) of lactose into its components, glucose and galactose, which unlike lactose can be absorbed by the small bowel mucosa. Thus, the lactose passes into the colon, where bacteria ferment it to produce fatty acids, methane, hydrogen, and carbon dioxide. These compounds produce the symptoms of lactose maldigestion, such as borborygmus, bloating, flatulence, abdominal discomfort, and diarrhea.

8. What other sugars or starches cause problems because of maldigestion or malabsorption in the proximal GI tract?

Sucrose is composed of fructose and glucose. A rare condition involving a congenital absence of sucrase results in problems similar to lactase deficiency.

Fructose absorption is facilitated when it occurs in conjunction with glucose absorption from the hydrolysis of sucrose, but when fructose is presented as a monosaccharide to the small bowel brush-border, its absorption is much slower. Consequently, consumption of large amounts of foods with high fructose content (pears, figs, prunes, grapes, soft drinks) can result in symptoms from fermentation of the nonabsorbed fructose in the colon.

Sorbitol, which is found in fruits (pears, prunes) and is used to give a sweet taste to "sugarless" products, may also produce symptoms from its fermentation in the colon.

Stachyose and **raffinose** are indigestible oligosaccharides found in beans. Malabsorption of a portion of the starch contained in wheat and other grains, due to interaction with fiber or the protein in the grain, may account for symptoms of gas, bloating, and diarrhea with ingestion of these foods. The clinical significance of these types of malabsorption disorders is that they can be confused with irritable bowel syndrome.

9. In what clinical setting should one suspect a protein-losing enteropathy? How would it be diagnosed?

Excess protein loss from the GI tract occurs in many conditions, but the two major reasons are intestinal lymphatic obstruction and breakdown of the enterocyte barrier. Conditions that can cause a protein-losing enteropathy include congenital lymphangiectasia, lymphoma, sarcoidosis, tuberculosis, right heart failure or constrictive pericarditis, Whipple's disease, Crohn's disease, Menetrier's disease, eosinophilic gastroenteritis, lupus, sprue, and some parasitic diseases. Patients with this condition are usually hypoalbuminemic with edema and possibly even ascites. Other serum proteins, such as fibrinogen, α_1-antitrypsin, and gamma globulins can also be low.

Protein-losing enteropathy was diagnosed previously by measuring the amount of radioactivity in the stool after injecting a patient with albumin radiolabeled with ^{51}Cr or [125]I. Currently, it is diagnosed by measuring the clearance of α_1-antitrypsin into the stool. A 24-hour stool specimen and a blood sample are collected with measurement of α_1-antitrypsin levels in both specimens. Clearance should be <13 ml/day (concentration in stool $\times$ 24-hr stool volume/serum concentration).

10. How can the Schilling test be used to diagnose the causes of malabsorption?

If a standard Schilling test is abnormal, then:

1. The patient lacks intrinsic factor from the stomach which is necessary for B12 (cobalamin) absorption in the ileum (pernicious anema).
2. The patient has insufficient pancreatic enzymes to digest the ingested B12 from R-protein which binds to it in the stomach. R-protein prevents B12 absorption, and if it is not removed from the B12, the B12 cannot bind to intrinsic factor, which facilitates its absorption in the ileum.
3. The patient has too many bacteria in the proximal small bowel which bind to and use the B12 for themselves.
4. The patient has ileal disease which prevents proper absorption of B12.

The Schilling test can be conducted in various ways to determine which disorder is present. One of the easiest is to repeat the test with either intrinsic factor, pancreatic enzymes, or after a course of antibiotics. Dual-labeled Schilling tests are available to help clarify the cause of the B12 malabsorption.

11. How is the D-xylose test used to diagnose the causes of malabsorption?

The standard D-xylose test is used to determine if a patient has a defect in the mucosal absorptive surface of the small bowel. D-Xylose is absorbed like any other monosaccharide across the brush-border of the intestinal cells, but it is not fully metabolized, and thus, a large portion is excreted into the urine. After a patient ingests 5 or 25 gm of D-xylose, the serum level is measured in 1 hour or the patient's urine is collected and analyzed for D-xylose. Low levels of D-xylose in the serum or urine imply damage to the small bowel mucosa which is preventing normal absorption. However, bacteria in the proximal small bowel compete with the intestinal cells for the D-xylose, and patients with renal dysfunction clear it into the urine more slowly than normal, which can cause problems with interpreting the results.

12. Name the four breath tests used in the evaluation of malabsorption. What do they detect?

The **triolein breath test** is used to detect fat malabsorption due to most any etiology. Patients ingest ^{14}C-triolein, and their breath is collected. If they absorb the triglyceride properly, they produce [14]CO_2 in their breath because of metabolism of the labeled glycerol.

The **[14]C-D-xylose** test can be used to detect small bowel bacterial overgrowth. Because D-xylose is metabolized in the small bowel lumen by excess bacteria, patients excrete excess [14]CO_2 in their breath if overgrowth is present.

The **bile acid breath test** also is used to detect small bowel bacterial overgrowth. The patient ingests ^{14}C-glycocholic acid and then collects breath samples. Early excessive production of [14]CO_2 indicates small bowel bacterial overgrowth because the bacteria deconjugate the ^{14}C-glycine from the cholic acid, resulting in the glycine being absorbed and metabolized to [14]CO_2. A late rise in breath [14]CO_2 indicates rapid transit into the colon or ileal disease. Generally, in the first 5 hours after ingestion of ^{14}C-glycocholic acid <5% reaches the colon and is deconjugated by the bacteria there.

The **hydrogen breath test** uses various sugars (glucose, lactose, lactulose) to study events in the small bowel. After the patient ingests the sugar, breath samples are collected for analysis of H_2 content. Use of a sugar like lactulose is useful for mearsuring small bowel transit time because it cannot be absorbed in the small bowel; the sugar enters the colon, where it is metabolized by bacteria into H_2 which is absorbed and excreted in the breath. Thus, timing the first appearance of excess H_2 in the breath coincides with the small bowel transit time. If one uses lactose, there should be no rise in breath H_2 because all the lactose will be absorbed; however, if the patient is lactase-deficient, it will not all be absorbed, resulting in some lactose entering the colon where it is metabolized to H_2. If the patient has small bowel bacterial overgrowth, ingestion of any sugar will result in an early increase in breath H_2, due to the metabolism of the sugar into H_2 by the bacteria, with its subsequent absorption and excretion into the breath.

13. Can any other test be used to diagnose small bowel bacterial overgrowth?
The gold standard test for detecting small bowel bacterial overgrowth is to culture a small bowel specimen and quantitate the number of bacteria present. This test has some logistic problems, since one must obtain a sample that is not contaminated despite passing through the mouth and stomach with the collection devise. Greater than 10^5 bacterial-forming units/ml in the proximal small intestinal fluid is considered excessive.

14. What is the Chymex test, and what is it used for?
The Chymex test uses N-benzoyl-L-tyrosyl-p-aminobenzoic acid (bentiromide) to detect pancreatic insufficiency. The bond between the N-benzoyl-L-tyrosyl and the p-aminobenzoic acid (PABA) is chymotrypsin-sensitive. As a complete molecule, the bentiromide cannot be absorbed, but if it is split by chymotrypsin from the pancreas, the PABA will be absorbed and excreted unchanged into the urine. Excretion of >50% of the ingested amount of PABA within 6 hours in a patient with normal renal function indicates normal pancreatic function. The patient must not use acetaminophen, thiazides, sulfonamides, procainamide, chloramphenicol, lidocaine, benzocaine, phenacetin, or sun screens containing PABA for 3 days before the test because these interfere with the PABA assay.

15. Which test is considered the gold standard for assessing pancreatic function in malabsorption?
The secretin test. In an intubated patient, fluid is collected from the duodenum after stimulation of the pancreas with intravenous secretin alone or with secretin and cholecystokinin. The aspirated fluid is analyzed for volume, bicarbonate level, and enzyme levels. If done properly with good tube positioning, gastric aspiration, duodenal and/or gastric perfusion markers, and careful handling and analysis of the aspirated fluid, the secretin test is an excellent way to quantitate pancreatic exocrine function precisely. This method can detect subtle pancreatic dysfunction that is not detectable with any other (indirect) measure of pancreatic function.

16. What can you do with 3-day-old stool?
Collection of stools for 72 hours is the traditional test for detecting malabsorption, particularly fat malabsorption, but it does not define the cause. The test needs to be conducted during a time when the patient is ingesting about 100 gm of fat per day. Preferably, the patient should be on such a diet for a few days before starting the collection, to increase the test's accuracy. Noncompliance is one of the test's major drawbacks. Normal digestion results in <7 gm/day of fat in the stool when the patient is on a diet of 100 gm of fat per day.

17. Do any drugs play a role in malabsorption, and how do they cause it?
Many drugs interfere with absorption, though many only cause specific malabsorption for certain other drugs or substances. **Neomycin** causes reversible inhibition of disaccharidase activity, damages the mucosa of the small bowel, and adversely affects the luminal phase of fat absorption by interfering with micelle formation. **Colchicine** causes cells to arrest in metaphase and thus dam-

ages the normally rapidly dividing cells of the small bowel mucosa. **Cholestyramine** and **colestipol** bind with bile acids. Patients taking these agents have increaed fat malabsorption and may have greatly increased fat malabsorption if they have had a partial resection of the terminal ileum (these agents will deplete the bile acid pool in these patients). Fat-soluble vitamins are poorly absorbed, and osteomalacia has been documented in patients on long-term cholestyramine therapy without vitamin D and calcium supplementation. Large amounts of **aluminum-containing antacids** cause phosphate malabsorption, which can be severe enough to cause metabolic bone disease (osteomalacia) and renal dysfunction. Chronic excessive **laxative use or abuse** can result in a variety of malabsorption problems.

18. What parasitic infections can produce malabsorption problems?

Giardia lamblia colonize the upper small intestine and produce various problems with absorption. They compete with the small bowel mucosa for nutrients, they can deconjugate bile salts and thus interfere with fat absorption, and they can cause mucosal damage, especially in patients with immune deficiencies. Patients with IgA deficiency are particularly prone to have severe symptoms when infected with *Giardia* and have a difficult time eliminating these organism even with appropriate treatment.

Coccidia are intracytoplasmic parasites that can produce significant malabsorption and profound diarrhea in immunocompetent and immunodeficient patients. The usual human pathogen is *Isospora belli*. It can be difficult to diagnose with stool specimens alone, because the oocysts are rare. Small bowel biopsy may be necessary to identify this organism.

Parasitic worms have long been known to produce malabsorption problems. *Diphyllobothrium latum*, a tapeworm commonly acquired from raw fish, causes vitamin B12 deficiency. Large infestations with the nematode *Strongyloides stercoralis*, which are particularly common in immunocompromised patients, can produce steatorrhea and a protein-losing enteropathy. *Capillaria philippinensis* is a rare nematode found in the Philippines that causes significant malabsorption and protein loss, though the exact mechanism is unclear.

19. Do any viruses cause malabsorption problems?

The human immunodeficiency virus (HIV) has been implicated as a cause of malabsorption when it produces an enteropathic syndrome characterized by voluminous diarrhea and steatorrhea.

20. Excesses of which hormones cause steatorrhea, and how do they do it?

Gastrinomas (Zollinger-Ellison syndrome) secrete **gastrin** and thus greatly increase the volume of acid produced by the stomach. Though the usual presentation is peptic ulcer disease, 10% of gastrinomas present with diarrhea, and most of these patients have some degree of steatorrhea. In these patients, the excess acid from the stomach leads to irreversible denaturing of lipase in the duodenum and overwhelms the ability of duodenal and pancreatic bicarbonate to neutralize it.

Somatostatinomas produce excess amounts of **somatostatin,** which can produce steatorrhea by inhibiting pancreatic secretion of digestive enzymes.

21. What is short bowel syndrome?

Short bowel syndrome occurs when the patient has lost enough of the small intestine to result in a decreased absorptive surface, with resultant nutritional problems and other side effects. Though not short bowel in the strictest sense, resection of >100 cm of terminal ileum without loss of any more proximal bowel can produce many of the problems seen in the classic short bowel syndrome because of the inability to absorb bile salts or vitamin B12 after loss of so much ileum.

In the acute phase after loss of a large amount of small bowel, the patient often has hypergastrinemia and thus increased acid production with the potential for significant problems with ulceration. As time goes on, this problem lessens and the patient may have some adaptive hypertrophy of the small bowel, with improvement in absorption. Complications of short bowel syndrome include hyperoxaluria with development of calcium oxalate renal stones, excess water and electrolyte losses, vitamin and mineral deficiencies, bacterial overgrowth from changes in small bowel motility, gallstone development from bile salt malabsorption, metabolic bone disease, and fatty liver.

22. Describe the best way to evaluate patients with suspected malabsorption.

Historical features and physical findings may immediately point to a specific potential cause of malabsorption, but when evaluating these patients, it is prudent to organize the evaluation so that the fewest tests can be done to arrive at the correct diagnosis. The algorithm on the opposite page attempts to approach the problem of malabsorption logically. It is meant as a guide since each patient may have unique features or findings that can result in appropriate deviation from the outlined pathways.

23. Are there special treatment considerations based on the final diagnosis? What are they?

Specific Treatments for Malabsorption Disorders

DIAGNOSIS	TREATMENT
Celiac sprue	Gluten-free diet
Tropical sprue	Folate, B12, tetracycline
Collagenous sprue	Steroids
Whipple's disease	Penicillin G, streptomycin, TMP/SMX
Lactase deficiency	Lactase supplementation
Other disaccharidase deficiencies	Dietary restriction
Bacterial overgrowth	Rotating antibiotics
Abetalipoproteinemia	Low-fat diet and fat-soluble vitamin supplementation
Lymphangiectasia	Correct causative disease
Crohn's disease	Steroids, 5-aminosalicylates
Eosinophilic enteritis	Steroids, cromolyn
Amyloidosis	Correct underlying process
Pancreatic insufficiency	Pancreatic enzymes
Short bowel syndrome	Medium-chain triglycerides, low-oxalate diet, TPN
Giardia	Metronidazole, quinacrine
Isospora belli	TMP/SMX
Diphyllobothrium latum	Praziquantel
Strongyloides stercoralis	Thiabendazole

TMP/SMX = trimethoprim/sulfamethoxazole; TPN = total parenteral nutrition.

BIBLIOGRAPHY

1. Brasitus TA: Parasites and malabsorption. Am J Med 67:1058–1065, 1979.
2. Brugge WR, Goff JS, Allen NC, et al: Development of a dual-label Schilling test for pancreatic exocrine function based on the differential absorption of cobalamin bound to intrinsic factor and R-protein. Gastroenterology 78:937–942, 1980.
3. Goff JS: A two-stage triolein breath test differentiates pancreatic insufficiency from other causes of malabsorption. Gastroenterology 83:44–48, 1982.
4. Longstreth GF, Newcomer AD: Drug-induced malabsorption. Mayo Clin Proc 50:284–293, 1975.
5. Mee AS, Burke M, Vallon AG, et al: Small bowel biopsy for malabsorption: Comparison of the diagnostic adequacy of endoscopic forceps and capsule biopsy specimens. BMJ 291:769–772, 1985.
6. Perrault J, Markowitz H: Protein-losing gastroenteropathy and the intestinal clearance of serum α_1-antitrypsin. Mayo Clin Proc 59:278–279, 1984.
7. Riby JE, Fujisawa T, Kretchner N: Fructose absorption. Am J Clin Nutr 58(suppl):748S–753S, 1993.
8. Rubesin SE, Rubin RA, Herlinger H: Small bowel malabsorption: Clinical and radiologic perspectives. Radiology 184:297–305, 1992.
9. Rumessen JJ, Gudmand-Hoyer E, Bachman E, Justesen T: Diagnosis of bacterial overgrowth of the small intestine: Comparison of the ^{14}C-D-xylose breath test and jejunal cultures in 60 patients. Scand J Gastroenterol 20:1267–1275, 1985.
10. Sakura H, Miura S, Morishita T, et al: Endoscopic and histopathological study on primary and secondary intestinal lymphangiectasia. Dig Dis Sci 26:312–320, 1981.
11. Tanner AR, Robinson DP: Pancreatic function testing: Serum PABA measurement is a reliable and accurate measure of exocrine function. Gut 29:1736–1740, 1988.

MALABSORPTION ALGORITHM

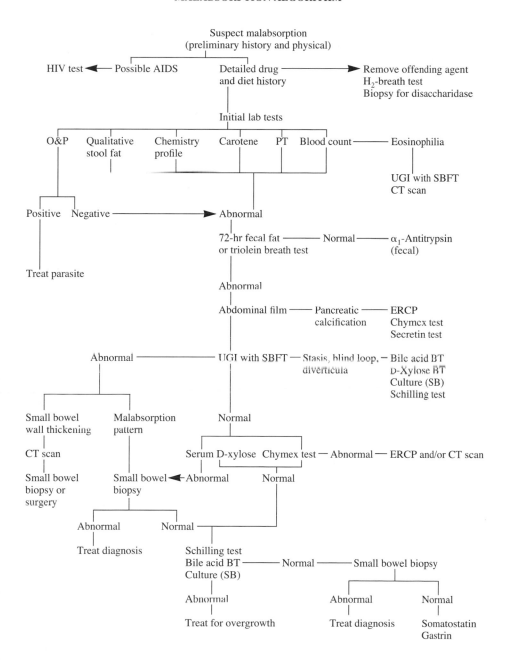

Algorithm of the evaluation of suspected malabsorption. (SBFT = small bowel follow-through; ERCP = endoscopic retrograde cholangiopancreatography; BT = breath test; O&P = ova and parasites exam; SB = small bowel.)

62. GI POTPOURRI: NAUSEA AND VOMITING, HICCUPS, BULIMIA/ANOREXIA, RUMINATION

Steven S. Shay, M.D.

NAUSEA AND VOMITING

1. How is vomiting distinguished from regurgitation? What disorders characteristically present with regurgitation?

Vomiting is characterized by the presence of nausea and autonomic symptoms, such as salivation, followed by the forceful abdominal and thoracic muscle contractions associated with retching. In contrast, **regurgitation** is the sudden, effortless return of small volumes of gastric or esophageal contents into the pharynx and implies cricopharyngeal relaxation or insufficiency.

Chronic regurgitation may result from oropharyngeal or esophageal disorders or gastroesophageal reflux. Zenker's diverticulum can accumulate secretions and food and may empty into the pharynx, especially at night. Structural lesions, such as esophageal cancer, may obstruct the esophagus. Esophageal diverticula may accumulate food particles and secretions and result in regurgitation when the contents are discharged into the esophageal lumen. Esophageal motility disorders, such as achalasia and primary esophageal spasm, may also be responsible for regurgitation.

2. What are the reflex pathways involved in the act of vomiting?

The **vomiting center,** located in the medulla, is comprised of many efferent nuclei in serial communication with each other. When the entire circuit is activated by afferent stimuli, the complete act of vomiting occurs. However, some stimuli trigger only individual components of the vomiting act and result in nausea or salivation.

Three afferent limbs carry stimuli to the vomiting center: (1) vagal and sympathetic afferents from the GI tract, vestibular system, and heart; (2) the chemoreceptor trigger zone (CTZ) in the area postrema of the floor of the fourth ventricle, which can be stimulated by emetogenic toxins or drugs, such as digitalis and chemotherapeutic agents; and (3) loci high in the central nervous system (CNS).

3. What disorders must be considered in acute nausea and vomiting?

Disorders Commonly Associated with Acute Nausea and Vomiting

Intra-abdominal disorders	Metabolic disorders
Gastrointestinal	Renal failure
Mechanical obstruction	Ketoacidosis (e.g., diabetes)
Stomach	Addison's diseae
Small bowel	
Pseudo-obstruction	
Peritonitis	CNS disorders
Acute pancreatitis	
Acute cholecystitis	Vestibular disorders
Infections or toxins	Pregnancy
Infection	
Epidemic: Norwalk agent, etc.	Drugs
Viral hepatitis	Narcotics
Toxin	Digitalis
Staphylococcus aureus	
Bacillus cereus	Aminophylline
Clostridium perfringens	Chemotherapeutic drugs

4. Should any specific associated symptoms or characteristics of vomiting be sought to narrow the differential? How do you confirm the etiology of nausea and vomiting?

The presence of **abdominal pain** strongly suggests an intra-abdominal process as the cause of acute nausea and vomiting, and the character of the pain, physical findings, and initial routine diagnostic laboratory tests (amylase, liver tests, complete blood count) will direct the subsequent diagnostic evaluation. Suspicion for peritonitis requires recumbent and upright abdominal x-rays, including the diaphragm, to exclude the presence of free air under the diaphragm. In contrast, the abdominal x-ray in the presence of colicky pain may confirm the presence of obstruction (mechanical or pseudo-obstruction). Suspicion of biliary colic or acute cholecystitis requires ultrasound and/or HIDA scan, whereas pancreatitis is typically first suspected because of an increased amylase.

The presence of **systemic symptoms** such as fever or diarrhea suggests the possibility of food poisoning with one of several toxins or an infection. Other systemic symptoms, such as polyuria and polydipsia, suggest a metabolic disorder, and a chemistry screen should be obtained to exclude these disorders.

The presence of **abnormal mental status,** headache, meningismus, or a preceding head injury suggests the possibilty of a CNS etiology and should be appropriately investigated. A history of vertigo or the presence of nystagmus suggests a motion disorder rather than CNS disease.

If there are no systemic symptoms, abdominal complaints, or CNS symptoms or signs, several other considerations should be entertained. The possibility of **pregnancy** should be considered early in any evaluation of nausea and vomiting, and serum and/or urine human chorionic gonadotropin obtained, as one wants to avoid tests utilizing radiation. Finally, all medications should be reviewed to exclude the possibility of **drug-associated** nausea and vomiting.

5. What are the major etiologic considerations for chronic vomiting? How are they evaluated?

Disorders that typically present with chronic nausea and vomiting are (1) functional gastric outlet obstruction (gastroparesis), (2) small bowel dysmotility, and (3) psychogenic vomiting. One historical clue is that all these disorders typically present with repeated postprandial vomiting.

Gastroparesis is defined as an impairment in gastric emptying in the absence of mechanical obstruction in the stomach or small bowel. This may be seen with certain drugs (e.g., narcotics), after gastrectomy, in patients with diabetes, scleroderma, or amyloidosis, or for no apparent reason (idiopathic). It is often difficult to distinguish idiopathic gastroparesis from psychogenic vomiting. Radionuclide solid-food gastric emptying, most commonly using a radiolabeled fried-egg sandwich, is the most helpful test in making the diagnosis.

Intestinal pseudo-obstruction, as the name suggests, requires that no obstruction be present by appropriate diagnostic tests, especially small bowel follow-through, performed during recovery from an episode. Other signs, such as abdominal distention, pain, changes in bowel habits, orthostatic hypotension, or bladder symptoms, may be present. Intestinal pseudo-obstruction may be seen with certain medications or systemic disorders, most commonly scleroderma, diabetes, and amyloidosis. These systemic disorders, as well as jejunal diverticulosis, must be specifically excluded with appropriate diagnostic studies. When these diagnoses have been excluded, primary small bowel myopathy or neuropathy may be present. Esophageal motility may suggest the diagnosis when aperistalsis is found. If these disorders are suspected and esophageal motility is normal, consideration of small bowel motility and/or small bowel biopsy at laparotomy will need to be made on an individual basis. This is best done in a referral center with expertise in these disorders.

Psychogenic vomiting is a cause of recurring vomiting, especially in young women, with an underlying emotional disturbance. However, it is occasionally a manifestation of major depression or a conversion reaction. Though a diagnosis of exclusion, certain characteristics suggest the diagnosis, including vomiting that has been present for a long time, especially during emotional strain. Moreover, vomiting is typically seen after the meal rather than delayed, and it can be suppressed if necessary. Finally, the vomiting may be of surprisingly little concern to the patient and of more concern to family members. Abdominal pain may be a major associated symptom. The diagnosis needs to be considered so that extensive diagnostic procedures or abdominal surgery be avoided, which could worsen and complicate the issue.

6. Can consequences of vomiting be anticipated and treated?

One needs to be vigilant for metabolic derangements. Because of the loss of hydrogen ions in the vomitus and contraction of the extracellular fluid volume, **alkalosis** commonly develops. Secondly, **potassium deficiency** is common due to the loss of potassium in the vomitus and wasting from the kidneys. Therefore, the clinical features of potassium deficiency, including muscle weakness, nocturia, and cardiac arrhythmias, may be present.

Another major consequence of vomiting is an **emetogenic injury.** With protracted or forceful vomiting, a Mallory-Weiss laceration or, rarely, Boerhaave's syndrome (transmural tear of the esophagus) may occur. These complications need to be considered in the patient with vomiting who develops a subsequent GI bleed, odynophagia, or catastrophic chest pain.

7. How do you treat the patient with nausea and vomiting? What medications are available?

In patients with severe acute nausea and vomiting, the metabolic derangements need to be sought as well as signs of dehydration. If present, these will usually require hospitalization, where initial therapy will be no intake by mouth and usually a nasogastric tube.

The best therapy for nausea and vomiting is prompt diagnosis and treatment of the primary disorder. However, specific treatment of the nausea and vomiting is often required to control symptoms.

Drugs Available to Treat Neausea and Vomiting

Antihistamines (H$_1$ antagonist)	Trimethobenzamide (Tigan)
Dimenhydrinate (Dramamine)	
Promethazine (Phenergan)	Dopaminergic antagonists
Meclizine (Antivert)	Metoclopramide (Reglan)
Cyclizine (Marezine)	Domperidone
Anticholinergic	Cisapride (Propulsid)
Scopolamine	
	Erythromycin
Phenothiazines	
Prochlorperazine (Compazine)	Serotonin receptor antagonists
Chlorpromazine (Thorazine)	Ondansetron (Zofran)
Butyrophenone	
Haloperidol (Haldol)	

The antihistamines (H$_1$ antagonist) and anticholinergics (scopolamine) are primarily used for patients with nausea and vomiting secondary to vestibular disorders or motion sickness. The anticholinergics commonly cause dry mouth as a side effect. The phenothiazines, haloperidol, and trimethobenzamide all act primarily via the chemoreceptor trigger zone, although there is also some information that they decrease input via visceral afferents. A common side effect of these drugs is sedation. Rare but serious side effects include blood dyscrasias, jaundice, and extrapyramidal signs.

8. When are the prokinetic agents, erythromycin, and serotonin antagonists used in patients with nausea and vomiting?

Metoclopramide has a central dopamine antagonist effect; however, the peripheral dopamine antagonist effect is responsible for the prokinetic activity. It has been used in gastroparesis and, in much larger doses, for prophylaxis against chemotherapy-associated nausea and vomiting. Common side effects include anxiety, lethargy, and increased prolactin levels. Rare side effects include depression and dystonia, particularly in older patients. **Domperidone** has a prokinetic effect, but because it does not readily cross the blood-brain barrier, it has less CNS effect. Side effects are uncommon. Domperidone is not yet available in the United States.

Cisapride works by direct stimulation of the cholingeric nerves, rather than an anti-dopaminergic effect. It is effective in gastroparesis and has a variable effect in pseudo-obstruction syndromes. **Erythromycin** interacts with motilin receptors on GI smooth muscle membranes in an action independent of its antibiotic effect. It is effective acutely in gastroparesis, though there is less evidence that it is effective on a prolonged basis.

The newest agents for the treatment of nausea and vomiting are the serotonin antagonists. **Ondansetron** is an antagonist to the $5-HT_3$ receptor, which is one of three serotonin receptors that have been identified. This receptor is present in both the CNS and the GI tract. Ondansetron is available only in a parenteral form and has been used primarily as prophylaxis against chemotherapy-associated nausea and vomiting. It appears to have only rare adverse affects.

HICCUPS

9. What are hiccups?
Hiccups are spasmodic, involuntary contractions of the muscles of inspiration (not just the diaphragm) near-simultaneous with closure of the glottis. The latter component is responsible for the audible sound. Hiccups are usually short-lived, typically occur postprandial or following alcohol ingestion, and subside without treatment or with simple measures such as breath-holding, water ingestion, or Valsalva maneuvers.

10. When are hiccups pathologic? What are the consequences?
An episode of hiccups lasting 48 hours or recurring episodes of protracted hiccups are defined as chronic. Some unfortunate individuals have prolonged episodes of hiccups or constant hiccups for years. When chronic, hiccups can be disabling, resulting in chronic fatigue, sleep deprivation, interference with normal eating, and depression. Thus, chronic hiccups requires diagnostic evaluation and prompt treatment. However, even acute hiccups in certain situations, such as in the early postmyocardial infarction period or postoperatively, can be devastating and require prompt treatment.

11. What causes chronic hiccups?
Because the afferent limb of the hiccup reflex includes the vagus and phrenic nerves, as well as sympathetic fibers T6–12, a wide variety of intra-abdominal and intrathoracic disorders have been associated with hiccups. In contrast, because hiccups results in physiologic changes (such as a decrease in lower esophageal sphincter pressure), some abnormalities, such as reflux esophagitis, usually are a result of hiccups rather than the cause. A variety of CNS disorders also have been found to cause chronic hiccups. Lastly, metabolic diseases, such as chronic renal failure and especially diabetes mellitus, are associated with chronic hiccups.

12. Describe the diagnostic evaluation for patients with chronic hiccups.
Fluoroscopy of the diaphragm should be performed. If the diaphragm shows unilateral involvement only (usually the left hemidiaphragm), the diagnostic evaluation should focus on the course of the phrenic nerve of the affected side. Bilateral diaphragmatic motion suggests an afferent or central origin.

Because there is a wide variety of intra-abdominal and intrathoracic disorders associated with chronic hiccups, unless associated symptoms point toward a specific organ system, one should begin with laboratory tests (complete blood count, chemistry screen), abdominal flat plate (mechanical obstruction), endoscopy (peptic ulcer disease, gastric cancer, infiltrating diseases), and chest x-ray. If negative, one should consider abdominal and chest CT scans and an MRI of the brain.

Unfortunately, a thorough evaluation may be negative or find only an abnormal condition that may be coexisting (gastritis) or secondary to the hiccups (esophagitis, for example).

13. What therapies are available for chronic hiccups?
The best therapy is directed toward the etiology. Unfortunately, this may not be possible, and therapy may have to be directed toward the hiccups themselves. Simple measures, such as breath-holding, swallowing water, Valsalva maneuvers, or rebreathing into a bag, are rarely helpful for protracted hiccups. Instead, more vigorous mechanical approaches or drug therapy is usually necessary, and occasionally phrenic nerve ablation should be considered. In my experience, the best way to stop an episode of hiccups is firm digital stimulation of the posterior pharynx, often with a nasogastric tube in place and after removing gastric contents. This is unpleasant for patients and is primarily useful for those with long intervals between isolated episodes of hiccups. For those whose hiccups recur a short time after cessation, this is not a feasible approach.

14. Which drugs can cure hiccups?
A wide variety of drugs have been proposed as effective therapy for hiccups, but experience with each is usually limited to just a few cases. Chlorpromazine, metoclopramide, and nifedipine all have advocates proclaiming their efficacy in chronic hiccups. In my experience, and that of others, the single most effective medication is baclofen, a GABA derivative used as an antispasticity agent in patients with tics or dystonias. Occasionally, complete cessation of hiccups occurs, but in most patients, there is a variable decrease in the frequency of episodes. Nevertheless, for some unfortunate patients who suffer near-daily hiccups for a large proportion of their day, this partial response can be gratifying. Dosage begins at 5 mg three times a day and is increased in a step-wise fashion to a maximum dose of 25 mg three times a day. Side effects include somnolence and fatigue. One should not discontinue the medication suddenly, but taper it over a period of time.

15. When is a surgical approach indicated?
When unilateral involvement is demonstrated at fluoroscopy and other measures have been exhausted, phrenic nerve intervention should be considered. Because respiratory function may be significantly impaired after diaphragmatic paralysis, pulmonary function tests should be obtained prior to intervention. Temporary diaphragmatic paralysis confirmed by fluoroscopy and concomitant cessation of hiccups should be demonstrated before permanent ablation of the phrenic nerve is considered.

EATING DISORDERS

16. If the eating disorders are psychiatric illnesses, why should an internist be aware of them?
Anorexia nervosa and bulimia nervosa, the two major well-defined eating disorders, are relatively common. The internist or gastroenterologist needs to be aware of these disorders, because the patient's family may first bring the individual to the physician with concern that profound weight loss, vomiting, or associated symptoms (constipation, abdominal pain, dyspepsia, etc.) suggest a GI disorder. Successful management requires: (1) early suspicion that an eating disorder is present; (2) evaluation for complications; (3) exclusion of a GI (e.g., Crohn's disease) or systemic (e.g., AIDS) disorder responsible for the symptoms; and then (4) prompt referral to an individual experienced in treating these disorders.

17. List the criteria required for the diagnosis of anorexia nervosa according to the Diagnostic Statistical Manual of Mental Disorders (DSM-IV).
  a. Refusal to maintain body weight at or above a minimally normal weight for age and height.
  b. Intense fear of gaining weight or becoming fat, even though underweight.
  c. Disturbance in the way in which one's body weight or shape is experienced, undue influence of body weight or shape on self-evaluation, or denial of the seriousness of the current low body weight.
  d. In postmenarcheal females, amenorrhea (i.e., the absence of at least three consecutive menstrual cycles).

18. What other characteristics of anorexia nervosa may aid in its diagnosis?
Females are overwhelmingly affected, with only 5–10% of patients being male. The onset in most is in late adolescence and early adulthood, at a mean age of 17 years. The onset is often associated with a stressful life event, such as going to college. There is a high incidence of sexual abuse among these individuals. Associated symptoms include a depressed mood, obsessive-compulsive acts (such as a preoccupation with food or food hoarding), and an over-controlling behavior resulting in a typically inflexible attitude in most life situations. Physical examination is dominated by the patient's emaciated state, but other clues include an increased size of the salivary glands (especially the parotids gland) and signs of recurring vomiting, such as decreased dental enamel and callouses on the dorsum of the hand.

19. Should any complications be anticipated in patients with anorexia nervosa?
Patients will have findings related to their starvation. They may have a mild leukopenia and normocytic anemia; moreover, endocrine evaluation may reveal hyperadrenocorticism and regression of the hypothalamic-pituitary-gonadal axis to a prepubertal pattern.
There may be sequela of vomiting and purging, if this specific type is present. Repeated vomiting may cause an emetogenic injury. Electrolyte disturbances, especially hypokalemia, may be present and especially profound in those patients using large amounts of laxatives for purging. Rare patients who use Ipecac may have a cardiac and skeletal myopathy. Lastly, amylase may be elevated in these individuals, though it is typically of salivary isoamylase type.

20. Discuss the differential diagnosis for patients with suspected anorexia nervosa.
When the patient has many of the characteristic findings of an eating disorder, it should be the working diagnosis, and only a few disorders need to be considered and expeditiously excluded. GI disorders to consider are inflammatory bowel disease (especially Crohn's disease), celiac sprue, pancreatic insufficiency, or recurring mechanical obstruction Non-GI disorders include primarily endocrine disorders (especially panhypopituitarism, Addison's disease, or hyperthyroidism), occult neoplasm, or AIDS.
Concomitant with considering the differential diagnoses should be a nutritional assessment. This should include transferrin, albumin, triceps skinfold, and an anergy panel. A prognostic nutritional index has been proposed for patients with anorexia nervosa that determines the need for aggressive nutritional support.

21. What is the natural history of anorexia nervosa?
The course of anorexia nervosa varies markedly, and the spectrum ranges from individuals with one episode with subsequent recovery, to those who have repeated relapses, to others with an unremitting course leading to death. Of patients admitted to a university hospital, long-term mortality has been reported to be 10%, due to starvation, suicide, or electrolyte imbalance.

22. How are patients with anorexia nervosa managed?
Because of the variable and serious nature of anorexia nervosa, treatment requires a primary physician experienced in these patients who can integrate a multiphasic treatment regimen. Medical management is required to restore weight and correct metabolic problems. In general, patients with moderate (65–80% of ideal body weight) and severe (<65% of ideal body weight) weight loss or low prognostic nutritional index scores require nutrition supplementation, and hospitalization is required for the severely malnourished.
A psychological approach also should be devised that uses one or a combination of:
1. Behavioral therapies, such as operant conditioning
2. Cognitive therapy, such as assessing and examining distortions in thought processes
3. Family counseling
4. Pharmacotherapy, such as chlorpromazine or antidepressants.

23. What are the DSM-IV diagnostic criteria for bulimia nervosa?
    a. Recurrent episodes of binge eating, characterized by both of the following:
       (1) Eating an amount of food that is definitely larger than most people would eat during a similar period of time and under similar circumstances.
       (2) A sense of lack of control over eating during the episode.
    b. Recurrent inappropriate compensatory behavior to prevent weight gain, such as self-induced vomiting; misuse of laxatives, diuretics, enemas, or other medications; fasting; or excessive exercise.
    c. Binge eating and compensatory behaviors both occur, on average, at least twice a week for 3 months.
    d. Self-evaluation is unduly influenced by body shape and weight.
    e. The disturbance does not occur exclusively during episodes of anorexia nervosa.
Although some argue that these patients are too similar to those with anorexia nervosa to differentiate, they have less body-image distortion, have more insight into therapy, and are more accepting of therapy.

24. What other characteristics of bulimia nervosa may aid in its diagnosis?
    The vast predominance of females and age of onset mirror anorexia nervosa. However, bulimia nervosa is more common and, in various studies, has been reported in 1–3% of the adolescent and young adult female population.
    Characteristically, patients try to conceal their binging or purging behavior, which tends to occur during periods of stress. Vomiting rarely occurs in public, as patients can control their vomiting until they get in a private location. Though vomiting is the most common compensatory behavior, occuring in 80–90%, approximately one-third use laxatives. The vomiting initially may be forceful, but later in the disease it becomes nearly effortless. Rare individuals use Ipecac.
    These individuals characteristically have difficulty in developing personal relationships, and unlike patients with anorexia nervosa, they may have chemical dependencies, especially alcohol. One-third have associated personality disorders.
    Physical findings are not obvious. Because they are not malnourished, bulemics generally appear healthy, and other individuals who know the patients well, even their family, may not be aware of the disorder. The physical findings characteristic of patients with repeated vomiting may be present, as noted for anorexia nervosa. The complications that occur are related to the compensatory vomiting and purging behavior and are the same as those for anorexia nervosa.

25. What is the natural history of bulimia nervosa? What therapy is available?
    The course of bulimia nervosa varies among individuals. In some, it is chronic; in others, it is intermittent with relapses lasting varying intervals. The long-term course is unknown.
    Bulimia nervosa can be managed on an outpatient basis. A program that includes both cognitive recognition of the patient's abnormal behavior as well as therapy directed at the abnormal behavior itself is the approach of choice. Antidepressants are useful as an adjunct but not as sole therapy.

26. What about other individuals with a suspected eating disorder who may not meet the strict criteria for anorexia nervosa or bulimia nervosa?
Certain individuals have some, but not all, of the features of anorexia nervosa or bulimia nervosa. DSM-IV defines several other presentations as nonspecific eating disorders.

RUMINATION

27. What is rumination, and how often does it occur?
    Rumination is the regurgitation of mouthfuls of recently ingested food, with subsequent remastication and reswallowing, when there is no apparent organic disease. Usually, rumination begins 15–20 minutes postprandial and continues until the stomach contents become sour as a re-

sult of acid, between 20–60 minutes later. As many as 20 episodes per meal is not uncommon. Patients do not describe it as distressful and are often embarrassed and attempt to hide the symptom. Rumination is facilitated by eating large volumes of food quickly and with a lot of liquids.

Rumination is uncommon in adults, though it is under-reported because patients are unlikely to discuss a symptom they consider embarrassing. Men predominate, and though no consistent intellectual or social characteristics are present, physicians and scientists are highly represented in various reviews.

28. What is the mechanism of rumination?

On observation, most individuals with rumination have abdominal and thoracic movements that precede and accompany the process. Gastroesophageal manometry performed postprandially in ruminating individuals has found that Valsalva maneuvers occur simultaneously with regurgitation, and in one report, this occurred repeatedly over a low lower esophageal sphincter and with a pharyngeal maneuver that preceded the upper esophageal sphincter relaxation. Thus, there is a voluntary component to rumination, and this has led to behavioral therapy and biofeedback becoming the therapy of choice in these individuals. No case has been reported in which rumination was accompanied by reverse peristalsis, as described in ruminant animals.

29. Can complications occur with rumination?

Heartburn may occur starting many years after the onset of rumination, suggesting that an acid-sensitive esophagus develops from repeated acid contact during ruminating. Rare reports of GI bleeding and hemorrhagic esophagitis at endoscopy have been published.

30. What should be the therapeutic approach?

Behavioral therapy is the treatment of choice for adults. Changing the composition of food, slowing the speed of eating, and giving less water with the meal have been effective approaches in some reports, and biofeedback directed against the increased intra-abdominal pressure that always precedes regurgitation episodes also has been effective. Aversive therapies, such as ingesting foods that are distasteful if regurgitated, should be avoided.

BIBLIOGRAPHY

 1. Amarnath RP, Abell TL, Malagelada J: The rumination syndrome in adults. Ann Intern Med 105:513–518, 1986.
 2. Drossman DA: Anorexia: A comprehensive approach. Adv Intern Med 28:339, 1983.
 3. Eating disorders: Anorexia nervosa and bulimia. Ann Intern Med 105:790–794, 1986.
 4. Eating disorders. In American Psychiatric Association: Diagnostic and Statistical Manual of Mental Disorders, 4th ed. Washington, DC, American Psychiatric Assoc, 1994, pp 539–550.
 5. Geffen N: Rumination in man. Am J Dig Dis 11:963–972, 1966.
 6. Hanson JS, McCallum RW: The diagnosis and management of nausea and vomiting: A review. Am J Gastroenterol 80:210–218, 1985.
 7. Katelaris PH, Jones DB: Chronic nausea and vomiting. Dig Dis 7:324–333, 1989.
 8. King M: Update: Eating disorders. Compr Ther 17(3):35–40, 1991.
 9. Launois S, Bizec JL, et al. Hiccup in adults: An overview. Eur Respir J 6:563–575, 1993.
10. Lewis JH: Hiccups: Causes and cures. J Clin Gastroenterol 7:539–552, 1985.
11. Malagelada JR, Camilleri M: Unexplained vomiting: A diagnostic challenge. Ann Intern Med 101:211–218, 1984.
12. Psychogenic vomiting—A disorder of gastrointestinal motility? Lancet 339:279, 1992.
13. Ramirez FC, Graham DY: Treatment of intractable hiccup with baclofen. Am J Gastroenterol 87:1789–1791, 1992.
14. Shay SS: Regurgitation and rumination. In Castell DO (ed): The Esophagus. Boston, Little, Brown, 1992, pp 571–579.
15. Shay SS, Myers RL, Johnson LF: Hiccups associated with reflux esophagitis. Gastroenterology 87:204–207, 1984.

63. FOREIGN BODIES AND THE GASTROINTESTINAL TRACT

Michael F. Lyons, II, M.D. and Amy M. Tsuchida, M.D.

1. How common are foreign bodies in the GI tract?

Most authors agree that millions of foreign bodies enter the oral or anal GI tract annually, and somewhere between 1500 and 2750 people die every year from these objects. However, only about 10–20% of foreign bodies require therapeutic intervention, and the rest pass through the alimentary tract without incident.

2. Are specific populations at risk for foreign-body ingestion?

The pediatric population accounts for approximately 80% of foreign-body ingestions, but foreign bodies inserted into the rectum are almost all described in adult populations. Other groups at increased risk for foreign-body ingestion include psychiatric patients, inmates, and individuals who frequently use alcohol or sedative-hypnotic medications. Also at risk are elderly subjects, who may have poorly fitting dentures, impaired cognitive function due to medications, or dementia or dysphagia following a stroke. Intentional ingestion of foreign objects is well described in individuals smuggling illicit drugs, jewels, or other valuable items.

3. Which areas of the GI tract lead to problems in the passage of foreign bodies?

Several areas of anatomic as well as physiologic narrowing exist along the lumen of the gut where foreign bodies will impact. The natural narrowings of the esophagus include the cricopharyngeal muscle of the proximal esophagus, extrinsic compression of the middle esophagus from the aortic arch and left mainstem bronchus, and the lower esophageal sphincter at the junction of the esophagus and stomach. The pylorus at the gastroduodenal junction, the C-loop, and the ligament of Treitz are other problematic areas in the foregut. The ileocecal valve at the junction of the small intestine and colon, the hepatic and splenic flexures of the colon, the valves of Houston in the rectum, and the anal sphincters complete the obstacles that must be negotiated. In addition, numerous anatomic and physiologic abnormalities, such as strictures or tumors, can lead to difficult passage of foreign bodies.(See table at top of opposite page.)

4. What are the common objects ingested?

Although the list of foreign objects ingested is as varied as the imagination, the most common object ingested by children is a coin. Meat boluses impacted above an esophageal stricture account for most adult cases. Accidental loss of sexual-stimulant devices account for over half of foreign objects introduced through the anus.

5. What is a typical clinical presentation for foreign-body ingestion?

Adults will relate a specific meal, foreign body, or food that has led to the onset of their symptoms. Children, on the other hand, may present up to months after their ingestion. Individuals with anorectal foreign bodies impart a wide variety of medical histories to account for their predicament, ranging from accidents or assault to medical remedies.

6. If respiratory symptoms develop related to foreign-body ingestion, what does this imply?

Patients presenting with wheezing, stridor, cough, or dyspnea following foreign-body ingestion suggest entrapment in the hypopharynx, trachea, pyriform sinus, or Zenker's diverticulum.

Anatomic and Physiologic Defects of the GI Tract Contributing to Foreign Body Obstruction

INTESTINAL SITE	ANATOMIC DEFECT	PHYSIOLOGIC DEFECT
Esophagus	Stenosis, atresia, rings, webs, benign/malignant stricture, diverticuli, vascular anomalies	Scleroderma, achalasia, Chagas' disease
Stomach	Pyloric stenosis (congenital, acquired), gastric malignancy	Gastroparesis (uremia, diabetes, postoperative)
Intestine	Postoperative adhesion, Meckel's diverticulum, strictures (ischemic, anastomotic, Crohn's disease), malignancy	Idiopathic intestinal pseudo-obstruction, scleroderma
Colon	Strictures (ischemic, anastomotic, ulcerative colitis, Crohn's disease, radiation, trauma, postinfection, postsurgical), diverticular disease, malignancy	Cathartic colon, idiopathic constipation, familial megacolon, idiopathic intestinal pseudo-obstruction
Anus	Stenosis (hemorrhoids, Crohn's disease, trauma, radiation, postinfection, postsurgical)	Hirschprung's disease

7. Do ingested sharp objects perforate the intestine?

Yes. This perforation is the exception, however. Sharp objects such as pins, needles, nails, and toothpicks certainly raise concern for both the patient and physician. It is important to realize, however, that 70–90% of the time, these objects pass through the alimentary tract without complication.

Two phenomena occur in the intestine to allow safe passage. Foreign bodies pass with axial flow down the lumen. Additionally, reflex relaxation and slowing of peristalsis cause sharp objects to turn around in the lumen so that the sharp end trails down the intestine. In the colon, the foreign object is centered in the fecal bolus which further protects the bowel wall.

8. Why is it important to identify the type of foreign body ingested?

Although most foreign bodies traverse the GI tract without complication, there are specific exceptions. Button batteries cause coagulation necrosis of the esophageal mucosa (but once in the stomach, gastric acid neutralizes this risk). Sharp objects can perforate any part of the alimentary tract. Objects longer than 6 cm frequently get lodged in the postbulbar C-loop of the duodenum. Large bolus objects can obstruct various parts of the GI tract (usually the esophagus).

9. How much urgency is there to remove a foreign body following ingestion?

Any object that has a high risk for complication should be endoscopically removed as soon as possible. Button batteries need to be removed emergently due to the severe trauma continuously incurred in the esophagus. If sharp objects can be reached with an endoscope, they should be removed immediately as well. Long objects (>6 cm) should be removed when identified. Finally, large bolus objects usually lead to an inability to handle oral secretions, and these objects should be removed urgently to reduce the risk of aspiration.

10. Describe the signs and symptoms of a complication related to a foreign-body ingestion.

Respiratory symptoms suggest entrapment of the foreign body in the hypopharynx, trachea, pyriform sinus, or Zenker's diverticulum (*see* Question 6). Sharp objects may penetrate, obstruct, or perforate the esophagus or intestines, presenting with chest, neck, or abdominal pain that varies from discomfort to acute abdomen. Injury to the esophagus can lead to hematemesis, fever, tachycardia, neck swelling, and crepitus. Massive hematemesis has been reported following an aortoesophageal fistula. Excessive drooling, inability to swallow saliva, and recurrent vomiting are seen with obstruction. Abdominal distention and hyperactive bowel sounds suggest intestinal obstruction. Hypoactive or absent bowel sounds, guarding, rebound, and abdominal pain are seen with luminal penetration or perforation. Aortoenteric fistula has led to exsanguination following ingestion of a sharp foreign body.

11. How should foreign bodies be removed?
Most foreign bodies pass without intervention, but some will not. Once identified, nearly all objects can be removed endoscopically by a skilled endoscopist. Other modalities also have been employed with variable success, though major complications have been reported. Consultation with a surgeon is appropriate for cases in which perforation or other major complications are probable.

BIBLIOGRAPHY

1. Lyons MF, Tsuchida AM: Foreign bodies of the gastrointestinal tract. Med Clin North Am 77:1101–1114, 1993.
2. Webb WA: Management of foreign bodies of the upper gastrointestinal tract: Update. Gastrointest Endosc 41:39–51, 1995.
3. Ginsberg GG: Management of ingested foreign objects and food bolus inpactions. Gastrointest Endosc 41:33–38, 1995.
4. Barone JE, Yee J, Nealon TF Jr: Management of foreign bodies and trauma of the rectum. Surg Gynecol Obstet 156:453–457, 1983.
5. Busch DB, Starling JR: Rectal foreign bodies: Case reports and a comprehensive review of the world's literature. Surgery 100:512–519, 1986.

64. EXERCISE AND THE GASTROINTESTINAL TRACT

Frank M. Moses, M.D.

1. Why is so little known about the effect of exercise on the GI tract?

Over the last 15 years, an increase in the medical literature has paralleled the public interest and participation in both recreational and competitive sports. A great deal of research has been performed to optimize rehydration in athletic events, focusing on the ability of the stomach to empty fluids and calories during strenuous exercise. However, the basic pathophysiology of the GI tract during exercise is in large part undefined. Exercise places additional stresses on the GI tract, and knowledge of this field could aid in the understanding of basic digestive processes in a way similar to the study of digestive diseases produced by toxins or infections.

Until recently, little attention was paid to exercise-associated digestive processes, either in health or disease. Whole texts are devoted to diseases of the GI tract, but the pathophysiology is almost exclusively evaluated at rest. Any experimental stress to the GI tract has been produced by disease or drugs, due in part to current experimental methods that are designed to be used at rest and are not easily converted for use during exercise. GI physiologists are not accustomed or trained to evaluate exercising subjects. Exercise physiologists, on the other hand, have shown little interest in GI function, except for optimizing gastric emptying in competitive athletes.

2. What physiologic changes occur in the GI system during exercise?

A great deal of the basic GI physiology associated with exercise is unexplored. However, it has been shown that **visceral blood flow** is diverted to exercising muscle groups and may decrease to 50–80% of control/resting values. These changes in blood flow may be compounded by hyperthermia, dehydration, and medications such as nonsteroidal anti-inflammatory drugs (NSAIDs). The **autonomic nervous system** is altered during acute exercise. With stress, the sympathetic system predominates. With habitual exercise the autonomic system adapts, and the parasympathetic is more prominent. Variable changes in **GI hormones** are known to occur with exercise and could affect GI motility, absorption, and other functions. **Mechanical effects** of running and jumping and other intra-abdominal pressure changes may alter GI function as well. Certain digestive organs, such as the stomach and colon, also appear to be particularly sensitive to the ischemic effects of severe exercise.

3. What GI symptoms are most frequently seen with exercise?

Surveys show a high prevalence of GI symptoms associated with exercise. Early surveys confirmed that distance runners were the most likely to suffer GI symptoms. Heartburn, abdominal cramps, urge to have a bowel movement, and loss of appetite following races are frequent.

A larger survey of marathoners found that nearly half had occasional loose stools, and 13% had three or more bowel movements per day. The urge to defecate was the most common symptom experienced by runners. Heartburn occurred in up to 9.5% and was prominent during running. Nausea and vomiting were more common with hard runs. Women suffered from GI symptoms more frequently than men. A small percentage reported bloody bowel movements with

GI Symptoms Associated with Exercise Among Runners and Triathletes

Loss of appetite	Abdominal cramps
Heartburn	Urge to defecate
Chest pain	Bowel movement with exercise
Belch	Diarrhea
Nausea	Rectal bleeding
Vomiting	

running. These symptoms may be more common among women and younger male runners and more frequent in those runners who become dehydrated and lose >4% body weight or drink the least fluids during a race. Symptoms such as stomach ache and intestinal cramps were also substantially greater with marathons than with a shorter race. A similar pattern, with predominantly lower GI symptoms more notable in faster runners, has also been reported.

Triathletes may suffer more upper abdominal symptoms during competition than runners. In a survey of international distance triathletes, dyspeptic symptoms, such as the loss of appetite, heartburn, nausea, and bloating, occurred in 25–35%. Triathletes tend to consume more food and drink during races than runners, which may affect their symptoms.

GI symptoms, particularly nausea, vomiting, and abdominal pain, may be manifestations of dehydration, electrolyte disturbances, or hyperthermia and should be suspected in the appropriate clinical setting. Some common symptoms, such as "side stitch," are not frequently discussed. Pancreatitis also has been associated with moderate running. GI symptoms with exercise are not typically severe unless they occur during circumstances in which the subject will not discontinue or substantially reduce the athletic stress, usually during competitive events and with military-style training.

4. Is the esophagus a common cause of exercise-associated chest pain?

Esophageal disorders commonly manifest as chest pain or heartburn secondary to gastroesophageal reflux (GER) or esophageal dysmotility. Chest pain, when it occurs in association with athletics or other exertion, should initiate an evaluation for cardiac disease. Several notable deaths of celebrities have shown that athletic participation, while indicative of a healthy lifestyle, does not confer immunity against coronary artery disease. Furthermore, there is some experimental evidence suggesting that GER may aggravate angina.

5. How commonly is heartburn provoked by exercise?

Heartburn is relatively common in the general population and in athletes, being reported in about 10% of runners' surveys. Ambulatory esophageal pH monitoring has determined that GER in normal controls is more frequent during exercise than rest. The type and intensity of exercise probably are important in determining the amount of GER.

Although GER is enhanced with cycling, a comparison study of seven men and five women with ambulatory esophageal pH monitors while undergoing sequential 15-minute periods of stationary bicycling, indoor track running, and a weightlifting routine versus a comparable rest period found that running induced the greatest amount of GER. Both the number of reflux episodes and the time of acid exposure increased with running. Most reflux events were associated with belching, and GER was accentuated postprandially. Patients with GER disorder have not been systematically evaluated with exercise.

6. What therapy is effective for exercise-induced heartburn?

Esophageal symptoms suffered by runners are frequent, but they are usually not severe. Treatment is often accomplished with dietary changes, fasting before runs, and, occasionally, medical therapy with antacids or histamine H_2 antagonists. Ambulatory pH monitoring performed in 14 runners at rest and during a 1-hour near-maximal run, with and without ranitidine, showed that ranitidine decreased the acid exposure time. Antacid and Gaviscon, an aluminum/magnesium antacid, also reduce esophageal acid exposure with running.

7. Does exercise affect esophageal motility?

Esophageal motility changes probably occur with exercise and may lead to some cases of noncardiac chest pain. However, interpretation of the literature is difficult. Most diagnostic manometry instrumentation is designed to be used at rest and is not able to filter out movement artifact and respiratory pressure changes produced by exercise.

Using standard esophageal motility at rest before, immediately after, and 1 hour after a submaximal treadmill run, an early study found no change in peristaltic amplitude or duration. Lower esophageal sphincter pressure, however, increased slightly from 24 to 32 mm Hg after exercise and then returned to 27 mm Hg at recovery. Most recently, Soffer et al., using solid-state manometry in trained and untrained cyclists, noted decreases in duration, amplitude, and frequency of esophageal contractions with increasing exercise intensities up to 90% VO_{2max}. The clinical relevance of these changes in esophageal motility is uncertain, and the mechanism is speculative. The subjects were not symptomatic. Some data have suggested that hyperventilation and stress can alter esophageal motility as well.

8. How does exercise affect the stomach?

Nausea and vomiting occur during or after racing, and exercise-induced abnormalities in gastric emptying can severely limit athletic performance, particularly during endurance events. Because of these problems, the stomach has been the major digestive focus for exercise physiologists. William Beaumont, observing the gastric fistula caused by a musket wound to the abdomen of a patriot soldier named Alexis St. Martin, noticed that exercise changed the appearance and function of the stomach. Disorders of gastric physiology may manifest as abnormalities in gastric emptying, with nausea, bloating, or vomiting or changes in acid secretion with mucosal damage and ulceration. Drugs such as NSAIDs, commonly used to alleviate musculoskeletal discomfort, may also affect gastric function and cause mucosal damage.

9. How does exercise alter gastric emptying (GE)? Does the type of food or exercise matter?

The major factors controlling GE are the characteristics of the meals. Liquid meals empty differently from solids. Increasing calories and fat in the meal progressively delay GE. Temperature, osmolality, and volume of the meal also affect emptying. In addition, the athlete's hydration status and body temperature may affect GE. Exercising in warm environments inhibits GE. Other factors such as sex, menstrual cycle, smoking, and time of day may influence GE. For these reasons, comparing different published exercise protocols and different meals is difficult.

Because athletes generally tolerate liquids during prolonged competition, GE of liquids has been investigated more thoroughly. Several studies found that light or moderate levels of exertion accelerated GE. One compared water GE during walking and running and found that GE increased with light to moderate exercise but not running at 74% VO_{2max}; the authors theorized that increased intra-abdominal pressures accelerated GE. Most other protocols have found that moderate exercise has little significant effect on GE of water, glucose, or electrolyte solutions. It has been noted that runners are more troubled by gastric symptoms than bicyclists and most other athletes, but when compared directly, both exercise modes produced slower emptying than that at rest, and no difference was noted between running and cycling.

Solid-meal GE is more dependent on gastric motility, and exercise might be expected to affect the solid-meal GE differently. An early study, using scintigraphy to compare GE of a mixed solid meal at rest versus mild exercise on a bicycle ergometer, found that exercise was associated with mildly accelerated emptying; this finding has subsequently been confirmed by others. Another study used scintigraphy of a mixed solid meal and compared trained distance runners at rest and with a 90-minute run with sedentary controls at rest; they found that the runners had significantly accelerated basal GE when compared to controls but that exercise had no effect on their GE.

10. Does exercise influence abnormal gastric emptying seen in gastroparesis or diabetes?

Several studies have suggested that mild- to moderate-intensity exercise accelerates GE of liquids and solids. An interesting thought is that exercise may improve the GE of patients with gastroparesis. We have followed one patient with idiopathic gastroparesis refractory to standard prokinetic medications who normalized GE by walking at an uncontrolled but moderate pace during a standard scintigraphic GE test. No formal studies of this kind have been published.

11. Does exercise affect gastric acid secretion?

Gastric secretion may be affected by exercise. However, the clinical importance is uncertain, and the question has received little attention. Feldman and Nixon found gastric acid secretion relatively unchanged in five healthy controls who exercised for 45 minutes on a bicycle at 50 or 70% VO_{2max}. The effect of exercise in duodenal ulcer patients has been contradictory.

12. What therapy is effective for gastric symptoms associated with exercise?

Treatment for disorders of gastric emptying are primarily preventive. Athletes should avoid fluids and foods in the diet known to delay gastric emptying and consume fluids early and often enough to avoid dehydration and hyperthermia, which could aggravate gastric stasis. Medications are probably of limited value. Some athletes stress that it is possible to adapt themselves to tolerate increased food and fluids by incremental training.

13. Does exercise alter intestinal transit?

Exercise-associated small bowel dysfunction may be responsible for runners' diarrhea, abdominal bloating, and pain. Furthermore, routine daily exercise seen in active patients could alter transit and absorption of oral medications. Physiologic changes caused by exercise could include either accelerated or slowed transit time. Published studies have used several investigational methods, and results are mixed. In general, the changes noted are small, and it is unlikely that changes in small bowel transit are responsible for any clinical changes. (See table on opposite page.)

14. Is intestinal absorption altered by exercise?

Small bowel absorption of water, electrolytes, and nutrients may be affected by exercise, mediated perhaps by altered motility, decreased blood flow, or neurohormonal changes. The investigative techniques are more cumbersome, and thus absorption has been infrequently investigated. Several studies using triple-lumen perfusion technique to assess absorption with exercise have found either no effect on the absorption rate of water, electrolytes, glucose, xylose, or urea or markedly depressed water and electrolyte absorption when glucose was omitted from the test solution. In a more recent study, volunteers underwent exercise at 42, 61, or 80% of VO_{2max} for 30–40 minutes and consumed a solution of water (with ^2H_2O), glucose, and electrolytes . The rate of ^2H appearance in the plasma was measured and was greater at rest than with exercise at low, mid, or high intensity. It appears unlikely that the small degree of change in intestinal transit noted in these studies could exceed the normal ability of absorption.

Carbohydrate absorption was evaluated in six men walking 4.8 km/hr for 4.5 hrs. While absorption of xylose was not altered, absorption of 3-*o*-methyl glucose was decreased, and an abnormality in active but not passive absorption with exercise was postulated.

Intestinal permeability might be affected by exercise. In an abstract, permeability to polyethylene glycol (PEG) 400 was altered in 17 men at rest and with a 90-minute treadmill run. When normalized for water flow, urinary PEG-400 excretion increased with exercise, indicating a relative increase in permeability with exercise. The clinical significance is uncertain, but the effect may contribute to increased antigen presentation to the gut immune system, some digestive symptoms, and cases of exercise-induced anaphylaxis.

15. Can exercise cause permanent intestinal damage?

One recently published case documents transmural small bowel ischemia of 1 m of distal ileum due to nonocclusive mesenteric infarction in a 65-year-old physician who presented with abdominal pain following a 6-km training run. This was an experienced runner who had previous episodes of explosive watery diarrhea following running but no other known associated conditions or risk factors. The ischemic section was surgically removed, and the patient recovered but has not resumed running.

16. What is the effect of exercise on the colon?

The most frequent GI symptoms among runners are the urge to defecate, defecation with running, abdominal cramping, and diarrhea. In a recent study of a running club, "nervous" diarrhea before

Effects of Exercise on Small Bowel Transit

SUBJECTS	MEAL/MARKER	EXERCISE	METHOD	RESULTS	CONCLUSION
1M/6F volunteers	Solid, 630 kcal, 405/gm No marker	Cycle for 60 min at 33 rpm HR = 117/bpm	BH2 q10 min	~ 300 min No change	No effect on OCTT
12 M volunteers	Liquid, 350 ml, 360 kcal Lactulose, 30 gm	TMW for 120 min at 5.6 km/hr HR = 109/bpm	BH2 q10 min modified	Rest 66 min Exer 44 min	Exercise decreases OCTT
7M/14F volunteers	Water, 150 ml Lactulose, 10 gm	TMW for 60 min at 4.5 km/hr HR = 106/bpm	BH2 q10 min	Rest 55 min Exer 89 min	Exercise increases OCTT
9 M volunteers	Water, lunch Nuc-tagged capsules	Varied min–hard, up to 5 hr HR to 160/bpm	Scintigraphy	4.1–5.4 hr No change	No effect on transit
10 M volunteers	Water Lactulose, 15 gm	2-hr TM run at 65% VO2	BH2 q10 min	Rest 68 min Exer 102 min	Exercise increases OCTT
10 M volunteers	Glucose polymer drink Lactulose, 15 gm	2-hr TM run at 65% VO2	BH2 q10 min	Rest 81 min Exer 123 min	Exercise increases OCTT
8 trained cyclists	860-kcal meal Lactulose, 10 gm	cycle 20 min at 80% VO2	BH2 q10 min	Rest 152 min Exer 159 min	No effect on transit

BH2 = breath hydrogen test;
TMW = treadmill walk;
OCTT = oral-cecal transit time.

the race was seen in 43%, and 62% stopped at some time during practice runs to defecate. More significantly, 47% had experienced diarrhea during racing, often with severe cramps, nausea, and vomiting. Rectal bleeding occurred in 16% and fecal incontinence in 12%.

17. Does exercise influence colonic transit or constipation?

The effects of exercise on colonic transit have been studied in several different manners, and the results generally support a slightly decreased transit time. In a controlled setting, subjects were confined to a metabolic laboratory during a 9-week training period in which diet was rigidly controlled. No change was found in fecal transit time as measured by radioisotope markers, fecal weight, fecal solids or pH, ammonia, or nitrogen. However, the training regimen was moderate, the subjects remained asymptomatic, and the inter- and intrasubject variation of colonic transit data was high.

In another study of colon transit, six men and four women were evaluated in a crossover trial in which the subjects either exercised ($\sim$50% VO_{2max}) on a treadmill or bicycle ergometer or rested for 1 hour in a chair daily for 1 week. Transit was measured by single-dose radiopaque markers. Stool frequency and weight were recorded. Diet and fiber intake were monitored by 24-hour diet record once weekly, and lifestyle was otherwise unchanged. Transit time decreased from 51.2 hours at rest to 36.6 hours when cycling and 34 hours when jogging. However, stool weight and frequency did not change, and no subject developed diarrhea with running.

Newer scintigraphic techniques of whole gut transit may offer an improved investigative modality for evaluating the effects of exercise on intestinal transit in symptomatic individuals.

18. Is there effective therapy for runners' diarrhea?

Colonic symptoms may be treated in a variety of ways. "Nervous" prerace diarrhea is generally self-limited and may respond to low-residue diets. Others have used antidiarrheal medications prophylactically. Ultramarathoners report that it is feasible to "train the gut" by reducing exercise duration and intensity to subsymptomatic levels and gradually increasing the exercise. Prerace cathartics should be avoided. Severe race-associated diarrhea may respond to reduction in effort.

19. What changes are seen in the liver enzymes with exercise?

Physically active individuals often are suspected of liver disorders because of incidentally noted abnormal enzymes, including bilirubin, AST, ALT, and alkaline phosphatase. These changes are not uncommon in long-distance runners and may mimic the patterns seen in myocardial infarction or chronic hepatitis. The changes are usually due to damaged muscle tissue. Hepatic damage may occur as part of the spectrum of shock, heat, and rhabdomyolysis which may be secondary to prolonged endurance events but is probably rare.

20. Is there a relationship between physical activity and gastrointestinal cancer?

Over the past decade, several epidemiologic studies have suggested that decreased physical activity or sedentary lifestyle is associated with an increased risk of colon cancer. Most of these studies evaluated job-related physical activity, but some have suggested that recreational aerobic activity is associated with a decreased incidence of other cancers. A small prospective trial and some animal work have also been suggestive.

Whereas the mechanisms for these changes are speculative, there have been some interesting data generated to support the hypotheses. Exercise may be associated with shortened colonic transit time, and several studies have shown that the incidence of colon cancer is reduced in people with shortened transit time. People who exercise on a regular basis frequently consume a diet higher in fiber and calories than sedentary individuals. Diets of this type are associated with a reduced gut transit time. Furthermore, data suggest that fecal bile acids, while quantitatively unchanged, are present in the stool at a lower concentration in exercising individuals. The ratio of secondary to primary fecal bile acids may be changed as well.

Colon cancer is also associated with obesity and elevated cholesterol levels which are usually reduced in populations of regular exercisers. The regular use of NSAID medications, frequently seen in habitual exercisers, has been associated with a decreased risk of colorectal cancer in some series.

21. Is exercise associated with anemia and GI bleeding?

Anemia and/or iron deficiency in athletes is probably uncommon but not rare, particularly in women athletes. Several series, in adults and children, have demonstrated anemia and iron deficiency in up to one-third of competitive athletes. **Runner's anemia** may be a pseudoanemia or artifact caused by plasma volume expansion or due to blood loss from intravascular hemolysis, hematuria, increased iron loss in sweat, decreased dietary iron intake or absorption, or GI bleeding.

GI bleeding has the greatest potential for iron loss. The incidence of GI bleeding in athletes is difficult to ascertain. Examples of acute upper or lower GI bleeding have been published as case reports or small series. A presumptive diagnosis of acute appendicitis manifested by abdominal pain in one case led to exploratory surgery, and the operative findings were consistent with ischemia.

The incidence of GI bleeding in runners has been studied by surveys and prospective collections of stool guaiac and is summarized in the table below. HemOccult positive rates of 8–85% following competitive races are demonstrated. The HemoQuant assays demonstrate increases in fecal blood loss with running and suggest that bleeding peaks 24–48 hours following the event. Bleeding probably is proportional to athletic intensity.

Studies of GI Bleeding in Marathon Runners

RACE DISTANCE	SUBJECTS	METHOD	RESULTS
Marathon	39	Post-race HemOccult	8% positive conversion
Marathon	707	Survey	1.2–2.4% report blood per rectum at times
Marathon	63	Pre/post-race HemOccult	13% positive conversion
Marathon	24	Pre/Post-race HemoQuant	Pre: 0.99 mg Hgb/gm stool
			Post: 2.25 mg Hgb/gm stool
Marathon	125	Pre/Post-race HemOccult	21% positive conversion
Marathon	32	Pre/Post-race HemOccult	22% positive conversion
100 mile Ultramarathon	34	Pre/Post race HemOccult	85% positive conversion

22. What is the source of bleeding?

Hemorrhagic gastritis is the most commonly noted endoscopic lesion associated with GI bleeding and exercise. In most cases, it is transient, resolving spontaneously within 72 hours, but may recur with repetitive stress. In one case hemorrhagic gastritis recurred in a young woman with running and resolved either with rest or with treatment with cimetidine while continuing to run. Histologic changes of submucosal hemorrhage and edema in the gastric antrum may be associated with running even in the absence of obvious endoscopic damage. The prevalence of gastric mucosal lesions associated with exercise is unknown. Prospective endoscopic surveys of runners have been inadequate to answer this question.

The second most commonly observed location of GI bleeding among athletes is the colon. Several cases have been published of presumed **ischemic colitis** following strenuous running or other athletic events and seen both endoscopically and at laparotomy. The colitis is commonly limited to the cecum and ascending colon and may be associated with ischemic and heat-related damage to other organ systems. Ischemic colitis may develop after only moderate levels of exertion, such as cycling 33 km at a nonstrenuous pace.

No instances of esophagitis or esophageal ulcer causing bleeding have been observed to date. A single case of infarction of the small bowel after running has been reported recently. Anorectal disorders, such as hemorrhoids and fissures, are common and may cause bleeding in some runners and bicyclists, although the incidence is unknown.

23. Discuss the pathophysiology of exercise-associated GI bleeding.

Ischemia is felt to be the etiology of exercise-induced hemorrhagic gastritis and colitis. Exercise induces a fall in visceral blood flow to 20–50% of baseline values. These values rival those of shock and may last for prolonged periods. During prolonged endurance events in which the athlete must eat, digestion of food increases the demand for visceral blood flow, compounding the relative decrement in blood flow caused by exercise and explaining why most ultramarathon runners convert to HemOccult positive.

Experimentally, hemorrhagic shock induces gastric mucosal damage that is mediated, in part, by gastric lumenal acid and may be prevented by acid neutralization. In one case, recurrent hemorrhagic gastritis was prevented with cimetidine. Prospective trials using cimetidine to prevent GI bleeding in runners have not been conclusive. In an initial trial, cimetidine reduced the percentage of HemOccult-positive conversion following an ultramarathon from 85% to 12.5%. Subsequent double-blinded trials using similar doses of cimetidine suggested a reduction in bleeding following marathon and ultramarathon distance races but were not statistically significant. Direct trauma to the proximal stomach from vigorous descent of the diaphragm may contribute to the observed mucosal damage.

The etiology of exercise-associated **hemorrhagic colitis** is felt by most authors to also be ischemia. The proximal colon is felt to be more susceptible to shock-induced ischemia in individuals without underlying vascular lesions. Lesions may also develop in the classic "watershed" regions of the splenic flexure and sigmoid colon, though they are less frequently noted. NSAIDs, while inconsistently associated with GI blood loss in runners, may contribute to colitis as well. It has been postulated that NSAIDs are more damaging in the face of ischemia and may exacerbate damage in runners. Runners, because of their thin bodies, may be susceptible to cecal volvulus and other forms of intra-abdominal trauma which could also cause bleeding and abdominal pain. Trauma could contribute to anal-rectal bleeding lesions.

Running and exercise are generally considered part of a healthy lifestyle. It does not confer immunity from underlying diseases that may manifest with GI bleeding. This is particularly true and more concerning if the athlete is older. Standard evaluations, such as a search for colon cancer, should be performed on individuals at risk for these diseases or any athlete who develops recurrent GI bleeding of an uncertain etiology.

24. Is there effective therapy for exercise-induced GI bleeding?

The therapy for exercise-associated GI bleeding depends to some degree on the location and severity of the bleed. Acutely, the athlete is treated as any patient presenting with GI bleeding. Most cases appear to be self-limited and resolve spontaneously upon cessation of exercise.

Some cases of **hemorrhagic gastritis** that recur repeatedly may be treated by reducing the level of exertion below symptomatic levels and gradually increasing the intensity over time, allowing the body to make appropriate adjustments. There is precedent to treat recurrent hemorrhagic gastritis with cimetidine (or presumably, an alternative H_2 receptor antagonist or omeprazole).

Treatment for **hemorrhagic colitis** is uncertain. Reduction in the level of exertion and "training through" may be successful in some. This condition appears to recur less often than the gastritis. Elemental diets may be helpful. Endurance athletes frequently use liquid meals during prolonged endurance events.

BIBLIOGRAPHY

1. Bartram HP, Wynder EL: Physical activity and colon cancer risk?: Physiological considerations. Am J Gastroenterol 84:109–112, 1989.
2. Bingham SA, Cummings JH: Effect of exercise and physical fitness on large intestinal function. Gastroenterology 97:1389–1399, 1989.
3. Brouns F, Saris WHM, Rehrer NJ: Abdominal complaints and gastrointestinal function during long-lasting exercise. Int J Sports Med 8:175–189, 1987.
4. Carrio I, Estorch M, Serra-Grima R, et al: Gastric emptying in marathon runners. Gut 30:152–155, 1989.
5. Clark CS, Kraus D, Sinclair J, Castell D: Gastroesophageal reflux induced by exercise in healthy volunteers. JAMA 261:3599–3601, 1989.
6. Clausen JP: Effective physical training on cardiovascular adjustment to exercise in man. Physiol Rev 57:779–815, 1977.

7. Cooper DT, Douglas SA, Firth LA, et al: Erosive gastritis and gastrointestinal bleeding in a female runner: Prevention of bleeding and healing of the gastritis with H2-receptor antagonist. Gastroenterology 92:2019–2023, 1987.
8. Ertan A, Schneider FE: Acute pancreatitis in long-distance runners. Am J Gastroenterol 90:70–71, 1995.
9. Feldman M, Nixon JV: The effect of exercise on post prandial gastric secretion and emptying in humans. J Appl Physiol Respir Envir Exer Physiol 53:851–854, 1982.
10. Fogoros RN: Runners trots: Gastrointestinal disturbances in runners. JAMA 243:1743–1744, 1980.
11. Holm L, Perry MA: Role of blood flow in gastric acid secretion. Am J Physiol 254:G281–G293, 1988.
12. Houmard JA, Egan PC, Johns RA, et al: Gastric emptying during 1 h of cycling and running at 75% VO_{2max}. Med Sci Sports Exer 23:320–5, 1991.
13. Kam LW, Pease WE, Thompson PD: Exercise-related mesenteric infarction. Am J Gastroenterol 89:1899–1900, 1994.
14. Kraus B, Sinclair J, Castell D: Gastroesophageal reflux in runners. Characteristics and treatment. Ann Intern Med 112:429–433, 1990.
15. Maughan RJ, Leiper JB, McGaw BA: Effects of exercise intensity on absorption of ingested fluids in man. Exp Physiol 75:419–421, 1990.
16. Moses FM: Gastrointestinal bleeding and the athlete. Am J Gastroenterol 88:1157–1159, 1993.
17. Moses FM, Baska RS, Peura DA, Deuster PA: The effect of cimetidine on marathon-associated gastrointestinal symptoms and bleeding. Dig Dis Sci 36:1390–1394, 1991.
18. Murray R: The effects of consuming carbohydrate-electrolyte beverages on gastric emptying and fluid absorption during and following exercise. Sports Med 4:322–351, 1987.
19. Neufor PD, Young AJ, Sawka MN: Gastric emptying during walking and running: Effects of varied exercise intensity. Eur J Appl Physiol 58:440–445, 1989.
20. Oettle GJ: Effect of moderate exercise on bowel habit. Gut 32:941–944, 1991.
21. Rehrer NJ, Beckers EJ, Brouns F, et al: Effects of dehydration on gastric emptying and gastrointestinal distress while running. Med Sci Sports Exer 22:790–795, 1990.
22. Sarna SK: Physiology and pathophysiology of colonic motor activity. Dig Dis Sci 36:998–1018, 1991.
23. Scobie BA: [Letter] N Z Fed Sports Med 6:31, 1978.
24. Soffer EE: Ambulatory recording of lower esophageal sphincter pressure: Adding the missing link. Gastroenterology 108:289–291, 1995.
25. Soffer EE, Merchant RK, Duethman G, et al: Effect of graded exercise on esophageal motility and gastroesophageal reflux in trained athletes. Dig Dis Sci 38:220–224, 1993.
26. Soffer EE, Wilson J, Duethman G, et al: Effect of graded exercise on esophageal motility and gastroesophageal reflux in nontrained subjects. Dig Dis Sci 39:193–198, 1994.
27. Williams JH, Mager M, Jacobson ED: Relationship of mesentric blood flow to intestinal absorption of carbohydrates. J Lab Clin Med 63:853–862, 1964.

65. FUNCTIONAL GASTROINTESTINAL DISORDERS AND IRRITABLE BOWEL SYNDROME

D. Michael Jones, M.D.

1. Why are the functional GI disorders important?

The functional GI disorders comprise a group of heterogeneous conditions that are common in most countries, from western society to the third world. Because these disorders are ubiquitous and manifest with a wide range of symptoms, patients may present to most medical and surgical specialists and to primary care providers. The cumulative cost of these disorders is enormous. Functional disorders account for about 50% of referrals to gastroenterologists.

2. What is the spectrum of functional GI symptoms?

Functional disorders may involve every segment of the GI tract, from esophagus to anorectum. Symptoms are varied and may include globus sensation, rumination, functional dyspepsia, gallbladder and/or sphincter of Oddi dysfunction with biliary type pain, and anorectal symptoms. The **irritable bowel syndrome,** which is one type of functional GI disorder, may cause abdominal pain or discomfort, altered stool frequency or consistency, abdominal bloating, difficult defecation, or increased mucus in the stools.

3. Discuss the epidemiology of functional GI disorders.

Irritable bowel syndrome (IBS) is the most common of the functional GI disorders. A national survey of 400,000 households in the United States in 1990 showed that two-thirds of the population has one or more functional GI symptoms, but most individuals do not seek medical attention. Symptoms that most often cause patients to seek care include pain and incontinence. A greater proportion of individuals seek care who have syndromes of functional chest pain, functional dyspepsia, IBS, chronic functional abdominal pain, and functional biliary pain. Conditions that occur more commonly in women include IBS, functional constipation, and functional biliary pain.

The frequency of health-care-seeking behavior for functional GI symptoms decreases with age and increases among lower-income groups. The presence of functional GI disorders is associated with more physician visits for non-GI diagnoses (e.g., headache and musculoskeletal complaints).

4. What are the potential problems in diagnosing functional GI disorders?

The medical history provides the most important information in diagnosing and classifying functional GI disorders. In IBS, the history *alone* reveals the information essential to the diagnosis—the physical findings are normal, as are laboratory and imaging studies.

Functional disorders have their basis in **abnormal physiology** (i.e., function). Anatomy (i.e., structure) is normal unless the chronic physiologic abnormality has resulted in secondary anatomic changes, such as hemorrhoids or diverticula in chronic IBS. Physicians are expert at investigating and treating anatomic disorders, because the radiographic and endoscopic imaging technologies are well-developed, but physiologic testing in the GI tract is less well developed. Thus, the diagnosis of functional disorders depends primarily on clinical (subjective) rather than laboratory (objective) data.

Finally, functional disorders are chronic and exacerbate and remit over time. Symptomatic control, rather than cure, is the focus of treatment. Because symptoms tend to recur and objective criteria for diagnosis are lacking, the diagnosis falls into question each time the patient's symptoms flare. Redundant and unnecessary workups are performed. Physicians often resist the finality and accuracy of a functional diagnosis for these reasons.

5. What causes functional gastrointestinal symptoms?

Before the 1980s, **disordered GI motility** was the usual explanation for functional symptoms. As techniques for measuring GI motility developed, it became apparent that abnormal or increased gut contractility was often not present when patients reported pain or symptoms. Conversely, when abnormal motility was recorded, patients often remained asymptomatic. The correlation between symptoms and abnormal motility is weak.

Without a motility-based explanation, theories of a **psychogenic influence** were proposed during the 1980s. However, most people who meet the criteria for irritable bowel syndrome who do *not* seek health care for their symptoms are psychologically similar to healthy controls. Psychological theories alone are insufficient to explain these disorders.

During this decade, the prevailing theory is that patients with functional symptoms have an **altered perception of nociceptive stimuli,** which they interpret as pain or other symptoms. Cultural, social, psychological, and interpersonal factors may influence their perception of pain. This theory is consistent with the biopsychosocial model of illness, in contrast to the traditional biomedical model of disease.

6. How are the functional gastrointestinal disorders classified?

Until recently, the functional GI disorders accounted for such a chaotic array of symptoms and syndromes that research efforts were impeded because study populations were ill defined and heterogeneous. In 1988, the 13th International Congress of Gastroenterology convened a panel of experts in Rome to establish criteria for the diagnosis of irritable bowel syndrome. The following year, the Second Rome Working Group classifed all functional GI disorders, proposed criteria for diagnosis, and proposed a management plan for each.

Many patients meet criteria for more than one functional disorder, and symptoms may overlap in some patients, making it difficult to classify symptoms into a single category. For example, IBS commonly coexists with functional esophageal pain or functional dyspepsia. Patients with functional disorders often present to many different medical and surgical disciplines, from cardiology to gynecology to primary care.

Functional Gastrointestinal Disorders

A. Esophageal disorders	D. Functional abdominal pain
A1. Globus	D1. Functional abdominal pain syndrome
A2. Rumination syndrome	D2. Unspecified functional abdominal pain
A3. Functional esophageal chest pain	E. Biliary disorders
A4. Functional heartburn	E1. Gallbladder dysfunction
A5. Functional dysphagia	E2. Sphincter of Oddi dysfunction
A6. Unspecified functional esophageal disorder	F. Anorectal disorders
B. Gastroduodenal disorders	F1. Functional incontinence
B1. Functional dyspepsia	F2. Functional anorectal pain
B1a. Ulcer-like dyspepsia	F2a. Levator ani syndrome
B1b. Dysmotility-like dyspepsia	F2b. Proctalgia fugax
B1c. Unspecified dyspepsia	F3. Dyschezia
B2. Aerophagia	F3a. Pelvic floor dyssynergia
C. Bowel disorders	F3b. Internal anal sphincter
C1. Irritable bowel syndrome (IBS)	dysfunction
C2. Functional abdominal bloating	F4. Unspecified functional
C3. Functional constipation	anorectal disorder
C4. Functional diarrhea	
C5. Unspecified functional bowel disorder	

7. What are symptom-based criteria? Why are they important?

Symptom-based criteria are specific groupings of symptoms that are used to diagnose and classify functional GI symptoms. Therefore, taking a **quality history** is of paramount importance. Symptom-based criteria target patient groups for management strategies based on symptoms. The outcomes of various management strategies can then be assessed from a well-defined population.

The traditional approach to patients with functional symptoms has been to perform excessive laboratory and imaging workups—not just once, but repeatedly—in patients whose problems are usually physiologic rather than anatomic. Research using symptom-based criteria allows investigators to test the predictive value of the symptom groups for identifying patients with functional disorders, to refine diagnostic and management approaches, and to minimize invasive, expensive, and unnecessary investigations.

8. What are the symptom-based criteria for diagnosis of irritable bowel syndrome?

Patients must exhibit the following criteria for at least 3 months (either continuously or recurrently):

1. Abdominal pain or discomfort that is:
   a. relieved with defecation, and/or
   b. associated with change in frequency of defecation, and/or
   c. associated with change in consistency of the stool.
2. *Plus* two or more of the following (which occur at least one-quarter of the time):
   a. altered stool frequency
   b. altered stool form (too hard, too soft)
   c. altered stool passage (straining, urgency, incomplete evacuation)
   d. passage of mucus
   e. bloating of abdominal distention

9. Describe the various clinical presentations of irritable bowel syndrome.

IBS typically exhibits two clinical patterns, cyclic and spastic. The **cyclic pattern** is most common and ranges in severity from very mild to functionally debilitating. Patients repeatedly exhibit transitions from very firm to very soft or watery stools, often with periods of urgency, abdominal pain, or bloating. Cyclicity may be irregular or variable in intensity, making the history challenging to elicit. Bowel cycles may parallel the menstrual cycle.

Spastic symptoms are probably caused by a hypercontractile, hyperreactive bowel, typically the left colon. Spastic features may be superimposed on the cyclic pattern, making these patients more challenging to diagnose and treat than the purely cyclic patients.

10. What are the special characteristics of cyclic IBS?

IBS is often described as cyclic, constipation-predominant or diarrhea-predominant. The Rome criteria categorize functional constipation and diarrhea separately from IBS.

As illustrated in the figure, during phase A of the cycle, the patient considers stool frequency and volume to be normal. During phase B, frequency and volume become sluggish. Although the term "constipation" is often used to describe this phase, it is a misnomer because patients may continue to have stools daily or every other day. The stools may become firm or scybalous, and defecation may seem incomplete. The sluggish phase may persist from 1–2 to many days.

Eventually, the sluggish phase B gives way to a rapid evacuation or "blowout" phase C, usually lasting 1–2 days. Solid stool and gas may be followed by soft or watery stool, which the patient may characterize as "diarrhea"—also a misnomer. Transient abdominal cramping may be present during phase C.

The cyclic pattern may be regular or irregular, with lengthy intervening periods of normal bowel function. The sluggish phase may be associated with upper GI satiety, intolerance of fatty foods, emotional lability, and impaired concentration. Following the blowout phase, patients anticipate variable periods of normalcy until the cycle recurs.

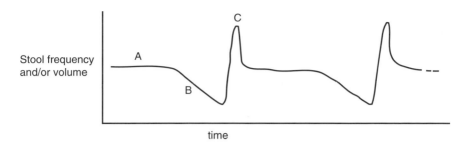

Time course of cyclic IBS.

11. What factors may exacerbate cyclic IBS?

Provocative factors include **changes** in diet, stress levels, activity level, job requirements, financial status, or family/domestic status. Cyclic IBS is better controlled with a predictable routine in daily living. Often, no provocative factors can be identified to explain deterioration in cyclic IBS. This inability to control defecatory patterns and other associated symptoms is frustrating to IBS patients, especially those with type A personalities, to whom "control" is important.

Patients should be encouraged to establish a daily routine for meals, exercise, work, social/family activities, and defecation. Reduction or elimination of highly fatty foods from the diet may help.

12. What is the treatment strategy for cyclic IBS?

In functional bowel syndromes, loose stools are a blessing, sluggish stools are a curse. . .

The goal for therapy is to reduce the variation (amplitude) of the cyclic pattern, resulting in increased regularity of defecatory patterns. Preventing the sluggish phase by adequate bulking is the primary strategy.

A **psyllium** or **methylcellulose**-based bulking agent is given daily. The osmotic action of these drugs holds water in the fecal stream, preventing hard stools and facilitating GI transit. The bulking agent should be taken within an hour of the major meal of the day or in divided doses to allow blending with the fecal stream. One to two tablespoons per day is usually sufficient, but the dose can be varied by the patient to produce a stool which is always soft and bulky. Adequate bulking *alone* is usually sufficient treatment. Bulking agents initiated during the sluggish phase often cause gastric satiety and discomfort; therefore, a laxative should be given prior to bulking in patients who are sluggish.

Occasionally, bulking agents soften the stool but do not facilitate gut transit, thereby exacerbating bloating, satiety, and pain. Such patients require periodic **laxative** use. For patients who require frequent or daily purgatives in addition to bulk, 1 pt to 1 qt of **polyethylene glycol** (PEG) solution is usually sufficient. Because the solution deteriorates after mixing, the required amount should be prepared daily.

Anticholinergic and analgesic drugs reduce gut motility and promote constipation. Although they may transiently improve pain, they aggravate the sluggish gut and should not be prescribed to patients who are inadequately bulked.

13. What symptoms suggest a spastic component to IBS?

Sigmoid colon hyperreactivity may be associated with urgency or tenesmus, desire to strain, ribbon-thin stools, left lower quadrant pain, and incomplete defecation requiring several attempts at stooling to evacuate the colon. Over time, anatomic changes may be associated with spastic IBS, including sigmoid muscular hypertrophy, hemorrhoids, and diverticuli. A prominent gastrocolic reflex may be noted by some patients, causing urgency during meals.

These symptoms tend to be alarming to some patients, causing those with spastic symptoms to seek medical attention more readily. Spastic symptoms may be clinically difficult to distinguish from distal inflammatory colitis, but the distinction is easily made by flexible sigmoidoscopy.

14. How is spastic IBS treated?

As with cyclic IBS, a standardized daily routine and bulking are helpful. Absolute avoidance of nicotine is essential. After adequate bulking, addition of spasmolytic drugs (**anticholinergics**) is appropriate, taking care to avoid constipation with higher doses. Dicyclomine (Bentyl), 20 mg at bedtime as the initial dose, is often effective. The dose can be increased to 20 mg twice daily if necessary. Once begun, spasmolytic drugs should be used consistently (daily) to prevent spasm and pain rather than sporadically in an attempt to abort painful attacks. The latter approach is generally ineffective and results in dosages that cause constipation and exacerbate symptoms.

The treatment regimen for each patient with IBS must be customized, requiring the physician to follow the thereapeutic response closely. Furthermore, both cyclic and spastic IBS patients must be educated to adjust their dose of bulking agent, laxatives, and spasmolytics as symptoms evolve. Such education requires the investment of time and patience by both physician and patient. During the initial visit, patients should be reassured that symptomatic improvement is possible; they should also be warned that there is no quick fix for IBS and that their sustained active participation in the treatment regimen is essential.

15. How intensive a workup should the IBS patient undergo?

The workup in patients with typical cyclic or spastic IBS should follow a "minimalist" approach. The diagnosis of IBS is made on symptom-based criteria rather than an exhaustive exclusionary workup.

Patients under age 35 who have a good response to treatment require no further investigation. Complete blood count and flexible sigmoidoscopy should complete the workup in patients aged 35 and older who have a good response to treatment and in all patients who respond incompletely to treatment.

Additional investigations are appropriate in patients who have symptoms or signs atypical for IBS. Weight loss and anemia necessitate at least imaging of the bowel and thyroid function testing. Persistent loose stools require investigations for infectious and inflammatory etiologies. Troublesome bloating warrants a search for giardia and lactose intolerance.

Whatever the initial workup entails, once the diagnosis of IBS is made, it should be viewed as *final*, not tentative. Repetitious imaging of the GI tract for recurrent exacerbations of functional symptoms rarely reveals anatomic abnormalities.

16. Are additional considerations necessary in patients with constipation-predominant or diarrhea-predominant functional disorders?

Patients with **functional constipation** are often the most difficult to treat. They have usually seen many physicians, may be frustrated or angry, and are often manipulative. Several weeks may pass between stooling events, resulting in bloating and pain with palpable stool in the colon. Confirmation of functional constipation may be achieved using radiopaque markers.

The initial step in this treatment is vigorous and complete purging of the patient. Several polyethylene glycol (PEG) purges on successive days may be required. Bulking agents alone are ineffective, and daily PEG solution is usually required for maintenace therapy. Spasmolytic and analgesic drugs that reduce colonic motility are best avoided in this group. Despite some reports to the contrary, these patients respond poorly to segmental colon resection. The role of the physician should be to encourage the patient, develop a regimen that facilitates evacuation, and keep the patient off the operating table.

Diarrhea-predominant IBS requires an exlusionary workup for causes of chronic diarrhea. True functional diarrhea often responds well to tricyclic or other antidepressant medications.

17. What is the prognosis for functional GI disorders and IBS?

Long-term prognosis depends on the specific functional disorder diagnosed. In general, patients with functional abdominal pain are the most difficult to treat and have more frequent encounters with health care providers. Some anorectal disorders may also cause pain or troublesome incontinence that is difficult to control.

IBS can be effectively managed, and most patients can be restored to full function with minimal debility. Prognosis is heavily dependent on the knowledge and skill of health care providers in recognizing IBS and approaching management methodically.

BIBLIOGRAPHY

1. Drossman DA, et al: Identification of subgroups of functional bowel disorders. Gastroenterol Int 3:159, 1990.
2. Drossman DA: Psychosocial factors in the care of patients with gastrointestinal diseases. In Yamada T (ed): Textbook of Gastroenterology. Philadelphia, J.B. Lippincott, 1991, 546–561.
3. Drossman DA, Thompson WG: The irritable bowel syndrome: Review and a graduated multicomponent treatment approach. Ann Intern Med 116:1009, 1992.
4. Drossman DA, et al: U.S. householder survey of functional GI disorders: Prevalence, sociodemography and health impact. Dig Dis Sci 38:1569, 1993.
5. Drossman DA, et al (eds): The Functional Gastrointestinal Disorders. Boston, Little, Brown, 1994.
6. Thompson WG: Irritable bowel syndrome. In Bayless TM (ed): Current Therapy in Gastroenterology and Liver Disease, 4th ed. St. Louis, Mosby, 1994, 205–209.

66. ENDOSCOPIC CANCER SCREENING AND SURVEILLANCE

Scot M. Lewey, D.O., and Peter R. McNally, D.O.

ESOPHAGUS

1. What is the risk of esophageal cancer in patients with achalasia?

A long-term follow-up study of patients with achalasia has reported the incidence of esophageal cancer to be 7%. The pathogenesis of esophageal cancer in these patients is unknown, but chronic stastis is believed to play a role. The mean interval between diagnosis of achalasia to the development of cancer is 17 years. When cancer occurs, 90% are of the squamous cell type, and the remainder are adenocarcinomas. The risk for malignancy is not completely eliminated by medical or surgical treatment of the achalasia. Esophageal cancer is usually far advanced before obstruction of the dilated esophagus occurs and symptoms manifest; hence, the 5-year survival is <5%.

2. Can endoscopic surveillance detect early esophageal cancer in patients with long-standing achalasia?

Yes, and there are examples of long-term survival after surgery. The recommended schedule for endoscopic surveillance begins 15–20 years after initial symptoms or 10–15 years after medical or surgical treatment. The esophagus should be cleaned of debris prior to endoscopic examination. Surface abnormalities of the esophagus should be biopsied. Generally, endoscopic surveillance should not be conducted more frequently than every 1–3 years.

3. What is the malignant potential of Barrett's esophagus?

Barrett's esophagus is a premalignant condition with a reported cancer prevalence of 10–40%. Endoscopic screening studies suggest the cancer incidence of 1 in 52 to 175 patient-years. Surgical and medical treatment of gastroesophageal reflux has not been shown to reduce the incidence of cancer.

4. What are the clinical determinants of relative risk for carcinoma in patients with Barrett's esophagus?

Only specialized, "intestinal-type" Barrett's epithelium is associated with risk for adenocarcinoma. Cancer may develop in Barrett's segments of any length, but patients with segments of metaplasia ≥6 cm in length appear to be at greater risk. Histologic evidence of high-grade dysplasia is a good indicator for cancer risk.

A histologic classification consisting of high-grade dysplasia (HGD), low-grade dysplasia (LGD)/indefinite, and no dysplasia is a useful and reproducible system, with an 86% interobserver agreement among expert pathologists for the diagnosis of HGD. Collective reports show a high correlation between HGD and carcinoma (32% of resected specimens). The significance of LGD is uncertain.

Because foci of HGD and cancer may be small and scattered throughout the Barrett's segment, their detection requires extensive surveillance biopsies. Quadrant sampling of the metaplastic segment at 2-cm intervals is recommended. Exfoliative brush cytology may be especially helpful when less rigorous surveillance biopsies are obtained.

Changes in mucosal DNA content as detected by flow cytometry may provide useful information in the surveillance of Barrett's esophagus, but the technique is demanding, expensive, and still under evaluation. The role of endoscopic ultrasound in Barrett's patients is unknown.

5. Outline the recommendations for endoscopic surveillance in patients with Barrett's esophagus.

An extensive endoscopic cancer surveillance program for Barrett's esophagus is most appropriate for those patients considered to be candidates for surgical cure if HGD or cancer is found.

Index endoscopy: Aggressive antireflux therapy should be initiated before a surveillance program is begun, due to the difficulty in distinguishing inflammatory dysplasia from neoplasia. Extensive sampling of the entire Barrett's segment should be performed, particularly of any areas with macroscopic abnormalities. A proven method involves quadrant biopsies with large particle forceps taken at 2-cm intervals starting 1 cm below the esophagogastric junction and extending to 1 cm above the squamocolumnar junction. Additional management should be guided by the histologic findings, as follows:

Cancer	Review biopsies with an experienced pathologist.
	If the histologic diagnosis is confirmed and the patient is a surgical candidate, then recommend operation after complete staging. If the histologic diagnosis is uncertain, then urgent rebiopsy.
High-grade dysplasia	Review biopsies with an expert pathologist.
	If the diagnosis is confirmed and there is no endoscopic esophagitis or histologic inflammatory atypia, then recommend surgery for the "fit" patient. If the surgical risk is considered excessive, then frequent endoscopic surveillance should be performed.
	If esophagitis or inflammatory atypia is considered responsible for the dysplasia, then institute aggressive antisecretory therapy for 4–8 weeks and repeat surveillance biopsies.
Low-grade dysplasia indefinite	Review biopsies with an expert pathologist.
	If the histologic diagnosis is confirmed and there is no endoscopic esophagitis or histologic inflammatory atypia, then surveillance biopsies every 12 months.
	If "indefinite" due to extensive inflammatory atypia, then institute aggressive antisecretory therapy for 8–12 weeks and repeat surveillance biopsies.
No dysplasia	Serial endoscopy with surveillance biopsies every 24 months.
	A shorter (12-month) surveillance period is reasonable in patients with long-segment Barrett's ≥6 cm.

6. What is the risk of esophageal cancer in patients with a prior history of caustic ingestion?

The risk has been estimated to be 1000 times greater than the risk in the general population. The cumulative results of four series have characterized the findings associated with lye-related esophageal cancer:

- Mean age at onset of cancer, 47 years
- Interval from caustic ingestion to development of cancer, 14–47 years (mean, 40 yrs)
- Location of cancers, mostly mid-esophagus

Malignancy appears to develop after a shorter interval if the corrosive injury occurs later in life. The periesophageal fibrosis caused by the corrosive injury decreases esophageal compliance, and therefore, cancer usually presents at an earlier stage. The resectability rate and 5-year survival for lye-associated esophageal carcinoma are 85% and 33%, respectively.

7. How frequently is endoscopic surveillance needed in patients with a prior history of caustic ingestion?

Begin endoscopic surveillance 15–20 years after the caustic ingestion. Generally, endoscopic examination should not be conducted more frequently than every 1–3 years. The threshold to evaluate swallowing problems with endoscopy should be low.

8. What is tylosis? What is the risk for esophageal malignancy?
Tylosis is an uncommon genetic disorder characterized by hyperkeratosis of the palms and soles. It is transmitted in an autosomal dominant pattern and associated with a predisposition for development of esophageal cancer. The prevalence of esophageal cancer in patients with tylosis can be >90% by 65 years of age. Death from esophageal cancer has been reported in tylosis patients as young as 30 years. A prospective endoscopic surveillance program has been initiated for a large family cohort in England.

9. Give the recommendations for endoscopic surveillance for patients with tylosis.
Start surveillance endoscopy at 30 years of age. Symptoms of dysphagia or swallowing difficulties should be evaluated promptly. Generally, endoscopic examination should not be conducted more frequently than every 1–3 years.

STOMACH AND SMALL BOWEL

10. What is the risk for malignancy among patients with gastric polyps?
In America, gastric polyps are uncommon. The risk of malignant transformation of a gastric polyp depends on the polyp histology. Most gastric polyps (70–90%) are hyperplastic, and their risk for malignant transformation is low (<4.0%). Adenomatous gastric polyps are true neoplams, and their risk for malignant transformation is as high as ~ 75%. Fundic gland polyps have no malignant potential but may suggest the diagnosis of familial polyposis syndrome and the need for ampullary and lower GI endoscopic surveillance.

11. What are the recommendations for endoscopic surveillance for patients with gastric polyps?
Begin surveillance endoscopy 1 year after removing all gastric polyps, evaluating for recurrence and new or previously missed polyps. If this exam is negative, then surveillance endoscopy should be repeated no more frequently than at 3–5 year intervals for patients with adenomatous polyps.

12. Who is at risk for ampullary and small bowel adenomas and frank malignancy?
In familial polyposis syndromes, the relative risk of duodenal adenocarcinoma and ampullary carcinoma is increased. Adenomatous changes and carcinoma have been reported in the ampulla and in the lower pancreatic and bile ducts. Adenomatous change of the ampulla may not be endoscopically apparent. Periampullary adenomas have a high risk of dysplasia. No treatment has been shown to be effective in reducing adenomas, although the efficacy of ablative therapy or chemotherapy using sulindac is under investigation. Although prophylactic duodenectomy has been considered, a risk/benefit analysis has not been done. Endoscopy therefore is necessary for detection of polyps and surveillance for dysplasia.

13. What endoscopic surveillance of the upper GI tract is necessary in patients with familial polyposis syndrome?
Once familial polyposis syndrome is diagnosed, periodic surveillance endoscopy should be initiated with both an end-viewing and side-viewing instrument. Antral lesions and duodenal polyps should be biopsied. Endoscopic retrograde cholangiopancreatography should be considered when the ampulla appears deformed or abnormal. Recognition of high-grade dysplasia necessitates further therapy, although the type of therapy is not fully defined yet. Studies are needed to ascertain the effectiveness of therapeutic programs such as sulindac, ablative polypectomy, and possibly, more extensive surgical procedures.

14. What is the risk for malignancy in the gastric remnant after gastrectomy surgery (gastric stump carcinoma)?
Gastric stump carcinoma is defined as carcinoma arising from the gastric remnant at least 5 years after surgery for benign disease. Cumulative analysis of over 50 studies indicates a two- to four-

fold increased incidence of gastric carcinoma beginning 15 years after the original surgery. Endoscopic surveillance studies have detected gastric stump carcinoma in 4–6% of these patients, and the progression from dysplasia to cancer has been shown to occur. Symptoms are an unreliable predictor of early gastric cancer, and multiple random biopsies are necessary to identify dysplasia, as the macroscopic abnormalities may be inapparent. The mean interval between gastric surgery and cancer is ~ 20 years. The variation in the reporting of gastric cancer risk among patients with pernicious anemia may be due to exposure to dietary nitrosamines, genetic factors, *Helicobacter pylori* infection, and/or alcohol and tobacco use.

15. How frequently should these patients undergo endoscopic surveillance for stump carcinoma?
Initiate surveillance endoscopy 15–20 years after gastric surgery. Multiple biopsies should be taken and examined for dysplasia. Periodic endoscopic surveillance every 1–3 years is reasonable. When mucosal dysplasia is identified, more frequent surveillance is indicated.

16. Is there risk for gastric carcinoma among patients with pernicious anemia?
Yes. Pernicious anemia (PA) is associated with type A gastritis and is thought to arise from chronic autoimmune injury to the gastric mucosa. The reported incidence of gastric cancer in patients with PA ranges from 2–10%. The coincidence of gastric polyps and PA is common. A study of 152 Minnesota residents with PA documented only a single case of gastric cancer during a 30-year period and tempered the enthusiasm for surveillance endoscopy; however, a recent, large population-based cohort study in Sweden and a retrospective study of over 30,000 veterans identified the subsequent risk of gastric malignancy after the diagnosis of PA to be increased by at least two-fold. Curiously, the gastric malignancy usually occurred within 1–2 years from initial diagnosis of PA.

17. Give the recommendations for endoscopic surveillance in patients with pernicious anemia.
Surveillance endoscopy is not currently recommended for these patients. However, index endoscopy at the time of the diagnosis of PA to evaluate for other risk factors for gastric cancer, such as gastric polyps, is appropriate.

COLON

18. After removal of an adenomatous colorectal polyp, how often should surveillance colonoscopy be performed?
After endoscopic resection of a large (>2 cm) polyp, multiple polyps (5), or any villous adenomas, colonoscopy should be repeated after 1 year, and thereafter at 3–5 year intervals unless large, multiple, or villous adenomatous polyps are identified.

When colon preparation is poor or large polyps are removed by piecemeal technique, it is prudent to reexamine the colon at 1 year or at 3–6 months, respectively. When no polyps are detected at the 3-year anniversary, the interval between colonoscopic surveillance examinations may be lengthened to 5 years.

These recommendations are based on the results of several studies that have shown the likelihood of finding cancer in individuals undergoing colonoscopy 1–3 years after adenoma removal is very low, even though the yield for detection of adenomas is approximately 30% (range, 12–60%). The polyps found at follow-up, however, tend to be small (<1 cm) and unlikely to have high-grade dysplasia or invasive cancer. Further support for these recommendations is provided by the results of the National Polyp Study, which demonstrated that colonoscopy performed 3 years after removal of adenomatous polyps was just as effective for detecting important colonic neoplasia as colonoscopy at 1 and 3 years. Surveillance colonoscopy with removal of adenomatous polyps does reduce the incidence of and mortality from colorectal cancer and therefore should be offered to patients with colorectal adenomas.

19. What is the recommendation for colonoscopic surveillance for a patient who has undergone resection of colorectal cancer?
Prior to resection, the yield for synchronous colorectal cancer and adenomatous polyps at initial clearing colonoscopy is ~ 2% and 25%, respectively. If a clearing colonoscopy was performed

preoperatively, then the yield of surveillance colonoscopy performed 6 months to 2 years after resection is 2–3% for anastomotic recurrence, 3–4% for metachronous cancer, and 25–33% for adenomas (similar to postadenoma removal). Colonoscopy should be performed 1 year from the date of surgery and repeated at 3–5-year intervals thereafter.

20. Patients with long-standing ulcerative colitis have a markedly increased risk for the development of colorectal cancer over the general population. What are the current recommendations for colonoscopic surveillance?

The risk for colorectal cancer in patients with ulcerative colitis is estimated to be 6–15 times greater than that of the general population. The risk increases significantly after 8–10 years of pancolitis or >14 years of left-sided colitis. The yield for cancer or high-grade dysplasia on initial colonoscopic surveillance in long-standing ulcerative colitis may be as high as 12% and 8%, respectively.

After 8–10 years of pancolitis and 15 years of left-sided colitis, surveillance colonoscopy should be performed annually. Neoplasia and dysplasia are often not endoscopically evident, and hence random biopsies are taken from the cecum to the rectum, >4 biopsies for every 10-cm segment, and examined histologically. Any abnormal areas of mucosa or mass lesions should also be biopsied. It has been estimated that approximately 64 biopsies are needed to accurately detect the highest grade of dysplasia with a 95% probability. Weinstein has recommended taking 4 biopsies every 10 cm to the sigmoid, then every 5 cm to the rectum.

21. Describe the management strategies according to histologic findings.

Cancer	Review biopsies with an experienced pathologist. If the histologic diagnosis is confirmed and the patient is a surgical candidate, then recommend proctocolectomy after complete staging. If the histologic diagnosis is uncertain, then urgent rebiopsy.
High-grade dysplasia (HGD)	Review biopsies with an expert pathologist. If the diagnosis is confirmed, then recommend surgery.
Dysplasia-associated lesion or mass (DALM)	Proctocolectomy is recommended when DALM is identified, because the risk for malignancy is estimated at >50%.
Low-grade dysplasia (LGD)/indefinite	Review biopsies with an expert pathologist. If the histologic diagnosis is confirmed and there is no endoscopic colitis or histologic inflammatory atypia, then consider colectomy or more intensive surveillance biopsies every 3–6 months.
No dysplasia	Serial endoscopy with surveillance biopsies every 12 months.

22. What about the risk of colorectal cancer among patients with Crohn's disease? Should these patients undergo an endoscopic surveillance program?

There appears to be an increased risk of colorectal cancer in Crohn's disease as well, about six times that of the general population. When Crohn's disease is confined to the ileum, the colorectal cancer risk appears to be similar to that of the general population. The current recommendations are less firmly established than those for ulcerative colitis. Biannual colonoscopy with multiple biopsies after 10 years of disease is reasonable.

23. What are the colorectal surveillance recommendations for patients with familial adenomatous polyposis syndromes?

Familial adenomatous polyposis is an autosomal dominant trait with universal penetrance. In persons inheriting this gene, the colon is often "carpeted" with hundreds to thousands of polyps by the age of 10 years. Annual sigmoidoscopic surveillance is initiated at age 10–12 years, and when any polyps are identified, full colonoscopy is recommended. Once multiple adenomas are documented, then colectomy is recommended.

24. For hereditary colorectal cancer, what are the recommendations for surveillance?

Lynch syndrome I, also known as hereditary nonpolyposis colorectal cancer (HNPCC), is characterized by an autosomally inherited predisposition to colorectal cancer. Lynch syndrome II, also known as family cancer syndrome, is characterized by an autosomally inherited risk for several cancers, including colorectal cancer. In both Lynch syndromes, colorectal cancer develops at a much younger age than do sporadic colon cancers occurring in the general population. These tumors also are more commonly found in the right colon.

Colonoscopy is recommended every 2–3 years beginning 10–15 years earlier than the youngest age of cancer development in a relative with colon cancer or beginning at age 20 if this information is not known. For individuals with a single first-degree relative with colorectal cancer diagnosed at > age 60 years, the risk may be equal to the general population's and may not support more than standard screening recommendations (annual fecal occult blood test and flexible sigmoidoscopy every 3–5 years), but beginning at age 40 instead of 50. For those whose first-degree relative developed colorectal cancer below age 50–55 years or those with multiple affected first-degree relatives, then colonoscopy every 3–5 years is recommended.

BIBLIOGRAPHY

1. Aggestrup S, Holm JC, Sorensen IIR: Does achalasia predispose to cancer of the esophagus? Chest 102:1013–1016, 1992.
2. Appleqvist P, Salmo M: Lye corrosion carcinoma of the esophagus. Cancer 45:2655, 1980.
3. Armbrecht U, Stockbrugger RW, Rode J, et al: Development of gastric dysplasia in pernicious anemia: A clinical endoscopic follow up study of 80 patients. Gut 31:1105–1109, 1990.
4. Bigelow NH: Carcinoma of the esophagus developing at the site of lye stricture. Cancer 6:1159, 1953.
5. Bond JH: Polyp guideline: Diagnosis, treatment, and surveillance for patients with nontamilial colorectal polyps. Ann Intern Med 119:836–843, 1993.
6. Chuong JJH, DuBovik S, McCallum RW. Achalasia as a risk factor for esophageal carcinoma: A reappraisal. Dig Dis Sci 29:1105–1108, 1984.
7. Dent TL, Kukora JS, Buinewicz BR: Endoscopic screening and surveillance for gastrointestinal malignancy. Surg Endosc 69:1205–1225, 1989.
8. Dent J, Bremmer CG, Collen MJ, et al: Barrett's oesophagus: Working Party Reports of World Congress of Gastroenterology. Melbourne, Blackwell Scientific, 1990, pp 17–26.
9. Eckardt VF, Junginger T, Gabbert HE, Bettendorf U: Superficial esophageal carcinoma in achalasia, detected by endoscopic surveillance. Z Gastroenterol 30:411–414, 1992.
10. Fleischer DE, Goldberg SB, Browning TH, et al: Detection and surveillance of colorectal cancer. JAMA 261:580–585, 1989.
11. Ginsberg G, Al-kawas F, Fleischer D, et al: Should all gastric polyps be removed? Am J Gastroenterol 87:1268, 1992.
12. Hameeteman W, Tytgat GNJ, Houthoff HJ, Van Den Tweel JG: Barrett's esophagus: Development of dysplasia and adenocarcinoma. Gastroenterol 96:1249–1256, 1989.
13. Hopkins RA, Postlethwait RW: Caustic burns and carcinoma of the esophagus. Ann Surg 194:146–148, 1982.
14. Howel-Evans W, McConnell RR, Clarke CA, Sheppard PM: Carcinoma of the esophagus with keratosis palmaris et tylosis (tylosis). Q J Med 27:413–429, 1958.
15. Hsing AW, Hansson LE, McLaughlin JK, et al: Pernicious anemia and subsequent cancer: A population-based cohort study. Cancer 71:745–750, 1993.
16. Jagelman DG, Petras RE, Sivak MV, McGannon E: Gastric and duodenal polyps in familial adenomatous polyposis: A prospective study of the nature and prevalence of upper gastrointestinal polyps. Gut 28:306–314, 1987.
17. Johan G, Offerhaus A, Giardiello M, et al: The risk of upper gastrointestinal cancer in familial adenomatous polyposis. Gastroenterol 102:1980–1982, 1992.
18. Just-Viera JO, Haight C: Achalasia and carcinoma of the esophagus. Surg Gynecol Obstet 128:1081–1095, 1969.
19. Leape LL, Ashcraft KW, Scarpelli DG, et al: Hazard to health—liquid lye. N Engl J Med 248:232–235, 1971.

20. Levine DS, Haggitt RC, Blount PL, et al: An endoscopic biopsy protocol can differentiate high-grade dysplasia from early adenocarcinoma in Barrett's esophagus. Gastroenterol 105:40–50, 1993.

21. Luk GD: Cancer surveillance strategies. In: Sleisenger MH, Fordtran JS, eds: Gastronintestinal Disease: Pathophysiology, diagnosis, management. Philadelphia, WB Saunders, 1993, pp 115–126.

22. Marger RS and Marger D. Carcinoma of the esophagus and tylosis: A lethal genetic combination. Cancer 72:17–9, 1993.

23. Morson BC, Sobin LH, Grundmann E, et al: Precancerous conditions and epithelial dysplasia in the stomach. J Clin Pathol 33:711–721, 1980.

24. Peracchia A, Segalin A, Bardini R, et al: Esophageal carcinoma and achalasia: Prevalance, incidence and results of treatment. Hepatogastroenterology 38:514–516, 1991.

25. Reid BJ, Haggitt RC, Rubin CE, et al: Criteria for dysplasia in Barrett's esophagus: A cooperative consensus study. Gastroenterol 88:1552A, 1985.

26. Reid BJ, Weinstein WM, Lewin KJ, et al: Endoscopic biopsy can detect high-grade dysplasia or early carcinoma in Barrett's esophagus without grossly recognizable neoplastic lesions. Gastroenterol 94:81–90, 1988.

27. Schafer LW, Larson DE, Melton LJ III, et al: The risk of gastric cancer after surgical treatment for benign disease. N Engl J Med 309:1210–1213, 1983.

28. Schafer LW, Larson DE, Melton LJ III, et al: Risk of development of gastric carcinoma in patients with pernicious anemia: A population based study in Rochester, Minnesota. Mayo Clin Proc 60:444–448, 1985.

29. Schnell T, Sontag S, Chejfec G, et al: Does length of Barrett's esophagus (BE) correlate with age, cigarette or alcohol consumption, or risk of adenocarcinoma (AdCa). Gastroenterology 98:120A, 1990.

30. Sjoblom SM, Sipponen P, Jarvinen H: Gastroscopic follow up of pernicious anemia patients. Gut 34:28–32, 1993.

31. Sonnenberg A, Massey BT, McCarty DJ, Jacobsen SJ: Epidemiology of hospitalization for achalasia in the United States. Dig Dis Sci 38:233–244, 1993.

32. Spechler SJ: Endoscopic surveillance for patients with Barrett's esophagus: Does the risk justify the practice. Ann Intern Med 106:902–904, 1987.

33. Stalnikowicz R, Benbassat J: Risk of gastric cancer after gastric surgery for benign disorders. Arch Intern Med 150:2022–2026, 1990.

34. Talley NJ, Zinsmeister AR, Weaver A, et al: Gastric adenocarcinoma and *Helicobacter pylori* infection. JNCI 83:1734–1739, 1991.

35. Winawer SJ, Zauber AG, O'Brien MJ, et al: Randomized comparison of surveillance intervals after colonoscopic removal of newly diagnosed adenomatous polyps. N Engl J Med 328:901–906, 1993.

36. Wychulis AR, Woolman GL, Anderson HA, Ellis FH Jr: Achalasia and carcinoma of the esophagus. JAMA 215:1638–1641, 1971.

67. RHEUMATOLOGIC MANIFESTATIONS OF GASTROINTESTINAL DISEASES

Sterling G. West, M.D.

ENTEROPATHIC ARTHRITIS

1. What bowel diseases are associated with inflammatory arthritis?
- Idiopathic inflammatory bowel disease (ulcerative colitis, Crohn's disease), pouchitis
- Microscopic colitis and collagenous colitis
- Infectious gastroenteritis
- Whipple's disease
- Gluten-sensitive enteropathy (celiac disease)
- Intestinal bypass arthritis

2. How often does an inflammatory peripheral or spinal arthritis occur in patients with idiopathic inflammatory bowel disease?

	ULCERATIVE COLITIS	CROHN'S DISEASE
Peripheral arthritis	10%	20%
Sacroiliitis	15%	15%
Sacroiliitis/spondylitis	5%	5%

3. What are the most common joints involved in ulcerative colitis and Crohn's disease patients with an inflammatory peripheral arthritis?

Upper extremity and small joint involvement is more common in ulcerative colitis than

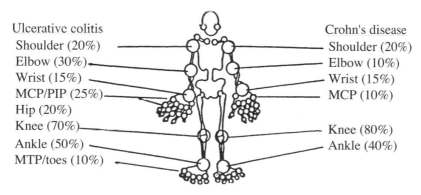

Ulcerative colitis
Shoulder (20%)
Elbow (30%)
Wrist (15%)
MCP/PIP (25%)
Hip (20%)
Knee (70%)
Ankle (50%)
MTP/toes (10%)

Crohn's disease
Shoulder (20%)
Elbow (10%)
Wrist (15%)
MCP (10%)
Knee (80%)
Ankle (40%)

Crohn's disease. Both ulcerative colitis- and Crohn's-related arthritis affect the knee and ankle predominantly.

4. Describe the clinical characteristics of the inflammatory peripheral arthritis associated with idiopathic inflammatory bowel disease (IBD).

The arthritis occurs equally in males and females, and children are affected as often as adults. The arthritis is typically acute in onset, migratory, and asymmetric, and it usually involves <5 joints (i.e., pauciarticular). Synovial fluid analysis reveals an inflammatory fluid with up to 50,000 WBC/mm^3 (predominantly neutrophils) and negative findings on crystal examination and cultures. Most arthritic episodes resolve in 1–2 months and do not result in radiographic changes or deformities.

5. What other extraintestinal manifestations commonly occur in patients with idiopathic IBD and inflammatory peripheral arthritis?

　　*P*yoderma gangrenosum (< 5%)
　　*A*phthous stomatitis (< 10%)
　　*I*nflammatory eye disease (acute anterior uveitis) (5–15%)
　　*N*odosum, erythema (< 10%)

6. Do the extent and activity of IBD correlate with the activity of the peripheral inflammatory arthritis?

Patients with ulcerative colitis and Crohn's disease are more likely to develop a peripheral arthritis if the colon is extensively involved. Most arthritic attacks occur during the first few years following onset of the bowel disease. The episodes coincide with flares of bowel disease in 60–70% of patients. Occasionally, the arthritis may precede symptoms of IBD, especially in children with Crohn's disease. Consequently, lack of GI symptoms and even a negative stool quaiac test does not exclude the possibility of occult Crohn's disease in a patient who presents with a characteristic arthritis!

7. What are the clinical characteristics of the inflammatory spinal arthritis occurring in idiopathic IBD?

The clinical characteristics and course of spinal arthritis in IBD are similar to those of ankylosing spondylitis. Inflammatory spinal arthritis occurs more commonly in males than females (3:1). Patients complain of back pain and prolonged stiffness, particularly at night and upon waking. This pain and stiffness improve with exercise and movement. Physical examination reveals sacroiliac joint tenderness, global loss of spinal motion, and, sometimes, reduced chest expansion.

8. Which points in the history and physical examination are helpful in separating inflammatory spinal arthritis from mechanical low back pain in an IBD patient?

On the basis of history and physical examination, 95% of patients with inflammatory spinal arthritis can be differentiated from patients with mechanical low back pain.

Clinical Differentiation of Inflammatory Spinal Arthritis (SA)
and Mechanical Low Back Pain (LBP)

	INFLAMMATORY SA	MECHANICAL LBP
Onset of pain	Insidious	Acute
Duration of morning stiffness	> 60 min	< 30 min
Night-time pain	Yes	Infrequent
Exercise effect on pain	Improvement	Worsen
Sacroiliac joint tenderness	Usually	No
Range of back motion	Global loss of motion	Abnormal flexion
Reduced chest expansion	Sometimes	No
Neurologic deficits	No	Possible
Duration of symptoms	> 3 mos	< 4 wks

9. Does the activity of inflammatory spinal arthritis correlate with the activity of the IBD?

No. The onset of sacroiliitis or spondylitis can precede by years, occur concurrently, or follow by years the onset of the inflammatory bowel disease. Furthermore, the course of the spinal arthritis is completely independent of the course of IBD.

10. What human leukocyte antigen (HLA) occurs more commonly than expected with inflammatory arthritis secondary to IBD?

Frequency of HLA B27 in Inflammatory Bowel Disease

	CROHN'S	ULCERATIVE COLITIS
Sacroiliitis/spondylitis	55%	70%
Peripheral arthritis	Same as normal healthy control population	Same as normal healthy control population

Eight percent of normal healthy whites have the HLA B27 gene. Thus, a patient with IBD who possesses the HLA B27 gene has a 7–10 times increased risk of developing inflammatory sacroiliitis or spondylitis compared to IBD patients who are HLA B27-negative.

11. Describe the typical radiographic features of inflammatory sacroiliitis and spondylitis in IBD patients.

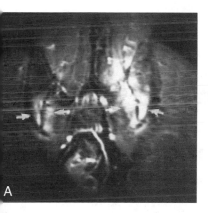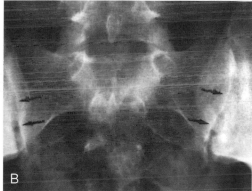

Figure 1. **A,** MR image of the sacroiliac joints showing inflammation (*arrows*) (T2-weighted image, TE50, R 2500). **B,** Radiograph showing early bilateral sacroiliitis (*arrows*).

The radiographic abnormalities in IBD patients with inflammatory spinal arthritis are similar to those seen in ankylosing spondylitis. Patients with early inflammatory **sacroiliitis** frequently have normal plain radiographs. In these patients, magnetic resonance (MR) imaging of the sacroiliac joints demonstrates inflammation and edema. Over several months to years, patients develop sclerosis and erosions in the lower two-thirds of the sacroiliac joint. Some patients may completely fuse these joints.

Patients with early **spondylitis** may also have normal radiographs. Later, radiographs may show "shiny corners" at the insertion of the annulus fibrosis, anterior squaring of the vertebrae, and syndesmophyte formation (*see* Figure 2). Syndesmophytes are thin, marginal, and bilateral. Some patients also show fusing of their facet joints and calcification of their supraspinous ligament.

12. What is a "bamboo" spine?

Bamboo spine describes the radiographic appearance of a spine that demonstrates bilateral syndesmophytes traversing the entire spine (lumbar, thoracic, and cervical) (*see* Figure 2B). This occurs in only 10% of patients with sacroiliitis or spondylitis. Patients who develop inflammatory hip disease may be at increased risk for subsequently developing a bamboo spine.

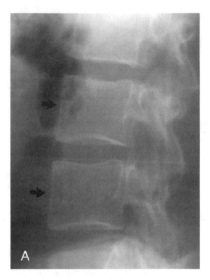
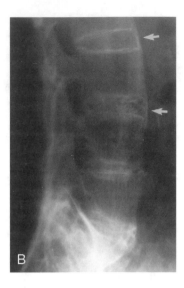

Figure 2. **A,** Radiograph showing anterior squaring of the vertebrae in a patient with early inflammatory spondylitis. **B,** Radiograph showing thin, marginal syndesmophytes (*arrows*) causing bamboo spine in a patient with Crohn's disease with advanced inflammatory spondylitis.

13. What other rheumatic problems occur with increased frequency in IBD patients?
- Achilles tendinitis/plantar fasciitis
- Clubbing of fingernails (5%)
- Hypertrophic osteoarthropathy
- Psoas abscess or septic hip from fistula formation (Crohn's disease)
- Osteoporosis secondary to medications (i.e., prednisone)
- Vasculitis
- Amyloidosis

14. Can treatment alleviate the symptoms of inflammatory peripheral arthritis and/or spinal arthritis in IBD patients?

	PERIPHERAL ARTHRITIS	SACROILIITIS/SPONDYLITIS
NSAIDS	Yes	Yes
Intra-articular corticosteroids	Yes	Yes (sacroiliitis)
Sulfasalazine	Yes	Maybe
Immunosuppressives	Yes	No
Bowel resection		
Ulcerative colitis	Yes	No
Crohn's disease	No	No

Nonsteroidal anti-inflammatory drugs (NSAIDs) may exacerbate IBD.

15. What rheumatic disorders are associated with pouchitis, microscopic (lymphocytic) colitis (MC), and/or collagenous colitis (CC)?

	POUCHITIS	MC	CC
IBD-like peripheral inflammatory arthritis	Yes	Yes	Yes (10%)
Rheumatoid arthritis	No	Yes	Yes
Ankylosing spondylitis	No	Yes*	No
Thyroiditis/other autoimmune disease	No	Yes	Yes

*Up to 50% of patients with ankylosing spondylitis have asymptomatic MC/Crohn's-like lesions on right-sided colon biopsies.

Controversy

16. Why are patients with IBD more prone to develop an inflammatory arthritis?
Environmental antigens capable of inciting rheumatic disorders enter the body's circulation by traversing the respiratory mucosa, skin, or GI mucosa. The human GI tract has an estimated surface area of 1000 m^2 and functions not only to absorb nutrients but also to exclude potentially harmful antigens. The gut-associated lymphoid tissue (GALT), which includes Peyer's patches, the lamina propria, and intraepithelial T cells, constitutes 25% of the GI mucosa and helps to exclude entry of bacteria and other foreign antigens. Although the upper GI tract is normally not exposed to microbes, the lower GI tract is constantly in contact with millions of bacteria (up to 10^{12}/g of feces).

Inflammation, whether from idiopathic inflammatory bowel disease or from infection with pathogenic microorganisms, can disrupt the normal integrity and function of the bowel, leading to increased gut permeability. This increased permeability may allow **nonviable bacterial antigens** in the gut lumen to enter the circulation more easily. These microbial antigens could either deposit directly in the joint synovia, leading to a local inflammatory reaction, or cause a systemic immune response, resulting in immune complexes that then deposit in joints and other tissues.

REACTIVE ARTHRITIS

17. What is a reactive arthritis?
A reactive arthritis is a **sterile** inflammatory arthritis that occurs within 1–3 weeks after an antecedent extra-articular infection (usually of the GI or genitourinary tracts).

18. What GI pathogens have been implicated in causing reactive arthritis?
Yersinia enterocolitica or *Y. pseudotuberculosis*
Salmonella enteritidis or *S. typhimurium*
Shigella dysenteriae or *S. flexneri*
Campylobacter jejuni

19. How commonly does reactive arthritis occur following an epidemic outbreak of infectious gastroenteritis?
Approximately 1–3% of patients who get an infectious gastroenteritis during an epidemic subsequently develop a reactive arthritis. It may be as high as 20% in *Yersinia*-infected individuals.

20. Which joints are most commonly involved in a reactive arthritis following a bowel infection (i.e., postenteritic reactive arthritis)?

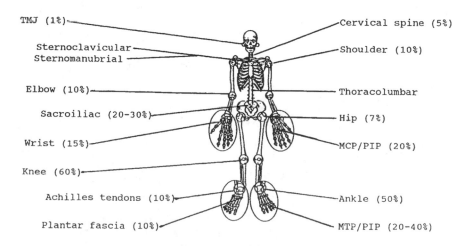

TMJ (1%)

Cervical spine (5%)

Sternoclavicular
Sternomanubrial

Shoulder (10%)

Elbow (10%)

Thoracolumbar

Sacroiliac (20–30%)

Hip (7%)

Wrist (15%)

MCP/PIP (20%)

Knee (60%)

Achilles tendons (10%)

Ankle (50%)

Plantar fascia (10%)

MTP/PIP (20–40%)

21. **Describe the clinical characteristics of postenteritic reactive arthritis.**
    Demographics — Males≥females; average age, 30 years
    Onset of arthritis — Abrupt, acute
    Distribution of joints — Asymmetric, pauciarticular; lower extremity involved in 80–90%,
        sacroiliitis in 30%
    Synovial fluid analysis — Inflammatory fluid (usually 10,000–50,000 WBC/mm^3), no crys-
        tals, negative cultures
    Course and prognosis — 80% resolve in 1–6 mos; 20% have chronic arthritis with x-ray
        changes of peripheral and/or sacroiliac joints

22. **What extra-articular manifestations occur in postenteritic reactive arthritis?**

Sterile urethritis (15–70%)	Erythema nodosum (5% of *Yersinia* infections)
Conjunctivitis	Circinate balanitis (25% of *Shigella* infections)
Acute anterior uveitis	Keratoderma blennorrhagicum
Oral ulcers (painless or painful)	

23. **How commonly do patients with postenteritic reactive arthritis have the clinical fea-**
tures of Reiter's syndrome?
The inflammatory arthritis, urethritis, conjunctivitis/uveitis, and mucocutaneous lesions which
characterize Reiter's syndrome may develop 2–4 weeks after an acute urethritis or diarrheal illness. The frequency varies with the causative enteric organism: *Shigella*, 85%; *Salmonella*,
10–15%; *Yersinia*, 10%; *Campylobacter*, 10%.

24. **How do the radiographic features of inflammatory sacroiliitis and spondylitis due to**
postenteritic reactive arthritis differ from those in IBD patients?

Radiologic Comparison of Spinal Arthritis in Postenteritic Reactive Arthritis vs. IBD

	REACTIVE ARTHRITIS	IBD
Sacroiliitis	Unilateral, asymmetric	Bilateral, sacroiliac involvement
Spondylitis	Asymmetric, nonmarginal, jug-handle syndesmophytes	Bilateral, thin, marginal syndesmophytes

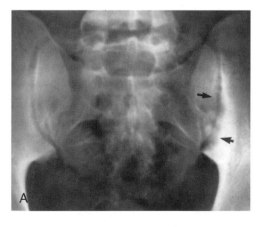 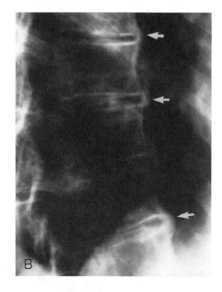

Figure 3. **A,** Radiograph showing unilateral sacroiliitis
(*arrows*) in a patient with reactive arthritis. **B,** Radiograph showing large, nonmarginal syndesmophytes (arrows) of the spine in a patient with reactive arthritis.

25. Discuss the relationship of HLA B27 positivity in patients with postenteritic reactive arthritis compared to a normal healthy population.
- Reactive arthritis patients, 70–80% HLA B27-positive; normal healthy controls, 4–8% HLA B27-positive.
- Whites and patients with radiographic sacroiliitis are more likely to be HLA B27-positive.
- A person who is HLA B27-positive has a 30–50 times increased risk of developing a reactive arthritis following an episode of infectious gastroenteritis compared to a person who does not have the HLA B27 gene.
- Only 20–25% of all HLA B27-positive individuals who get an infectious gastroenteritis from *Shigella, Salmonella,* or *Yersinia* go on to develop a postenteritic reactive arthritis.

26. Explain the current theory for the pathogenesis of a postenteritic reactive arthritis.
Bacterial lipopolysaccharide antigens from the pathogens (*Yersinia, Salmonella*) causing the infectious gastroenteritis are deposited in the joints of patients who develop a postenteritic reactive arthritis. These bacterial cell wall components are felt to incite inflammation in the joint. The role that HLA B27 plays in the pathogenesis is debated. One possibility is that the HLA B27 molecule presents these bacterial antigens to the immune system in a unique way, leading to inflammation. Another postulate is that there is molecular mimicry between the HLA B27 molecule and the bacterial antigens, causing an aberrant immune response. It is important to note that intact viable organisms cannot be cultured from the joint of a patient with reactive arthritis.

27. Is any therapy beneficial for postenteritic reactive arthritis?

Treatment of Postenteritic Reactive Arthritis

Treatment	PERIPHERAL ARTHRITIS		Sacroiliitis
	Acute	Chronic	
NSAIDs	Yes	Yes	Yes
Corticosteroids			
Intra-articular	Yes	Yes	Yes
Oral	Only if used in high doses		No
Antibiotics			
2-week course	No	No	No
3-month course	NA	Maybe	No
Sulfasalazine	NA	Yes	Maybe
Methotrexate	NA	Yes	No

*NA = not applicable

WHIPPLE'S DISEASE

28. Who was Whipple?
George Hoyt Whipple, M.D., in 1907 reported the case of a 36-year-old medical missionary with diarrhea, malabsorption with weight loss, mesenteric lymphadenopathy, and migratory polyarthritis. He named this disease "intestinal lipodystrophy," but it is now known as Whipple's disease. Dr. Whipple also became a Nobel Laureate in Physiology in 1934 and founder of the University of Rochester Medical School.

29. What are the multisystem manifestations of Whipple's disease?

Wasting/weight loss	**D**iarrhea
Hyperpigmentation (skin)	**I**nterstitial nephritis
Intestinal pain	**S**kin rashes
Pleurisy	**E**ye inflammation
Pneumonitis	**A**rthritis
Lymphadenopathy	**S**ubcutaneous nodules
Encephalopathy	**E**ndocarditis
Steatorrhea	

30. Describe the clinical characteristics of the arthritis associated with Whipple's disease.
Whipple's disease occurs most commonly in middle-aged white men. Seronegative oligoarthritis or polyarthritis is the presenting symptom in 60% of patients and may precede the intestinal symptoms by years. Over 90% of patients will develop an arthritis at some time during their disease course. Arthritis is inflammatory, often migratory, and does not correlate with intestinal symptoms. Sacroiliitis or spondylitis occurs in 5–10% of patients, especially in those who are HLA B27-positive (33% of patients). Synovial fluid analysis shows an inflammatory fluid with 5000–100,000 cells/mm^3. Radiographs usually remain unremarkable.

31. What is the etiology of Whipple's disease?
Multiple tissues show deposits that stain with periodic acid-Shiff (PAS). These deposits contain rod-shaped free bacilli seen by electron microscopy. Recently, these bacilli have been shown to be a new organism, a gram-positive actinomycete called *Tropheryma whippelii.*

32. How is Whipple's disease best treated?
Tetracycline, penicillin, erythromycin or trimethoprim/sulfamethoxazole (TMP/SMX) for > 1 year. Relapses can occur (30%). Chloramphenicol or TMP/SMX is recommended if the central nervous system is involved.

OTHER RHEUMATIC DISEASES

33. What rheumatic manifestations have been described in patients with celiac disease (gluten-sensitive enteropathy)?
- **Arthritis**—Symmetric polyarthritis involving predominantly large joints (knees and ankles > hips and shoulders); may precede enteropathic symptoms in 50% of cases.
- **Osteomalacia**—Due to steatorrhea from severe enteropathy.
- **Dermatitis herpetiformis**

34. Which HLA type is more common in patients with celiac disease than in normal healthy controls?
HLA DR3, frequently in association with HLA B8, is seen in 95% of patients with celiac disease compared to 12% of the normal population.

35. What is the treatment for the arthritis secondary to celiac disease?
The arthritis responds dramatically to a gluten-free diet.

36. Describe the intestinal bypass arthritis-dermatitis syndrome.
This syndrome occurs in 20–80% of patients who have undergone intestinal bypass surgery for morbid obesity. The arthritis is inflammatory, polyarticular, symmetric, and frequently migratory, and it affects both upper and lower extremity joints. Radiographic findings usually remain normal, despite 25% of patients having chronic recurring episodes of arthritis. Up to 80% develop dermatologic abnormalities, the most characteristic of which is a maculopapular or vesiculopustular rash.

The pathogenesis involves bacterial overgrowth in the blind loop, resulting in antigenic stimulation that purportedly causes immune complex formation (frequently cryoprecipitates containing bacterial antigens) and deposit in the joints and skin. Treatment includes NSAIDs and oral antibiotics, which usually improve symptoms. Only surgical reanastomosis of the blind loop can result in complete elimination of symptoms.

RHEUMATIC SYNDROMES AND PANCREATIC DISEASE

37. What pancreatic diseases have been associated with rheumatic syndromes?
Pancreatitis, pancreatic carcinoma, and pancreatic insufficiency.

38. What are the clinical features of the pancreatic panniculitis syndrome?
Pancreatic panniculitis is a systemic syndrome occurring in some patients with pancreatitis or pancreatic acinar cell carcinoma. Its clinical manifestations include:

- Tender, red nodules, usually on the extremities, which are frequently misdiagnosed as erythema nodosum but really are areas of panniculitis with fat necrosis.
- Arthritis (60%) and arthralgias, usually of the ankles and knees. Synovial fluid is typically noninflammatory and creamy in color, and it contains lipid droplets that stain with Sudan black or oil red O.
- Eosinophilia
- Osteolytic bone lesions from bone marrow necrosis, pleuropericarditis, fever

A good way to remember the manifestations is the mnemonic PANCREAS:

Pancreatitis
Arthritis
Nodules secondary to fat necrosis
Cancer of the pancreas
Radiographic abnormalities (osteolytic lesions of bone)
Eosinophilia
Amylase, lipase and trypsin elevations
Serositis including pleuropericarditis

39. What causes the pancreatic panniculitis syndrome?

Skin and synovial biopsies show fat necrosis, which is caused by release of trypsin, amylase, and lipase from the diseased pancreas.

40. What musculoskeletal problem can occur with pancreatic insufficiency?

Osteomalacia due to fat-soluble vitamin D malabsorption.

BIBLIOGRAPHY

1. Chakravarty K, Scott DGI: Oligoarthritis—a presenting feature of occult coeliac disease. Br J Rheumatol 31:349–350, 1992.
2. DeVos M, Cuvelier C, Miclants H, et al: Ileocolonoscopy in seronegative spondyloarthropathy. Gastroenterology 96:339–344, 1989.
3. Fleming JL, Wiesner RH, Shorter RC: Whipple's disease: Clinical, biochemical, and histopathologic features and assessment of treatment in 29 patients. Mayo Clin Proc 63:539–552, 1988.
4. Ganfors K, Jalkanen S, Von Essen R, et al: Yersinia antigens in synovial-fluid cells from patients with reactive arthritis. N Engl J Med 320:216–221, 1989.
5. Ganfors K, Jalkanen S, Lindberg AA, et al: Salmonella lipopolysaccharide in synovial cells from patients with reactive arthritis. Lancet 335:685–688, 1990.
6. Inman RD: Reactive arthritis after infectious enteritis. In Schumacher HR (ed): Primer on the Rheumatic Diseases, 10th ed. Atlanta, Arthritis Foundation, 1993, pp 166–167.
7. Inman RD, Johnston ME, Hodge M, et al: Postdysenteric reactive arthritis: A clinical and immunogenetic study following an outbreak of salmonellosis. Arthritis Rheum 31:1377–1383, 1988.
8. Keat A: Reiter's syndrome and reactive arthritis in perspective. N Engl J Med 309:1606–1615, 1983.
9. Mielants H, Veys EM, Goemaere S, et al: A prospective study of patients with spondyloarthropathy with special reference to HLA-B27 and to gut histology. J Rheumatol 20:1353–1358, 1993.
10. Relman DA, Schmidt TM, MacDermott RP, et al: Identification of the uncultured bacillus of Whipple's disease. N Engl J Med 327:293–301, 1992.
11. Roubenoff R, Ratain J, Giardiello I, et al: Collagenous colitis, enteropathic arthritis, and autoimmune diseases: Results of a patient survey. J Rheumatol 16:1229–1232, 1989.
12. Scofield RH, Warren WL, Koelsch G, et al: A hypothesis for the HLA B27 immune dysregulation in spondyloarthropathy: Contributions from enteric organisms, B27 structure, peptides bound by B27, and convergent evolution. Proc Natl Acad Sci USA 90:9330–9334, 1993.
13. Thomson GTD, DeRubeis DA, Hodge MA, et al: Post-Salmonella reactive arthritis: Late clinical sequelae in a point source cohort. Am J Med 98:13–21, 1995.
14. Wands JR, LaMont TJ, Mann BS, et al: Arthritis associated with intestinal bypass procedure for morbid obesity: Complement activation and characterization of circulatory cryoproteins. N Engl J Med 294:121–124, 1976.
15. Weiner SR, Clarke J, Taggart NA, et al: Rheumatic manifestations of inflammatory bowel disease. Semin Arthritis Rheum 20:353–366, 1991.
16. Wollheim FA: Enteropathic arthritis. In Kelley WK, Harris ED, Ruddy S, Sledge CB (eds): Textbook of Rheumatology, 4th ed. Philadelphia, W.B. Saunders, 1993, pp 985–997.

68. HEMATOLOGIC MANIFESTATIONS OF GASTROINTESTINAL DISEASE

Arlene J. Zaloznik, M.D.

1. Describe the etiology of postgastrectomy iron-deficiency anemia.

Iron-deficiency anemia is a frequent postoperative complication of gastric surgery, including both total gastrectomy and partial gastrectomy. In the early postoperative period, the anemia results from the depletion of iron stores secondary to preoperative blood loss. Chronic iron deficiency develops later due to reduced gastric acidity and impaired iron absorption. Both ferrous and ferric iron are soluble in an acid pH. As the pH increases, ferric iron is converted to insoluble ferric hydroxide. Because iron is actively absorbed in the duodenum, the rapid intestinal transit that follows the loss of the reservoir function of the stomach may lead to decreased absorption. Iron deficiency is more common when the duodenum is surgically bypassed. Recurrent bleeding at the anastomotic site may also contribute to the development of the postgastrectomy iron-deficiency anemia.

2. What is the mechanism of vitamin B12 deficiency after a total or subtotal gastrectomy?

After a **total gastrectomy,** vitamin B12 deficiency is inevitable over time. The loss of the intrinsic factor-secreting cells and the hydrochloric acid- and pepsin-secreting cells leads to an inability to absorb cobalamin (vitamin B12). The average time to develop the anemia is 5 years (range, 2–10 yrs).

During the first several years after a **partial gastrectomy,** vitamin B12 deficiency is uncommon. With time, atrophic gastritis develops in the gastric remnant and is the etiology of late vitamin B12 deficiency.

Vitamin B12 deficiency is commonly seen in patients after Billroth II surgery who develop a **bacterial overgrowth** syndrome. The bacteria take up cobalamin and reduce the amount available for absorption in the ileum. Folate is produced by the abundant bacteria, so folate deficiency is uncommon. High serum or red cell folate levels in the absence of folate supplements suggest small bowel bacterial overgrowth.

3. How should patients with postgastrectomy anemia be evaluated?

The evaluation of anemia in patients after surgery for peptic ulcer disease requires the measurement of serum ferritin and vitamin B12 levels. The stool should be examined for occult blood. The administration of intramuscular vitamin B12 and oral or intravenous iron may be required if deficiencies are documented. If patients have had Billroth II surgery and a bacterial overgrowth syndrome is present, antibiotic therapy may be indicated.

4. What are the etiologies of the anemia seen in the small intestinal malabsorption syndromes?

Celiac disease, tropical sprue, Whipple's disease, regional enteritis, and any other disorder that alters the integrity of the small bowel can lead to a malabsorption of iron, folate, and vitamin B12. Folate deficiency is the most common cause of anemia seen in the small intestinal malabsorption syndromes involving the proximal small bowel. Vitamin B12 deficiency is uncommon unless there is extensive involvement of the distal ileum. Iron-deficiency anemia secondary to chronic GI blood loss is commonly seen in the inflammatory bowel diseases.

The hematologic consequences of small bowel resection depend on the area resected. If > 100 cm of ileum is removed, vitamin B12 deficiency results. Although the duodenum is the primary site of iron absorption, the distal small bowel also has a limited capacity to absorb iron. Iron deficiency usually does not occur unless there is extensive small bowel resection. Folate deficiency rarely occurs unless a large portion of the small intestine is removed.

5. What is a potentially life-threatening sequela of acute viral hepatitis?

Pancytopenia with an aplastic or hypoplastic marrow is a rare, potentially fatal complication of viral hepatitis, occurring in 0.1–0.2% of patients. The risk of aplastic anemia appears to be greatest after non-A, non-B hepatitis. The average age of onset is 18 years, and males are affected more often than females. The aplastic anemia occurs within 6 months of the onset of hepatitis, often developing as the hepatitis is improved or resolved. There is no relation between the severity of the hepatitis and the occurrence of the aplasia. Although the pathogenesis of the aplasia is unknown, the most plausible explanation is an irreversible viral-induced hematopoietic stem cell injury. Fatality rates in post-hepatitis aplastic anemia are >80%, with a mean survival after the onset of pancytopenia of 10 weeks. Bone marrow transplantation is the treatment of choice for severe aplasia.

6. Why do patients with chronic liver disease develop a chronic, mild spherocytic hemolytic anemia?

A small population of spherocytic red blood cells are present in the peripheral circulation. These spherocytes reflect the splenic conditioning of red cells by the congested spleen. The spherocytes are ultimately destroyed in the spleen. In most patients with liver disease, target cells form due to an excess of cholesterol and phospholipid in the red cell membrane. Increases in membrane lipid correlate with increases in membrane surface area. These target cells are the opposite of the spherocytes and are not as easily destroyed by the spleen and thus minimize the hemolysis of liver disease.

7. What is Zieve's syndrome?

A syndrome has been described in which alcohol-induced fatty liver is associated with both hypertriglyceridemia and hemolysis. There is no evidence that the red cell survival is influenced by the hypertriglyceridemia. The genesis of the hemolysis is not well understood.

8. What is spur cell anemia?

The syndrome of spur cell anemia represents an abnormality of red cell changes in membrane lipids. Spur cells contain increased amounts of cholesterol and lecithin, resulting in an increased cholesterol/phospholipid ratio. The red cells are bizarrely spiculated and undergo premature destruction in the spleen.

Spur cell anemia, usually associated with hemolysis, is estimated to occur in 3% of patients with cirrhosis. Splenomegaly is a constant feature of this disorder and often associated with ascites and hepatic encephalopathy. In many patients, spur cell anemia occurs within weeks or months of death. Transfusion therapy is of limited value because transfused cells acquire the spur cell abnormality. Splenectomy may lead to the slowing of the hemolytic process but carries a high surgical risk in these patients with end-stage liver disease, portal hypertension, and coagulopathy.

9. What etiologic factors (other than hemolysis) are involved in the development of anemia in patients with chronic liver disease?

Anemia is a frequent manifestation of chronic liver disease. Hypervolemia secondary to an increased plasma volume is frequently seen in patients with cirrhosis and results in a dilutional anemia. Hematocrit values may be as low as 20% in the presence of a normal red cell mass. The anemia of chronic liver disease is usually normochromic and normocytic unless complicated by an iron or folate deficiency.

The presence of macrocytic red cells on blood smears and an elevated erythrocyte mean cell volume (MCV) are common findings in alcoholic patients. The macrocytosis may be the result of:

- Folate-deficiency megaloblastic anemia
- Reticulocytosis
- Macrocytosis of liver disease
- Macrocytosis of alcoholism

Megaloblastic anemia resulting from folate deficiency is the most common cause, occurring in almost 40% of patients. Classic findings include an elevated erythrocyte MCV, hypersegmented neutrophils and macro-ovalocyte on the peripheral smear, increased serum unconjugated bilirubin, markedly elevated serum lactic dehydrogenase (LDH), and megaloblastic erythroid and myeloid precursors in the bone marrow associated with low serum and erythrocyte folate concentrations. Folate deficiency develops commonly in drinkers of wine and whiskey, which contain little or none of the vitamin. It is seen less frequently in those who prefer beer, which is rich in the vitamin.

Ethanol ingestion directly affects the bone marrow, causing megaloblastic changes. The degree of macrocytosis is typically modest, with MCVs no higher than 110 fl. Anemia is frequently absent or very slight. On the blood smear, the macrocytes are characteristically round and neutrophil hypersegmentation is absent. With abstention, the macrocytosis clears in 1–4 months.

10. Describe the diagnostic approach to anemia in the alcoholic patient.

The most common causes of anemia in patients with cirrhosis are folate deficiency, iron deficiency, blood loss, and spur cell hemolytic anemia. The initial diagnostic approach to anemia in the alcoholic patient should include the MCV, reticulocyte count, serum ferritin, and peripheral blood smear. Folate and vitamin B12 deficiency should be ruled out if the MCV is >110 fl, if neutrophil hypersegmentation is present, and if > 3% macro-ovalocytes are present. If reticulocytosis is present and there is no evidence of bleeding loss or recovery from megaloblastic anemia, then the patient should be evaluated for hemolysis.

Serum ferritin levels are frequently increased in patients with alcoholic liver disease. When iron-deficiency anemia is present, serum ferritin levels will be in the lower end of normal range rather than decreased. The serum ferritin is the best noninvasive screening test for iron-deficiency anemia in alcoholics.

11. What is the function of the liver in normal coagulation?

The liver is the principal site of synthesis and regulation of all the coagulation proteins (fibrinogen and the vitamin K-dependent factors II, VII, IX, X; factors V and VIII; contact factors XI and XII; and fibrin-stabilizing factor XIII), with the exception of von Willebrand factor and the fibrolytic proteins (tissue plasminogen activator and urokinase-type plasminogen activator). The liver also synthesizes protease inhibitors, such as antithrombin III, protein C, and heparin cofactor II, which modulate the coagulation cascade. In addition, the liver clears activated clotting factors, activation complexes, and end-products of the fibrinogen-to-fibrin conversion from the blood.

12. What coagulation abnormalities are associated with chronic liver disease?

Cholestatic liver disease leads to an inadequate excretion of bile salts into the gut, with malabsorption of vitamin K and consequent deficient hepatic synthesis of factors II, VII, IX, and X. In **fulminant** hepatic failure or **decompensated cirrhosis,** blood levels of all factors fall in proportion to their biologic half-life. Factor VII, with a half-life of 2–6 hours, drops first. As the liver disease progresses, the other factor levels also decrease. Only von Willebrand factor and factor VIII:C levels are unaffected. Fibrinogen concentrations are usually lower than normal. These changes result in the prolongation of the activated partial thromboplastin time, prothrombin time, and thrombin clotting time. An increase in fibrinolytic activity may be manifest as disseminated intravascular clotting. Both qualitative and quantitative platelet abnormalities occur. Defective platelet aggregation correlates with the severity of the liver disease and results in prolonged bleeding times. Thrombocytopenia is often the result of increased platelet pooling in an enlarged spleen associated with portal hypertension.

13. How should the hemostatic defects of chronic liver disease be managed?

The management of a patient with cirrhosis and a hemostatic defect is dependent on the nature of the defect and the degree and site of bleeding. Patients with a prolonged prothrombin time should receive parenteral vitamin K. Fresh frozen plasma (FFP) contains all the components of the clotting and fibrinolytic system except platelets. While FFP is the best treatment modality, volume overload may become a problem. Six to eight units of FFP are sufficient in most cases to correct severe clotting factor defects. Cryoprecipitate should be considered for patients with low fibrinogen concentrations. Platelet concentrates are indicated when patients have quantitative or qualitative platelet defects.

14. What are the causes of thrombocytopenia in the alcoholic liver disease?

Thrombocytopenia occurs in both the acutely ill, hospitalized alcoholic patient and in chronic alcoholics. Megakaryocytes are typically normal to increased in numbers in the bone marrow. A rapid return to normal typically occurs within 1 week of alcohol withdrawal. Failure of the platelet count to increase within 5–7 days indicates the presence of an underlying disorder. A rebound thrombocytosis usually occurs during the second week of abstinence. The pathogenesis of the thrombocytopenia is most likely due to ineffective thrombopoiesis and a decrease in platelet survival. In addition, folate deficiency, hypersplenism, sepsis, and disseminated intravascular coagulation associated with shock, sepsis, or cirrhosis may also cause thrombocytopenia. Bone marrow aspiration for estimation of megakaryocyte numbers is not helpful, because all of the listed conditions are associated with normal to increased numbers of megakaryocytes.

Most cases of alcohol-induced thrombocytopenia can be managed by expectant observation of the platelet count. Patients with serious hemorrahge and platelet counts <20,000/µl should be given platelet transfusions.

15. Do hepatobiliary complications occur in sickle cell disease (SS)?

Yes. Hepatic crisis, gallstones, viral hepatitis, and hepatic failure. Patients with SS may have abnormal liver function tests in the absence of hepatic crisis, viral hepatitis, biliary disease, or other known causes of liver disease. Hepatomegaly develops in early childhood, with progression to cirrhosis in adults. Patients with sickle cell trait are not at an increased risk for hepatobiliary disease.

16. What is the clinical picture of hepatic crisis in patients with sickle cell disease?

The most common hepatic complication of SS is the hepatic crisis, occurring in 10% of patients. This syndrome, which resembles acute cholecystitis, presents with RUQ pain, fever, leukocytosis, and variable elevations in serum transaminases and bilirubin levels. Often, there is a preceding upper respiratory infection or vaso-occlusive crisis without hepatic involvement. The liver is enlarged and tender in most instances. The course is variable, but the disorder usually resolves in 1–2 weeks. Patients are managed with intravenous fluids and antibiotics. Each hepatic crisis leaves patches of ischemic necrosis, fibrosis, and nodular regeneration.

An uncommon but virulent form of hepatic crisis is **diffuse intrahepatic cholestasis.** Massive intrasinusoidal sickling precipitates severe RUQ pain, hepatomegaly, and liver failure with hepatic encephalopathy. Treatment includes exchange transfusions, but patients usually die of hepatic failure.

17. How should gallstones be managed in patients with sickle cell disease?

Gallstones are found in 50–70% of adults with homozygous sickle-cell disease and are asymptomatic in two-thirds of the adults. The incidence increases with age. The diagnosis of acute cholecystitis is often difficult because the clinical picture resembles hepatic crisis.

The management of asymptomatic gallstones remains controversial. The risk of surgery must be considered in determining the benefit. Complications of elective surgery, including pneumonia, pulmonary infiltrates, and atelectasis, are significant but not prohibitive. Emergency surgery on patients in crisis carries high morbidity and mortality. The course of asymptomatic gallstones in SS is unknown, and cholecystectomy does not prevent future hepatic crisis. Cholecystectomy should be reserved for patients with demonstrated gallstones in whom there is difficulty in differentiating recurrent abdominal crisis from cholecystitis and those patients whose abdominal symptoms are clearly related to biliary disease.

18. What are the hematologic paraneoplastic syndromes associated with GI malignancies?

Mucin-producing adenocarcinomas, such as gastric cancer, have been associated with **microangiopathic hemolytic anemia.** The anemia is characterized by red blood cell fragments in the peripheral blood, thrombocytopenia, and disseminated intravascular coagulation. The prognosis of patients who have MAHA and cancer is poor, with an average survival time of 3 weeks. There is no effective therapy.

Tumor-associated erythrocytosis is uncommon but has been reported with hepatocellular carcinomas.

Migratory superficial thrombophlebitis (**Trousseau's syndrome**) is characterized by recurrent thrombophlebitis in the absence of apparent predisposing factors. Mucin-producing adenocarcinomas of the GI tract, particularly pancreatic cancer, are most frequently associated with this thrombosis. Trousseau's syndrome mainly involves multiple superficial and unusual vessels. The migratory thrombophlebitis may occur before or after the diagnosis of malignancy. Although acute episodes require heparin therapy, treatment of the underlying malignancy is the mainstay of therapy.

19. What are indications for red blood cell transfusion?

The goals of blood transfusion are to increase the red cell mass and, as a result, to increase oxygen transport while restoring and maintaining the blood volume. The decision to transfuse a patient with red blood cells should be made after careful consideration of the cause and severity of anemia, physiologic adjustments to anemia, the patient's hemodynamic status, available alternatives to blood transfusion, and possible risks of transfusion therapy. Patients with acute blood loss can develop hypotension, tachycardia, and shock. Those patients with chronic stable anemia or gradually developing anemia often tolerate very low levels of hemoglobin.

Patients with a hemoglobin >10 gm/dl and no symptoms rarely need a transfusion. If the hemoglobin is 6–10 gm/dl, transfusion is indicated when symptoms are present; the asymptomatic patient may not need a transfusion. Once the hemoglobin is <6 gm/dl, symptoms are usually always present, and red blood cells are usually needed. An exception would be in those patients with a chronic stable anemia, such as the anemia of chronic disease or pernicious anemia.

BIBLIOGRAPHY

1. Cooper R: Hemolytic syndromes and red cell membrane abnormalities in liver disease. Semin Hematol 17:103–112, 1980.
2. Doll DC, Weiss RB: Neoplasia and the erythron. J Clin Oncol 3:429–446, 1985.
3. Jain R: Use of blood transfusion in management of anemia. Med Clin North Am 76:727–744, 1992.
4. Lindenbaum J: Hematologic complications of alcohol abuse. Semin Liver Dis 7:169–181, 1987.
5. Luzzatto G, Schafer AI: The prethrombotic state in cancer. Semin Oncol 17:147–159, 1990.
6. Mammen EF: Coagulation defects in liver disease. Med Clin North Am 78:545–554, 1994.
7. Phillips DL, Keefe EB: Hematologic manifestations of gastrointestinal disease. Hematol/Oncol Clin North Am 1:207–228, 1987.
8. Schubert TT: Hepatobiliary system in sickle cell disease. Gastroenterology 90:2013–2021, 1986.
9. Zeldis JB, Dienstag JL, Gale RP: Aplastic anemia and non-A, non-B hepatitis. Am J Med 74:64–68, 1983.

69. DERMATOLOGIC MANIFESTATIONS OF GASTROINTESTINAL DISEASE

James E. Cremins, M.D.

1. What is a "spider angioma"? How is it related to gastrointestinal disorders?

Spider angiomas gradually form as an arteriole becomes more prominent near the surface of the skin and radiates capillaries (see figure below). The arteriole represents the spider's body, and the capillaries, its legs. Although these lesions occur in normal adults and are frequently found in healthy children, they appear with increased frequency during pregnancy and in patients with chronic liver disease. Spider formation is probably stimulated by higher than normal estrogen concentrations. With central pressure applied to a spider angiomata, blanching occurs. When the pressure is removed the spider legs fill from the central arteriole. This feature distinguishes spider angiomata from telangiectasias that are not associated with chronic liver disease. Other physical findings that may suggest the presence of chronic liver disease include jaundice, clubbed fingers, palmar erythema, gynecomastia, testicular atrophy, loss of axillary and pubic hair, and multiple ecchymoses.

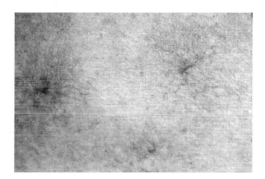

2. A 28-year-old woman presents with recent-onset diarrhea and bruise-like skin lesions on her shins. What is the skin lesion?

The lesion is **erythema nodosum,** a tender, nodular erythematous eruption usually confined to the extensor aspect of the extremities. These nodules are the result of inflammation in the subcutaneous fat and probably represent a hypersensitivity reaction to an antigen in the septal vessels of the fat lobule. Prodromal symptoms of fatigue and malaise may precede the eruption by 1–3 weeks, and the nodules usually last from 3–6 weeks. The nodules most commonly affect the anterior lower extremities (shins) in a symmetrical fashion. Other associated signs and symptoms include fever, arthritis, and arthralgias.

3. With which GI disorders is erythema nodosum most frequently associated?

Erythema nodosum is a well-known extraintestinal manifestation of **ulcerative colitis, Crohn's disease,** and **infectious colitis** (e.g., *Salmonella* and *Yersinia* enterocolitis). Its incidence in patients with ulcerative colitis was 7% in one large series but is lower in Crohn's disease.

All patients with erythema nodosum and GI symptoms should be fully evaluated for enteric infection (stool cultures, to include *Yersinia* and *Salmonella*) and inflammatory bowel disease. It often parallels the activity of the inflammatory bowel disease.

Causes and Common Associations of Erythema Nodosum

DRUGS	INFECTIONS	MALIGNANCY	OTHER
Estrogens	Bacterial	Hodgkin's disease	Behçet's disease
Oral contraceptives	Streptococci	Leukemia	Ulcerative colitis
Sulfonamides	*Salmonella*		Crohn's disease
Bromides	*Yersinia*		Sarcoidosis
	Tuberculosis		Pregnancy
	Chlamydia		Reiter's disease
	Fungal		
	Coccidioidomycosis		
	Histoplasmosis		
	Viral		
	Protozoan		

4. What is pyoderma gangrenosum?

Pyoderma gangrenosum (PG) is an uncommon, severe, ulcerating cutaneous disease of unknown origin. More than 50% of patients with PG do not have an associated disease. However, the best-known associated clinical disorder is inflammatory bowel disease, and this diagnosis should be considered and excluded in every patient with PG. The lesion begins as a tender, erythematous macule or nodule, frequently on the lower legs. Pustules or vesicles soon occur, and the surrounding skin becomes dusky red and indurated. Fully evolved lesions have a dusky purple undermined border, tend to be persistent, and heal with scarring (see figure below). PG lesions demonstrate pathergy (rapid extension after trauma); thus, surgical therapy is not recommended. PG has been reported to occur in patients with ulcerative colitis, Crohn's disease (UC > CD), rheumatoid arthritis, chronic active hepatitis, hematologic and lymphoreticular malignancies, and monoclonal gammopathy.

The diagnosis of PG is a clinical diagnosis of exclusion: infections, vasculitic syndromes, and neoplasia must be ruled out. Treatment modalities include corticosteroids (intravenous, oral, and intralesional), dapsone (300–400 mg/day orally), minocycline (300 mg/day orally), clofazimine (300 mg/day orally), intravenous cyclosporine, and intralesional cromolyn sodium. In patients with PG related to ulcerative colitis, colectomy is usually followed by spontaneous healing of the skin lesion. In general, the most successful mode of treatment is treatment of the underlying disorder.

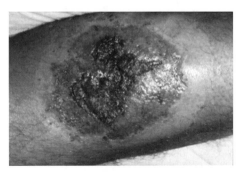

5. A patient has extensive calluses on his palms and soles. What is the lesion, and how does it relate to diseases of the digestive system?

The lesion is keratosis palmaris et plantaris, or tylosis. In 1958, investigators described two English families in whom tylosis was associated with the development of esophageal carcinoma, before the age of 65. A total of 18 cases of esophageal carcinoma occurred in the two families. Prior to 1958, tylosis had not been linked to internal malignancy or any significant disease process. In 1981, a third family, in the United States, was identified with hereditary tylosis and a GI malignancy—this time, adenocarcinoma of the colon.

The condition is due to a single autosomal dominant gene. Tylosis has multiple causes, and there are several individual case reports of tylosis associated with malignancy *without* a family history. However, in patients with long-standing skin lesions and a family history of cancer, strong consideration should be given to prompt screening for GI malignancy.

6. What skin lesion is associated with Gardner's syndrome?

Epidermal inclusion cysts are associated with Gardner's syndrome, a syndrome of multiple intestinal polyps first described in 1953. It is indistinguishable from familial adenomatous polyposis (FAP), except for the presence of extraintestinal tumors. The syndrome is inherited in an autosomal dominant fashion and occurs in 1 of 14,025 births. Gardner's syndrome consists of a triad of findings:

1. Multiple intestinal polyps—100% of patients have colonic adenomas, and 10% have small intestine polyps. In 50% of patients, these polyps occur by age 16. The lifetime risk of colon cancer is the same as in FAP (100%).

2. Soft tissue tumors—Epidermal inclusion cysts, lipomas, fibromas, and desmoid tumors.

3. Bone tumors—Most often osteomas.

Patients with Gardner's syndrome develop multiple epidermal inclusion cysts in their teenage years. Desmoid tumors are locally aggressive, nonmetastasizing tumors of fibrous tissue that often affect the abdominal wall and can become difficult surgical problems. Osteomas often occur in the mandible or maxilla and may be detectable on dental films. Other less common lesions in these patients include supernumerary teeth and congenital hypertrophy of the retinal pigmented epithelium (CHRPE). Associated extracolonic malignancies include papillary thyroid carcinoma, adrenal carcinoma, hepatoblastoma, and periampullary or duodenal carcinoma (occurring in up to 10%).

When a diagnosis of Gardner's syndrome is being considered, workup should include bone radiographs (including jaw or dental series), retinal exam, and panendoscopy (EGD and colonoscopy). Given the 100% lifetime risk of colon cancer, proctocolectomy is the treatment of choice. After colectomy, the rectal mucosal remnant and upper GI tract should be monitored regularly. Strong consideration should also be given to screening for associated extracolonic malignancies.

7. What is Peutz Jeghers syndrome?

This autosomal dominant condition is characterized by small intestine hamartomatous polyps and hyperpigmented macules of the lips and buccal mucosa. Most polyps occur in the jejunum and ileum, but they may also occur in the stomach, duodenum, and colon. The intestinal lesions may present in childhood as intussusception, obstruction, or GI bleeding.

The melanotic macules begin in infancy and most commonly affect the lips, but also the palms, soles, digits, periorbital skin, anus, and buccal mucosa. All except the buccal lesions fade with age. Most patients are asymptomatic. Diagnosis is made by association of small bowel polyps with the characteristic pigmented lesions of the lips and mouth. In general, no treatment is necessary. If symptoms from polyps occur, the treatment of choice is segmental resection.

8. What is the malignant potential of polyps in Peutz-Jeghers syndrome?

The risk is much less than in FAP, but the risk is real. Adenocarcinomas in the stomach, small bowel, and colon may arise from the hamartomas (most commonly in the stomach and duodenum). The incidence of attributable GI malignancy ranges from 2–13%.

Extraintestinal neoplasia associated with this syndrome include breast carcinoma (which is often bilateral), cervical adenocarcinoma, and benign ovarian and testicular tumors. Although guidelines for surveillance of intestinal and extraintestinal malignancy associated with Peutz-Jeghers syndrome have not been established, one should consider regular breast exam, mammogram, pelvic exam, and ovarian ultrasonography in affected women, patients, as well as periodic GI examination in all patients.

9. Does Cowden's disease involve an increased risk for cancer?

Cowden's disease, also known as multiple hamartoma syndrome, is a rare, autosomal dominant disorder of which < 100 cases have been reported. Recognition of this syndrome is based on the characteristic mucocutaneous findings that include "cobble-stoning" of the oral mucosa and gingiva (see figure below left) and verrucous, hyperkeratotic papules called trichilemmomas (see figure below right). Trichilemmomas have an acral and facial distribution. They range in size from pinpoint to pea-sized and develop insidiously around the second decade. Approximately 35% of patients develop hamartomatous polyps, which can be present throughout the GI tract. However, these patients are not at increased risk for GI cancers, and symptoms from these polyps are rare.

The clinical significance of Cowden's disease relates to its non-GI pathology. Two-thirds of affected patients have goiter, with a 10% risk of thyroid carcinoma. Among female patients, 75% have breast lesions (fibrocystic breast disease or fibroadenomas), with a 50% incidence of breast carcinoma, frequently at a young age (mean age, 41 yrs). Recognition of Cowden's disease is important so patients can be aggressively screened for thyroid and breast malignancy. GI investigation is unnecessary unless symptoms are present.

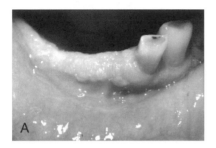 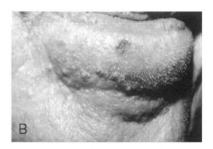

10. A 54-year-old black women presents with abnormal-appearing, darkened skinfolds. What is this skin lesion, and what underlying disease processes could have caused it?

Acanthosis nigricans is a symmetric, smooth, thickening and darkening of the skin that appears in intertriginous areas. The most common sites include the axillae and neck (see figure below). It is a nonspecific process that is usually idiopathic or associated with obesity, diabetes mellitus with insulin resistance, impaired glucose tolerance, Cushing's syndrome, and Stein-Leventhal syndrome. Acanthosis nigricans, however, also is associated with internal malignancy. Suspicion for malignancy should arise when acanthosis nigricans occurs in nonobese, nondiabetic patients.

Adenocarcinoma, specifically gastric, pancreatic, and bronchogenic, is associated with this lesion. Malignancy appears in synchrony with the skin lesions in approximately 60% of cases; in 20–30% of cases, acanthosis nigricans can precede the malignancy. In patients with a history of abdominal adenocarcinoma who subsequently develop acanthosis nigricans, an aggressive search for metastatic disease or recurrence should be pursued. The development of malignancy-associated acanthosis nigricans is believed to be related to growth factors released by the tumor. The skin lesions remit after the tumor is removed.

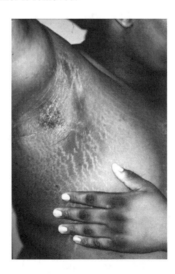

11. What is necrolytic migratory erythema (NME)?

NME is the classic cutaneous manifestation of the glucagonoma syndrome. The eruption typically involves perioral, lower abdominal, and perineal locations. The skin lesions are initially scaly and erythematous, but they soon evolve into raised, bullous lesions and eventually desquamate. Stomatitis and angular cheilitis may accompany the lesion.

The glucagonoma syndrome, which occurs with a glucagon-secreting islet cell tumor of the pancreas, consists of diabetes mellitus, glossitis, anemia, weight loss, and the characteristic skin lesion (NME). Despite the well-defined clinical syndrome and a very indolent growth pattern, approximately 70% of patients present with advanced disease not amenable to surgical cure. Many of the symptoms of the syndrome (i.e., anemia, weight loss, diabetes) are nonspecific and can be associated with other endocrine disorders or chronic disease states. However, virtually all patients have hyperglucagonemia, and the vast majority have NME. Thus, a vigorous search for a tumor is indicated when typical skin lesions occur in a patient with suggestive symptoms and elevated glucagon.

The ideal treatment is surgical removal of the tumor. Chemotherapeutic agents have been employed to help reduce the glucagon concentration and often cause the skin rash to regress prior to surgical intervention. With smaller or localized lesions, surgical removal alone is adequate therapy.

12. Name two skin lesions that are signs of GI hemorrhage.

Cullen's sign is a bluish discoloration of the skin around the umbilicus that often occurs with intraperitoneal hemorrhage (see figure below). This sign is also seen in acute hemorrhagic pancreatitis and following rupture of the uterine tube in ectopic pregnancy.

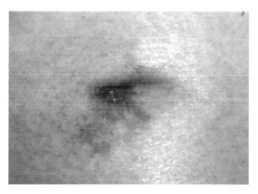

Grey Turner's sign is another dermatologic clue to acute hemorrhagic pancreatitis. It is an ecchymotic discoloration of the left flank that results from retroperitoneal hemorrhage tracking into the flank. Its color is blue-red, blue-purple, or green, depending upon the degree of degradation of hemoglobin in the tissue. Patients' coagulation parameters are usually normal. Grey Turner's sign can also be seen in strangulated bowel and extravasation of hemorrhage from an abscess.

13. A 50-year-old white man has mild anemia, documented steatorrhea, and a burning, blister-like skin lesion. What is the skin lesion, and what underlying GI disorder may he have?

The lesion is **dermatitis herpetiformis** (DH), a papular, vesicular lesion that is pruritic and burning. Classically, it symmetrically involves the elbows, knees, sacrum, and shoulders. Pathologically, the lesion is the result of IgA deposition in the dermal papillae. Approximately 20% of patients with DH have celiac disease (nontropical sprue). Celiac disease can be clinically silent or present with diarrhea and malabsorption, anemia, and DH. Two-thirds of patients with DH have an abnormal small bowel histology similar to sprue, which perhaps represents latent sprue. Characteristic changes in the small bowel include a mixed lymphocytic and plasma cell infiltrate and villous atrophy.

DH associated with celiac disease responds to dapsone (100–200 mg orally each day) and a gluten-free diet. Even in the absence of GI symptoms, strict observance to a gluten-free diet will help heal the skin lesions and minimize the need for medical therapy. Dapsone alone can effectively treat patients with DH (and no celiac disease). Burning vesicular skin lesions in a patient with steatorrhea and anemia should hint at the diagnosis of DH and celiac sprue. Such a clinical scenario should prompt evaluation of the small bowel, specifically esophagoduodenoscopy with small bowel biopsies.

14. A 55-year-old male presents with recent history of melena. His physical exam reveals multiple oral and buccal telangiectasias. How does this relate to the GI tract?

The patient has **hereditary hemorrhagic telangiectasias** (HHT), an autosomal dominant disease that is characterized by multiple telangiectasias of the skin, mucous membranes, and various internal organs. Telangiectasias can occur on any mucocutaneous surface but are most common on the lips, tongue, face, hands, chest, and feet. They have been described in all parts of the alimentary canal, liver, lungs, brain, and retina.

Epistaxis is the most common cause of morbidity in this disease. The GI tract is the second most frequent site of hemorrhage, with GI bleeding occurring in 13–44% of patients. Localization of the GI bleeding site is of paramount importance, especially with therapeutic endoscopy. Bleeding from telangiectasias can occur anywhere in the GI tract, but the predominant location seems to be gastroduodenal. The exact role of therapeutic endoscopy (electrocautery, laser coagulation) in GI bleeding is not well-defined. Actively bleeding lesions are often difficult to identify, and therapy aimed at "potential" sources may do more harm than good. The precise use of therapeutic endoscopy may only be defined after controlled studies are done.

15. Name the types of liver involvement seen in HHT.

Liver disease in HHT can range from none at all to severe with cirrhosis and portal hypertension. Patients can develop disease in different ways, and combinations of the presentations also occur. Hepatic iron overload is the most common reason for liver disease in HHT.

1. Peliosis hepatis, hepatic adenoma, or hepatocellular carcinoma secondary to prolonged estrogen therapy
2. Acute hepatitis followed by chronic hepatitis, and even cirrhosis secondary to multiple transfusions
3. Iron overload secondary to transfusions and/or iron therapy
4. Macroscopic or microscopic telangiectasias directly involving the liver
5. Congestive hepatopathy secondary to high-output congestive heart failure from chronic anemia and arteriovenous shunting

16. What is the sign of Leser-Trélat?

Leser-Trélat's sign is the abrupt appearance of multiple **seborrheic keratoses** or a sudden increase in the number or size of preexisting lesions in association with an internal malignancy. The sign is credited to two European surgeons, Edmund Leser and Ulysse Trélat, who reported cases in 1890.

In most cases, cutaneous manifestations and internal malignancy clinically appear at about the same time. In some cases, the cutaneous signs may precede or follow the diagnosis of malignancy. Usually, the tumor has metastasized by the time of diagnosis. In about one-third of cases, the skin lesions parallel the course of malignancy, regressing after tumor removal.

Seborrheic keratoses seen with the sign of Leser-Trélat are identical to the sporadic lesions. They occur most commonly on the trunk and less frequently on the extremities. They are sharply demarcated brownish lesions, with a "stuck-on" appearance.

Most patients with Leser-Trélat's sign harbor an adenocarcioma, stomach and colon being frequently involved, with the rectum an unusual primary site. Adenocarcinoma of the kidney, breast, lung, gallbladder, bile ducts, duodenum, pancreas, uterus, ovaries, and prostate also have been reported. Lymphoproliferative malignancies include bronchogenic carcinoma, hepatoma, osteogenic sarcoma, neurofibrosarcoma, leiomyosarcoma, germinoma, and ductal carcinoma of the breast.

17. A 28-year-old HIV-positive patient has diarrhea and multiple lesions of Kaposi's sarcoma over his legs. What, if any, involvement of the GI tract can occur?

Kaposi's sarcoma (KS) is a vascular neoplasm that often appears on the lower extremities (see figure on following page). Until the AIDS epidemic, it was rarely seen in the United States and Europe outside of elderly Jewish, Greek, or Italian men. Progression was usually slow, and many patients died from other causes. In HIV-infected patients, KS is rapidly progressive and of-

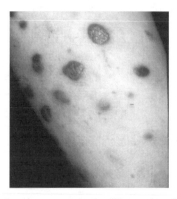

ten affects internal organs. Lesions can occur in the GI tract, involving the small intestine, stomach, esophagus, colon, and peritoneum. The liver can also be involved. Most GI lesions are silent, with the patients remaining asymptomatic. However, GI bleeding can occur, and malabsorption of protein and fat (protein-losing enteropathy, with edema, ascites, and anasarca) is also seen. KS has masqueraded as an intra-abdominal abscess (acute appendicitis) and acute abdomen (duodenal perforation).

18. You have been asked to evaluate a 40-year-old woman with brisk rectal bleeding and yellow skin papules about the neck. What is the diagnosis?

The patient has **pseudoxanthoma elasticum** (PXE), a disorder characterized by yellowish papules and plaques that produce a "chicken-skin" appearance and associated vascular lesions. Degenerated and calcified elastic fibers are found within the skin lesions and within the media and intima of blood vessels. Resultant vascular complications include hypertension, intermittent claudication, angina, retinal damage ("angioid streaks" on opthalmoscopic exam), and GI bleeding.

GI involvement can manifest as upper or lower GI bleeding. Endoscopy demonstrates yellow "cobble-stone" changes. Hemorrhage is usually recurrent. The pathogenesis of PXE is unknown, and treatment is primarily focused on its complications.

BIBLIOGRAPHY

1. Bennion SD, Patterson JW: Keratosis punctata palmaris et plantaris and adenocarcinoma of the colon. J Am Acad Dermatol 10:587–591, 1984.
2. Cappell MS, Gujral N: Diseases of the peritoneum and mesentery in patients with the acquired immunodeficiency syndrome. Pract Gastroenterol 18:15–20, 30–31, 1994.
3. Cohn MS, Claussen RF: The sign of Leser-Trelat associated with adenocarcinoma of the rectum. Cutis 51:255–257, 1993.
4. Edney JA, et al: Glucagonoma syndrome is an underdiagnosed clinical entity. Am J Surg 160:625–629, 1990.
5. Habif TP (ed): Clinical Dermatology—A Color Guide to Diagnosis and Therapy, 2nd ed. St. Louis, C.V. Mosby, 1990.
6. Harper PS, Harper RMJ, Howel-Evans AW: Carcinoma of the esophagus with tylosis. Q J Med 155:317–333, 1970.
7. Reilly PJ, Nostrant TT: Clinical manifestations of hereditary hemorrhagic telangiectasias. Am J Gastroenterol 79:363–367, 1984.
8. Sudduth RH, et al: Small bowel obstruction in a patient with Peutz-Jeghers syndrome: The role of intraoperative endoscopy. Gastrointest Endosc 38:69–72, 1992.
9. Vase P, Grove O: Gastrointestinal lesions in hereditary hemorrhagic telangiectasias. Gastroenterology 91:1079–1083, 1986.
10. White JW: Erythema nodosum. Dermatol Clin 3:119–127, 1985.
11. Yamada T (ed): Textbook of Gastroenterology, 2nd ed. Philadelphia, J.B. Lippincott, 1995.

ACKNOWLEDGMENT

Special thanks to Col. James Fitzpatrick, M.D. for contributing figures to this chapter.

70. ENDOCRINE DISORDERS AND THE GASTROINTESTINAL TRACT

John A. Merenich, M.D.

1. What are the common gastrointestinal complaints of patients with diabetes mellitus?

Common Symptoms in Diabetes Mellitus

Constipation	60%
Nausea and vomiting	30%
Abdominal pain	30%
Diarrhea	20%
Fecal incontinence	20%
Dysphagia	5%

GI complaints are reported by as many as 75% of patients with diabetes mellitus. Although hyperglycemia, altered hormone production, increased susceptibility to secondary infections, and microangiopathy contribute to the development of these alterations in GI tract function, visceral autonomic neuropathy appears to play a critical role in most of the disorders.

2. Are esophageal motility abnormalities a common source of complaints in patients with diabetes mellitus?

Manometry and scintigraphy show that abnormalities of the esophagus are present in most patients with diabetes mellitus, but accompanying clinical symptoms are infrequent. Symptomatic gastroesophageal reflux, when it occurs, is most often observed in patients with peripheral/sensory neuropathy or symptomatic diabetic gastroparesis. Dysphagia and odynophagia are also distinctly unusual; their occurrence in patients with diabetes should prompt further evaluation for another source. There is one notable exception to this generalization: because of their impaired immune status, patients with diabetes are more prone to *Candida* esophagitis, which can occasionally cause difficulty or pain with swallowing. Fiberoptic esophagoscopy is often required to make the diagnosis because the presence of absence of oral *Candida* does not predict or rule out esophageal infection.

3. What are the causes of gastroparesis in diabetic patients, and how should it be treated?

Reduced amplitude of fundic contractions, decreased amplitude and frequency of antral contractions, and pylorospasm all contribute to a delay of gastric emptying (solids > liquids) in patients with diabetes. In addition to worsening nausea and vomiting and early satiety, delayed gastric emptying may contribute to erratic glucose control in some individuals.

Treatment of Gastroparesis in Diabetes Mellitus

MANEUVER	COMMENTS
Avoid agents that impair gastric emptying	Especially anticholinergics and antidepressants: if needed, use agents with minimal anticholinergic properties, like desipramine and fluoxetine
Adjust diet	Decrease fiber and fat intake; give frequent small meals; increase liquid supplements
Use prokinetic agents (30 min before meals and at bedtime)	Metoclopramide, 5–20 mg Cisapride, 10–20 mg Erythromycin, 250 mg
Consider feeding jejunostomy	For refractory patients with severe malnutrition and volume depletion

4. Describe the mechanisms of chronic diarrhea in diabetes mellitus and their treatments.
Chronic diarrhea in patients with diabetes mellitus is usually related to either chronic autonomic dysfunction or associated diseases that are more prevalent in the diabetic population.

Causes and Treatment of Chronic Diarrhea in Diabetes Mellitus

CAUSES OF DIABETIC DIARRHEA	TREATMENT
Intestinal bacterial overgrowth	Tetracycline, metronidazole, cephalosporins, quinolones (10–14 days each month on a rotating basis)
Celiac disease	Gluten-free diet
Use of dietetic foods	Avoid sorbitol products
Pancreatic exocrine deficiency	Pancreatic enzyme
Bile acid malabsorption	Cholestyramine (4–12 gm/day) or aluminum hydroxide
Abnormal colonic motility	Loperamide, diphenoxylate, clonidine (0.1–0.6 mg/day)
Altered intestinal secretion	Octreotide (50–75 µg, sc, before meals)
Anorectal dysfunction	Biofeedback

5. Explain the clinical implications of impaired GI motility in patients with hypothyroidism.
Delayed gastric emptying, prolonged intestinal transit time, and decreased amplitude and frequency of sigmoid colon and rectal muscular contractions have been documented in patients with hypothyroidism. Intestinal ischemia, myopathy, and neuropathy may all contribute to dysmotility. Decreased frequency of bowel movements (< 1 every 48 hours) is reported in about 12% of patients with hypothyroidism. Elderly patients, especially, may complain of severe constipation refractory to laxatives; in severe cases, ileus progressing to pseudo-obstruction has been observed. Because of its insidious onset, intestinal dysmotility of hypothyroidism is sometimes misdiagnosed as functional bowel disease.

6. What autoimmune gastrointestinal abnormalities are more prevalent in patients with autoimmune thyroiditis?
Immune gastritis and pernicious anemia coexist with hypothyroidism in about 10% of patients with autoimmune thyroiditis. Moreover, anti-parietal cell antibodies are detected in up to one-third of patients with primary hypothyroidism. Autoimmune liver disease is also more prevalent in patients with thyroid disease; hypothyroidism occurs in 16% and thyroid antibody titers are elevated in 26% of patients with primary biliary cirrhosis. Indeed, primary biliary cirrhosis and chronic active hepatitis should be considered if the serum transaminase elevation commonly observed in hypothyroid patients is severe (> 2–3 times normal) or persists after thyroid hormone replacement.

7. What are the gastrointestinal manifestations of thyrotoxic storm?
Thyrotoxic storm refers to a rare, life-threatening syndrome resulting from extreme accentuation of the usual manifestations of thyrotoxicosis. The diagnosis is entirely clinical, but the disorder almost always includes some evidence of severe GI dysfunction. Nausea, vomiting, and abdominal pain are common. Hyperdefecation commonly observed in many patients with thyrotoxicosis may progress to severe diarrhea that can significantly compromise volume status. Hepatic dysfunction characterized by hepatomegaly, abdominal tenderness, and elevated serum transaminase concentrations is also a frequent component of thyroid storm; hyperbilirubinemia and jaundice indicate advanced disease and are associated with a high rate of mortality. The exact nature of hepatic inflammation, steatosis, necrosis, and cirrhosis described at autopsy in patients dying from thyrotoxicosis is unclear. The combination of increased metabolic demand without compensatory increase in hepatic blood flow results in relative ischemia that may account for some of the clinical and histologic findings.

8. Name the metabolic causes of acute pancreatitis.
Hypertriglyceridemia and **hypercalcemia** are the two metabolic disturbances that can cause acute pancreatitis. Triglyceride concentration in excess of 1000 mg/dl has been reported in one-fourth to one-third of patients presenting with acute pancreatitis. Although excessive ethanol use may account for both pancreatitis and secondary triglyceride elevation, a direct causative or ex-

acerbating role of hypertriglyceridemia in the development of pancreatic inflammation in many individuals has been postulated. Acute pancreatitis has been reported in association with hypercalcemia of any cause, but it is most often observed in patients with hyperparathyroidism. Less than 1% of patients with acute pancreatitis, however, have documented hyperparathyroidism.

9. Discuss the three key steps in the management of pancreatitis associated with hypertriglyceridemia.
    1. Recognition: Hypertriglyceridema should be considered in all patients with pancreatitis, especially those with "idiopathic" pancreatitis or recurrent episodes of inflammation. Serum triglyceride concentrations should be measured early in the course of pancreatitis, because clearance of chylomicrons (triglyceride-rich lipoprotein particles believed responsible for the syndrome) may be cleared within a few days of an acute attack, especially in fasting patients.
    2. Management of the acute attack: Decreasing the triglyceride concentration to <500 mg/dl is a primary concern and is usually associated with prompt cessation of abdominal pain. Initial fasting, followed by low-fat diet, is absolutely necessary to achieve this goal. Lipid-lowering agents, such as fibrates and nicotinic acid, are usually ineffective until serum triglyceride levels are reduced to 1000–1500 mg/dl. Administration of large doses of pancreatic enzymes may also help suppress nausea and abdominal pain. Because excess glucose serves as substrate for endogenous triglyceride production, appropriate insulin therapy to achieve euglycemia should be instituted as soon as possible in patients with diabetes mellitus.
    3. Prevention of recurrent hyperchylomicronemia: Restricted fat intake, avoidance of alcohol, weight loss, and exercise help prevent redevelopment of excessive chylomicrons. Patients should avoid agents known to increase serum triglycerides, including estrogens, vitamin A, retinoic acid, B-blockers, and thiazide diuretics. Patients with diabetes should be evaluated regularly to ensure adequate glycemic control. Triglyceride-lowering agents, such as niacin, gemfibrozil, and fish oils, may also help if fasting triglyceride concentrations remain elevated.

10. How can gastrointestinal and hepatic disturbances cause hypoglycemia?
Hypoglycemia (<50 mg/dl) can occur in both the absorptive and postabsorptive state. Postabsorptive (fasting) hypoglycemia includes processes characterized by underproduction or overutilization of glucose, the latter being either insulin-dependent or insulin-independent. GI and hepatic disturbances, therefore, may result or contribute to the development of hypoglycemia at many levels (see figure below).

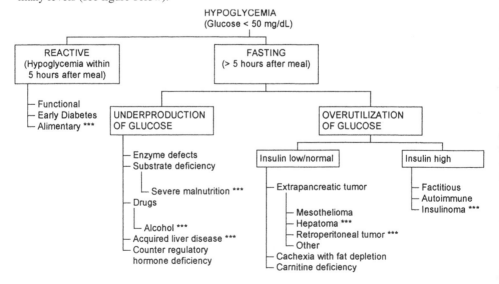

Cause of hypoglycemia. Asterisks (***) identify the GI-related causes.

11. What is alimentary hypoglycemia?
Alimentary hypoglycemia refers to hypoglycemia that results from rapid emptying of the gastric contents into the small intestine. It occurs most often in patients who have undergone previous gastric surgery, such as subtotal gastrectomy, vagotomy, or pyloroplasty. Hyperinsulinism and increased production of gastric inhibitory polypeptide, prompted by the initial accelerated glucose absorption, result in the characteristic "overshoot" hypoglycemia that occurs 2–3 hours after eating. Ingestion of small, frequent meals containing low quantities of simple carbohydrates effectively alleviates symptoms in most patients. Alimentary hypoglycemia is sometimes referred to as "late dumping syndrome." True dumping syndrome, however, is characterized by abdominal distention, nausea, tachycardia, diarrhea, and flushing that results from the osmotic effects of rapid transit of food into the small bowel, coupled with the elaboration of various vasoactive hormones.

12. How does ethanol cause hypoglycemia?
The oxidation of ethanol by alcohol dehydrogenase and aldehyde dehydrogenase requires NAD as a cofactor. As the NADH/NAD ratio increases, gluconeogenesis, which is also NAD-dependent, is impaired. As shown in the figure below, ethanol also inhibits hepatic uptake of key gluconeogenic precursors. Glycogenolysis, however, is not impaired by alcohol. Suppression of adrenocorticotropic hormone (ACTH), potentiation of insulin-induced hypoglycemia, and increased insulin secretion in response to an oral glucose load have all been observed after ethanol ingestion and may predispose prone individuals to reactive hypoglycemia.

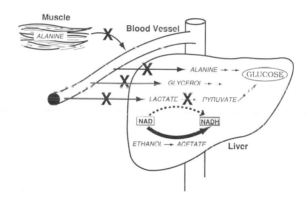

Ethanol inhibition of gluconeogenesis. Sites of inhibition are indicated by X's.

13. Do gastrointestinal malignancies occur more frequently in patients with acromegaly?
Several epidemiologic and retrospective analyses suggest an increased prevalence of GI malignancies in patients with acromegaly. Esophageal and gastric cancer may occur more frequently, but the association of colon cancer with growth hormone excess is most consistent; overall, there appears to be a 3- to 8-fold excess risk of colon cancer or premalignant polyps in acromegalic patients. Colon lesions tend to occur more frequently in men, those >50 years of age, and patients with a family history of colon cancer. The presence of three or more skin tags is also associated with increased cancer risk. The precise mechanisms causing GI malignancies are uncertain. Growth hormones may increase the expression of the c-*myc* proto-oncogene, and insulin-like growth factor-I stimulates cellular proliferation. From a clinical perspective, all patients with acromegaly should be screened with colonoscopy at 5-year intervals. More frequent screening is indicated in high-risk patients.

14. What are the gastrointestinal consequences of hypercalcemia?
Nausea and vomiting are frequent manifestations of hypercalcemia. Consequent fluid loss and poor intake contribute to diminished renal plasma blood flow and decreased glomerular filtration rate, further worsening the hypercalcemia. Constipation and anorexia are also observed in patients

with chronic hypercalcemia. Acute pancreatitis has been reported in association with hypercalcemia of any cause. Peptic ulcer disease is a manifestation of patients with hyperparathyroidism.

15. When should gastrointestinal surgery be considered in patients with severe obesity?

Although life-altering and expensive, surgical intervention may be helpful in severely obese patients (> 100 lbs above ideal body weight) with major medical complications resulting from their obesity. Reduction of 30–40% of presurgical weight within 6–12 months can be expected. Without long-term commitment to behavioral modification, diet adjustment, and exercise, however, many patients regain most of their lost weight within a few years.

16. Which surgical procedures are usually performed for treatment of severe obesity?

The most widely used procedure has been jejunoileal bypass. This procedure is associated with an operative mortality of about 5%, bile acid malabsorption, diarrhea, fat-soluble vitamin deficiency, arthritis, calcium oxalate nephrolithiasis, and liver disease. More recently, gastric plication (gastroplasty) and gastric bypass have gained favor because of their fewer complications and operative mortality <1%. Deficiency of iron, thiamine, and vitamin B12 can result after these procedures.

17. Do all patients with multiple endocrine neoplasia (MEN) syndromes have pancreatic tumors?

Pancreatic islet cell tumors are the second most prevalent manifestation (80%) of the MEN type 1 syndrome, an inherited autosomal dominant trait with high penetrance. Parathyroid hyperplasia (95–100%) and pituitary tumors/hyperplasia (60%) are the other classic components of the MEN 1 syndrome; nodular thyroid disease, adrenal cortical hyperplasia, and foregut carcinoid tumors are occasionally observed. Pancreatic tumors are *not* features of MEN type 2a (medullary carcinoma of the thyroid, parathyroid hyperplasia, pheochromocytoma) or MEN 2b syndrome (medullary cancer of the thyroid, pheochromocytoma, mucosal neuromas, colon polyps).

18. Which pancreatic tumors are observed in MEN 1 syndrome?

Although a particular cell line predominates in most MEN 1 patients with pancreatic tumors, hyperplasia of several cell types is often observed. Pancreatic polypeptide, for example, is cosecreted in most patients with MEN 1 and may be a useful tumor marker, but the hormone does not result in any clinical symptoms. The distribution of the symptom-producing pancreatic tumors in patients with MEN 1 syndrome is as follows:

Gastrinoma	60%
Insulinoma	30%
VIPoma	3%
Somatostatinoma	1%
Glucagonoma	5%
Other	1%

19. List the major clinical manifestations of the pancreatic endocrine tumors.

Pancreatic Endocrine Tumors and Their Clinical Manifestations

TUMOR TYPE	CLINICAL MANIFESTATIONS
Glucagonoma	Hyperglycemia, anorexia, glossitis, anemia, necrolytic migratory erythema
VIPoma (watery diarrhea syndrome)	Watery diarrhea, hypokalemia, hypochlorhydria, hypercalcemia, acidosis
Gastrioma	Recurrent peptic ulcer, refractory esophagitis, diarrhea
Insulinoma	Fasting hypoglycemia, weight gain, hunger, neuroglycopenia (altered mental status, disorientation, seizure, coma, etc.)
Pancreatic polypeptidoma	None
Somatostatinoma	Diabetes mellitus, cholelithiasis, diarrhea, steatorrhea

20. What is carcinoid syndrome?

Carcinoid syndrome consists of explosive diarrhea and abdominal cramping, episodic flushing of the face and torso, predominantly right-sided heart valvular disease, and (occasionally) bronchospasm. The diarrhea and cardiac lesions are mediated by serotonin; tachykinins, bradykinins, histamine, and prostaglandins probably account for the cutaneous and pulmonary manifestations. Because most carcinoid tumors are small and their products are effectively metabolized by the liver, only about 5–10% of patients with carcinoid tumors manifest the syndrome. Large, bulky tumors with hepatic metastasis or small carcinoid tumors outside the portal circulation (e.g., bronchial carcinoid) are most often associated with the syndrome. Hindgut carcinoid tumors (distal colon and rectal origin) almost never cause the syndrome.

21. Outline the treatment of carcinoid syndrome.

I. General measures
   a. Niacin supplementation (most tryptophan is diverted to serotonin production)
   b. High-protein diet (malabsorption common)
   c. Avoid stress, sympathomimetics, and alcohol (may worsen or precipitate attacks)
II. Treatment of flushing
   a. Somatostatin analogs
   b. Interferon
   c. H_1 and H_2 blockers (esp for gastric carcinoids)
   d. Phenoxybenzamine
III. Treatment of diarrhea
   a. Loperamide and diphenoxylate
   b. Somatostatin analogs
   c. Antiserotonin agents (methysergide and cyproheptadine)
   d. Cholestyramine (when bile acid malabsorption is prominent)
IV. Treatment of asthma and bronchospasm
   a. Methylxanthine bronchodilators
   b. Glucocorticoids
   c. *Not* β-agonists or epinephrine (may precipitate or worsen attacks)
V. Reduction of tumor burden
   a. Surgery (debulking or wedge resection)
   b. Hepatic artery embolization or ligation
   c. Chemotherapy
      1. Streptozocin and fluorouracil
      2. Methotrexate and cyclophosphamide
      3. Interferon

22. Discuss the possible therapeutic uses of somatostatin analogs for gastrointestinal diseases.

Somatostatin analogs, such as octreotide, have a longer half-life than somatostatin, can be administered subcutaneously, and have potent antisecretagogue effects. They are helpful in the management of patients with unresectable neuroendocrine tumors, especially carcinoid, VIPoma, insulinoma, and glucagonoma. They have not been helpful in the prevention or treatment of acute or chronic pancreatitis but may be effective adjuncts in the treatment of pancreatic fistula, ascites, and pseudocyst. Secretory diarrhea resulting from short bowel syndrome, ileostomy, amyloidosis, diabetes, and AIDS is reduced when somatostatin is administered 15–30 minutes before meals. The agent has provided relief for some patients with intestinal fistula, dumping syndrome, and irritable bowel syndrome. Finally, recent evidence suggests that somatostatin may be as potent as vassopressin in treatment of esophageal variceal bleeding.

23. What is the most prominent gastrointestinal manifestation of medullary cancer of the thyroid?

Diarrhea, sometimes severe, occurs in 30–50% of patients. Vasoactive intestinal polypeptide, kinins, and prostaglandins (not calcitonin) account for the diarrhea in most patients with the tumor. ACTH and serotonin may also be elaborated by the tumor, causing Cushing's syndrome and carcinoid syndrome, respectively.

24. What is the "rule of 10s" regarding insulinoma?

10% of insulinomas are associated with MEN 1 syndrome

10% are malignant

10% are bilateral

10% are <2 cm in size

10% occur in patients <30 years of age

BIBLIOGRAPHY

1. Arky RA: Hypoglycemia associated with liver disease and ethanol. Endocrinol Metab Clin North Am 18:75, 1989.
2. Braverman LE, Utiger RD: The Thyroid, 6th ed. Philadelphia, J.B. Lippincott, 1991.
3. Delcore R, Friesen SR: Gastrointestinal neuroendocrine tumors: J Am Coll Surg 178:187, 1994.
4. Kahn CR, Weir GC: Joslin's Diabetes Mellitus, 18th ed. Philadelphia, Lea & Febiger, 1994.
5. Modlin IM, Basson MD: Clinical applications of gastrointestinal hormones. Endocrinol Metab Clin North Am 22:823, 1993.
6. Molitch ME: Clinical manifestations of acromegaly. Endocrinol Metab Clin North Am 21:597, 1992.
7. Shulkes A, Wilson JS: Somatostatin in gastroenterology. BMJ 308:1381, 1994.
8. Steinberg W, Tenner S: Acute pancreatitis. N Engl J Med 330:1198, 1994.
9. Toskes PP: Hyperlipidemic pancreatitis. Gastroenterol Clin North Am 19:783, 1990.
10. Valdovinos MA, Camilleri M, Zimmerman BR: Chronic diarrhea in diabetes mellitus: Mechanisms and an approach to diagnosis and treatment. Mayo Clin Proc 68:691, 1993.
11. Vassilopoulou-Sellin R, Ajani J: Neuroendocrine tumors of the pancreas. Endocrinol Metab Clin North Am 23:53, 1994.
12. Wilson JD, Foster DW: Williams Textbook of Endocrinology, 8th ed. Philadelphia, W.B. Saunders, 1992.
13. Yang R, Arem R, Chan L: Gastrointestinal tract complications of diabetes mellitus. Arch Intern Med 144:1251, 1984.

71. ALLERGIC MANIFESTATIONS OF GASTROINTESTINAL DISEASE

P. Dennis Dyer, M.D.

1. How does an adverse reaction to food differ from actual food-induced anaphylaxis? What are the different possible mechanisms for adverse reactions to foods?

An adverse reaction to food refers broadly to a clinically abnormal response to ingested foods or food additives. This is a broad category that can be divided into two major groups: immunologic-mediated food reactions and nonimmunologic food reactions.

Adverse Reactions to Food

IMMUNOLOGIC (ALLERGY)	NONIMMUNOLOGIC (INTOLERANCE)
Food anaphylaxis	Food toxicity
Delayed reactions	Pharmacologic food reaction
Gluten-sensitive enteropathy	Metabolic food reaction
Intestinal cow's milk allergy	

The term **food allergy** can be used synonymously with **immunologic-mediated reactions** to foods, of which food anaphylaxis is the most concerning. *Anaphylaxis* involves symptoms of urticaria, angioedema, asthma, laryngeal edema, nausea and vomiting, hypotension, and possible cardiovascular collapse with death. The onset of symptoms is usually immediate or within 1–2 hours of the ingestion of the responsible food. Other immunologic food reactions include gluten-sensitive enteropathy and intestinal cow's milk allergy of infancy, which are characterized by a delayed onset.

Nonimmunologic food reactions are often referred to as **food intolerance** and include food poisoning or toxicity, pharmacologic reactions, and metabolic reactions. **Food poisoning** or **food toxicity** is caused by the direct action of the food or food contaminant that results in significant symptoms; for example, scombroid fish poisoning results from the ingestion of fish containing histamine that accumulates during the breakdown of the spoiled fish. The symptoms include flushing, nausea, vomiting, diarrhea, headache, and possible hypotension. **Pharmacologic food reactions** result from direct pharmacologic effect of the food or food additive, which causes a well-defined symptom—for example, patients with migraine headaches may experience precipitation of migraines from chocolate or cheese, both of which contain phenylethylamine, a vasoactive monoamine. An example of **food metabolic disorders** is lactose deficiency, which causes intestinal reactions to milk ingestion.

2. The diagnosis of food anaphylaxis is facilitated by the onset of symptoms following the ingestion of the incriminated food. What additional studies can be done to confirm this diagnosis?

The onset of anaphylaxis immediately with food ingestion simplifies the diagnosis of food anaphylaxis, but often the patient has consumed several foods during a meal or 1–2 hours may pass prior to the onset of symptoms. To establish a particular food as the inciting agent, **food prick skin testing** can be accomplished to establish the diagnosis. The history dictates which foods should be chosen for the food test panel. Prick tests at a concentration of 1:20 w/vol are used and judged positive only in light of the history. False-positive food skin tests are common, and a positive skin test does not necessarily connote food allergy. A properly performed negative food skin test is highly predictive for the absence of specific IgE and the absence of future reactions.

Radioallergosorbent testing (RAST), an in vitro technique to detect circulating specific IgE, is rarely required in the diagnosis of food allergy but may be indicated in a patient with exquisite food allergy. Exquisite food allergy has been documented, especially to peanuts, where the mere opening of a jar of peanut butter has caused symptoms. Such patients are at risk for anaphylaxis from skin testing, and the in vitro RAST is safer.

Occasionally, patients with positive skin tests to multiple foods cannot ascertain which food was responsible for the anaphylaxis, or the diagnosis of anaphylaxis may be in question. In these situations, a cautious oral challenge to include an open food challenge or a double-blind, placebo-controlled food challenge is warranted to verify the diagnosis. This test should only be performed by a specialist familiar with the challenge procedure and experienced with treatment of anaphylaxis.

3. Certain foods are notorious for causing anaphylaxis. What are they?

Adults	Children
Peanuts	Milk
Tree nuts	Egg
Crustacea	Peanut
Fish	Soy
	Wheat
	Fish

In adults, the most common foods causing anaphylaxis include peanuts, tree nuts, crustacea (shrimp, crab, and lobster), and fish. Foods that cause anaphylaxis in children include peanuts, milk, egg, soy, wheat, and fish. Peanut is well established as a sensitivity that is not lost with time, so it is common for both adults and children. Besides these common foods, any consumable food can induce anaphylaxis, including the unlikely candidates of cottonseed and sesame seed. Most patients are usually sensitive to only one or two foods, and multiple food sensitivities are unlikely.

4. In the management of food anaphylaxis, what guidelines should be provided to the patient besides avoidance of the incriminated food?

Once the food causing anaphylaxis is identified, guidelines besides strict avoidance are in order.

1. **Maintain epinephrine in an injectable form** to self-administer in case of accidental ingestion of the incriminated food. This occurs especially in restaurants or when food is eaten away from home. Individuals should self-administer epinephrine at the onset of symptoms of anaphylaxis and should also consider taking oral antihistamines. These items should be carried by the food-allergic patient when dining away from home. These individuals should receive nursing instruction on the administration of epinephrine and should have an organized plan once a reaction is encountered to include accessing emergency medical care.

2. **Read labels on prepared foods,** especially candies. Certain candies and candy bars contain peanuts and nuts that are not obvious from reading the name or description of the product.

5. If a patient is allergic to peanuts, will ingestion of walnuts also cause anaphylaxis?

There is a distinct difference between tree nuts and the legume peanut, so there is no cross-reactivity between them. Peanut-allergic patients can consume tree nuts, such as pecans and walnuts. Also, peanut- and soy-allergic individuals can consume peanut oil and soy oil without difficulty. There is in vitro cross-reactivity between crustacea, so shrimp-allergic individuals should avoid lobster and crab until complete testing is performed.

6. Is there a connection between the reactions to radiocontrast media and anaphylactic reactions to seafood?

Systemic reactions to radiocontrast media are often labeled as "iodine allergy," and the patient is instructed to avoid seafood. **Seafood allergy** in the strict sense is an IgE-mediated reaction leading to symptoms of anaphylaxis and is induced by consumption of either crustacea or mollusks (oysters and clams). The most common and well-described reaction is to shrimp. Several in vitro studies have demonstrated the actual proteins that are the responsible allergens for shrimp-induced anaphylaxis; serum IgE to that shrimp protein induces the anaphylaxis, and this allergen is not iodine.

Radiocontrast media reactions develop after administration of the iodinated high-osmolality contrast agents, leading to systemic symptoms suggestive of anaphylaxis. The reaction stems from the high osmolality of the agent, which causes direct histamine release and activation of complement with resultant systemic symptoms. The reaction is not from IgE to iodine or to the iodinated contrast media and is not a real "iodine allergy." The term iodine allergy is only a useful way to communicate to patients a radiocontrast reaction. Thus, there is no relation between reactions to radiocontrast media and food-induced anaphylaxis to shrimp or other seafood.

7. Sufferers of seasonal allergic rhinitis often complain of oral and pharyngeal pruritus following ingestion of fresh fruits. What is this disease entity, and what association does it have with allergic rhinitis?

Sufferers of ragweed induced-allergic rhinitis have long complained of symptoms of oral and pharyngeal pruritus with the ingestion of watermelon. This is now described as the **oral allergy syndrome** and consists of pruritus of the lips, tongue, palate, and oral pharynx and occasionally angioedema of the same area. This reaction is rarely associated with systemic symptoms and is usually short-lived without sequelae. Individuals with ragweed hayfever may have symptoms with the ingestion of watermelon or cantaloupe, and birch pollen-allergic individuals have symptoms with apples, celery, and carrots. Other fresh fruits and vegetables, including peaches, pears, and potatoes, may also cause these symptoms. Overall, the oral allergy syndrome is self-limited and can be identified by its existence in individuals with allergic rhinitis.

8. Does food allergy play a role in the irritable bowel syndrome?

The irritable bowel syndrome continues to be a common GI disease without any clear etiology, except for some evidence for alterations in intestinal motility. Several studies have examined food allergy as the basis for the irritable bowel syndrome, but the studies have failed to show any association. Certain foods, such as milk products, can precipitate symptoms in these patients if there is concomitant lactase deficiency, but true food hypersensitivity does not cause or precipitate irritable bowel syndrome.

9. What chronic gastrointestinal disease can exacerbate bronchial asthma?

Gastroesophageal reflux commonly occurs in asthmatics, and the reflux may worsen the asthma and complicate its treatment. In addition, theophylline, used in the treatment of chronic asthma, can decrease lower esophageal sphincter pressure and compound the existing reflux in asthmatics. The purported mechanisms are vagally mediated reflex bronchoconstriction from acid in the proximal esophagus and microaspiration of gastric acid that causes direct irritant bronchoconstriction. Asthmatics with gastroesophageal reflux symptoms, those with moderate nocturnal asthma, and difficult-to-control asthmatics are most likely to have their asthma complicated by reflux.

In evaluating asthmatics for gastroesophageal reflux, the most definite study would be a **reflux asthma study,** in which peak flows or spirograms are repeated at frequent intervals with simultaneous esophageal pH monitoring to demonstrate associated drops in airflow and esophageal pH. In such patients, treatment with H_2 blockers or omeprazole may significantly improve symptoms and reduce the need for asthma medication. Otherwise, the demonstration of reflux in asthmatics with pH monitoring or radiographic studies does not itself establish a causal relationship. In this case, a trial of an antireflux regimen may be warranted to determine the significance of reflux in aggravating the patient's asthma. The endpoint of this trial should use objective criteria to establish causation, such as improved spirometry, reduction in nocturnal symptoms, or a reduction in as-needed β-agonist.

10. Which intestinal parasitic infections should be considered in a patient with eosinophilia?

The association of eosinophilia with parasitic infections has been long established, but the most representative example is the helminth parasites and not protozoa. Tissue invasion by the parasite is the primary prerequisite for the induction of eosinophilia, and strict intraluminal parasites, such as *Enterobius* (pinworm) and *Trichuris* (whipworm), usually do not induce peripheral eosinophilia. Strongyloidiasis, schistosomiasis, ascariasis, and filariasis are examples of parasites invading different tissue with resultant eosinophilia. Because tissue invasion is the determining criteria, examination of stool for ova and parasites may be insufficient in the evaluation of peripheral eosinophilia. If a parasitic infection is suspected, a more directed approach to include other body fluids and tissue biopsy may be needed to diagnose the infection.

11. Eosinophilic gastroenteritis is also associated with peripheral eosinophilia. What clinical symptoms suggest this disease?

This uncommon disease is characterized by peripheral eosinophilia, eosinophilic infiltration of the GI tract, and various GI symptoms depending on the site and depth of mucosal involvement. The more common symptoms include postprandial nausea and vomiting, cramping, abdominal pain, diarrhea, and weight loss, which are the typical symptoms for mucosal involvement. Other more advanced symptoms include fecal blood loss, iron-deficiency anemia, protein-losing enteropathy, and growth retardation. With infiltration of the muscular layer of the GI tract, symptoms of gastric or small bowel obstruction may develop. Serosal involvement will lead to ascites, which will contain eosinophils.

With these symptoms and peripheral eosinophilia, gastric and small bowel biopsies are needed to confirm the diagnosis. The antrum of the stomach is often involved and may be a good starting point for biopsy. Also, multiple biopsies of the small bowel may be required because of possible patchy involvement. The demonstration of eosinophilic infiltration with the biopsies clinches the diagnosis.

12. What screening test should be ordered to evaluate a patient with recurrent angioedema and recurrent bouts of small bowel obstruction?

Patients presenting with recurrent angioedema, which is not associated with pruritus and urticaria, can be evaluated with a C4 level to detect **hereditary angioedema.** Patients with the more common urticaria and angioedema are not candidates for screening, because they do not have the characteristic of only angioedema. A low C4 level suggests ongoing complement activation secondary to C1 esterase inhibitor deficiency. If the C4 level is low, measurement of a C1 inhibitor serum level and functional assay will diagnose hereditary angioedema, if the C1 inhibitor is low or dysfunctional.

Patients with hereditary angioedema usually have a family history of angioedema and have a history of recurrent angioedema, typically of the lips, periorbital area, extremities, or genitalia. The angioedema may involve the GI tract, leading to the symptoms of vomiting, diarrhea, abdominal colic, and small bowel obstruction. A history of angioedema with lack of both fever and leukocytosis during acute GI symptoms suggests this diagnosis. Some patients may have primarily recurrent small bowel obstruction as their *forme fruste* of this disease, and obtaining a C4 level clarifies this diagnosis. By far the most concerning symptom is laryngeal edema, which can be fatal, and prompt action to preserve the airway is critical.

13. Describe the gastrointestinal mucosal immune system. Which immunoglobulin is increased in production in this system?

The mucosal immune system of the GI tract consists of organized mucosal lymphoid tissue collectively referred to as **gut-associated lymphoid tissue,** or GALT (see figure below). This lymphoid tissue is responsible for receiving antigen across the mucosa via specialized epithelial cells called membranous cells (M cells). The M cells are responsible for transporting vesicles of macromolecules from the gut lumen across the cell to the subepithelial tissues. These cells overlie the areas of lymphoid follicles referred to as **Peyer's patches,** and within these follicles are germinal centers containing B lymphocytes. The uniqueness of these B cells is the increased number of IgA-bearing B cells, which are predestined to produce **IgA.**

Besides the lymphoid aggregates, there is also a diffuse net of **lymphoid tissue** throughout the mucosa of the GI tract. This tissue gives rise to two interesting populations of lymphocytes: (1) intraepithelial lymphocytes that reside within the epithelial layer and are composed mainly of T cells, and (2) lamina propria lymphocytes that contain a mixed population of B and T cells. The B cells of the lamina propria lymphocyte population are also dominated by IgA-bearing B cells.

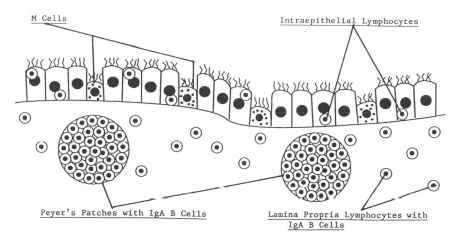

Components of gut-associated lymphoid tissue and lymphocyte populations.

14. Giardiasis in association with recurrent sinopulmonary infections suggests which humoral immunodeficiency states?

Recurrent sinopulmonary infections are suggestive of immunodeficiencies resulting from hypogammaglobulinemia, which can be diagnosed by obtaining serum immunoglobulin levels. In adults, **acquired hypogammaglobulinemia** or **common variable immunodeficiency** is a heterogeneous disorder of B-cell differentiation, with resultant failure to secrete immunoglobulins. Besides recurrent pneumonia and sinusitis, these patients develop giardiasis as a consequence of their immunodeficiency. They usually present with diarrhea and can also develop malabsorption secondary to the giardiasis. The giardiasis is treatable with standard medical regimens, and the institution of monthly gammaglobulin replacement infusions should lessen the frequency of giardiasis and other infections. In contrast, patients with **selective IgA deficiency** usually do not experience infections with *Giardia,* and only a minority develop recurrent sinopulmonary infections.

15. What GI manifestations are highly suggestive of chronic granulomatous disease?

A male infant presenting with hepatomegaly from a liver abscess, ulcerative stomatitis, diarrhea, and perianal abscess, along with lymphadenopathy, osteomyelitis, and pneumonia is suspect for chronic granulomatous disease (CGD). Along with these manifestations, infections with unusual organisms of *Staphylococcus aureus* and *S. epidermidis, Serratia marcescens, Pseudomonas, Candida,* and *Aspergillus* are also suggestive of CGD. CGD is a rare disorder inherited primarily in an X-linked recessive pattern, but autosomal patterns have been described. Defective phagocytic respiratory burst secondary to the faulty NADPH oxidase results in ineffective neutrophil killing of bacterial and fungal organisms intracellularly. The abnormal oxidase results from the absence or dysfunction of cytochrome *b,* but other defects are now being described in this important oxidase.

16. What relative immunodeficiency disorders can develop from a protein-losing enteropathy? Which laboratory tests are needed to confirm this diagnosis?

Inflammatory diseases of the bowel can lead to loss of immunoglobulins and other proteins in the stool, which is referred to as **protein-losing enteropathy.** Low serum immunoglobulin levels confirm this diagnosis, and because this protein loss is nonspecific, hypoalbuminemia is also found with the hypogammaglobulinemia. The protein-losing enteropathy can be caused by a variety of GI diseases, including severe Crohn's disease, ulcerative colitis, gluten-induced enteropathy, and protein-losing gastropathy of Menetrier's disease.

In addition to protein loss, lymphocytes may also be lost in the GI tract, especially with diseases that affect the intestinal lymphatics, including intestinal lymphangiectasia. A **lymphocyte count** showing lymphopenia and **delayed-type hypersensitivity test** showing anergy would confirm significant lymphocyte loss. Fortunately, both of these relative immunodeficiencies are not significantly associated with increased infections.

17. Describe the gastrointestinal manifestations of acute graft-versus-host disease.
Acute graft-versus-host disease (GVHD) develops when immunocompetent donor lymphocytes attack host tissues, primarily after bone marrow transplantation. In acute GVHD, the skin, GI tract, and liver are primary areas of involvement. The GI hallmark of acute GVHD is the onset of severe diarrhea and abdominal cramping several weeks after transplantation. This may develop into a large-volume diarrhea with resultant protein and electrolyte loss. The liver involvement can vary from subclinical hyperbilirubinemia to jaundice and hepatomegaly. The onset of a maculopapular skin rash along with the diarrhea and hyperbilirubinemia is helpful in diagnosing GVHD versus infectious or other causes of the GI symptoms. Interestingly in chronic GVHD, patients can develop esophageal disease, including dysphagia, odynophagia, and esophageal strictures. Chronic GVHD usually develops months later and also includes chronic skin disease and liver disease.

18. Two major epidemics associated with peripheral eosinophilia have developed following the ingestion of two different substances. What were the disease entities, and what were the ingestants?
The two epidemics were the toxic-oil syndrome and eosinophilia-myalgia syndrome. The **toxic-oil syndrome** occurred in Spain in 1981 and consisted of symptoms of cough, dyspnea, fever, pulmonary infiltrates, peripheral eosinophilia, vomiting, diarrhea, and rash, with eventual paralytic neuromuscular symptoms. This syndrome was associated with consumption of an illegally sold cooking oil that contained a high proportion of rapeseed oil and eventually affected up to 20,000 individuals.

The **eosinophilia-myalgia syndrome** developed around 1989 in the United States and consisted of the acute onset of myalgias, peripheral eosinophilia, rash, and fever, with certain individuals developing a chronic neuromuscular phase. The ingestion of large amounts of L-tryptophan, which contained an impurity, was the culprit in this syndrome. The L-tryptophan was easily available at health food stores for the treatment of insomnia and various other ailments.

BIBLIOGRAPHY

1. Anderson JA: The establishment of common language concerning adverse reactions to foods and food additives. J Allergy Clin Immunol 78:140–144, 1986.
2. Atkins FM, Steinberg SS, Metcalfe DD: Evaluation of immediate adverse reactions to foods in adult patients: 1. Correlation of demographic, laboratory, and prick skin test data with response to controlled oral food challenge. J Allergy Clin Immunol 75:348–355, 1985.
3. Crowe SE, Perdue MH: Gastrointestinal food hypersensitivity: Basic mechanisms of pathophysiology. Gastroenterology 103:1075–1095, 1992.
4. Kilbourne EM, Rigau-Perez JG, Heath CW, et al: Clinical epidemiology of toxic-oil syndrome: Manifestations of a new illness. N Engl J Med 309:1408–1414, 1983.
5. Metcalfe DD, Sampson HA (eds): Workshop on experimental methodology for clinical studies of adverse reactions to foods and food additives. J Allergy Clin Immunol 86:421–442, 1990.
6. Metcalfe DD, Sampson HA, Simon RA (eds): Food Allergy: Adverse Reactions to Foods and Food Additives. Boston, Blackwell Scientific Publications, 1991.
7. Morrow JD, Margolies GR, Rowland J, Roberts LJ: Evidence that histamine is the causative toxin of scombroid-fish poisoning. N Engl J Med 324:716–720, 1991.
8. Ortolani C, Ispano M, Pastorello E, et al: The oral allergy syndrome. Ann Allergy 61:47–52, 1988.
9. Sachs MI, O'Connell E: Cross-reactivity of foods—mechanisms and clinical significance. Ann Allergy 61:36–40, 1988.
10. Sampson HA: Adverse reactions to foods. In Middleton E, Reed CE, Ellis EF, et al (eds): Allergy Principles and Practice, vol II, 4th ed. St. Louis, C.V. Mosby, 1993, pp 1661–1680.
11. Shanahan F, Targan SR: Gastrointestinal manifestations of immunologic disorders. In Yamada T, Alpers DH, Owyang C, et al (eds): Textbook of Gasteroenterology, vol II. Philadelphia, J.B. Lippincott, 1991, pp 2157–2171.
12. Strober W, James SP: The mucosal immune system. In Stites DP, Terr AI, Parslow TG (eds): Basic & Clinical Immunology, 8th ed. Norwalk, CT, Appleton & Lange, 1994, pp 541–551.
13. Wershil BK, Walker WA: The mucosal barrier, IgE-mediated gastrointestinal events, and eosinophilic gastroenteritis. Gastroenterol Clin North Am 21:387–404, 1992.
14. Yunginger JW, Sweeney KG, Sturner WO, et al: Fatal food-induced anaphylaxis. JAMA 260:1450–1452, 1988.
15. Zwetchkenbaum J, Burakoff R: The irritable bowel syndrome and food hypersensitivity. Ann Allergy 61:47–49, 1988.

IX. Gastrointestinal Radiology

72. PLAIN ABDOMINAL X-RAY AND CONTRAST RADIOGRAPHY

John Charles Lemon, M.D.

1. What information should be on an x-ray requisition?

State the answer you expect from the x-ray study. Note where the pain is located, particularly which side. Include a prior history of surgery, noting *what* the operation was and *when*.

2. Why perform plain abdominal x-rays?

To get prompt information inexpensively and with little patient discomfort.

Characteristic X-ray Findings in Common GI Diseases

DISEASE	FINDINGS
Gallbladder	15% of stones are radiodense; air in gallbladder lumen or wall
Nephrolithiasis, urolithiasis	80% of calculi are radiodense
Pancreatitis	Chronic pancreatitis: calcification of the pancreas
	Acute pancreatitis: "sentinel" loop of jejunum; transverse colon gas, none of left colon ("colon cut-off")
Closed loop obstruction	Soft tissue mass
Intussusception	Soft tissue mass
Abscess	Patchy radiolucencies like feces, but outside colon lumen
Diverticulitis	Similar to abscess but usually in sigmoid area
Appendicitis	Fecalith within an 8-cm radius of appendiceal base; air-fluid levels of cecum and ileum
Trauma	Many findings — **do not delay CT**
Inflammatory bowel disease	Small bowel obstruction; renal and gallbladder stones increased in patients with ileal disease or resection; mass effect seen with abscess; evaluate for toxic megacolon
Ischemia of bowel	Paralytic ileus; thumb-printing; gasless abdomen; portal vein gas — plain films usually not helpful
Gallstone ileus	Women > male; pneumobilia; small bowel obstruction; RLQ calcification (stone)
Ascites	"Ground-glass" density of abdomen; centrally packed loops; blurred right hepatic lobe tip

3. What are the main considerations in pneumoperitoneum?

Free air is seen in 75% of perforations and 58% of postoperative patients. An erect chest film can identify 1.0 ml of subdiaphragmatic air, and a left lateral decubitus x-ray can detect 10 ml of air lateral to the right hepatic lobe. The patient should be maintained in these positions for 10 minutes before filming. In two-thirds of cases, free air is seen on supine films. Findings of pneumoperitoneum include:

1. Air on both sides of the bowel wall (Rigler's sign);
2. RUQ air anterior to the liver;
3. Subhepatic air (straight oblique radiolucency along the inferomedial edge of the liver);
4. Density of the falciform ligament outlined by air;
5. A lucent triangle of air between three bowel loops.

The presence of a large amount of air 4–5 days postoperatively is suspicious for perforation, particularly in children or obese persons. Thin patients may exhibit free air for as long as 3–4 weeks postop.

Among conditions that masquerade as **pneumoperitoneum** are basilar pulmonary atelectasis, subdiaphragmatic extraperitoneal fat, and apposition of air-filled loops appearing as Rigler's sign. Unlike true pneumoperitoneum, these impostors do not move with positional changes.

4. What are the important plain film considerations in small intestinal obstruction (SBO)?

Paralytic ileus shows air in dilated small bowel within the "picture frame" of a dilated colon. Mechanical SBO shows confluent dilated loops (> 3.0 cm) with scanty or absent colon gas. Fluid-filled loops may appear as "gasless abdomen" in SBO. Colon obstruction may have colon gas decompressed into small bowel and hides the possibility. Normally, the right colon absorbs fluid so efficiently that copious fluid proximal to the hepatic flexure strongly suggests left colon obstruction. A cecal diameter of 15 cm is reason to do a prompt contrast study and hasten surgical decompression when colon obstruction is identified. Because it is not usually possible to tell the "age" of an SBO from single study, follow-up plain films will help. With gastric outlet obstruction, the stomach dilates greatly and depresses the transverse colon.

5. Any "insider hints" about plain film diagnosis?

- A "blurry" film indicates **patient motion** and negates the worth of the exam.
- **Abscesses** are more common postoperatively than otherwise and occur in predictable locations: subdiaphragmatic, colon gutters, small bowel mesentery, and pelvis. Abscess look-a-likes are necrotic tumors and open abdominal wounds. Bizarre air collections may be due to retroperitoneal air from abscesses or retroperitoneal perforations.
- Gallstones and urinary stones and fecalith may be poorly calcified and hard to detect, so look hard!
- Cecal **volvulus** shows cecum in midabdomen or LUQ, and sigmoid volvulus has the dilated loop rising out of the pelvis with a central white line of the sigmoid walls in apposition (see Figure 1).

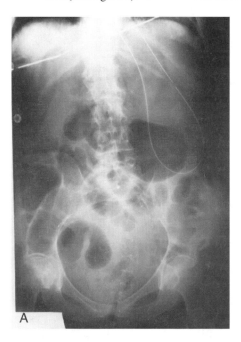
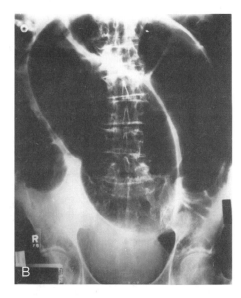

Figure 1. **A,** Cecal volvulus. Dilated, gas-filled cecum is seen overlying the vertebrae. Nasogastric tube confirms that the gas-filled structure is not the stomach. **B,** Dilated sigmoid colon loop in a sigmoid volvulus.

- The plain film is not usually reliable in distinguishing a paralytic ileus from mechanical obstruction in the first 10 days postoperatively.
- Ogilvie's syndrome can be distinguished from obstruction by turning the patient to the right decubitus, waiting, and then turning the patient prone to move the gas to the left colon and rectum.
- Step back from the film, and look for a *huge* mass. The trees may be obscuring the forest!

6. Is GI fluoroscopy ever needed?

Yes. It provides assessment of function, mobility, and presence of infiltrations or fixation. GI fluoroscopy quickly confirms a lesion or shows a worrisome area as normal. It is the *sine qua non* test to evaluate swallowing disorders and fistulae.

7. What do I need to know about GI contrast media?

Modern commercial barium sulfate is available in different weight/volume concentrations for specific studies: **e.g.,** double-contrast barium enema vs single-contrast barium enema. Each has additives for wetting, antifoaming, and suspension. Aqueous agents are used mainly for suspected perforation.

Advantages and Disadvantages of Radiocontrast Media

BARIUM	AQUEOUS AGENTS
Advantages	
• Preferred agent, provides the best mucosal detail and resists dilution	• Preferred agent in any suspected perforation
• Does not solidify in SBO	• Preferred enema agent in LBO, but limited use in SBO (will show complete SBO)
• May be used safely if aqueous contrast does not show perforation of esophagus	• Identifies large abnormalities well: extrinsic masses, colonic constrictions, most free perforations
• Little harm if tracheal aspiration occurs or if tracheoesophageal fistula suspected	
• Less expensive	
Disadvantages	
• May cause life-threatening mediastinitis and peritonitis if perforation present	• Agents are hyperosmolar and absorb water into small bowel, worsening complete SBO, so use cautiously in young and elderly
• Colon absorbs luminal water from barium and may convert partial colonic obstruction into complete obstruction	• Aspiration of ionic agents may cause severe pulmonary edema, nonionic agents safer but expensive
• Additives may cause allergies and cause patient discomfort	• Hyperosmolarity may have laxative effect and cause patient discomfort

COLON STUDIES

8. What is defecography?

Defecography, or evacuation proctography, provides an x-ray record of and a perspective on defecation. It is done with fluoroscopy with spot filming and videotaping as needed.

9. What is the importance of defecography?

It provides measurable information about constipation and incontinence. In the **constipated** patient, it yields findings that can be used to prevent pudendal neuropathy from straining and incontinence. As perineal lift is normal in the constipated patient, a perineal support device may prevent incontinence.

In patients with **incontinence** caused by prolapse, sphincter trauma, or neurogenic factors, defecography can demonstrate internal intussusception and changes of the anorectal angle amenable to surgery; it also can monitor healing after trauma.

10. Describe the difference between double-contrast and single-contrast barium enema examinations.

Double-contrast barium enema (DCBE) uses thick barium and air distention to provide fine mucosal detail. Single-contrast barium enema (SCBE) is performed with "thin" barium and higher kilovoltage to "see through" the column of contrast. SCBE is easier to perform in the debilitated patient and those with redundant colons. SCBE is preferred in cases of intussusception and severe diverticulosis.

11. What are some commonly encountered technical problems with barium enemas?
- Inadequate preparation with residual colonic feces.
- Incontinence (use intravenous glucagon and a retention balloon).
- Nonfilling of right colon by DCBE.
- Numerous diverticula can mask a cancer on DCBE study (use endoscopy or SCBE for restudy) (see Figure 2).

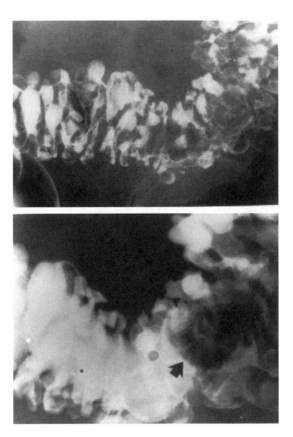

Figure 2. *Top,* Double-contrast barium enema showing many diverticula, but no tumor. *Bottom,* Single-contrast study outlines the polypoid carcinoma. (From Gore RM, Levine MS, and Laufer I: A Textbook of Gastrointestinal Radiology. Philadelphia, W.B. Saunders, 1994; with permission.)

12. Name an avoidable complication of barium enemas.
Perforation of the rectum (usually diseased). The radiologist should perform a digital exam before inserting the rectal tube. Proctoscopy or sigmoidoscopy should precede the barium enema when a low-lying obstruction is suspected.

13. What is the role of the barium exam in evaluation of inflammatory bowel disease?
Barium exam can differentiate Crohn's disease from ulcerative colitis in 80–90% of cases (see table on next page).

Ulcerative Colitis	Crohn's Disease
Disease is contiguous, confluent, circumferential	Distribution is patchy and asymmetric, skip areas common
Fine granular mucosal changes	
Starts in the rectum and spreads proximally	Ulceration common, may be superficial aphthoid or deep and fissuring
Anal and perianal involvement rare	Fistulae common
Ileocecal valve often patulous and fixed open	Often involves only the right colon
	Ileocecal valve often stenotic when involved

14. Can the barium enema differentiate other causes of intestinal inflammation?
There is too much overlap in appearance to distinguish bacillary enteritis from parasitic infection by barium exam. Tuberculous enteritis is suggested by combined ileal and cecal involvement. Amebiasis is often characterized by a cone deformity to the cecum and the absence of ileal involvement.

15. When is the barium enema useful in the evaluation of suspected acute diverticulitis?
Only in extraluminal extravasation.

16. List the advantages and disadvantages of the barium enema and colonoscopy in the evaluation of colon polyps.

Barium Enema	Colonoscopy
Less expensive, fewer complications, no need for sedation	Preferred test, provides best mucosal detail
May identify lesions in the "blind" areas behind folds, hepatic and splenic flexures, and tortuous sigmoid	Permits histologic sampling or removal of identified lesions
Inadequate preparation	Failure to reach cecum in 2–5% of patients
Unable to sample or remove identified lesions	Sedation necessary in most patients, may cause some cardiopulmonary suppression

When colonoscopic and barium findings are discordant, consultative review is mandatory. Repetition of one or both studies may be necessary.

17. Can barium enema determine which polyps are malignant?
No. Polyps on thin stalks are unlikely to be malignant. Nodular, irregular polyps and polyps with a contour defect are likely to be malignant. The size of polyps does correlate with the risk for malignancy:

Size (mm)	Malignant
< 5	0%
6–10	1%
10–20	10%
> 20	45%

18. Can barium enema differentiate larger colonic neoplasms?
The larger cancers and lymphomas look alike on barium exams. Endometrioses and metastatic invasion from prostate, cervical, or bladder sites appear similar.

19. Is barium study useful in benign tumor differentiation?
Lipomas—smooth, change shape with pressure.
Hemangioma—rare, but have phleboliths.
Villous adenoma—flat with crevices (50% malignant).

20. How is the barium enema used to evaluate the postoperative colon?
DCBE is the primary diagnostic procedure for detection of local and anastomotic recurrence and can show metachronous lesions. CT and magnetic resonance (MR) are the best follow-up studies in patients who have already been operated on for anastomotic recurrence.

21. What is role of the barium enema in appendicitis?
Little, currently. The barium exam can show the extrinsic mass of appendiceal abscess. However, 20% of normal appendices do not fill at barium exam. CT scan is more accurate in problematic cases.

22. How are polyps and diverticula differentiated on barium examination?
Figure 3 demonstrates how polyps can be distinguished from diverticula on a barium enema.
      A, B. On examination, the barium density fades away from the polyp (*panel A*), whereas the barium density fades inward in a diverticulum (*panel B*).
      C. The diverticulum is seen outside the lumen (*panel C*).
      D. The apex of the polyp points to center of the intestinal lumen, whereas the apex of a diverticulum points away from the center of the lumen (*panel D*).

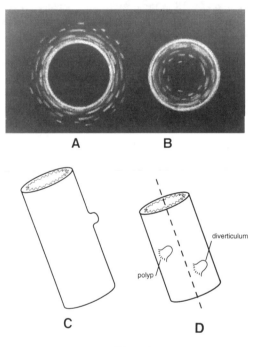

Figure 3.

ESOPHAGEAL STUDIES

23. What is the role of the x-ray esophagogram?
X-ray esophagography provides a simple functional assessment of esophageal motility. Webs, diverticula, rings, intrinsic and extrinsic masses, and strictures are seen clearly. It is probably the easiest way to distinguish between sliding and paraesophageal hernias (see Figure 4 on next page). Video esophagography is the best method to evaluate swallowing disorders or transfer dysphagia, although it will not detect mild esophagitis. The technique detects varices in only 50% of cases. In cases of chest pain, an abnormal esophagogram does not prove esophageal origin of the pain. Optimal technique for x-ray esophagography requires double contrast and full column study in the erect and horizontal positions and the administration of a 13-mm barium pill.

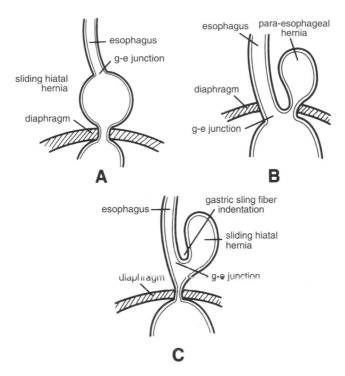

Figure 4. Esophagographic differentiation of sliding hiatal and paraesophageal hernias. **A,** Sliding hiatal hernia. The gastroesophageal (g-e) junction is seen above the diaphragm. **B,** Paraesophageal hernia. The gastroesophageal junction is below the diaphragm. **C,** Sliding hiatal hernia with gastric sling fiber indentation mimicking paraesophageal hernia. Note the gastroesophageal junction above the diaphragm.

24. How do hiatal hernia, reflux esophagitis, and x-ray examination relate?

Most patients with hiatal hernia do not have endoscopic evidence of reflux esophagitis, but 90% of patients with reflux esophagitis have hiatal hernia. The relation of the two is undecided.

On x-ray, findings of esophagitis include abnormal motility in 25–50% of patients with reflux esophagitis, mucosal nodularity, ulcers, thick folds, inflammatory polyps, distal webs, scarring, and strictures. The fine, transverse, "feline" folds are transient and commonly seen with reflux, but alone they do not indicate esophagitis. Acid barium administration is no longer used due to its high false-positive rate. Most strictures are smooth, long (2–4 cm) and tapered but cannot be distinguished from invasive cancer or Barrett's esophagus. Endoscopy and biopsy should be performed whenever esophageal strictures are detected. Nearly all patients with a 12-mm stricture are symptomatic, and use of the 13-mm barium pill will identify 95% of all symptomatic strictures. Only 20–40% of patients with proven reflux esophagitis by endoscopy will reflux barium during upper GI examination, so the absence of barium reflux does not exclude gastroesophageal reflux. The accuracy of single and double-centered studies in moderate and severe esophagitis, counting false positives, is 75%. Endoscopy and biopsy are the most reliable tests for reflux esophagitis.

25. What are the radiographic findings of the non-reflux causes of esophagitis?

The more specific radiographic appearances occur in candidal esophagitis, with its typical raised plaques, and in cytomegalovirus and herpes esophagitis, with their discrete ulcers on a normal background. The benign glycogenic acanthosis mimics candidiasis but is asymptomatic. Other multiple inflammations are drug-induced ulcers, mainly due to tetracycline or those caused by radiation, caustic ingestion, Crohn's disease, nasogastric tube trauma, and graft-vs-host disease. Some of these are suggested by radiographic appearance alone, but a clinical history usually will suggest the cause. Esophageal pseudodiverticulosis has a classical appearance, but its relation to inflammation of the esophagus is debated.

26. Is barium study useful in esophageal neoplastic disease?

Yes. Proper double-contrast technique is quite sensitive in detection of a large number of benign and malignant neoplasms of the esophagus, as well as cysts and hematomas. Benign lesions tend to be smooth and taper gradually, whereas malignant lesions are ragged with a bright shelf-like demarcation. Localized lesions of the esophagus should be biopsied. Use of effervescent granules in obstructing carcinomas has caused perforation, so an initial swallow without use of the gas distention is recommended when a history of severe dysphagia is elicited.

27. Are there any other useful indications for esophagography?

In a patient with a history of recent vomiting and chest pain, esophageal perforation (Boerhaave's syndrome) is suggested. A chest x-ray may show subcutaneous or mediastinal air or a unilateral pleural effusion. Only small quantities of aqueous contrast material should be administered to define the extent and location of the leak. If less opaque aqueous media fails to show a tear, then the study can be repeated with barium. Foreign-body impaction (toy or meat) is easily diagnosed. Use of a gas-forming agent to dislodge the foreign body should not be done with an obstruction of > 24 hours due to the danger of perforation. An esophagogram can distinguish a sliding hiatal hernia from a paraesophageal hernia (*see* Figure 4).

28. Compare the advantages and disadvantages of upper GI radiology versus endoscopy.

Comparison of Upper GI Radiology and Endoscopy

RADIOLOGY	ENDOSCOPY
Advantages	
Quick, well-tolerated, safe, cheaper	Better sensitivity, particularly in mild
Arguably best primary exam for esophagus	inflammation
More reliable in scirrhous tumors	Can provide biopsy, hence more accurate
Easy differentiation of hiatal hernias	Gold standard in workup of acute upper GI
	hemorrhage, with detection ~ 100%
Disadvantages	
Operator dependent	Operator dependent
Misses mild inflammations	Measurable morbidity and mortality (mortality,
Poor in the postop stomach	1:5000).
No place in acute workup (barium obscures	Costly relative to x-ray
both endoscopy and angiography)	Time-consuming

X-ray gives modest numbers of false-positive diagnoses. In a series of 199 cases when x-ray was done first and endoscopy as thought clinically necessary, *no* pathology was missed.

GASTRIC AND DUODENAL STUDIES

29. What are the x-ray findings in gastritis?

Morphologic patterns that have good specificity include erosions (ulcers < 5 mm), aphthous ulcers, emphysema of the gastric wall, and hyperplastic polyps. Fold thickening (> 1.0 cm) suggests gastritis. A differential diagnosis of fold thickening includes hypertrophic gastritis, Menetrier's disease, lymphoma, Zollinger-Ellison syndrome, amyloidosis, eosinophilic gastroenteritis, linitis plastica, and others.

30. Can x-ray films differentiate benign and malignant gastric ulcers?

Yes. There are three categories: **Benign ulcers** show ulcer beyond the stomach lumen, have uniform radial folds, and show Hampton's line. **Malignant ulcers** show ulcer inside the lumen, mass, and meniscus. **Equivocal** ulcers are not clearly benign or malignant.

Studies show that nearly all benign ulcers detected by upper GI x-rays are, in fact, benign when *strict* adherence to criteria is followed. Therefore, any ulcer not classically benign should be biopsied. Most clinicians advocate endoscopic confirmation of complete healing of all gastric ulcers.

31. What about barium study or endoscopy in gastric malignancy?

A recent study showed true-positive results in 79 of 80 patients (99%) when using modern double-contrast barium exam in gastric carcinoma. Endoscopy is 99% accurate. Endoscopy requires 6–10 biopsy sites and is less reliable in scirrhous carcinoma. Therefore, if endoscopy is negative in a primary exam, then the follow-up should include a barium study. Gastric lymphoma is often hard to differentiate by barium study and endoscopy; therefore, consider CT.

32. What facts are important in duodenal x-ray exam?

- Barium study detects 80% of duodenal ulcers > 5 mm in size and about 75% of duodenal ulcers < 5 mm. The identification rate is less in the presence of duodenal bulb scarring.
- Duodenal ulcer distal to the papilla should suggest Zollinger-Ellison syndrome.
- Duodenitis may be confidently diagnosed only in face of small erosions or markedly enlarged folds, but the milder forms escape detection. The rate of false-positive and false-negative results was 50% in a 1991 study.
- The thick, duodenal folds seen early in an upper GI exam that revert to a normal appearance later in same study are probably due to early incomplete filling of troughs between folds. Cold barium or irritation also may be factors.

33. What is the usefulness of barium study of the small bowel?

It is the primary diagnostic method to evaluate most small bowel pathology. Only the proximal jejunal and most distal part of ileum can be reached by endoscopy for biopsy. CT scan may be complementary to barium study.

34. How is it done?

1. **Radiographic follow-through:** Done with fluoroscopy only, without fluoroscopy, or compression. "Miss" rate is unacceptably high.

2. **Fluoroscopic follow-through:** Emphasizes palpation and loop separation, by an attentive radiologist.

3. **Enteroclysis:** A tube with or without occlusive balloon is passed into jejunum. Infusion of 0.5% methylcellulose permits double contrast and separation of folds.

4. **Retrograde small bowel enema:** Done by refluxing barium from colon to small bowel. Produces excellent detail, but not used frequently now. Mainly used to show location of suspected ileal obstruction.

35. List the advantages of enteroclysis.

1. Diminishes dilutional effect of gastric and small bowel secretions.
2. Fluid overload decreases motility of small bowel.
3. All the small bowel is seen at one time.
4. Done at one sitting, usually in 30 minutes, and therefore is easier on the patient, particularly the aged.
5. Safe, with only one report of duodenal perforation.
6. Produces distention.

To paraphrase Dr. Hans Herlinger, "Look at enteroclysis and follow-through studies, and ask which demonstrates morphology better." In one study, enteroclysis showed > 90% of proven tumors, and conventional follow-through only 33%; however, not all follow-throughs were done with fluoroscopy.

36. What are the indications for enteroclysis?

1. Malabsorption. The gold standard is biopsy and histologic study. Enteroclysis shows 2 patterns:
    a. Fairly specific appearance: Seen in bacterial overgrowth syndromes, adult celiac disease, adult cystic fibrosis, Zollinger-Ellison syndrome, and short bowel syndrome
    b. Low specificity: In Whipple's disease, lymphangiectasia, amyloidosis, mastocytosis.
2. Partial mechanical small bowel obstruction

3. Crohn's disease, to show morphology and extent
4. Obscure GI tract bleeding
5. To exclude small bowel disease, as clinically necessary (see Figure 5)

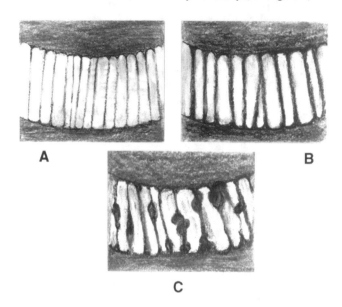

A   B

C

Figure 5. Differentiation of small bowel lumen findings on enteroclysis. **A,** Straight thin folds, dilated lumen. Seen in obstruction, sprue, and scleroderma. **B,** Thick ($\geq$ 3 mm) straight folds. Seen in bowel edema due to heart failure, hypoproteinemia, or chronic obstruction, or in intramural hemorrhage due to vascular occlusion or hemorrhagic diatheses. **C,** Thickened nodular folds suggest Crohn's disease, lymphoma, or Whipple's disease.

37. Any insider hints for barium small bowel study?
- Gastroduodenoscopy and enteroclysis can miss a duodenal loop lesion. Remember to inject duodenal loop after withdrawing enteroclysis tube.
- *Moulage,* a term for massive barium flocculation seen before modern barium preparations, is rarely seen now.
- Reglan may help intubate duodenum.
- Radiologic categorization into fold size, dilation, and nodularity plus history and clinical information permit the radiologist to suggest a diagnosis 75% of time.
- **Motivation is all. When asked how he found so much small bowel disease, Dr. Richard Marshak replied,** *"Because I look for it!"*

BIBLIOGRAPHY

1. Freeney P, Stevenson G (eds): Margulis and Burhenne's Alimentary Tract Radiology. St. Louis, Mosby-Year Book, 1994.
2. Goldberg HI, Sheft DJ: Abnormalities in small intestine contour and caliber: A working classification. Radiol Clin North Am 14(3), 1976.
3. Gore RM, Levine MS, Laufer I (eds): A Textbook of Gastrointestinal Radiology. Philadelphia, W.B. Saunders, 1994.
4. Taveras JM, Ferrucci JT (eds): Radiology. Philadelphia, J.B. Lippincott, 1995.

73. INTERVENTIONAL RADIOLOGY

Dale McCarter, M.D., and Keith Shonnard, M.D.

IMAGE-GUIDED BIOPSY

1. What imaging modalities are used for percutaneous biopsy?

Fluoroscopy, ultrasound (US), and computed tomography (CT) are the main imaging modalities utilized for percutaneous biopsy. Additionally, the superior soft-tissue characterization of magnetic resonance (MR) imaging has stimulated the development of several MR-compatible biopsy systems. These MR systems are not widely available now but undoubtedly will play an important role in the future. The primary factors influencing the choice of which modality to use include: (1) visibility of the lesion to be biopsied as well as adjacent vital structures, (2) accessibility of the lesion, and (3) need for performance in the intensive care unit (ICU).

CT, with it's superior tissue definition, is ideal for approaching retroperitoneal and small deep-seated lesions, especially those surrounded by vascular structures or bowel. Fluoroscopy and ultrasound offer continuous real-time monitoring of the biopsy process, are faster and less expensive than CT, and are ideal for the biopsy of larger superficial lesions (see Figure 1). Additionally, the portability of ultrasound makes it an attractive option in the critically ill ICU patient.

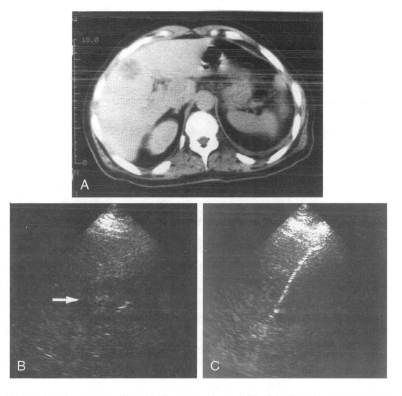

Figure 1. Metastatic colon cancer to liver. **A,** Contrast-enhanced CT of the liver demonstrates a 3-cm hypo-dense mass. **B,** Ultrasound of the liver reveals the mass to be primarily hypoechoic (*arrow*). **C,** The needle tract is conspicuously demonstrated during ultrasound-guided biopsy.

2. How is needle selection determined?
Biopsy needles vary in size from 15–23 gauge. The distinction is made by whether the interventional radiologist is obtaining a core of tissue for histologic examination or fine-needle aspirate (FNA) for cytopathologic examination. **Core biopsies** are obtained by using a 16–20-gauge, spring-activated biopsy gun. The specimen is usually adequate to make a specific histologic diagnosis. Core specimens should be obtained in patients with no known primary tumor. Fifteen-gauge needles are used if lymphoma is of clinical concern, as this larger core sample allows cell-type differentiation.

With **FNA**, a small skinny needle (21–23 gauge) is used to obtain an aspirate of cells from the target mass. Malignancy can usually be determined from the specimen, although cell-type classification can be difficult and requires an excellent cytopathologist. In patients with a known primary and possible metastatic disease, a skinny needle will usually suffice. Recent studies have shown complication rates from the use of fine needles and larger cutting needles to be equal.

3. What are the contraindications to percutaneous needle biopsy?
There are few contraindications to performing a needle biopsy. A safe pathway for needle placement from the skin to the target must be available, and any coagulopathy should be corrected prior to the procedure.

4. What are the potential complications of needle biopsy?
Complications of needle biopsy are relatively uncommon. Complication rates range from 0.3–0.8% and are predominantly due to hemorrhage, adjacent organ damage (pneumothorax), pancreatitis, or infection at the skin entry site. Tumor seeding of the needle tract does not occur.

ABDOMINAL ABSCESS

5. What imaging modality should be used in a patient suspected of having an intra-abdominal abscess?
Any inflammatory process involving a solid organ or bowel loop may lead to intra-abdominal abscess formation. The imaging modality of choice for a patient with suspected intra-abdominal abscess is CT scanning of the abdomen and pelvis (see Figure 2). Ultrasound is of limited utility in screening for abdominal abscess, although it may be helpful in evaluating the unstable ICU patient.

Intra-Abdominal Abscesses

Abscesses in Crohn's disease
Diverticular abscess
Periappendiceal abscess
Liver abscess
Renal/perinephric abscess
Pancreatic abscess
Splenic abscess
Pelvic inflammatory disease/pelvic abscess
Postoperative abscess

6. Which patients are not candidates for percutaneous abscess drainage (PAD)?
The only absolute contraindication for PAD is the absence of a safe route for placement of the drainage catheter. In these patients, surgery is recommended. Drainage of the abscess from a transperitoneal approach is preferable; however, access routes transversing a solid organ (liver) or the stomach can be used. Prior to any abscess drainage, broad-spectrum antibiotics are instituted to decrease the risk of septic shock during the procedure.

7. How successful is percutaneous abscess drainage?
Greater than 80% of patients with an intra-abdominal abscess are successfully treated by PAD. In 5–10%, PAD succeeds as a temporizing measure, stabilizing the patient prior to surgery (ruptured appendix or diverticulitis). Failure of PAD to initially treat the abscess or recurrence following treatment occurs in <5% of cases.

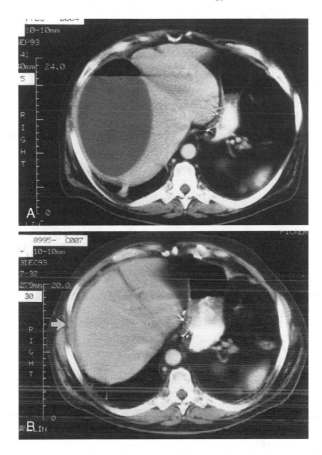

Figure 2. A 65-year-old man presented with fever and malaise 6 months following ventral hernia repair and cholecystectomy. **A**, CT demonstrates a large right subphrenic abscess. **B**, Follow-up CT demonstrates only minimal thickening adjacent to the liver capsule (*arrow*).

8. Can an abscess that communicates with the bowel be treated by percutaneous techniques?

Treatment of enteric fistulae is an especially challenging problem, both for the clinician and interventionalist. The mainstays of therapy are bowel rest, parenteral nutrition, and optional drainage and decompression of the fistulous tract. Percutaneous therapy has a lower morbidity and mortality than conventional surgical techniques. Placement of a drainage catheter in the fistula provides decompression and allows for subsequent healing of the tract. For high-output fistulae, this may require several months.

9. How is the therapeutic endpoint determined?

The prompt defervescence of fever and improvement in the patient's leukocytosis, malaise, and constitutional symptoms herald the initial success of PAD. The therapeutic endpoint is reached when the patient is clinically doing well, imaging modalities demonstrate complete resolution of the abscess, and catheter output is <10 ml/day.

10. Can an intrahepatic abscess be treated percutaneously?

Yes. The mainstay of therapy for intrahepatic abscess today is PAD along with intravenous antibiotics selected for the offending organism. Percutaneous drainage of pyogenic and amebic liver abscesses has a success rate of >95%. A relative contraindication to PAD is an intrahepatic echinococcal cyst, where leakage of contents has been linked to serious anaphylactic reactions. The therapeutic endpoint is similar to that for intra-abdominal abscess.

PANCREATIC INTERVENTIONS

11. How should pancreatitis be imaged?

Dynamic contrast-enhanced CT is the standard imaging modality for the diagnosis and evaluation of acute pancreatitis. Indications for performing the initial CT examination are:
(1) Patients in whom the clinical diagnosis of acute pancreatitis is in doubt;
(2) Patients with severe clinical pancreatitis;
(3) Patients with a Ranson score >3 or APACHE score >8;
(4) Patients who fail to improve clinically following 72 hours of conservative medical management;
(5) Patients who initially improve during medical management, then acutely deteriorate.

Ultrasound is an adjunctive imaging modality and is most useful in the serial follow-up of pancreatic fluid collections. The role of MR imaging in the diagnosis, evaluation, and staging of acute pancreatitis has not been fully explored yet.

12. Can CT imaging be used to stage pancreatitis?

Investigators have developed a staging system based on CT that can be used as a prognostic indicator of the severity of acute pancreatitis. With CT, one estimates the presence and degree of peripancreatic inflammation and/or fluid collections and the presence and extent of pancreatic necrosis. Combining the two CT prognostic indicators (fluid collections and necrosis) yields the CT severity index (CTSI), ranging from 1–10. Studies indicate patients with a CTSI of 0–2 have up to a 5% morbidity but 0% mortality, whereas a CTSI of 7–10 yields an approximate 90% morbidity and 15–25% mortality risk for the patient.

CT Severity Index (CTSI) in Acute Pancreatitis

GRADE	POINTS	DESCRIPTION
Pancreatic inflammation/fluid		
A	0	Normal
B	1	Focal or diffuse pancreatic enlargement
C	2	Pancreatic enlargement (B) plus peripancreatic inflammation
D	3	Single fluid collection
E	4	Two or more fluid collections or presence of gas
Pancreatic necrosis		
	0	No necrosis
	2	<30% necrosis
	4	30–50% necrosis
	6	>50% necrosis

13. What are the complications of pancreatitis?

With the elaboration of pancreatic secretions into the pancreatic and peripancreatic tissues, multiple complications can occur, including pancreatic necrosis (sterile or infected), acute pancreatic fluid collections (pseudocyst or abscess), or hemorrhage. **Pancreatic necrosis** is identified on dynamic contrast-enhanced CT as parenchyma demonstrating decreased enhancement (low attenuation) relative to the remaining pancreatic tissue. **Pancreatic abscess**, if it develops, occurs more acutely, whereas a **pseudocyst** usually forms 4–8 weeks following the onset of symptoms. Although **hemorrhage** can occur early in the course of acute pancreatitis, life-threatening retroperitoneal hemorrhage tends to occur late. The rupture of a pseudoaneurysm, usually of the splenic or superior mesenteric arteries, will lead to sudden, masssive hemorrhage, identified on CT as high-attenuation fluid within the peritoneal cavity, retroperitoneum, or preexisting fluid collection. The treatment of choice is emergent angiography and transcatheter embolization.

14. When should a pancreatic pseudocyst be percutaneously drained?

The mere presence of a pancreatic fluid collection does not warrant percutaneous drainage. More than 50% of acute fluid collections caused by pancreatitis, including pseudocysts <5 cm in size, resolve spontaneously and should therefore be managed conservatively. However, a pseudocyst that is enlarging, causing severe pain, infected, or obstructing the biliary tree or GI tract should be drained (see Figure 3). One exception to this is a pseudocyst with associated pancreatic necrosis. Because of the risk of catheter-introduced bacterial infection, the appropriate treatment is surgical debridement.

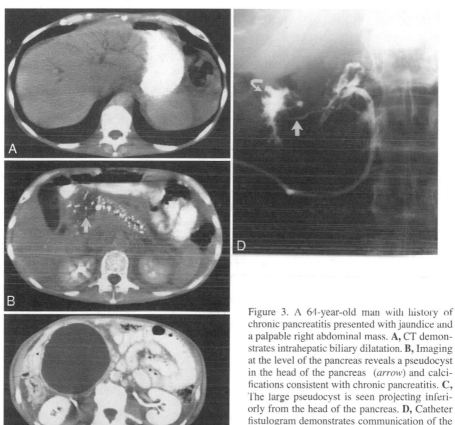

Figure 3. A 64-year-old man with history of chronic pancreatitis presented with jaundice and a palpable right abdominal mass. **A,** CT demonstrates intrahepatic biliary dilatation. **B,** Imaging at the level of the pancreas reveals a pseudocyst in the head of the pancreas (*arrow*) and calcifications consistent with chronic pancreatitis. **C,** The large pseudocyst is seen projecting inferiorly from the head of the pancreas. **D,** Catheter fistulogram demonstrates communication of the pseudocyst with the pancreatic duct (*arrow*) duodenum (*curved arrow*).

15. What is the success rate for percutaneous catheter treatment of pancreatic pseudocysts?

Success rates in excess of 90% are expected with percutaneous drainage of noninfected pseudocysts. This is equal to that of surgical therapy; however, the morbidity rate from percutaneous treatment is significantly less. To optimize successful treatment, the catheter is not removed until the communication with the pancreatic duct has closed and the cyst is collapsed (see panel D in Figure 3).

16. Is there a role for interventional radiology in the treatment of pancreatic abscess?

Pancreatic abscesses can be treated effectively with percutaneous catheter drainage. Successful drainage depends on the use of large-bore (20–24 F) catheters and sump systems. Traditional surgical techniques, usually adequate to drain the abscess, yield mortality rates ranging from 14–56%. No surgical options are lost if percutaneous treatment is initially attempted.

17. What is the treatment of choice for infected pancreatic necrosis?
It is important to distinguish pancreatic abscess from infected pancreatic necrosis. The mortality risk of infected necrosis is nearly double that of pancreatic abscess. Optimal treatment is **surgical necrosectomy** and **pancreatic bed debridement**. Percutaneous treatment of this condition would be controversial at best. Catheter therapy is limited in its ability to remove necrotic debris, which is paramount to successful treatment.

HEPATIC INTERVENTIONS

18. What is hepatic chemoembolization?
Hepatic chemoembolization (HCE) is a regional treatment for hepatic malignancy. The principal indications for HCE are nonresectability and tumor confined to the liver. This procedure combines the intra-arterial infusion of chemotherapeutic agents with embolization of the blood vessel supplying the tumor, a combination that leads to high local drug concentrations and tumor ischemia while decreasing systemic toxicity.

HCE is a relatively safe and effective therapy because liver tumors derive their blood supply from the hepatic artery. The unique dual blood supply to the liver (hepatic artery and portal vein) allows safe embolization of this vessel with little risk of hepatic ischemia.

19. Why would HCE be used to treat individuals with hepatic malignancy?
Surgical resection is the optimal treatment for individuals with hepatic malignancy. Unfortunately, most of these patients are not surgical candidates due to tumor extent, invasion of blood vessels, associated liver dysfunction, or distant metastases. Response to conventional treatments, such as systemic chemotherapy or radiation therapy, is also poor in these patients.

20. How effective is HCE?
Response rates are encouraging for hepatocellular carcinoma, metastatic carcinoid, and islet cell tumors, but less promising for colorectal metastases. This therapy has been effective in the palliation of symptoms, but increased survival rates have not been shown.

21. Is percutaneous transhepatic biliary drainage the primary method to treat biliary obstruction?
The role of percutaneous transhepatic biliary drainage (PTBD) in the management of benign and malignant biliary disease has significantly diminished with the advancement of interventional endoscopy. Currently, **endoscopic drainage** is the primary method for biliary decompression because of its relative lack of complications compared to the transhepatic approach and better patient tolerance. However, not all endoscopic drainages are successful, and PTBD continues to play an important, though diminished, role in the management of biliary disease. At our institution, biliary disease is managed by a team that includes an endoscopist, interventional radiologist, and surgeon. All patients are double-consented for ERCP and possible PTBD should the endoscopy be unsuccessful.

22. What are the indications for PTBD?
  • Unsuccessful endoscopic drainage
  • Biliary obstruction at the level of the porta hepatis
  • Biliary obstruction following biliary enteric anastomosis
  • Bile duct injuries following laparoscopic cholecystectomy
The most frequent of these indications is failed endoscopic drainage for any reason.
Hilar obstruction is a difficult area to treat for the endoscopist or interventionalist. This obstruction is usually secondary to cholangiocarcinoma or metastatic disease that involves the left and right biliary ducts, with frequent occlusion of intrahepatic segmental ducts. The multisegmental nature of these obstructions makes them difficult to drain by the endoscopist, and generally drainage is better accomplished by PTBD.

Success rates for endoscopic drainage in patients with **biliary obstruction** following biliary enteric anastomosis is ≤50%. This is due to the technical difficulty of negotiating the endoscope through the afferent loop. In these patients, PTBD may be necessary to evaluate for recurrent disease or anastomotic stricture.

Bile duct injuries secondary to laparoscopic cholecystectomy are due to inadvertent laceration or ligation of the biliary system. PTBD is directed at relieving the obstruction or, in patients with a bile leak, diverting the bile and stenting the injury. This allows healing and may be curative. Otherwise, elective surgery is performed once the patient's condition stabilizes. Endoscopic drainage can be difficult in these patients, as the bile duct may be severed.

23. Describe the classification system for bile duct injuries following laparoscopic cholecystectomy.

Class I	Laceration of the common hepatic duct (CHD)
Class II	Stricture/ligation
Class III	Segment of duct excised
Class IV	Injury to the right hepatic duct

Laparoscopic injuries are usually seen at the level of the proximal common hepatic duct (CHD) and occur when the CHD is mistaken for the cystic duct (class I, III) or during efforts to control bleeding (class II). Class IV injuries occur during the laparoscopic dissection. The most frequent of these injuries is Class III. Class I, III, and IV present with bile ascites or biloma, while Class II injuries present with jaundice. Any patient may be infected at the time of presentation.

24. Explain the advantages and disadvantages of using metallic stents for the treatment of biliary obstruction.

Metallic stents have supplanted plastic endoprostheses in the percutaneous treatment of malignant biliary obstructions (see Figure 4). Their primary advantage is the smaller-sized catheter used to deliver the stent compared to the much larger plastic endoprosthesis, thus decreasing patient discomfort and liver complications. Additionally, metallic stents expand to a larger internal diameter (1 cm), affording better drainage and longer patency rates. A disadvantage is the high cost, and should they occlude (tumor overgrowth, epithelial hyperplasia, or inspissated bile), reintervention of the biliary tract is necessary.

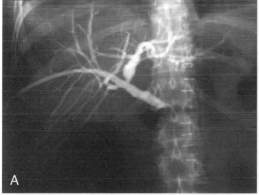
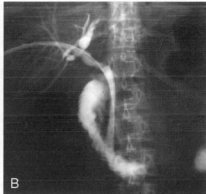
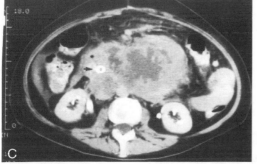

Figure 4. A 58-year-old woman presented with jaundice and abdominal mass. **A,** PTBD shows complete obstruction of the CBD. **B,** Following placement of a metallic stent, the CBD is widely patent. **C,** CT scan of the abdomen shows the large, poorly differentiated lymphoma encasing the biliary stent (*arrow*).

25. What are the indications for percutaneous cholecystostomy?

Percutaneous placement of a drainage catheter into the gallbladder is a well-established technique. Its two primary indications are (1) persistent and unexplained sepsis in the critically ill ICU patient with acalculous cholecytitis and (2) acute cholecystitis in patients too ill to undergo surgery. Less frequent indications include temporary treatment for gallbladder perforation, drainage for distant malignant biliary obstruction, and transcholecystic biliary intervention.

GASTROINTESTINAL BLEEDING

26 When does diagnostic angiography and percutaneous transcatheter therapy play a role in the management of gastrointestinal bleeding?

GI bleeding that is refractory to conservative management or invasive endoscopic techniques requires angiographic evaluation. For the interventional radiologist to identify the bleeding site:

    1. The patient must be actively bleeding at the time of the study.

    2. The bleeding must be brisk enough to be detectable during the angiogram, usually 1.5–2.0 ml/min. GI bleeding at lower rates is difficult to detect angiographically.

27. Is localization of the bleeding site before angiography important for the interventional radiologist?

Preangiographic localization of the GI bleeding site is extremely helpful. A visceral angiogram involves evaluation of the celiac, superior mesenteric, and inferior mesenteric arteries; selective catheterization of these vessels and the multiple angiographic projections required when looking for a bleeding site can make this a tedious and time-consuming procedure. If the preangiographic endoscopy has localized the bleeding, the vessel supplying this region should be studied first and thus shorten the procedure. If the exact site of bleeding is not known, determination of whether it is from the upper or lower GI tract is helpful and can guide the interventionalist as to which vessel is studied first. A ^{99m}/Tc-labeled red blood cell study may provide localizing information in this situation.

28. What are the two types of transcatheter therapy used for GI bleeding?

Transcatheter therapies for GI bleeding include pharmacologic agents and embolic materials. The **pharmacologic agent** of choice is **vasopressin** (Pitressin). This hypothalamic hormone acts directly on the smooth muscle of arterioles and capillaries to cause vasoconstriction. The superior mesenteric, gastroduodenal, left gastric, and gastroepiploic arteries are particularly sensitive to the intra-arterial administration of this agent. Following selective catheterization of the bleeding vessel, vasopressin is infused at 0.2 u/min (see Figure 5). A repeat arteriogram is performed after 30 minutes to assess the effectiveness of treatment. If bleeding persists, the dose may be doubled to 0.4 u/min. The infusion is continued for 12–24 hours, during which time the patient is monitored closely for side effects, which may prematurely terminate the therapy (myocardial, bowel, and extremity ischemia, water retention, hyponatremia, and cardiac arrhythmias). The patient is reevaluated clinically and angiographically. If the bleeding has stopped, the vasopressin is slowly tapered to normal saline with subsequent catheter removal.

GI bleeding can also be treated by **embolization** of the bleeding vessel. The catheter is selectively placed near the bleeding site for delivery of the embolic material. The embolic agents can be temporary or permanent. Temporary agents include Gelfoam and autologous blood clot, while the more numerous permanent agents include polyvinyl alcohol (PVA), coils, glues, alcohol, and hot contrast. Of these, Gelfoam and coils are the two characteristically used for bleeding in the GI tract. The availability of coaxial systems and microcatheters now permits superselective catheterization with accurate deposition of embolic material at the bleeding site. These advances have decreased the risk of bowel infarction, making this a relatively safe procedure even in the small bowel and colon.

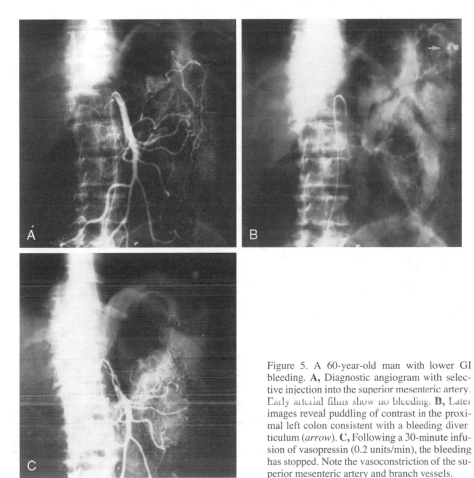

Figure 5. A 60-year-old man with lower GI bleeding. **A,** Diagnostic angiogram with selective injection into the superior mesenteric artery. Early arterial films show no bleeding. **B,** Later images reveal puddling of contrast in the proximal left colon consistent with a bleeding diverticulum (*arrow*). **C,** Following a 30-minute infusion of vasopressin (0.2 units/min), the bleeding has stopped. Note the vasoconstriction of the superior mesenteric artery and branch vessels.

TRANSJUGULAR INTRAHEPATIC PORTOSYSTEMIC SHUNT

29. What is TIPS? How is it performed?

TIPS, or transjugular intrahepatic portosystemic shunt, is a percutaneous technique that creates a shunt in the liver between the portal and hepatic veins to treat variceal bleeding secondary to portal hypertension (see Figure 6). The procedure is performed by accessing the central venous system via the right internal jugular vein. It is preferable to select the right hepatic vein for TIPS, although the middle hepatic vein may be used. A 16-gauge Colapinto transjugular needle is used to puncture through the liver from the hepatic vein into the portal vein. The transhepatic tract is dilated with a balloon catheter followed by the placement of a flexible metallic stent.

A successful TIPS results in a reduction of the portosystemic pressure gradient to 8–12 mm Hg. The stent is dilated until this is accomplished. The portosystemic gradient (PSG) is an important measurement with a strong correlation to portal venous hypertension. Bleeding from varices is rare in patients with a PSG of <12 mm Hg. The esophageal varices usually decompress once the TIPS has been created. If the varices continue to fill at portal venography, the interventionalist may elect to embolize them.

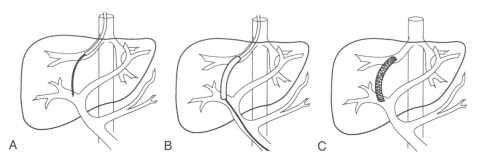

Figure 6. Diagram of the TIPS procedure. **A,** Following placement of a sheath in the right hepatic vein, a Colapinto needle is used to puncture through the liver to the portal vein. **B,** The liver parenchyma is dilated with a balloon catheter. **C,** A metallic stent is placed across the transhepatic tract, bridging the hepatic and portal veins.

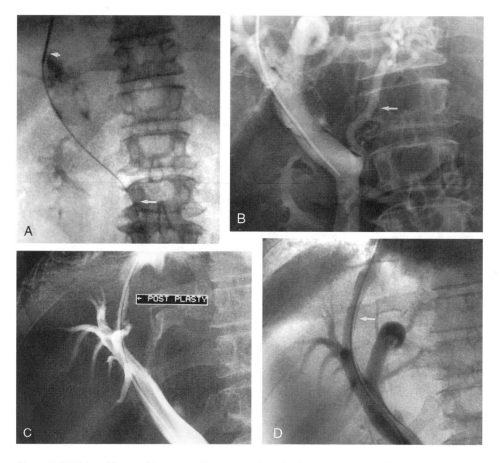

Figure 7. TIPS in a 52-year-old woman with cryptogenic cirrhosis and refractory variceal bleeding. **A,** The portal vein has been punctured with a Colapinto needle (*arrowhead*) and a guidewire placed into the superior mesenteric vein (*arrow*). The PSG was 28 mmHg. **B,** Portal venogram shows a large cardiac vein and esophageal varices (*arrow*). **C,** Following balloon dilation of the transhepatic tract, a suboptimal portal-systemic shunt is shown. **D,** A metallic stent (*arrow*) has been deployed across the transhepatic tract, allowing for greater luminal diameter. Postprocedural PSG was 10 mmHg.

30. What are the indications for TIPS?

The most important and frequent indication for TIPS is **refractory variceal hemorrhage** (see Figure 7). This may be on an acute basis (for active bleeding not controlled with sclerotherapy or pharmacotherapy) or chronic basis (for recurrent major hemorrhage despite a course of sclerotherapy). At this time, the procedure is not indicated for initial therapy of variceal hemorrhage, initial therapy to prevent recurrent variceal hemorrhage, or as a pre-operative procedure to reduce mortality during liver transplant. TIPS is particularly helpful when bleeding occurs from inaccessible intestinal or gastric varices or is the result of portal hypertensive gastropathy. Two potentially promising uses for TIPS currently under investigation are diuretic refractory ascites and hepatorenal syndrome.

31. Are there any contraindications to performing the TIPS procedure?

There are few absolute contraindications to TIPS. The procedure should not be performed in patients with polycystic liver disease. The risk of hemorrhage in these patients is significantly increased because the shunt tract may traverse the cysts rather than being contained by hepatic parenchyma. Also, being a portosystemic shunt, TIPS increases right-sided heart pressures and should not be performed in patients with right heart failure. Relative contraindications include systemic infection, portal vein thrombosis, biliary obstruction, and severe hepatic encephalopathy.

32. What is the technical success rate for TIPS and causes for failed procedures?

TIPS is probably the most technically challenging procedure that the interventional radiologist performs. Despite this, the technical success rate is >90%. Most failures are secondary to portal vein occlusion, where the occluded segment of portal vein could not be catheterized from the transjugular approach.

33. How effective is the TIPS procedure for controlling variceal hemorrhage?

TIPS is extremely effective in controlling acute variceal hemorrhage. It appears to be as effective as a surgical portacaval shunt without the added risk of hepatic injury from general anesthesia. Mid-term studies have found recurrent variceal bleeding following TIPS to be <10%. Nearly all of these patients were found to have shunt abnormalities, either stenosis or occlusion. Angiographic reevaluation with shunt revision (balloon dilation or additional stent placement) or placement of a second TIPS nearly always controls bleeding.

34. What is the morbidity and mortality for TIPS?

TIPS is generally accepted to have lower morbidity and mortality rates than surgically created portacaval shunts. Review of the four largest TIPS series in the radiologic literature shows a 30-day mortality rate of 7–20%. Most deaths were in Child-Pugh class C patients. Direct TIPS-related procedural mortality is <2%. These deaths were predominantly due to intraprocedural cardiac events or intraperitoneal hemorrhage following puncture through the liver capsule. Serious procedural complications occur in <10% of patients, and include self-limited peritoneal hemorrhage, myocardial infarction, transient renal failure, hepatic arterial injury, hepatic infarction, and pulmonary edema.

35. Describe the short-term and long-term complications seen with TIPS.

Acute thrombosis of the stent, although infrequent, may occur immediately or shortly after the TIPS procedure. The interventionalist treats this by removing or displacing the thrombus from the stent (i.e., shunt thrombectomy). Delayed **shunt stenosis** or **occlusion** is usually a result of pseudointimal proliferation within the stent or incomplete coverage of the parenchymal tract with the stent. Treatment is shunt revision. Primary shunt patency is 70% at 1 year and 55% at 2 years. Secondary patency rates (patency following shunt revision) are >90%.

The most significant long-term complication of TIPS is **hepatic encephalopathy**. New or worsened encephalopathy is seen in 20–30% of patients following TIPS. This usually can be treated with diet and lactulose administration. Clinical variables associated with an increased risk for developing post-TIPS encephalopathy include an etiology of liver disease other than alcohol, female sex, increasing age, and prior history of encephalopathy.

36. How is shunt patency followed? Is there a routine surveillance for these patients?
Shunt patency is followed by color Doppler ultrasound. A baseline study is obtained 24 hours following the procedure. In the asymptomatic patient, routine follow-up is performed at 3 and 6 months post-TIPS, then at 6-month intervals. Should the patient become symptomatic or significant interval change be seen on the ultrasound, angiographic reevaluation and therapeutic intervention may be performed to restore normal shunt function.

BIBLIOGRAPHY

1. Balthazar E, Freeny P, vanSonnenberg E: Imaging and intervention in acute pancreatitis. Radiology 193:297–306, 1994.
2. Balthazar E, Robinson D, Megibow A, Ranson J: Acute pancreatitis: Value of CT in establishing prognosis. Radiology 174:331–333, 1990.
3. Castaneda-Zuniga WR, Tadavarthy SM: Interventional Radiology. Baltimore, Williams & Wilkins, 1988.
4. Freedom A, Sanyal A, Tisnado J, et al: Complications of transjugular intrahepatic portosystemic shunt: A comprehensive review. Radiographics 13:1185–1210, 1993.
5. Hariri M, Slivka A, Carr-Locke D, et al: Pseudocyst drainage predisposes to infection when pancreatic necrosis is unrecognized. Am Gastroenterol 89:1781–1784, 1994.
6. Kadir S: Current Practice of Interventional Radiology. Philadelphia, B.C. Decker, 1991.
7. Laberge J, Ring E, Gordon R, et al: Creation of transjugular intrahepatic portosystemic shunts with the Wallstent endoprosthesis: Results in 100 patients. Radiology 187:413–420, 1993.
8. vanSonnenberg E, D'Agostino H, Casola G, et al: Percutaneous abscess drainage: Current concepts. Radiology 181:617–626, 1991.

74. NONINVASIVE GI IMAGING: ULTRASOUND, COMPUTED TOMOGRAPHY, MAGNETIC RESONANCE SCANNING

David W. Bean, Jr., M.D., Steven H. Peck, M.D., and Kevin M. Rak, M.D.

LIVER IMAGING

1. How is segmental liver anatomy defined?

Early descriptions of liver anatomy divided the organ into four lobes based on the surface configuration. More recently, the segmental anatomy has been based on the vasculature, primarily involving the hepatic veins (see Figure 1). The different hepatic segments are divided by intersegmental fissures, which are traversed or are in the same plane as the hepatic veins.

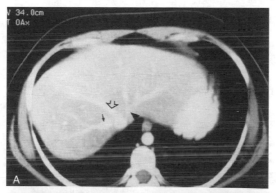

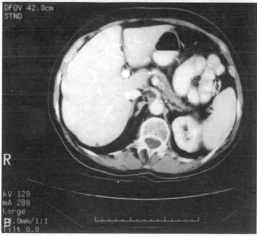

Figure 1. CT scans showing vascular anatomy of liver. **A,** The right hepatic vein (*black arrow*) divides the anterior and posterior segments of the right lobe of the liver. The middle hepatic vein (*open arrow*) divides the right lobe from the left lobe. The left hepatic vein (*arrowhead*) divides the medial and lateral segments of the left lobe of the liver. **B,** The falciform ligament (*white arrow*) divides the medial and lateral segments of the left lobe of the liver. The caudate lobe is marked by the *small arrow*.

The right and left lobes of the liver are divided by the main lobar fissure. This fissure is represented by a line from the gallbladder recess through the inferior vena cava (IVC); superiorly in the liver, this is represented by the middle hepatic vein. The anterior and posterior segments of the right lobe of the liver are divided by the right intersegmental fissure. This fissure is approximated by the right hepatic vein.

The left intersegmental fissure divides the medial and lateral segments of the left lobe of the liver. This fissure is marked on the external liver margin by the falciform ligament and internally has the ligamentum teres running within it. Superiorly within the liver, it is marked by the left hepatic vein. The caudate lobe is the portion of liver located between the IVC and the fissure of the ligamentum venosum.

2. What are the typical imaging features of liver metastases?

On **computed tomography** (CT), most of liver metastases are of low density when compared to the surrounding parenchyma (see Figure 2); however, high-density metastases can be seen with pancreatic islet cell carcinoma, renal cell carcinoma, carcinoid tumor, or thyroid carcinoma.

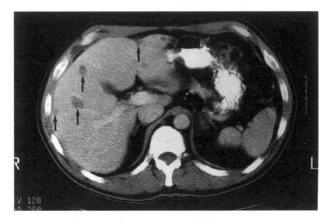

Figure 2. Liver metastases (*arrows*) in a patient with colon carcinoma present as hypodense lesions compared to the surrounding normal liver parenchyma.

3. How does vasculature determine the detection of liver metastases on CT?

Liver metastases are supplied by branches of the hepatic artery, and their detection is based on timing and the lesions' hypovascularity. The liver parenchyma receives 75% of its blood flow from the portal vein and 25% from the hepatic artery. Following a peripheral injection of intravenous contrast, organs with only an arterial supply (e.g., spleen, kidney) enhance brightly, but the liver enhances little, since the contrast from the hepatic artery is diluted by blood from the portal vein. Only after contrast circulates through the spleen and mesentery to reach the portal vein does the dominant contrast effect occur. This takes about 60 seconds; the spleen and kidney enhance 30 seconds earlier. CT imaging is best when performed during the portal venous contrast phase, because this is when the contrast between the enhancing liver and low-density metastases is greatest.

To increase liver enhancement without having contrast reach metastases, many medical centers place a catheter in the superior mesenteric artery for a contrast injection during CT scanning. **CT arterial portography** (as it is called) can increase the sensitivity of lesion detection to 91%. A standard contrast-enhanced CT scan has a sensitivity of 63–71%. The improved vascular contrast also improves localization of metastases to a specific subsegment. Improved localization and sensitivity are particularly helpful when contemplating partial hepatic resection for metastases secondary to colorectal carcinoma; by detecting more lesions, needless surgery can be avoided.

Other CT techniques experimented with, such as delayed contrast-enhanced CT, non-contrast-enhanced CT, and CT scanning during contrast injection through a hepatic artery catheter, have failed to match the success of CT arterial portography in clinical trials. About 5% of metastases contain calcification. These are usually from mucinous adenocarcinomas of the ovary or GI tract. Cystic metastatic lesions can arise from tumors of the pancreas and ovary or from necrosis of squamous cell carcinoma metastases.

The **ultrasound** (US) appearance of metastases varies greatly. Colon carcinoma and many others tend to produce hyperechoic metastases, but hypoechoic lesions are also common, particularly with lymphoma and cystic or necrotic metastases. Hypoechoic halos of edema surrounding hyperechoic metastases produce the common "bull's-eye" appearance. The sensitivity of ultrasound for detecting metastases is about 61%; however, intraoperative ultrasound can increase the sensitivity to 96% and may be the most sensitive modality available.

Researchers continue to evaluate the use of various **magnetic resonance** (MR) pulse sequences for detection of liver metastases; however, motion artifact from breathing continues to be a large problem. The sensitivity of MR is less than that of contrast-enhanced CT. In general, metastases are hypointense on T1-weighted images and hyperintense on T2-weighted images. Exceptions occur with hemorrhagic and malignant melanoma metastases, which are hyperintense to varying degrees on T1 weighted images.

4. What are imaging characteristics of hepatocellular carcinoma (HCC)?

HCC grows in one of three major patterns: a large solitary mass, multifocal HCC with a dominant mass and satellite lesions, or diffuse infiltration. In North America, underlying cirrhosis is seen in 60% of patients or hemochromatosis in 20%. HCC arising in normal livers tends to occur at a younger age (fibrolamellar HCC) and typically presents as a solitary, well-circumscribed mass.

Sonographic features of HCC are variable and may simulate metastatic disease. Small HCCs (< 3 cm) are often hypoechoic, whereas larger lesions are of mixed echogenicity. Fatty metamorphosis within the tumor may cause internal hyperechoic foci. Vascular invasion is common and suggestive of HCC. HCC invades portal veins more frequently than hepatic veins, and such tumor thrombus can be demonstrated with Doppler ultrasound.

By **CT,** underlying cirrhotic or hemochromatotic changes are commonly seen; 10% of HCCs calcify. Low attenuation areas due to central necrosis are common, and nonnecrotic areas are typically hyperdense after contrast administration (see Figure 3). Small HCCs may enhance similarly to liver parenchyma, making contour deformity or mass effect the only means of detection. Vas-

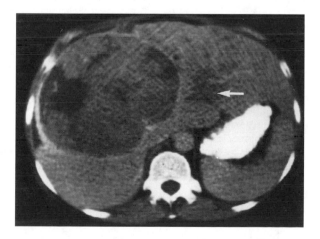

Figure 3. CT shows large necrotic hepatocellular carcinoma. The area of lower attenuation in the left lobe (*arrow*) is a separate focus of multifocal HCC.

cular invasion can be documented by CT, and hemoperitoneum due to rare spontaneous rupture can also be seen. A hyperdense, enhancing capsule is common. CT portography is more sensitive in detecting small lesions.

On **MR,** the mass may be iso-, hypo-, or hyperintense on T1 images, depending on the degree of fatty change and internal fibrosis. Encapsulated HCC typically has a hypointense rim on T1 images. Fibrolamellar HCC appears somewhat similar to focal nodular hyperplasia in that both have a central scar with multiple fibrous septae. However, fibrolamellar HCC has a high prevalence of calcification, and the central scar is typically hypointense on T2 images, whereas it is hyperintense in focal nodular hyperplasia.

5. Describe the imaging findings of hepatic hemangiomas.

Cavernous hemangiomas are the most common benign neoplasm of the liver. Most are ≤ 5 cm in size and solitary, although they can be multiple. They typically are located in a peripheral subcapsular location, commonly in the right lobe of the liver. Blood flow within cavernous hemangiomas is usually very slow, which accounts for some of its imaging characteristics.

US: Cavernous hemangiomas appear as well-defined hyperechoic masses. Doppler and color flow imaging do not show any detectable flow. They occasionally have a mixed or hypoechoic appearance.

CT: On unenhanced CT, hemangiomas are usually hypodense, well-defined lesions. They may appear iso- or hyperdense if they arise in a area of focal fatty infiltration. Following a bolus injection of intravenous contrast, they may have a characteristic enhancement pattern, showing initial peripheral enhancement followed by a slow filling of the center of the lesion. The enhancement pattern as it fills has been described as nodular or fingerlike and can take from 5–60 minutes to fill completely. Up to one-fourth of these lesions do not show this characteristic pattern of enhancement, and these lesions may show initial central or uniform enhancement, which may also be seen in malignant lesions.

MRI: A typical hemangioma is well-defined and has decreased signal intensity relative to normal liver on T1-weighted images. On T2-weighted images, hemangiomas have increased signal compared to the liver. The signal is equal to or greater than the signal of bile within the gallbladder. Using fast-scanning techniques and a bolus of gadolinium, a similar enhancement pattern to that of CT can be seen on MRI.

6. Outline the workup for a suspected cavernous hemangioma.

If a lesion has the typical **ultrasound** findings of a cavernous hemangioma and is ≤ 3 cm and if the patient has normal **liver function tests** (LFTs) and no history of a malignancy that could metastasize to the liver, then a followup ultrasound in 3–6 months is appropriate. If the lesion is atypical by ultrasound or if the patient has a known primary neoplasm or abnormal LFTs, then further workup is warranted. If the lesion is ≥ 2 cm, then a ^{99m}Tc-**tagged red blood cell** (RBC) **scan** is the next step. This nuclear medicine procedure is highly sensitive and specific for lesions of this size. If the lesion is < 2 cm, the RBC scan can be attempted, but the sensitivity and specificity decrease as the size of the lesion decreases. If the RBC scan is equivocal, the next study is **MRI,** preferably with rapid scanning techniques and gadolinium enhancement. In this scenario, **CT** should be a third-line choice or used if MRI is not available.

If the intial lesion is found by **CT** and follows the strict criteria of a hemangioma—a well-defined, low-density lesion on unenhanced images, with peripheral enhancement followed by complete filling of the lesion—further workup is probably not necessary. If the diagnosis needs further confirmation, a **tagged RBC study** or **ultrasound** would be a good choice. If the intial CT scan does not meet the strict criteria or the patient has abnormal LFTs, then a confirmatory **nuclear medicine** or **MRI scan** is appropriate. If the CT criteria are not met, it is typically due to incomplete filling of the lesion.

If these different studies do not confirm that a lesion is a cavernous hemangioma, **biopsy** may be necessary for the final diagnosis.

7. How can focal nodular hyperplasia (FNH) and hepatocellular adenoma (HCA) be differentiated?

Hepatic adenomas and FNH are more common in females, and both, particularly HCA, are associated with oral contraceptive use. FNH is benign, whereas HCA can cause morbidity and mortality due to its propensity to hemorrhage and rare malignant degeneration. Differentiation between these lesions may be difficult, and particularly in smaller lesions without hemorrhage, biopsy is required for differentiation.

FNH: The characteristic feature is the **central scar,** containing radiating fibrous tissue with vascular and biliary elements. However, the central scar is nonspecific, and it may also be seen with fibrolamellar HCC, hemangioma, and other lesions. By ultrasound, FNH is a well-demarcated hypoechoic mass, possibly with central scar. By CT, a central low-density scar may be seen in 20–40% of cases. The scar should be somewhat linear or branching to help distinguish it from central necrosis in a mass. On noncontrast images, FNH is hypodense without calcification. On post-contrast images, it commonly enhances similar to normal liver, except for the persisting central low-density scar. Thus, if there is no central scar, FNH may be missed by CT or may be seen only as deformity of the liver contour. On dynamic contrast-enhanced studies, FNH and its scar may have transiently higher attenuation than the liver due to vascular enhancement. By MR, FNH is isointense on T1 and iso- to hyperintense on T2. The central scar is hyperintense on T2 images and enhances with Gd-DTPA. Because of the presence of Kupffer cells, sulfur-colloid scintigraphy demonstrates normal uptake in 50%, decreased uptake in 40%, and increased uptake or hot-spots in 10%, probably due to Kupffer cell hyperplasia. However, HCA also may show normal sulfur colloid uptake in 20%.

HCA: Sonography typically shows a heterogeneous mass due to areas of internal hemorrhage. On noncontrast **CT,** a hypodense mass is seen; internal areas of higher attenuation may be present due to recent hemorrhage. **Hemorrhage** is a key distinguishing feature from FNH. After contrast administration, there may be centripetal enhancement similar to that in hemangiomas, though this hyperenhancement does not persist in adenomas as it does in hemangiomas. By MR, HCA may be hyperintense on T1, due to internal fat/glycogen, although similar findings may be seen in HCC. The lesions are commonly heterogeneous due to necrosis and internal hemorrhage.

8. What does an hepatic abscess look like on imaging?

US: On ultrasound, an hepatic abscess appears as a complex fluid collection, typically with septations (see Figure 4), an irregular wall, and debris or air within the fluid. Air is seen as a fo-

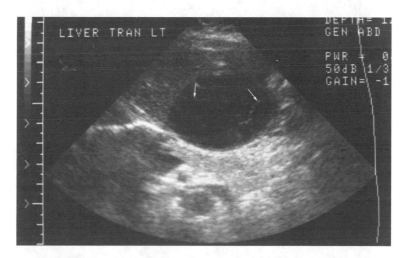

Figure 4. Ultrasound of an intrahepatic abscess. A hematoma may have a similar appearance. The *arrows* point to internal septations.

cal area of echogenicity and has posterior shadowing. Abscesses also can appear as simple fluid collections similar to a cyst.

CT: CT is the most sensitive imaging modality, with a sensitivity of ~ 95–98%. CT findings can vary depending on the size and age of the abscess. Generally, they appear as a low-density, well-defined mass. The cavity may have a smooth or irregular margin. Density values of the fluid may range from 2–40 Hounsfield units (HU) depending on the protein content of the fluid. Abscesses can be unilocular or multilocular and may contain internal septations. They usually have a well-defined wall which may enhance. The most specific sign is **air bubbles** within the abscess cavity, although this sign is seen in only 20% of cases.

MRI: An abscess appears as a well-defined lesion of low signal intensity on T1-weighted images and bright signal intensity on T2 images. The cavity may have homogeneous or heterogeneous signal, and septations may be seen. The capsule appears as a low-signal rim and may enhance with gadolinium.

Other causes of complex cysts, such as a focal hematoma, and necrotic or hemorrhagic neoplasm, may have similar appearances.

9. What are the imaging findings of fatty infiltration of the liver?

Fatty infiltration of the liver is due to deposition of triglycerides within the hepatocytes and is associated with many disorders, including ethanol abuse, obesity, excess steroids, hyperalimentation, diabetes, radiation or chemotherapy, and glycogen storage disease. It can cause slightly abnormal LFTs and hepatomegaly. Fatty infiltration may be diffuse or focal.

US: Fatty infiltration is seen as a focal or diffuse area of increased echogenicity. There is decreased or nonvisualization of intrahepatic vessels, the deeper posterior portions of the liver, and the diphragm posterior to the liver. Ultrasound will not show any mass effect on adjacent biliary structures or blood vessels. The finding of diffuse increased echogenicity of the liver is nonspecific and can be seen in hepatitis or cirrhosis.

CT: Fatty infiltration is seen as an area of decreased attenuation, which is easier to appreciate in the focal form where there is adjacent normal liver (see Figure 5). On an unenhanced CT scan, the normal liver is usually 8 HU greater in density than the spleen, but in fatty infiltration, less dense than the spleen. However, other lesions may also appear as an area of decreased density on an unenhanced CT, such as hepatomas and metastatic disease. In fatty infiltration, the he-

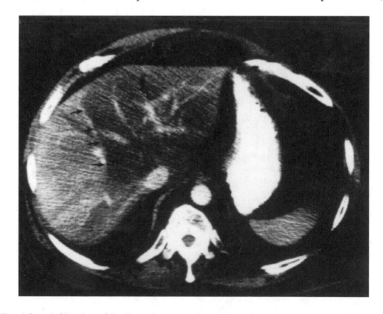

Figure 5. Focal fatty infiltration of the liver shown as a low-attenuation area next to normal liver (*arrows*).

patic vessels stand out and may appear as if they have contrast within them on an unenhanced scan. Also in focal fatty infiltration, the normal hepatic vessels traverse the area of decreased attenuation, a finding not seen in a malignant mass. Focal fatty infiltration tends to have linear margins and to be in a lobar distribution.

MRI: Fat tissue is typically bright on T1-weighted images and has dark or decreased signal on T2 images. Focal fatty infiltration usually does not show as dramatic of a change in signal as is seen in the subcutaneous fat; the signal changes may be very subtle. As with CT, it is important to see normal vessels in the area of signal abnormality and no mass effect on adjacent structures. Fat-suppression MRI scans are more sensitive than routine T1 and T2 scans and show fatty infiltration as areas of decreased signal intensity compared to normal liver.

10. Which imaging techniques are used to detect cirrhosis?

US: On sonography, cirrhosis is characterized by abnormal echotexture. The hepatic parenchyma is typically hyperechoic with "coarsened" echoes, making the liver somewhat heterogeneous. Intrahepatic vasculature is poorly defined. Unfortunately, these findings are nonspecific, as increased parenchymal echogenicity is also seen in fatty infiltration and heterogeneity may be due to infiltrating neoplasm. Furthermore, no direct correlation exists between the degree of hepatic dysfunction and the sonographic appearance. More specific sonographic features of cirrhosis include nodularity of the liver surface and selective enlargement of the caudate lobe (see Figure 8A below). A caudate: right lobe volume ratio of > 96% allows 96% confidence in diagnosing cirrhosis. In portal hypertension, the normal portal venous velocity is highly variable, but the Doppler detection of hepatofugal flow is diagnostic. Doppler also provides improved identification of portal collateral vessels, particularly the recanalized umbilical vein.

CT: Although early parenchymal changes may not be visible on CT, fatty infiltration, the initial manifestation of alcoholic liver disease, is well seen. The liver enlarges, and its attenuation becomes abnormally lower than that of the spleen. In later stages of cirrhosis, liver volume typically decreases. A nodular contour (due to regenerating nodules, scarring, and atrophy) may be seen, with somewhat heterogeneous enhancement. Regenerating nodules are isodense with liver and can only be inferred from contour deformity. The typical enlargement of the caudate lobe and lateral-segment left lobe are seen, as well as atrophy of the right lobe and medial-segment left lobe. Mesenteric fat develops a higher attenuation than retroperitoneal or subcutaneous fat. CT demonstrates varices, ascites, and splenomegaly associated with portal hypertension (see Figure 6B below). Unlike sonography, CT cannot determine the direction of vascular flow, but it is superior in delineating the full extent of varices and collateral vessels.

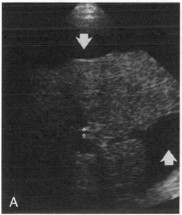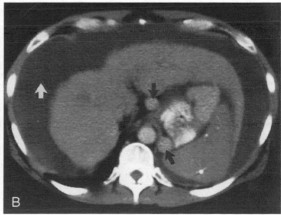

Figure 6. Cirrhosis. **A,** Ultrasound shows small, echogenic liver with nodular contour, compatible with cirrhosis. Low echogenicity ascites surrounds the liver (*arrows*). **B,** CT demonstrates small liver with nodular contour and enhancing varices (*black arrows*) and extensive ascites (*white arrow*).

MR: MR has little role in the diagnosis of cirrhosis but can help in distinguishing cirrhotic nodules from hepatocellular carcinoma. Regenerating nodules are low intensity on T2, owing to hemosiderin deposits, whereas hepatocellular carcinoma is hyperintense. Hyperplastic adenomatous nodules without atypia are hyperintense on T1 and hypointense on T2, again allowing differentiation from carcinoma.

11. Which is the most sensitive exam in detecting hemochromatosis?

MR and CT imaging rely upon the increased iron content of the liver and other organs to give the diagnosis of hemochromatosis. Ultrasound of the liver is normal despite iron deposition unless underlying cirrhosis exists. Increased attenuation of the liver on CT is due to the high atomic number of iron, but it is not specific finding; amiodarone, chemotherapy agents, and glycogen deposits can produce similar findings. Increased attenuation of the liver on CT scans is typically > 85 HU in hemochromatosis, compared to a normal attenuation of ~ 60 HU. With MR, the iron deposition causes decreased intensity due to paramagnetic effects. The findings are most striking on T2-weighted images but can be seen to a lesser extent on T1 images. MR appears to be more sensitive and specific than CT, and MR quantitation in the future may eliminate the need for some liver biopsies.

Primary hemochromatosis is an autosomal recessive disease in which patients absorb excessive amounts of dietary iron that accumulates in the parenchymal cells of the liver, heart, spleen, and pancreas. Secondary hemochromatosis, caused by multiple blood transfusions, results in iron deposition in the reticuloendothelial cells of primarily the liver and spleen. In cirrhosis or intravascular hemolysis, there is a mildly increased iron level in the hepatocytes. Neither MR or CT can distinguish which cells of a particular organ are overloaded with iron. However, the organ distribution of imaging abnormalities can sometimes provide valuable information.

12. What is a normal Doppler waveform?

The changing frequency of reflected sound waves from flowing blood allows ultrasound to calculate the velocity and direction of blood flow. A "normal" Doppler waveform is different for each artery or vein of the body. Veins have continuous low-velocity flow that frequently varies with respiration. In the portal vein flow is hepatopedal and generally ranges from 15–25 cm/sec (see Figure 7A). Flow velocity normally decreases during inspiration and increases during expiration. Arterial flow does not vary with respiration but varies dramatically with the cardiac cycle, showing high-velocity flow during systole and relatively high flow (i.e., low resistance) during diastole (see Figure 7B). In a fasting patient, the superior mesenteric artery has equally high systolic velocity, but minimal flow and even flow reversal during diastole (i.e., high resistance). Ingestion of a meal creates a lower resistance system by increasing the diastolic flow to the bowel with end arterial dilatation.

In both arteries and veins, color Doppler can be used readily to verify the presence and direction of flow. Flow in arteries and veins normally is different colors (red or blue) due to their opposing directions. Arteries demonstrate color pulsation due to rapidly changing speed of flow. The equipment operator determines whether blood flowing toward the transducer is blue or red, and blood flowing away from the transducer takes on the other color. Color Doppler can be a quick way to verify vessel patency and direction of blood flow. A tubular structure in the porta hepatis without color is either a duct or vessel with no flow or thrombus in it.

13. How are Doppler waveforms altered in portal vein thrombosis, portal hypertension, and Budd-Chiari syndrome?

In acute **portal vein thrombosis,** there is markedly diminished flow or no flow in the portal vein. In most instances, echogenic material is seen in the portal vein (see Figure 8A), although in a few cases, the portal vein may appear normal. Doppler analysis yields no waveform, and with color imaging, there is no color in the vessel. In the more chronic condition of cavernous transformation of the portal vein, the portal vein cannot be seen, but rather an echogenic structure in the porta hepatis represents a fibrotic remnant. The presence of multiple tubular channels in the

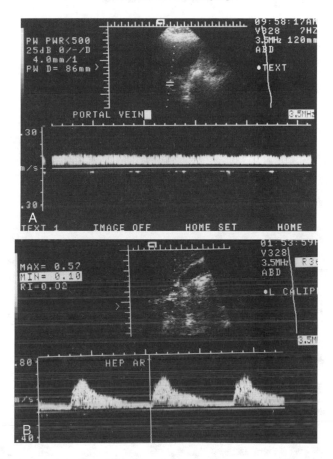

Figure 7. Doppler ultrasound. **A,** Normal blood flow in the portal vein. Flow registers above the baseline because it is traveling toward the ultrasound probe. **B,** Normal hepatic artery blood flow. Again, flow is toward the ultrasound probe. High-velocity flow represents systole, and lower-velocity flow represents diastole.

porta hepatis with demonstrable flow by color imaging or Doppler evaluation is virtually diagnostic of cavernous transformation.

Portal hypertension can be suggested on ultrasound by portal vein enlargement with decreased flow velocity. Enlargement to 13 mm has been suggested as indicating portal hypertension, although portal vein size is so variable that specific measurements are unreliable. **Retrograde (hepatofugal) flow** in the portal vein indicates advanced disease and is a very useful, but late, finding (see Figure 8B and C). Detection of portosystemic collaterals aids greatly in detecting portal hypertension. The easiest collateral to detect by ultrasound is the recanalized paraumbilical vein (see Figure 8D), which drains the left portal vein as it travels through the ligamentum teres to the abdominal wall. The coronary (left gastric) vein, another collateral vessel, originates at the portosplenic confluence and ascends to the gastroesophageal junction to feed esophageal varices. Detection of hepatofugal flow in the coronary is one of the best indicators of portal hypertension. Splenic varices are easily detected as tubular structures with flow in the splenic hilum. Other portosystemic collaterals include splenorenal shunts and retroperitoneal veins.

Budd-Chiari syndrome refers to obstruction of hepatic venous outflow. It can occur at a number of levels from the small hepatic venules to the inferior vena cava (IVC). Typically, the liver parenchyma is diffusely heterogeneous, but to make the diagnosis, one must observe

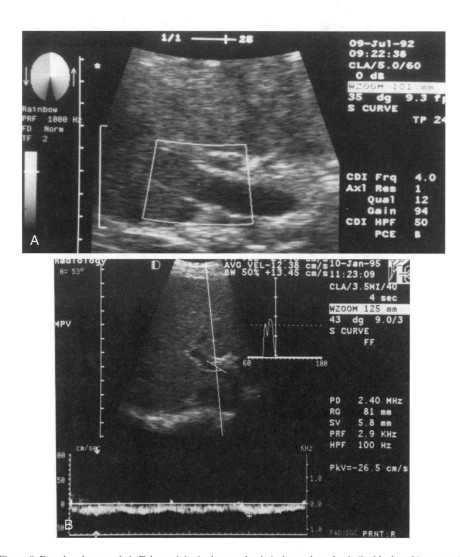

Figure 8. Doppler ultrasound. **A,** Echogenicity in the portal vein is due to thrombosis (inside the *white square*) in this patient with hepatocellular carcinoma invading the portal vein. **B,** Hepatofugal blood flow registers below the baseline in the portal vein of this patient with known portal hypertension.

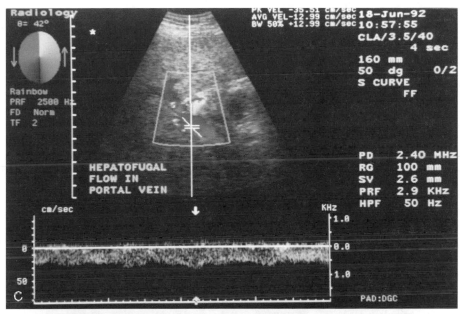

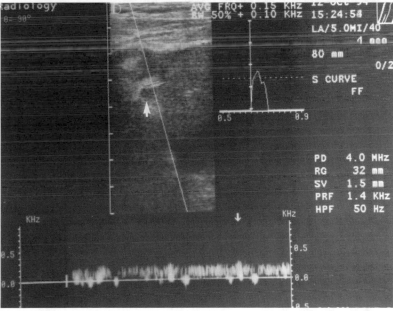

Figure 8 (*Continued*). Doppler ultrasound. **C,** Color Doppler image registers blue (retrograde) flow in the portal vein in this patient with portal hypertension and hepatofugal flow. If flow was normal in direction, it would be red. (Courtesy of Patrick Meyers, RT.) **D,** Doppler-identified blood flow in the falciform ligament (*white arrow*) is due to recanalized paraumbilical veins in another patient with portal hypertension. Note subhepatic ascites.

echogenic thrombi or absent flow in one or more hepatic veins or the suprahepatic IVC. Twenty percent of patients have associated portal vein thrombosis, and many others have ascites.

14. Discuss ultrasound's role in the evaluation of transjugular intrahepatic portosystemic shunts (TIPS).

The role of ultrasound in evaluating TIPS is still evolving as experience with the procedure grows. Currently, ultrasound is used for preprocedure evaluation and to assess shunt patency after the procedure.

The preprocedure examination is obtained 24–48 hours before the TIPS and assesses the liver and spleen parenchyma, splenic size, possible varices and ascites, flow characteristics of the hepatic vessels, and patency of the internal jugular veins.

After the procedure, a new baseline examination is obtained within 24–48 hours. Flow is documented within the shunt, and baseline velocity measurements are obtained at both ends and in the middle of the shunt. The flow in the shunt is usually of a high velocity and very turbulent, and there is a wide range of peak velocities in patent, well-functioning shunts (see Figure 9); this is why the initial baseline examination is so important. A decrease in the peak velocity, along with other signs of shunt failure, will prompt a portagram for further evaluation. Signs of a failing shunt include a decreased velocity in the shunt, reaccumulation of ascites, reappearance or increased

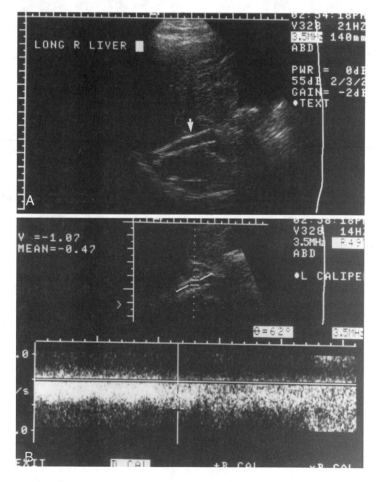

Figure 9. TIPS. **A,** Ultrasound appearance of a TIPS. **B,** Doppler ultrasound showing flow within a patent TIPS.

size of varices, and flow of blood away from the shunt. A peak shunt velocity of 50–60 cm/sec should prompt an angiographic study of the shunt to evaluate for stenosis.

BILIARY TRACT IMAGING

15. What is the significance of gallbladder wall thickening on ultrasound?

A wall thickness > 3 mm in a distended gallbladder is abnormal and must be explained. Abnormal wall thickness, combined with a sonographic Murphy's sign and gallstones, has a positive predictive value of > 90% for acute cholecystitis, the most common cause of pathologic wall thickening.

Many other conditions can cause gallbladder wall thickening. Congestive heart failure and constrictive pericarditis cause congestive hepatomegaly, which is often accompanied by a thickened, edematous gallbladder wall. Hypoalbuminemia, secondary to chronic liver dysfunction or nephrotic syndrome, results in a decrease in plasma oncotic pressure that produces generalized tissue edema, including edema of the gallbladder wall. Portal venous congestion from portal hypertension of any cause and hepatic veno-occlusive disease can produce gallbladder wall thickening. Inflammation of the gallbladder from nearby hepatitis or AIDS-related cholangitis may produce wall thickening. Chronic cholecyctitis, adenomyomatosis, primary sclerosing cholangitis, and leukemic infiltration are additional causes of wall thickening. Gallbladder carcinoma also causes wall thickening but is easily differentiated by its mass-like appearance and association with adenopathy and liver metastases.

16. What is the radiologic workup of suspected biliary tree obstruction?

Ultrasound is the screening examination of choice when biliary ductal disease is suspected. By ultrasound, normal nondilated intrahepatic ducts are 1–2 mm in diameter and are not usually visualized. The size of the common hepatic duct (CHD) is a sensitive indicator of the presence of biliary obstruction, being more sensitive than intrahepatic ducts in assessing early or partial biliary obstruction. The normal CBD is 4–5 mm in diameter, with > 6 mm indicating ductal dilatation (see Figure 10A). However, extrahepatic ductal diameter increases with age and may be increased in patients following cholecystectomy or with prior resolved obstruction. Thus, dilated ducts are not the equivalent of obstruction. Repeat scanning after an oral fatty meal or intravenous cholecystokinin may help distinguish dilatation from obstruction, as a dilated CBD that fails to decrease in size or increases after this provocative test indicates obstruction. In complicated cases, Doppler examination can readily differentiate the biliary ducts from vasculature in the portal triad. With intrahepatic ductal dilatation, tubular low-echogenicity structures are seen to parallel the portal veins, producing the "too many tubes" sign.

Although ultrasound is the best screening exam for biliary disease, once this is detected, **CT** is more efficacious in depicting the degree, site, and cause of obstruction. CT provides more complete delineation of the full length of the CBD, as bowel gas commonly obscures sonographic visualization of the distal CBD. Again, the normal CBD is up to 6 mm, whereas a 9 mm CBD is considered dilated (see Figure 10B).

Biliary ductal dilatation may also be diagnosed by **MR,** although this is not typically cost-effective, and the inferior spatial resolution often precludes complete evaluation. Endoscopic retrograde cholangiopancreatography (ERCP) or percutaneous transhepatic cholangiography provides a more detailed evaluation than ultrasound or CT but is invasive.

17. Describe the differential imaging features seen in the common causes of biliary obstruction.

Biliary obstruction may be related to biliary (choledocholithiasis, cholangitis, cholangiocarcinoma) or extrabiliary disease (pancreatitis, periampullary carcinoma). Intrahepatic ductal dilatation with a normal CBD suggests an intrahepatic mass or abnormality. Dilatation of the pancreatic duct typically localizes the obstruction to the pancreatic or ampullary level.

An abrupt transition from a dilated CBD to a narrowed or obliterated duct is more characteristic of neoplasm (or stone), whereas a gradual tapering of the CBD at the pancreatic head is typical of fibrosis associated with chronic pancreatitis.

Ultrasound is 60–70% accurate in detecting common duct stones; unlike gallbladder calculi,

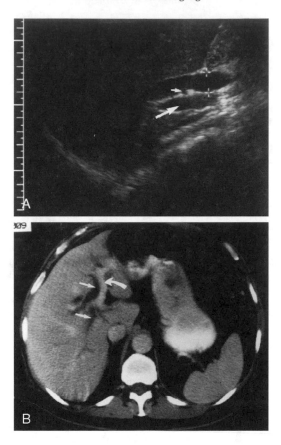

Figure 10. **A,** Ultrasound demonstrates a dilated common biliary duct, marked by calipers, measuring 15.7 mm in a patient with a CBD stricture. An hypoechoic portal vein (*long arrow*) and hepatic artery (*short arrow*) are seen posterior to CBD. **B,** CT demonstrates a dilated intrahepatic biliary tree (*straight arrows*) adjacent to an enhancing portal vein (*curved arrow*) in a patient with pancreatic carcinoma.

CBD stones do not necessarily cause acoustic shadowing. CT detection requires thin-section acquisition (≤ 5 mm). Depending on their composition, stones may be seen as soft tissue or calcific intraluminal densities.

Cholangiocarcinoma should be suspected when there is abrupt biliary obstruction but no visualized mass or stone. The primary mass is commonly difficult to identify by ultrasound or CT. Because cholangiocarcinoma often arises near or at the liver hilum (Klatskin tumor), it commonly presents with dilated intrahepatic ducts and normal-sized extrahepatic ducts.

An abrupt versus tapered appearance of the CBD can help differentiate pancreatic carcinoma from chronic pancreatitis. However, chronic pancreatitis can also present as a focal mass, and in such cases, biopsy may be required to differentiate these etiologies.

PANCREATIC IMAGING

18. How can acute pancreatitis be distinguished from chronic pancreatitis on imaging?

Acute pancreatitis: The classic sonographic appearance of acute pancreatitis is a hypoechoic, diffusely enlarged pancreas, although focal involvement may be seen in 18% of cases. Ultrasound is inferior to CT in evaluating acute pancreatitis for multiple reasons: (1) overlying bowel gas frequently limits complete visualization of the gland; (2) definition of extent of peripancreatic fluid collections is inferior to that of CT; and (3) ultrasound cannot diagnose pancreatic necrosis. Therefore, CT is the preferred study in patients with clinically severe pancreatitis. However, ultrasound is effective in follow-up of pseudocysts, which may be echo-free or have internal echogenicity due to hemorrhage or debris.

CT is typically performed with intravenous contrast, but if hemorrhagic pancreatitis is suspected, noncontrast images should be performed first to detect high-attenuation hemorrhage. With **mild** pancratitis, CT may be normal, whereas with **moderate** disease, the gland becomes enlarged and slightly heterogeneous, with inflammation causing peripancreatic fat to have higher attenuation ("dirty fat"). With **severe** disease, intraglandular intravasation of pancreatic fluid causes intrapancreatic **fluid collections,** and extravasation causes peripancreatic fluid collections, peripancreatic inflammation, and thickened fascial planes (see Figure 11A). Fluid collections are most common in the anterior pararenal space and lesser sac but can have wide extension.

Chronic pancreatitis: Sonography is 60–80% accurate in diagnosing chronic pancreatitis, and **dilatation of the pancreatic duct** is the most specific sonographic abnormality. Calcifications are seen as echogenic, shadowing foci within the gland. The gland may be enlarged early in the course but atrophic or focally enlarged later. Parenchymal echogenicity is variable.

Similar findings are noted with CT. Alteration of gland size is variable, and focal enlargement due to a chronic inflammatory mass may necessitate biopsy to exclude carcinoma. The pancreatic duct can be dilatated (> 3 mm) to the level of the papilla and may appear beaded, irregular, or smooth. **Calcifications** are the most reliable CT indicator of chronic pancreatitis and are seen in 50% of cases (see Figure 11B). Pseudocysts may be seen within or adjacent to the gland.

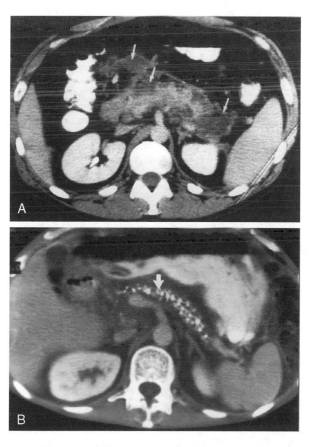

Figure 11. Pancreatitis. **A,** CT in acute pancreatitis demonstrates extensive peripancreatic fluid collections (*arrows*). **B,** CT shows multiple pancreatic calcifications (*arrows*) in a patient with chronic pancreatitis.

19. Describe the role of CT and ultrasound in assessing the complications of pancreatitis.

1. Pseudocysts evolve from fluid collections in about 30–50% of patients with acute pancreatitis. The development of a pseudocyst requires at least 4 weeks. More than half of these (measuring ≤ 5 cm) spontaneously regress. Pseudocysts failing to resolve or causing symptoms (pain, infection, hemorrhage, GI obstruction or fistula) require drainage. On CT, a pseudocyst appears as an oval fluid collection with a nonepithelialized enhancing wall. Ultrasound demonstrates an anechoic fluid collection with or without internal debris surrounded by a thin wall. Gas bubbles inside a pseudocyst relate to infection or fistula formation within the bowel.

2. Pancreatic ascites presents as free intraperitoneal fluid with high amylase levels in about 7% of patients with acute pancreatitis. These patients tend to have severe disease with obvious additional CT abnormalities, but rarely, the pancreas will appear normal; in these cases, percutaneous drainage of fluid and evaluation of amylase level is needed to establish the diagnosis.

3. Necrosis in acute pancreatitis can be detected by CT with a sensitivity of about 75–80%. Necrosis is defined as a lack of contrast enhancement in the expected location of pancreatic tissue, and it can develop early or late in the course of the patient's illness. The degree of necrosis is an important prognostic factor, in that patients who never develop CT evidence of necrosis have no mortality and a morbidity of only 6%, those with mild necrosis (< 30% of the total gland) exhibit no mortality but have a rate of complications of 40%, and patients with more severe necrosis (> 50%) have a morbidity rate of 75–100% and a mortality rate of 11–25%. Necrotic tissue can become secondarily infected, which is recognized on CT as bubbles of gas within areas of pancreatic gland necrosis (i.e., emphysematous pancreatitis). Infection more commonly does not contain gas, and under these circumstances, culture of a percutaneous aspirate verifies the diagnosis and identifies the organism.

4. Pancreatic abscesses occur secondary to liquefactive necrosis with subsequent infection. CT shows a focal low-attenuation fluid collection with thick enhancing walls. Gas bubbles may be present. On ultrasound, one sees a hypoechoic or even anechoic mass with a surrounding hyperechoic wall. Rates of abscess formation vary with the amount of pancreatic necrosis, and they usually occur 4 weeks after the onset of acute pancreatitis. The distinction between abscess and infected necrosis can be difficult, but it is an important one since the treatment alternatives are very different.

5. Pseudoaneurysms, resulting from enzymatic breakdown of the arterial wall, most commonly involve the splenic artery, followed by the gastroduodenal and pancreaticoduodenal arteries. Pseudoaneurysm rupture can cause massive hemorrhage and can occur into the retroperitoneum, peritoneal cavity, pancreatic duct, pseudocyst, or bowel, causing a GI tract bleed. CT is probably best for identifying pseudoaneurysms. High-density areas in or around a pseudoaneurysm represent either acute thrombus or hemorrhage. Ultrasound using color Doppler can be just as sensitive in detecting pseudoaneurysms and their complications, providing there is no overlying bowel gas.

6. Splenic vein thrombosis is detected by lack of normal enhancement in the expected region of the splenic vein on CT. Color Doppler can be used to make the same diagnosis. Thrombosis of the portal and superior mesenteric veins, although less common, is also well imaged by both modalities.

20. What are the imaging findings of pancreatic ductal adenocarcinoma?

1. Pancreatic enlargement: Although enlargement may be focal or diffuse, focal enlargement is more common. Diffuse enlargement is often secondary to pancreatitis caused by the neoplasm. Focal enlargement is better appreciated in the body and tail of the pancreas.

2. Distortion of the pancreatic contour or shape: Pancreatic cancer may also cause a focal bulge or irregularity of the organ surface. Involvement of the uncinate process of the pancreas may cause it to have a focal bulge or rounded appearance. Enlargement and contour distortion are the most frequent findings of pancreatic cancer.

3. Difference in density or echogenicity: On ultrasound, pancreatic cancer tends to be hypoechoic compared to normal pancreas; however, it may also appear isoechoic compared to normal pancreas. On CT, it is usually hypodense in comparison to normal pancreas, and this is better demonstrated with the use of intravenous contrast.

4. Pancreatic duct dilatation: This can be an important clue of a small neoplasm that may not be appreciated otherwise. It is more common when the neoplasm is located in the pancreatic head.

5. Biliary tract dilatation: Bile duct dilatation is more commonly seen with a neoplasm in the head of the pancreas. Isolated intrahepatic biliary ductal dilatation may be seen with pancreatic cancer that has spread to the porta hepatis.

6. Local invasion: Invasion into the peripancreatic fat is most commonly seen, but invasion into the porta hepatis, stomach, spleen, and adjacent bowel loops can also occur.

7. Regional lymph node enlargement: Pancreatic cancer may spread to the nodes in the porta hepatis, para-aortic region, and region around the celiac and superior mesenteric artery axis.

8. Liver metastasis: The liver is a common site of metastasis for pancreatic cancer. These appear as low-density lesions and may be single or multiple.

21. Which imaging modality is best for detecting and evaluating pancreatic cancer?
The two primary modalities to evaluate suspected pancreatic cancer are **ultrasound** and **CT**. CT is probably the best first-line imaging modality, but ultrasound is fairly equivalent in its ability to detect pancreatic cancer. CT is better at evaluating adjacent spread or nodal involvement, and it does not have the problem of incomplete evaluation of the body and tail of the pancreas, which occurs in up to 25% of ultrasound examinations. Overlying bowel gas can obstruct these areas on ultrasound. In a patient who presents with biliary obstruction, both ultrasound and CT are good first-line examinations.

22. What are the common cystic pancreatic neoplasms?
Serous (microcystic) and mucinous (macrocystic) cystic neoplasms. **Serous tumors** are more common in females, and 82% occur in persons age 60 or greater. They are almost always benign and predominate in the pancreatic head. Serous tumors calcify more commonly (50%) than any other pancreatic tumor and are typified by a **central stellate scar**, which frequently calcifies. They typically comprise many tiny (< 2 cm) cysts. On ultrasound, the multiple small cysts may not be individually resolved, so the mass commonly is hyperechoic. The hyperechoic central stellate scar and calcifications may be seen by ultrasound or CT, suggesting the diagnosis. The CT appearance also is varied; with innumerable minute cysts, it may appear as a solid tumor, whereas with multiple small but visible cysts, it has a honeycomb or "swiss-cheese" appearance. Soft-tissue components do enhance with contrast and the pancreatic contour may be lobulated.

Mucinous cystic neoplasms also have a strong female predominance but tend to occur in younger patients. They have a strong predilection for the pancreatic tail (85%), calcify in 30% of cases and must be considered malignant. They are larger lesions, averaging 12 cm, and are composed of unilocular or multilocular cysts > 2 cm. Ultrasound demonstrates **internal septations** that may be few or many and thick or thin. These septations are thicker than those in microcystic tumors, and the septations may calcify, which is better seen with CT. The tumor wall and organ of origin are better demonstrated with CT, whereas internal septations and solid excrescences are better seen by ultrasound. Differential diagnostic considerations include papillary cystic tumor, cystic islet cell tumor, cystic metastasis, pseudocysts or abscess.

ABDOMINAL AND PELVIC IMAGING

23. How is simple ascites distinguished from complicated ascites?
Simple ascites is a watery transudate that is usually secondary to major organ system failure—i.e., hepatic, renal, or cardiac failure. Because it is a transudate, simple ascites has a density similar to water on CT. Density measurements range from 0–20 HU. Generally, as the protein content of the fluid increases, so do the Hounsfield units. By ultrasound, simple ascites is anechoic, without internal echoes or septations, and demonstrates increased through transmission. Simple ascites is free-flowing and located in the dependent portions of the abdomen and pelvis.

It is often found in Morison's pouch, paracolic gutters, and pelvis. With large amounts of ascites, the bowel seems to float within the fluid, usually in the center of the abdomen. Simple ascites also has a sharp, smooth interface with other intra-abdominal contents. See Figure 12A and B.

Loculated ascites should not be considered as a simple fluid collection. Loculated fluid indicates the presence of **adhesions.** The reason for the adhesions may be relatively benign, as in prior surgery, but it may also be a sign of an infectious or malignant process. Loculated ascites is typically located in nondependent portions of the abdomen; it does not change position when the patient is scanned in a different position, and it often displaces adjacent bowel loops. A thick or nodular border may indicate an infectious or malignant process.

Complex ascites is usually secondary to an infectious, hemorrhagic, or neoplastic process. The findings of complex ascites include a density greater than water, internal debris or septations, air bubbles within the collection, or a thick or nodular border or capsule (see Figure 12C and D). Usually, the density measurements must be > 20 HU to be considered complex, reflecting the increased protein content of these collections. Not all complex fluid collections have these findings, and sometimes these look like simple fluid collections. In many cases, the only way to confirm if a collection is simple or not is to aspirate the fluid.

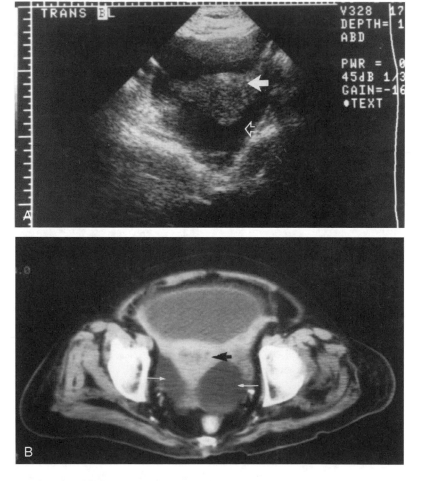

Figure 12. Ascites. **A** and **B,** Ultrasound and CT scan showing simple ascites (*arrows*) in the pelvis adjacent to the uterus (*arrowhead*).

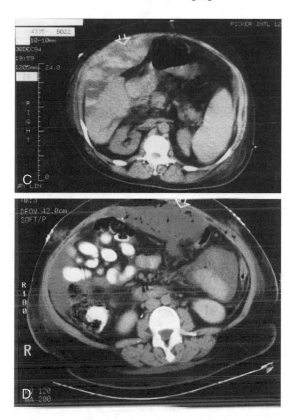

Figure 12 (*Continued*). **C,** Intra-abdominal hemorrhage presenting as a complex fluid collection. **D,** Intra ab dominal abscess presenting as a complex fluid collection with multiple air bubbles.

24. How do you differentiate abdominal fluid from pleural fluid?

Both ultrasound and CT are good modalities to ascertain if a collection is intra-abdominal or pleural. If the collection can be seen by ultrasound, it usually outlines the diaphragm, making the determination less confusing. By CT, certain signs have been described to make this differentiation:

1. Ascites is located anterior or lateral to the diaphragmatic crus, whereas pleural fluid is located posterior or medial to the crus.
2. Pleural effusion can extend medial to the crus and appear to touch the spine or aorta.
3. Abdominal fluid is often contiguous with other abdominal fluid collections.
4. Ascites has a sharp interface with intra-abdominal organs such as the liver and spleen. Pleural fluid has a less sharp interface because the diaphragm lies between the fluid and abdominal organs.
5. Ascitic fluid spares the bare area of the liver, which lies between the left and right coronary ligaments along the posterior border of the right lobe of the liver. These bare areas are peritoneal reflections that suspend the liver from the diaphragm; peritoneal fluid cannot pass through these ligaments to accumulate in the bare area. However, bare area is in contact with the diaphragm, so pleural fluid can accumulate behind the bare area.

25. When is CT used to evaluate the small bowel?

Conventional barium examinations remain superior to CT for evaluating intraluminal and mucosal disease, but CT is far better for evaluating the intramural component of small bowel as well as the adjacent mesentery, omentum, retroperitoneum, peritoneal cavity, and viscera. Successful visualization requires opacification and distention with oral contrast as well as intravenous contrast. With adequate distention by oral contrast, the thickness of the bowel wall is about 2 mm.

Smooth and concentric thickening of the bowel wall in the range of 7–11 mm is a typical appearance for nonmalignant disease, such as Crohn's disease, ischemic enteritis, ulcerative colitis, infectious enteritis, radiation enteritis, Shönlein-Henoch purpura, intramural hemorrhage, and bowel edema associated with portal hypertension. Extraintestinal findings are an important part of the exam. For example, with Crohn's disease, one should look for associated abscesses, fibrofatty proliferation, fistulas, and inflammation of the mesentery (see figure below). Thickening of the skin and increased density of the mesenteric and subcutaneous fat can accompany radiation enteritis, which typically involves bowel in the pelvis. Severe cases of ischemic enteritis can be accompanied by portal venous gas, intramural hemorrhage, or blood elsewhere in the peritoneal cavity.

Eccentric and irregular thickening of the bowel wall exceeding 2 cm with involvement of a short segment is suspicious for carcinoma. When this finding is associated with massive mesenteric or retroperitoneal adenopathy, lymphoma should be considered. When it is associated with liver lesions, adenocarcinoma should be considered. Benign small bowel tumors, such as neurofibromas and leiomyomas, are difficult to distinguish from malignant tumors. The exception is a lipoma, which is easily recognized by its low attenuation in the range of −90 to −120 HU. Small bowel carcinoids are typically located in the RLQ and can have a characteristic appearance of partial calcification and a surrounding desmoplastic reaction.

Enteroenteric intussusception is easily defined by the invaginated low-density mesenteric fat situated between the higher density of the inner intussusceptum and the outer receiving loop, the intussuscipiens. The underlying neoplasm may or may not be seen.

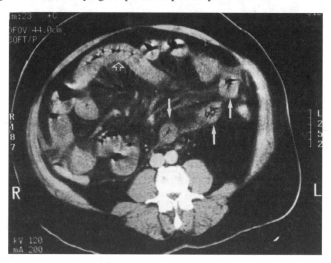

Figure 13. Thickening of multiple loops of small bowel due to ischemia in a patient with mesenteric infarction. Thickened loops are seen in both longitudinal (*open arrow*) and cross-sectional (*arrows*) planes.

26. How is CT used to evaluate the large bowel?

Optimal evaluation of the colon requires bowel preparation and luminal distention with rectal contrast or air to evaluate the true wall thickness. Normal wall thickness of a distended colon is < 3 mm. Indications for colonic distention include staging for colorectal or pelvic cancer, inflammatory bowel disease, diverticulitis, or appendicitis. Intravenous contrast facilitates evaluation of the bowel wall, solid organs, and vascular structures.

Sigmoid or cecal **diverticulitis** is well suited for evaluation with CT because it is a pericolic process rather than a disease of the lumen. Acute findings include increased density in the pericolic fat, thickening of the wall, and diverticula. CT is also excellent for imaging complications of abscess and fistula information in more severe cases. The differentiation between perforated sigmoid carcinoma and diverticulitis can be difficult or even impossible with CT alone. In cases in which the wall thickening is excessive (> 3 cm) or eccentric, one should consider sigmoid carcinoma.

Circumferential wall thickening (see Figure 14A below) is a nonspecific finding seen in numerous conditons, including Crohn's disease, ischemic colitis, pseudomembranous colitis, radiation colitis, neutropenic colitis, and inflammatory colitis due to cytomegalovirus or *Campylobacter* infection. Benign intestinal wall thickening of an involved segment can present either as homogeneous enhancing soft-tissue density or, less commonly, as concentric rings of high and low attenuation—termed the "double halo" or target sign (see Figure 14B below). Concentric rings result from hyperemic enhancement of the mucosa and serosa (high attenuation) and submucosal edema (low attenuation).

The etiology of wall thickening can sometimes be determined by location or associated findings. For example, arterial occlusion of the superior mesentric artery associated with bowel wall thickening in the region of the splenic flexure suggests ischemic disease. Distribution of disease in the rectosigmoid and in low-lying loops of pelvic small bowel suggests radiation enteritis. Inflammation adjacent to the large bowel can produce wall thickening mimicking a primary colonic process. For example, a ruptured appendicitis can produce cecal wall thickening, and severe pancreatitis can cause thickening of the transverse colon if inflammatory changes spread through the transverse mesocolon.

Irregular, eccentric, lobulated wall thickening is suggestive of **adenocarcinoma.** In some cases, an intraluminal polypoid mass can be seen. Local tumor extension is masslike, and in the absence of perforation, the surrounding pericolic fat maintains its homogeneous low attenuation unlike with inflammatory conditions. Tumor staging by the Dukes system with CT is accurate only about 50% of the time, but when present, findings of regional adenopathy, retroperitoneal adenopathy, or liver metastases confirm the diagnosis of bowel carcinoma. A large tumor mass usually enhances heterogeneously secondary to regions of necrosis. CT is useful in evaluating anastomatic recurrence from colorectal carcinoma, which can occur in the serosa beyond the reach of the endoscope.

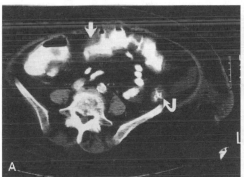

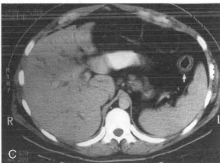

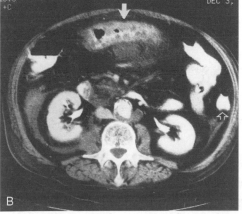

Figure 14. Large bowel. **A,** Large bowel wall thickening involves both the transverse (*straight arrow*) and descending colon (*curved arrow*) on an axial image of the lower abdomen in this patient with pseudomembranous colitis. **B,** Thickening of the left colon wall (*arrow*) displays the "double halo" sign in a patient with Crohn's disease. The dilated intrahepatic ducts are due to primary sclerosing cholangitis. **C,** Wall thickening of the transverse colon (*arrows*) seen in both longitudinal and cross-sectional planes, in a patient with severe pancreatitis.

Lymphoma of the colon presents differently than adenocarcinoma in that it thickens the wall to a much greater degree, often up to 4 cm. Lymphoma is rarely isolated to the colon and additional sites of involvement should be sought.

27. Describe the optimal radiographic work-up of diverticulitis.

CT is generally considered to be the most efficacious method for making the radiologic diagnosis of diverticulitis. Abdominal plain films are typically noncontributory. The barium enema depicts diverticula and may demonstrate fistulous tracts or extrinsic luminal defects related to the adjacent inflammatory process. CT is superior because it directly depicts the severity of the pericolic inflammation and the full degree of intraperitoneal or retroperitoneal extension. It is more sensitive than barium study in detecting abscesses and fistulae.

The hallmark of acute diverticulitis on CT is inflammation or increased attenuation of the pericolic fat, so-called **dirty fat** (see Figure 15). With greater degrees of inflammation, soft-tissue phlegmon may be seen, or fluid collections due to abscess may occur. Air bubbles may be seen in the fat or within abscesses or, with free perforation, they may be seen in the peritoneal cavity. Diverticula are seen and thickened colon wall (> 4 mm) is usually present, but this finding is nonspecific and may also be seen with diverticulosis. This wall thickening may occasionally be difficult to distinguish from colon cancer, but an abrupt transition zone is more suggestive of tumor and pericolic fatty inflammation suggests diverticulitis.

The assessment of the colon by CT is greatly improved with adequate colonic opacification or distention. This can be achieved with oral contrast or, if the patient has no peritoneal signs, with rectal air insufflation or water-soluble contrast per rectum.

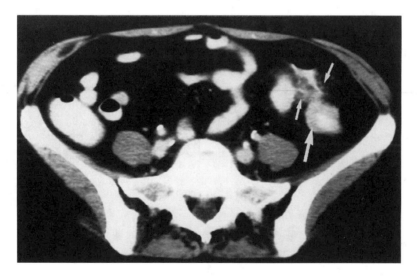

Figure 15. Typical CT appearance of diverticulitis, with stranding and increased density of the pericolic fat (*short arrows*) and thickening of the wall of the descending colon (*long arrow*).

28. What are the CT and ultrasound findings of acute appendicitis?

Ultrasound: Findings of acute appendicitis include a distended and noncompressible appendix, appendicolith, adjacent fluid collection, peritoneal fluid, and a focal mixed echogenic mass representing a phlegmon or abscess. The normal anteroposterior dimension of the appendix is 5–6 mm, with anything greater than this considered abnormal. See Figure 16.

CT: The findings are a distended and thick-walled appendix. An appendicolith may be seen in one-fourth of cases. Local signs of inflammation include increased density or stranding in the adjacent fat tissue, focal thickening of adjacent fascia, focal fluid collections, and adjacent phlegmon or abscess.

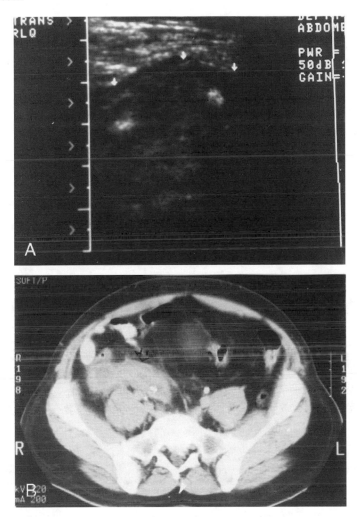

Figure 16. Acute appendicitis. **A,** Ultrasound shows a thickened appendix wall (*arrows*) and echogenic appendicoliths. **B,** CT shows a dilated fluid-filled appendix and a calcified appendicolith.

29. Which examination is better for diagnosing acute appendicitis?

The 96% sensitivity of CT is slightly superior to that of ultrasound (85–90%). The specificity is comparable at 90%. CT is better at showing a normal appendix and is better at showing the extent of adjacent inflammatory changes. The disadvantages of CT are its higher cost, use of ionizing radiation, and use of intravenous and contrast. Ultrasound is a good first choice in children, pregnant patients, and thin people. CT should be used for all other types of patients and is very effective in heavier patients.

30. Discuss the role of imaging in the assessment of intra-abdominal abscess.

US: In suspected intra-abdominal abscess, ultrasound has the advantage of being performed at the patient's bedside. It is best suited for evaluation of abscesses in the pelvis, RUQ, and LUQ, where the bladder, liver, and spleen, respectively, provide acoustic windows for sound transmission. However, assessment of the midabdomen is commonly impossible due to overlying bowel gas. Abscesses have a varied appearance but commonly are irregularly marginated, primarily hypoechoic, with internal areas of increased echogenicity.

CT: The entire abdomen and pelvis should be scanned, with administration of sufficient oral contast to opacify the bowel, as fluid-filled bowel loops can easily simulate an abscess; rectal contrast may also be helpful. The CT appearance of an abscess depends on its age or maturity. In the early stage, the abscess may appear as a soft-tissue density mass. As it matures and undergoes liquefactive necrosis, the central region has a near-water attenuation, possibly with internal air bubbles or an air-fluid level (see figure below). Granulation tissue forming the wall of the abscess typically enhances with intravenous contrast, providing a higher attenuation rim. Mass effect with displacement of surrounding structures may be seen, and there is commonly inflammation and increased density of adjacent fat.

Scintigraphy: Radionuclide imaging may be performed with gallium-67 citrate or indium-111-labeled white blood cells (WBCs). The advantage of scintigraphy is that it provides whole-body images and may detect infection in unsuspected sites. Gallium images, however, may require 48–72 hours for optimal interpretation, and normal colonic excretion of gallium may cause confusion in interpretation. Indium-labeled WBC imaging is more rapid than Ga-67, but uptake is somewhat nonspecific, and the liver and spleen are difficult to evaluate because of normal uptake in these organs.

Recommendations: Generally, CT is the imaging procedure of first choice for detecting abscess in the acutely ill patient. Ultrasound can be used as the initial exam if the abscess is suspected in the RUQ, LUQ, or pelvis or with suspected appendiceal abscess. In patients who are not acutely ill and have no localizing signs, radionuclide scintigraphy can be considered as the initial screening technique.

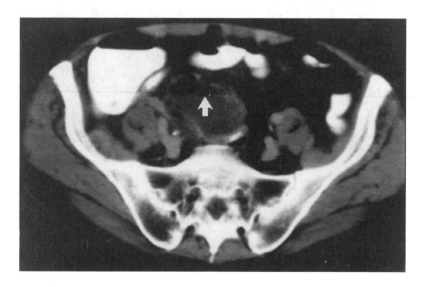

Figure 17. Abdominal abscess with air-fluid level (*arrow*) and internal debris.

AIDS-RELATED DISORDERS

31. What characteristic features of AIDS are seen in the biliary system?

Gallbladder and bile duct abnormalities, including gallbladder wall thickening, sludge, cholelithiasis, bile duct dilatation, bile duct wall thickening, pericholecystic fluid, and an ultrasonic Murphy's sign, can be seen in as many as 20% of AIDS patients during ultrasound. The most common abnormality, **gallbladder wall thickening,** is often asymptomatic and not related to intrinsic gallbladder disease, but rather to edema from hepatitis or hypoproteinemia. Gallbladder wall thickening associated with a positive Murphy's sign is suggestive of acalculous chole-cystitis, either secondary to cytomegalovirus or *Cryyptosporidium* infection.

AIDS-related cholangitis is also usually secondary to cytomegalovirus or *Cryptosporidium*. Ultrasound is the best noninvasive test for evaluating the extrahepatic ducts, but CT is better for evaluating the intrahepatic ducts. Endoscopic retrograde cholaniopancreatography (ERCP) displays the morphologic appearance of the entire ductal system better than either modality, and the findings of dilatated ducts, papillary narrowing, diffuse intrahepatic strictures, extrahepatic strictures, or any combination of these findings seen in AIDS-related cholangitis mimic those of sclerosing cholangitis, papillary stenosis, or both. Patients with papillary stenosis or isolated extrahepatic ductal involvement benefit most from sphincterotomy or common bile duct stents.

Biliary ductal dilatation can also be caused by obstruction from enlarged lymph nodes in the porta hepatis or retroperitoneum from Kaposi's sarcoma or lymphoma. Non-AIDS related conditions, such as biliary calculi, cholangiocarcinoma, or pancreatic carcinoma, may also be a consideration and a search for these entities should be made in the appropriate clinical setting.

32. Describe the imaging features of AIDS in the liver.

Hepatomegaly is seen in nearly 20% of AIDS patients. It is usually a nonspecific response to infection, hepatitis, fatty infiltration, or neoplastic infiltration from lymphoma or Kaposi's sarcoma. Approximately 10% of AIDS patients have diffusely increased liver echogenicity on ultrasound, due to either **fatty infiltration** caused by malnutrition (a fatty liver has decreased attenuation on CT) or **hepatic granulomatosis** caused by *Mycobacterium avium-intracellulare, M. tuberculosis, Cryptococcus, Histoplasma,* cytomegalovirus, *Toxoplasma,* or a drug reaction from sulfonamides. Infection in the liver can also take the form of single or multiple liver **abscesses.** On ultrasound, such lesions can have increased, decreased, or mixed echogenicity, but with CT they are generally low in attenuation. Microscopic involvement of the liver may show very little changes on CT and ultrasound, and a core biopsy may be the only method possible for diagnosis. When **infection** involves the liver of an AIDS patient, it is almost always secondary to disseminated disease, and one should search for associated abnormalities such as cholangitis, adenopathy, splenomegaly, and ascites.

Kaposi's sarcoma is the most common neoplasm in AIDS; however, the diagnosis of liver involvement is rarely made antemortem. The findings are variable because the tumor is multifocal. On ultrasound, one sees hepatomegaly and hyperechoic lesions in the parenchyma (often adjacent to the portal veins), whereas on contrast-enhanced CT, lesions are initially low in attenuation but enhance after time (4–7 min) to become either homogeneous with or more attenuated than the surrounding liver parenchyma. Kaposi's sarcoma is actually far more likely to present as adenopathy in the retroperitoneum, mesentery, or mediastinum than as lesions in the liver.

Lymphoma is more commonly extranodal in AIDS patients than in the general population, and the liver and spleen are two of the more common extranodal sites. Both CT and ultrasound will show one or more visceral lesions. With ultrasound, lesions are usually hypoechoic, and on CT, such lesions are generally low in attenuation. Organ involvement can be the sole manifestation, yet normally lymphoma is associated with bulky adenopathy of the retroperitoneum, mesentery, or mediastinum.

33. What extrahepatic manifestations of AIDS in the GI tract can be noted by imaging?

HIV-positive patients often demonstrate hepatosplenomegaly, and CT may demonstrate multiple, small (< 5-mm) mesenteric or retroperitoneal nodes. Proctitis may be seen as thickened rectal wall with increased attenuation of perirectal fat. Patients who have progressed to clinical AIDS often demonstrate opportunistic infection or opportunistic tumor on CT or ultrasound. Enlargement of lymph nodes suggests AIDS rather than HIV disease, and focal defects in solid organs suggest either abscess or tumor infiltration.

GI tract involvement with Kaposi's sarcoma (KS) is common (as is skin involvement), and submucosal nodules may be seen with barium studies anywhere in the GI tract. When the nodules become larger, they can be seen on CT, and nodular mural thickening of the gut suggests KS. Lymphadenopathy is usually absent or mild in KS, unlike lymphoma.

Lymphoma in AIDS is usually of B-cell type and aggressive, with a propensity for extra-nodular distribution. Lymphadenopathy is usually bulky, but an isolated node may be involved. Hepatic and splenic lesions are low attenuation on CT and hypoechoic by sonography. Bowel wall thickening may be a manifestation of GI tract involvement.

Opportunistic infections are manifold: *Candida,* herpes simplex, or cytomegalovirus (CMV) may cause esophagitis, possibly delineated with barium studies. CMV may involve any area of the gut, commonly the cecal region. CT may demonstrate thick-walled bowel with enhancing serosa and mucosa. *Mycobacterium-tuberculosis* may involve the ileocecal region, and wall thickening and low-density lymph nodes in the RLQ are typical on CT.

Mycobacterium avium intracellulare usually involves the small bowel, with multiple nodes having central low attenuation due to liquefaction. *Cryptosporidium* is characterized by profuse watery contents of small bowel on CT. *Pneumocystis carinii* abscesses are seen as multifocal small areas of low attenuation in liver, spleen, pancreas, kidneys, or lymph nodes. Calcifications are common early as well as late in abscess formation.

BIBLIOGRAPHY

1. Balthazar EJ: CT of the gastrointestinal tract: Principles and interpretation. AJR 156:23–32, 1991.
2. Balthazar EJ, Freeny PC, vanSonnenberg E: Imaging and intervention in acute pancreatitis. Radiology 193:297–306, 1994.
3. Dolmatch BL, Lang FC, Federle MP, et al: AIDS-related cholangitis: Radiographic findings in nine patients. Radiology 14:143–147, 1987.
4. Federle MP: Radiology of the immunocompromised host. Radiol Clin North Am 27:507–662, 1989.
5. Freeny PC: Radiologic diagnosis and staging of pancreatic ductal adenocarcinoma. Radiol Clin North Am 27:121–128, 1989.
6. Foshager MC, Ferral H, Finlay DE, et al: Color Doppler sonography of transjugular intrahepatic portosystemic shunts (TIPS). AJR 163:105–111, 1994.
7. Lee MJ, et al: Differential diagnosis of hyperintense liver lesions on T1-weighted MR images. AJR 159:1017–1020, 1992.
8. Gore RM, Levine MS, Laufer I (eds): Textbook of Gastrointestinal Radiology. Philadelphia, W.B. Saunders, 1994.
9. Lee JKT, Sagel SS, Stanley RJ (eds): Computed Body Tomography with MRI, 2nd ed. New York, Raven Press, 1989.
10. Moss AA, Gamsu G, Genant HK: Computed Tomography of the Body with Magnetic Resonance Imaging, 2nd ed. Philadelphia, W.B. Saunders, 1992.
11. Putnam CE, Ravin CE: Textbook of Diagnostic Imaging, 2nd ed. Philadelphia, W.B. Saunders, 1994.
12. Ros PR, Bidgood WD: Abdominal Magnetic Resonance Imaging. St. Louis, C.V. Mosby, 1993.
13. Schneiderman DJ: Hepatobiliary abnormalities of AIDS. Gastroenterol Clin North Am 17:615–630, 1988.
14. Smith FJ, et al: Abdominal abnormalities in AIDS: Detection at US in a large population. Radiology 192:691–695, 1984.
15. Teixidor HS, Godwin TA, Ramirez EA: Cryptosporidiosis of the biliary tract in AIDS. Radiology 180:51–56, 1991.

75. NUCLEAR MEDICINE STUDIES

Mike McBiles, M.D.

1. Outline the general advantages of nuclear medicine procedures compared with other imaging modalities.

In almost every case, nuclear medicine procedures derive their advantages from one or more of the following categories:

    a. **Functional information** is provided by them that either is not available by other modalities or is obtained at greater expense or patient risk.

    b. **Very high contrast** (target-to-background ratio) can be achieved in many instances by nuclear medicine techniques, allowing diagnostic studies despite poor spatial resolution.

    c. **Relatively noninvasive** studies are the rule in nuclear medicine, requiring only an injection of a radioactive dose or swallowing a substance followed by imaging.

2. What are the disadvantages of nuclear medicine procedures compared with other radiographic studies?

    a. **Spatial resolution,** usually on the order of 1–2 cm, is inferior to that of other imaging modalities.

    b. **Patient imaging time** can be long, sometimes up to 1 hour or more.

    c. **Radiation risk** is obviously greater than it is with magnetic resonance (MR) or ultrasound. However, when compared to plain film or computed tomographic (CT) imaging, the radiation risk from most nuclear medicine studies is equal to or less than that of an average CT study (gallium-67 or indium-111 white blood cell studies are the exceptions and average 2–4 times more radiation risk than other nuclear medicine studies). In some studies, such as gastric emptying and esophageal transit studies, radiation risk is insignificant compared to that with fluoroscopy.

    d. **Availability** is limited, with specialized procedures requiring radiopharmaceuticals or interpretation expertise not available in all centers.

3. What nuclear medicine tests are most helpful in GI medicine?

Nuclear medicine procedures have been used in the evaluation of practically every GI problem. However, improvements in and widespread use of endoscopy, manometry, pH monitoring, and other imaging techniques have limited nuclear medicine's application to specific clinical problems.

Uses of Nuclear Medicine Procedures in GI Diseases

TEST/STUDY	USEFUL IN DIAGNOSIS/EVALUATION
Cholescintigraphy (hepatobiliary imaging)	Acute cholecystitis
	Gallbladder dyskinesis
	Common duct obstruction
	Biliary atresia
	Sphincter of Oddi dysfunction
	Mass lesions
	Biliary leak
	Choleangiointestinal anastomosis patency
	Gastroenterostomy, afferent loop patency
Gastric emptying	Quantify gastric motility
Esophageal motility/transit	Quantify esophageal transit
	Evaluate/detect reflux
	Aspiration detection
Liver/spleen scan	Hepatic mass lesions
	Accessory spleen/splenosis
Heat-damaged RBC scan	Accessory spleen/splenosis

Table continued on following page

Uses of Nuclear Medicine Procedures in GI Diseases (Continued)

TEST/STUDY	USEFUL IN DIAGNOSIS/EVALUATION
Gallium scanning	Staging of many abdominal malignancies
	Abdominal abscess
^{131}I-MIBG, ^{111}In-octreotide	Neural crest tumor imaging
^{111}In-satumomab pentetide	Colorectal cancer staging
In WBC scanning	Evaluation of abdominal infection/abscess
^{99}mTc-HMPAO WBC scanning	Evaluation of sites of active inflammatory bowel disease
^{99}mTc-RBC scanning	GI bleeding localization
	Hepatic hemangiomas
Pertechnetate scanning	Meckel's diverticulum
	Retained gastric antrum
Sulfur-colloid injections	GI bleeding localization
Peritoneovenous shunt study	Peritoneovenous shunt patency
Hepatic arterial perfusion	Territory perfused by hepatic intra-arterial catheters
Shilling's test	Vitamin B12 malabsorption

RBC = red blood cell; MIBG = *m*-iodobenzylguanidine; HM-PAO = hexamethyl-propyleneamineoxime; WBC = white blood cell.

4. How is cholescintigraphy (hepatobiliary imaging) performed? What is a normal study?

The conduct of the basic cholescintigraphic study is the same for nearly all of its clinical indications (*see* Question 3). The patient is injected with a technetium-99m labeled imidodiacetic acid (IDA) derivative. Currently, commonly used compounds are DISHIDA, mebrofenin, and HIDA (hepato-IDA), the latter being the popular term used among clinicians for all these tests. Despite their excretion by the same mechanism as bilirubin, current compounds can provide diagnostic studies at very high bilirubin levels (>20 mg/dl).

After injection, sequential images, usually 1 minute in duration, are obtained for 60 minutes or longer. Normally, the IDA compound is rapidly cleared by the liver, and on images displayed at normal intensity, blood pool activity in the heart is faint or not discernible by 5 minutes after injection. Persistent blood pool activity and poor liver uptake are indications of hepatocellular dysfunction. Right and left hepatic ducts are frequently, but not invariably, seen by 10 minutes, and the common bile duct and small bowel are seen by 20 minutes. The gallbladder is usually seen by this time also but can be normally visualized for up to 1 hour, provided the patient has not eaten within 4 hours. By 1 hour, almost all activity is in the bile ducts, gallbladder, and bowel, and the liver is seen faintly or not at all.

In all the studies listed in Question 3, failure to see an expected structure at 1 hour (e.g., gallbladder in acute cholecystitis, small bowel in biliary atresia) requires delayed imaging for up to 4 hours. Sometimes, various manipulations, such as sincalide or morphine infusions, are performed after the initial 60-minute images and then imaging is continued for another 30–60 minutes.

5. In acute cholecystitis, how should the patient be prepared? What manipulations are used to shorten the study or increase its reliability?

Traditionally, acute cholecystitis is diagnosed on functional cholescintigraphy by noting a lack of filling of the gallbladder (usually due to a cystic duct stone) on the initial 60-minute study and on 4-hour images (positive study). All manipulations and preparations are performed to ensure that this lack of gallbladder visualization is a true-positive finding or to shorten this long, sometimes tedious study. Because food is a potent and long-lasting stimulus for endogenous cholecystokinin (CCK) release and subsequent gallbladder contraction, the **patient should not eat for 4 hours** prior to the study; otherwise a false-positive study may result. Prolonged fasting causes viscous bile formation in the normal gallbladder, which may impair its filling by the radio-pharmaceutical and cause a false-positive study. Most clinics now give the short-acting CCK analog **sincalide,** 0.01–0.04 μg/kg intravenously over 3 minutes, one-half hour before cholescintigraphy if the patient has fasted >24 hours, is on hyperalimentation, or is severely ill.

Despite these manipulations, the gallbladder may not fill during the 60-minute cholescintigraphic study. Rather than do reimaging at 4 hours, **morphine,** 0.01 μg/kg intravenously, may be given if the gallbladder is not seen but the small bowel is seen at 60 minutes; following morphine administration, imaging is then continued for 30 additional minutes. Because morphine causes sphincter of Oddi contraction, which results in increased biliary tree pressure, a functional obstruction of the cystic duct will be overcome by this manipulation. If the gallbladder still is not seen, delayed imaging is not necessary and acute cholecystitis is diagnosed (see Figure 1). Concern has been voiced that both sincalide and morphine interventions may cause perforation of a gangrenous gallbladder, but this complication has never been reported.

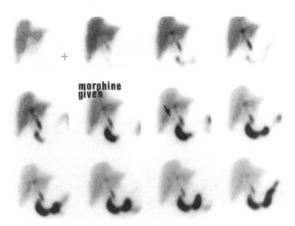

Figure 1. Acute cholecystitis. Hepatobiliary study with ^{99}mTc- mebrofenin, acquired every 5 minutes after ^{99}mTc-mebrofenin injection, shows rapid clearance and uptake by the liver, with rapid excretion into the common bile duct and small bowel. Note the absence of gallbladder (*arrow* points to the area usually occupied by gallbladder). Morphine, 1 mg intravenously given at the 30-minute image, failed to fill the gallbladder in an additional 30 minutes of imaging. Alternatively, a 4-hour delayed image could have been obtained instead of injecting morphine, but this step would have prolonged the study unnecessarily.

6. If acute cholecystitis is a possibility, should hepatobiliary scintigraphy be used?
Hepatobiliary scintigraphy is the most accurate method of diagnosing acute cholecystitis, with a sensitivity and specificity of 95%. However, it should not be used in every instance when acute cholecystitis is suspected. If, for example, the pretest probability of acute cholecystitis is very low (<10%) then a positive study in a low-probability (screening) population is likely to be a false-positive; likewise, if the pretest probability is high (>90%), then a negative study in a high-probability population is likely to be a false-negative. In subgroups such as those with acalculous cholecystitis or hyperalimentation and in the critically ill, there is a significant false-positive rate, and correlative imaging with ultrasound or CT may be necessary.

7. How is cholescintigraphy used to diagnose and manage biliary leak?
Cholescintigraphy is highly sensitive and specific for detecting biliary leak (see Figure 2). Because nonbile fluid collections are common after surgery, anatomic studies have a poor specificity. Cholescintigraphy has poor spatial resolution, and so the exact site of the leak may not be documented; endoscopic retrograde cholangiopancreatography (ERCP) or percutaneous transhepatic cholangiography (PTC) may be necessary for anatomic definition. Cholescintigraphy can also be used noninvasively to document resolution of a bile leak.

8. How is cholescintigraphy used in diagnosing common bile duct obstruction?
Ductal dilatation seen on ultrasound may be a nonspecific finding if there has been previous biliary surgery, and acute obstruction (<24–48 hours old) may not show ductal dilatation. Cholescintigraphy will show a lack of gallbladder and small bowel visualization, and frequently lack

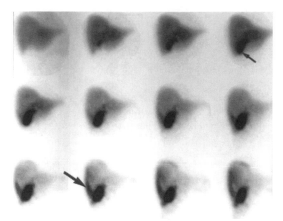

Figure 2. Bile leak. After percutaneous liver biopsy, the patient developed severe RUQ pain. Ultrasound was not helpful. Sequential 5-minute images after ^{99m}Tc-mebrofenin injection show leakage of a thin rim of bile along the inferior and lateral liver edge (*large arrow*). Note gallbladder filling early in the study (*small arrow*) and the lack of small bowel activity, implying preferential flow of bile to the gallbladder and site of leakage.

of biliary tree visualization, on the 4-hour delayed images in common duct obstruction, and with very high sensitivity and specificity (see Figure 3). Cholescintigraphy is reliable even at high bilirubin levels. It can be used to distinguish obstructive from nonobstructive jaundice.

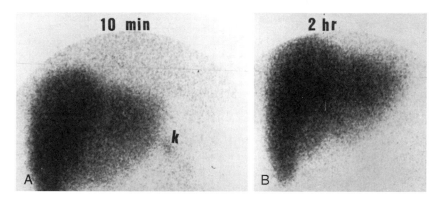

Figure 3. Common bile duct obstruction. After injection of the hepatobiliary agent, there is no visible activity in the intrahepatic ducts or small bowel on 10-minute (*panel A*) or 2-hour (*panel B*) images. Ultrasound did not show dilated ducts, and a common duct stone was not seen, a common occurrence in acute common duct obstruction. Activity to left of liver (*K*) is the radiopharmaceutical agent excreted in the urine in an alternate pathway to biliary excretion.

9. What is cholescintigraphy's role in diagnosing biliary atresia?

By the same rationale as outlined in Question 8, cholescintigraphy is sensitive and highly specific for the diagnosis of biliary atresia if the patient is properly prepared. The major differential diagnostic possibility in the neonate is severe neonatal hepatitis. Ultrasonographic findings are insensitive: ultrasound may show ductal dilatation in biliary atresia, but dilatation is usually absent. The main scintigraphic problem is a false-positive study caused by a lack of biliary secretion in severe hepatitis. Premedication of the neonate with oral phenobarbital, 5 mg/kg/day for 5 days, stimulates bile flow and eliminates this problem. The importance of therapeutic serum levels of phenobarbital cannot be overemphasized. If radioactivity in the small bowel is seen on delayed images, biliary atresia is ruled out (see Figure 4).

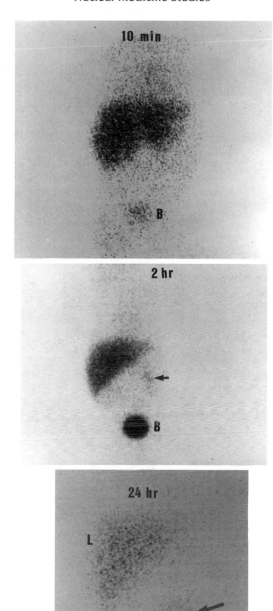

Figure 4. Neonatal hepatitis in a patient with suspected biliary atresia. This difficult diagnosis can be made with an hepatobiliary agent. In this case, ^{99}mTc-mebrofenin was injected after a 5-day preparation with phenobarbital. Note the continued blood pool activity in the heart on the 2-hour image and excretion into the bladder *(B)*, suggesting hepatocellular dysfunction with abnormal excretion of the hepatobiliary agent in to the alternate urinary pathway. At 4-hours there is a subtle focus *(arrow)* in the abdomen that may be in the bowel or radiopharmaceutical excreted by the alternate urinary pathway. The 24-hour image with the bladder catheterized shows ill-defined activity in the LLQ *(arrow)*, inferolateral to liver *(L)*, confirming excretion of the radiopharmaceutical agent into the bowel and ruling out biliary atresia.

10. How is sphincter of Oddi dysfunction assessed by cholescintigraphy?

A significant number of patients continue to have pain following cholescintigraphy, and sphincter of Oddi dysfunction may be the cause. Although manometry during ERCP is diagnostic, this study is invasive and not without complications. An empiric scintigraphic scoring system looking at quantitative parameters of bile movement and liver function has been developed. Very high correlation with biliary tree manometric findings has been demonstrated.

11. When can cholescintigraphy be helpful in evaluating obstruction in gastroenterostomies?

Afferent loops are difficult to evaluate with barium studies because the afferent loop must be filled antegrade with barium. By cholescintigraphy, afferent loop obstruction can be reliably excluded if there is afferent and efferent loop activity 1 hour after radiopharmaceutical injection, and it is diagnosed if there is persistent accumulation in the afferent loop with little or no efferent loop activity at 2 hours.

12. What is gallbladder dyskinesia? How does cholescintigraphy evaluate the emptying of the gallbladder?

A significant number of patients have normal imaging and clinical workups, yet have pain referable to the gallbladder, as evidenced by relief of symptoms upon cholecystectomy. The poorly understood and heterogeneous entity of gallbladder dyskinesia has been proposed as an etiology of this pain. It is thought that poorly coordinated contractions between the gallbladder and cystic duct can cause pain. It has been proposed that gallbladder dyskinesia may be manifested by an abnormally low ejection of bile under the stimulus of cholecystokinin (sincalide).

After the gallbladder is filled during traditional cholescintigraphy, gallbladder contraction is stimulated by an infusion of sincalide, 0.01 μg/kg over 30–45 minutes. The amount of gallbladder emptying over 30 minutes reflects the gallbladder ejection fraction (GBEF; normal >35–40%). This protocol has demonstrated an impressive correlation of both normal and abnormal GBEF with surgical and medical follow-up and can reliably separate normals from abnormals.

13. What is a nuclear medicine gastric emptying study?

Both liquid and solid gastric emptying studies can be performed under nuclear medicine examination. Liquid studies are usually performed on infants and consist of giving a mixture of ^{99}mTc-sulfur colloid with milk or formula at normal feeding time, imaging every 15 minutes for 60 minutes, and calculating an emptying half-time. In adults a solid-phase emptying is usually performed after an overnight fast by mixing ^{99}mTc-sulfur colloid–labeled scrambled eggs with a standard meal, performing anterior and posterior imaging every 15 minutes for 90 minutes, and calculating the percentage of emptying. The meal has not been standardized, and normal values are dependent on the meal composition. Using a 300-calorie meal of scrambled eggs, bread, and butter, solid gastric emptying is 63% at 1 hour (± SD of 11%).

14. In what clinical situations is a nuclear medicine gastric emptying study useful?

Symptoms related to problems of abnormal gastric motility can be nonspecific, and barium studies are not quantifiable and are nonphysiologic. On the one hand, gastric emptying studies are semiqualitative, show less than optimal reproducibility, and are not standardized. Nevertheless, a rough estimate of emptying in clinically important groups (such as diabetics and partial- gastrectomy patients) is possible and can be helpful in explaining nonspecific symptoms or suggesting another etiology if the results are clearly normal or abnormal (see Figure 5).

15. What nuclear medicine esophageal studies are available, and how are they used?

Three studies have been used clinically: esophageal motility, esophageal reflux, and pulmonary aspiration studies.

Esophageal motility study: This study is performed by rapid sequential imaging of the

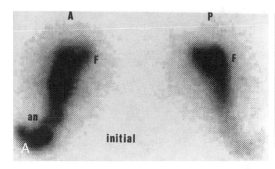

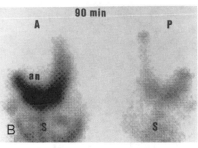

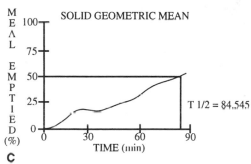

Figure 5. Normal gastric emptying study. **A,** Initial anterior *(A)* and posterior *(P)* images after ingestion of ^{99}mTc-sulfur colloid–labeled scrambled eggs in beef stew show activity in the fundus *(F)* on posterior images and extending to the antrum *(an).* **B,** At 90 minutes, there is little radiopharmaceutical agent left in the fundus, a significant amount in the antrum *(an),* and noticeable activity distributed throughout the small bowel *(S).* **C,** At 84.5 minutes, 50% of the meal had emptied (normal, 35–60% using this type of meal).

esophagus during swallowing of ^{99}mTc-colloid in water. Although it provides a precise and reproducible quantitation of esophageal function, barium studies usually provide adequate definition of the anatomic or functional problem. Esophageal motility studies are useful as an easily performed study in the noninvasive follow-up of therapy for dysmotility and achalasia.

Esophageal reflux study: This study is performed by serial imaging of the esophagus after the patient drinks acidified orange juice containing ^{99}mTc-colloid and during serial inflation of an abdominal binder. Although less sensitive than 24-hour pH monitoring, the test is more sensitive than barium studies and can be used as an easily performed screening study or to evaluate response to therapy in known reflux.

Pulmonary aspiration studies: These are performed by imaging the chest after oral administration of ^{99}mTc- colloid in water. Activity in the lungs is diagnostic of aspiration. Although the study sensitivity is low, it is probably higher than that of radiographic contrast studies, and also the test has the advantage of easy serial imaging to detect intermittent aspiration.

16. What is the role for nuclear medicine studies in evaluating hepatic mass lesions?

The traditional "liver/spleen scan" using an intravenous injection of the Kupffer cell–seeking ^{99}mTc-sulfur or -albumin colloids has largely been replaced by ultrasound and CT because these latter studies have superior resolution and are able to evaluate adjacent structures. However, in the occasional patient in whom other studies are equivocal, such as those with fatty infiltrate (see Figure 6), radionuclide functional imaging can be helpful.

Focal nodular hyperplasia (FNH) appears warm or hot on liver/spleen imaging because of its predominance of Kupffer cells but cold on hepatobiliary scintigraphy because of its relative lack of hepatocytes. The combination of these findings is very specific for FNH. Conversely, **hepatic adenomas** are usually composed mostly of hepatocytes and so appear warm or hot on hepatobiliary imaging and cold on liver/spleen imaging. This combination is also a specific finding. Hepatomas also appear warm or cold (but not hot) on cholescintigraphy, and the great majority of hepatomas avidly accumulate gallium-67. This combination of findings is also specific, except in the uncommon gallium-avid metastasis to the liver *(see* table).

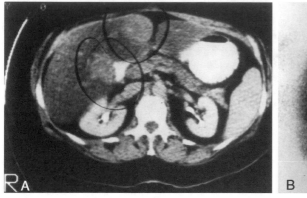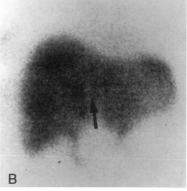

Figure 6. Evaluation of mass lesion. **A,** Contrast-enhanced CT scan of the liver shows diffuse fatty infiltration with two areas of relatively normal-appearing liver *(circles)* in this patient with colon cancer treated with 5-fluorouracil. Regenerating liver nodules and metastatic disease are the diagnostic possibilities. **B,** Given the large size of these lesions and their anterior location, metastatic lesions would be readily seen as a photopenic defect on hepatobiliary imaging *(arrow)*. Because no defects are seen, these are regenerating nodules.

Differential Diagnosis of Hepatic Mass Lesions by Nuclear Medicine Studies

	99mTc-Sulfur Colloid	Delayed Images, Hepatobiliary Agent	99mTc-RBCs	Gallium-67
Adenoma	Cold or decreased	Normal to increased	Normal	Decreased to normal
Hepatoma	Cold	Decreased, normal, or increased	Decreased to normal	Normal to increased; markedly increased is diagnostic*
Hemangioma	Cold	Cold	Markedly increased is diagnostic	Cold
Metastasis	Cold	Cold	Normal to slightly increased	Decreased, normal, slightly increased
Focal nodular, hyperplasia	Normal to increased	Decreased to normal	Normal	Normal

*Except in occasional gallium-avid metastasis to liver. Normal indicates lesion intensity same as liver.

17. Which nuclear medicine procedure is diagnostic for hepatic hemangiomas?

Often CT, MRI, and ultrasound are nondiagnostic for a hemangioma. Delayed SPECT imaging (single-photon emission computed tomography, three-dimensional scintigraphic images similar to CT) of these blood-filled lesions with 99mTc- labeled RBCs provides the most sensitive and specific diagnosis of hemangiomas >2.5 cm (see Figure 7). The positive predictive value of SPECT for hemangioma on smaller lesions, even < 1 cm, is also very high. This is because of the very high target-to-background ratio in these lesions, a result of their uniquely high proportion of blood to other tissue. Delayed SPECT imaging is the procedure of choice in these situations. In lesions near large vessels, however, it may be difficult to differentiate the vessel from the hemangioma, and other imaging modalities should be used. Also, the unusual clot-filled or fibrotic lesions will not be detected with high sensitivity.

18. Describe the vitamin B12 absorption (Schilling's) test and its use.

The Schilling's test measures the ability of the body to absorb and excrete vitamin B12. Because there are many causes of vitamin B12 malabsorption, the workup is usually performed in stages, each designed to evaluate in sequence the most clinically prevalent causes of vitamin B12 deficiency. Al-

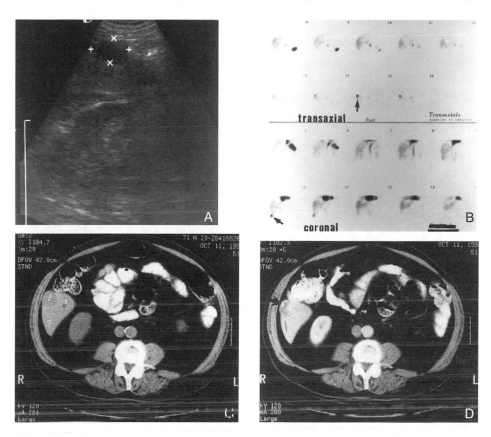

Figure 7. Liver hemangioma. **A,** Ultrasound shows a 3-cm hypoechoic lesion with internal echoes, consistent with hemangioma but a nonspecific finding. **B,** A [99]mTc-RBC study obtained at 2 hours with SPECT shows an intense focus in the inferior right lobe of the liver on transaxial and coronal images *(arrows)*. **C,** CT scan without contrast shows a lesion in this same area *(box 1)*. **D,** CT with contrast shows centripetal, nodular filling of this lesion *(arrow)*, confirming the diagnosis of hemangioma made on the [99]mTc- RBC study.

though some clinicians treat all B12-deficient patients without searching for a cause, the etiology can be important in many patients because of associated or unsuspected problems that should be recognized.

It is not necessary, nor in fact desirable, for the patient with severe vitamin B12 deficiency to abstain from vitamin B12 therapy prior to the Schilling's test. In stage 1 and all subsequent stages, non-radiolabeled vitamin B12, 1 mg intramuscularly, is given to bind B12 receptors 2 hours after the patient takes a pill containing radioactive-cobalt–labeled vitamin B12. It is extremely important that the patient not eat for 3 hours before and after taking the pill (to prevent the radiolabeled B12 from being bound by food) and that a 24–48-hour urine be accurately collected. Urinary creatinine and volume should be determined. Less than normal 24-hour urinary creatinine levels suggest inadequate collection that would artifactually decrease the amount of vitamin B12 excreted in the urine. The collected urine is analyzed for radioactive cobalt. Normally, >10% of the radioactive oral dose is excreted by 24 hours. If the excretion of vitamin B12 at 24 hours is normal, then this implies normal GI absorption.

If the results of stage 1 are abnormal, then the patient undergoes stage 2, which is a repeat of stage 1 except that oral intrinsic factor is given together with the radioactive B12 pill. Stage 3 has several variations that depend on the clinical suspicion of the etiology of B12 malabsorption (see Figure 8). A normal stage-2 excretion of vitamin B12 after an abnormal stage 1 excretion implies a diagnosis of pernicious anemia.

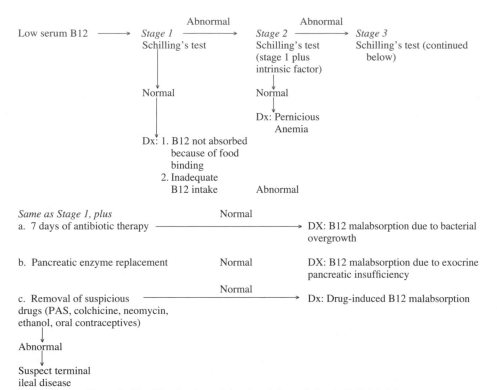

Figure 8. Algorithm for determining the etiology of vitamin B12 deficiency.

19. How can nuclear medicine procedures assist in detecting ectopic gastric tissue?

As a source of pediatric GI bleeding, **Meckel's diverticulum** almost always contains gastric tissue. Because ^{99m}Tc-pertechnetate is concentrated and extracted by gastric tissue, this agent is an ideal one to localize these sources of GI bleeding, which can be very difficult to detect with traditional contrast studies.

The study is performed by injecting pertechnetate intravenously and imaging the abdomen for 45 minutes. Typically, ectopic gastric mucosa appears at the same time as stomach tissue and does not move during imaging. The test's sensitivity is 85% for detecting bleeding Meckel's diverticula. Manipulations to increase the sensitivity of the study include pretreatment with cimetidine (to block pertechnetate excretion into the bowel lumen) and/or glucagon (to inhibit bowel motility so that ^{99m}Tc-pertechnetate is not washed away). A similar procedure can be performed to identify a **retained gastric antrum** after surgery for peptic ulcer disease and has a sensitivity of 73% and specificity of 100%.

20. Can accessory splenic tissue or splenosis be detected via nuclear medicine procedures?

After splenectomy as treatment of idiopathic thrombocytopenia, treatment failure is associated with unremoved accessory spleen. Unrecognized splenosis may also be a cause of unexplained abdominal pain. The most sensitive imaging procedure for localization of small foci of splenic tissue is the **heat-damaged 99mTc-red blood cell (RBC) scan,** because damaged RBCs localize in splenic tissue intensely and specifically. This is the procedure of choice, especially if SPECT is used. However, the RBC-damaging process requires exquisite laboratory technique and may not be readily available in many centers. It is therefore reasonable to perform a liver/spleen scan as an initial study and, if it is positive for splenic tissue, institute appropriate therapy (see Figure 9). If it is negative, a heat-damaged RBC study should be performed.

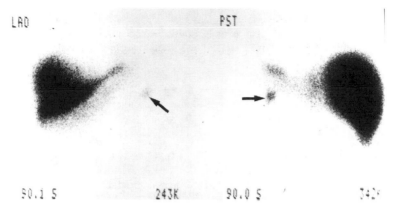

LAO   PST

Figure 9. Accessory spleen in a patient after splenectomy for idiopathic thrombocytopenic purpura. The very high contrast achieved with ^{99}mTc-sulfur colloid can detect a small remnant *(arrow)* and direct surgical exploration. Left anterior oblique (LAO) and posterior (PST) images of the abdomen are shown. If ^{99}mTc-sulfur colloid studies are negative, even higher contrast, specificity, and target-to-background ratios can be obtained by using scanning with heat-damaged RBCs, which preferentially accumulate in splenic tissue and demonstrate an almost identical scintigraphic pattern as ^{99}mTc-sulfur colloid.

21. What nuclear medicine studies help in the management of inflammatory bowel disease and abdominal abscesses?

Gallium-67, ^{99}mTc-HMPAO–labeled white blood cells (WBCs) and indium-111-labeled WBCs have all been used to image abdominal infections.

Gallium-67 is normally excreted into the bowel, and a small amount of ^{99}mTc-HMPAO dissociates from the WBCs and is excreted into the bowel; therefore, these agents are less useful for imaging **abdominal inflammation**. With gallium-67, it may be necessary to image for up to 1 week to allow for bowel activity to move so that suspicious abdominal foci can be adequately characterized. This disadvantage of gallium-67 is offset slightly by its low cost, despite its higher dosimetry (equal to the radiation of 2–4 abdominal CT scans). ^{99}mTc- HMPAO and ^{111}In-labeled WBC studies are expensive and require special labeling expertise.

^{111}In-labeled WBCs, which normally accumulate only in the liver, spleen, and bone marrow, are the agent of choice in localizing **abdominal infection** in cases in which CT, MRI, and ultrasound are nondiagnostic. The normal WBC uptake in the liver and spleen is a minor drawback and can be overcome by dual-isotope imaging with ^{99}mTc-colloid (liver/spleen scanning), because intra/perisplenic or liver abscess will be cold on liver/spleen scanning and hot on the ^{111}In-WBC study. The necessity for delayed 24-hour imaging to maximize sensitivity is also a drawback.

One-hour postinjection ^{99}mTc-HMPAO WBC imaging also correlates well with the degree of inflammation and localization of **inflammatory bowel disease** seen on other imaging modalities, and thus it can be used for noninvasive follow-up in these patients. This agent is preferable to ^{111}IN-WBC studies because of higher sensitivity and lower dosimetry.

22. Which nuclear medicine procedures are useful in localizing lower GI bleeding?

The difficulty of localizing acute lower GI bleeding is well recognized. The precise nature of the bleeding lesion is frequently immaterial to patient management, because the final common therapeutic pathway often involves partial bowel resection anyway. Even acute and rapid bleeding is intermittent and so frequently is not detected on angiography, or the culprit lesion is obscured by luminal blood during endoscopy. Small bowel bleeding distal to areas reachable by upper endoscopy is notoriously difficult to localize.

Two nuclear procedures have been used to localize GI bleeding sources: short-term imaging after ^{99}mTc-colloid injection, and extended imaging after ^{99}mTc-tagged RBC injection. Despite the theoretical advantage of ^{99}mTc-colloid's being able to detect smaller bleeds, this technique shares angiography's limitation of a short intravascular residence time (few minutes) of the contrast material. ^{99m}Tc-RBC imaging has assumed dominance because the very long intravascular residence time (limited by radioactive decay) allows detection of intraluminal radioactive blood accumulation if extended imaging is employed.

The study is begun by performing an in vitro tag of RBCs with Tc-99m. In vitro tagging is an important step because poor tagging in vivo will cause urinary and gastric excretion artifact. The radiolabeled RBCs are injected, and multiple sequential computer images are obtained for 90 minutes or longer. Computer acquisition is important because sensitivity for localization is higher when the study is displayed in a cine-loop.

23. Are nuclear medicine procedures clinically useful in localizing GI bleeding, or are simpler techniques adequate?

^{99m}Tc-RBC studies are more sensitive, in general, than angiography in detecting intermittent bleeding (see Figure 10). Early claims that the nuclear medicine GI bleeding study should always

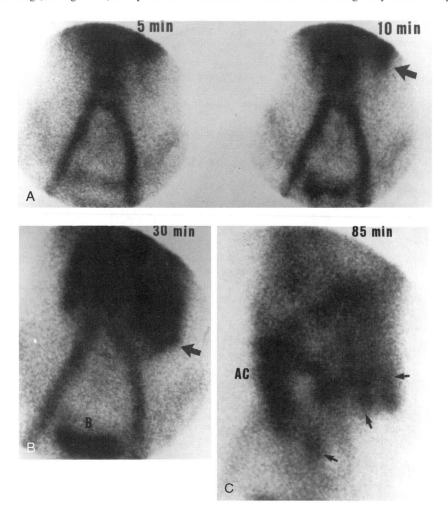

Figure 10. GI bleeding from the small bowel. After negative upper endoscopy and continued bleeding, a ^{99m}Tc-labeled RBC scan shows a focus of bleeding near the spleen *(large arrows)*. Continued imaging at 85 minutes demonstrates serpiginous transit through the small bowel *(small arrows)* toward the RLQ, confirming a proximal, small bowel origin. At surgery, a bleeding distal duodenal ulcer was found. *(B, bladder; AC, ascending colon.)*

be used as a screening study prior to angiography may not be defensible. However, with rigorous technique and attention to rigid diagnostic criteria for bleeding localization, the bleeding study is helpful in many difficult cases. Knowledge of the advantages and disadvantages of each technique allows one to select the most appropriate study as the clinical situation dictates.

24. Is there a nuclear medicine technique that is helpful in placement of arterial perfusion catheters?

Placement of hepatic arterial perfusion catheters is hampered by the existence of occasional unrecognized systemic shunting, catheter dislodgement, and unintended perfusion of an area not suitable for highly toxic chemotherapeutic drugs. Arterial catheter injection of ^{99}mTc-macroaggregated albumin (MAA) will result in microembolization at the arteriolar level and provide an imaging map of the true area of perfusion of the catheter, especially if SPECT is used. This imaging cannot be done reliably with radiographic contrast because of its rapid dilution at the arteriolar level.

25. How can nuclear medicine assess peritoneovenous shunt patency?

Increasing abdominal girth in the presence of a peritineovenous (LeVeen or Denver) shunt can be a diagnostic challenge because shunt obstruction, increased ascites production, and loculation can all be etiologies. Radiographic studies are not possible if the shunt is radiopaque, and in any event, such studies would require shunt cannulation. Because a one-way valve is located at the abdominal origin of the shunt, it is therefore difficult to evaluate the shunt in a retrograde manner. Patency can be readily evaluated by injecting ^{99}mTc-MAA intraperitoneally and imaging the chest for one-half hour. The shunt tube may not be visualized, but trapping of the ^{99}mTc-MAA in lung arterioles is defacto evidence of shunt patency.

Comparison of Methods for Localizing GI Bleeding

STUDY	ADVANTAGES	DISADVANTAGES
^{99}mTc-sulfur or albumin colloid	Can be rapidly performed upon request If negative, patient is not actively bleeding Can detect very small bleeds Relatively noninvasive	Blind areas around liver and spleen May not detect site of intermittent bleeding unless multiple sequential injections are used
^{99}mTc-tagged RBCs	Most sensitive for intermittent bleeding Can scan and rescan for up to 24 hours Relatively noninvasive	Requires lengthy (20–45 min) tagging process Rescanning may not accurately localize bleed because luminal blood may move rapidly Blind areas around liver and spleen
Angiography	May be therapeutic (vasopressin, Gelfoam)	Insensitive unless there is brisk bleeding at time of contrast injection Invasive

26. Can abdominal malignancies be evaluated with nuclear medicine studies?

Traditionally, **gallium-67**, a nonspecific tumor and infection marker, has been used to evaluate suspicious malignancy. It is not useful in staging of tumors, but rather its usefulness is in evaluating for recurrence in hepatomas and Hodgkin's and non-Hodgkin's lymphomas, where anatomic studies have difficulty separating necrosis and scar from recurrent tumor. Its utility is hampered by variable tumor avidity and by interfering GI activity caused by its excretion into the large bowel. The problem of separating GI activity from target lesion activity can be partially overcome by SPECT imaging and serial imaging for up to 1 week, to allow for elimination of gallium-67 excreted into the bowel.

Recent FDA approval of ^{111}In-pentreotide and ^{131}I- MIBG for imaging of neural crest tumors has opened up new possibilities in evaluating these difficult-to-image tumors. **^{131}I-MIBG,** a dopamine analog, is particularly useful in complementing CT and MRI in staging and detecting carcinoid tumors, neuroblastoma, paragangliomas, and pheochromocytomas. [111]**In-octreotide,** a somatostatin analog, is also highly sensitive and specific for a variety of neural chest tumors that express somatostatin receptors. It will frequently detect occult lesions not seen by other modalities and can lend specificity to questionable GI lesions found on MRI and CT, including gastrinoma, glucagonoma, paraganglioma, pheochromocytoma, carcinoid, and Hodgkin's and non-Hodgkin's lymphoma.

The radiolabeled antibody [111]**In-satumomab** has also been approved recently by the FDA and is extremely useful in evaluating colon cancer in patients with an elevated carcinoembryonic antigen level and an otherwise negative diagnostic evaluation, patients with known recurrent disease presumed isolated and amenable to surgical resection, and patients in whom the standard diagnostic workup provides equivocal information. ^{111}In-satumomab frequently detects occult disease and significantly affects therapy in almost half of patients in these important clinical groups.

BIBLIOGRAPHY

1. Corman M, Galandiak S, Block G, et al: Immunoscintigraphy with ^{111}In-satumomab pentetide in patients with colorectal adenocarcinoma: Performance and impact on clinical management. Dis Colon Rectum 37:129–137, 1994.
2. Davis L, McCarroll K: Correlative imaging of the liver and hepatobiliary system. Semin Nucl Med 26:208–216, 1994.
3. Mettler F, Guiberteau M: Essentials of Nuclear Medicine Imaging, 3rd ed. Philadelphia, W.B. Saunders, 1991, pp 177–208.
4. Pawels S, Leners N, Fiasse R, Jamar F: Localization of gastroenteropancreatic neuroendocrine tumors with [111]indium-pentetreotide scintigraphy. Semin Oncol 12(suppl 13):15–20, 1994.
5. Shapiro M: The role of the radiologist in the management of gastrointestinal bleeding. Gastroenterol Clin North Am 23:123–181, 1994.
6. Sodee D, Velchik M, Noto R, et al: Gastrointestinal system. In Early P, Sodee D (eds): Principles and Practice of Nuclear Medicine. St. Louis, C.V. Mosby, 1995, pp 476–579.
7. Sostre S, Kalloo A, Spiegler E, et al: A noninvasive test of sphincter of Oddi dysfunction in postcholecystectomy patients: The scintigraphic score. J Nucl Med 33:1216–1222, 1992.
8. Weissmann H, Gliedman M, Wilk P, et al: Evaluation of the postoperative patient with [99]mTc-IDA cholescintigraphy. Semin Nucl Med 12:27–52, 1982.
9. Yap L, Wycherley, Morphett A, Toouli J: Acalculous biliary pain: Cholecystectomy alleviates symptoms in patients with abnormal cholescintigraphy. Gastroenterology 101:786–793, 1991.
10. Arndt J, Van der Sluys, Veer A, Blok D, et al: Prospective comparative study of technetuim-99m-WBCs and indium-111-granulocytes for the examination of patients with inflammatory bowel disease. J Nucl Med 34:1052–1057, 1993.

76. ENDOSCOPIC ULTRASOUND

Peter R. McNally, D.O.

1. When was intraluminal GI ultrasound first performed?

The use of ultrasound to image the GI tract began in 1956, when Wild and Reid performed the first rectal ultrasound. For the last decade, there has been a revitalized interest in the use of GI ultrasound. Intraluminal ultrasound permits precise definition of the gut wall layers and examination of adjacent structures of the chest and abdomen. The proximity of the ultrasound transducer and the high scanning frequencies used in ultrasound provide incomparable morphologic detail of the gut wall and the extraintestinal anatomy.

2. How do ultrasound waves visualize the GI tract?

Ultrasound pulses represent longitudinal waves that are propagated through soft tissues or fluid by motion of molecules within the conducting media. The ultrasound wavelength is the distance between two waves of compression and rarefaction. Ultrasound is defined as frequency > 20,000 cycles/sec (20 Hz); most diagnostic ultrasound utilizes frequencies ranging from 2–20 million cycles/sec (2–20 MHz). The velocity of sound transmission through soft tissues is a constant 1540 m/sec and is independent of frequency. Transmission of ultrasound within a medium is dependent on the compressibility and density of the medium, two properties that tend to be inversely proportional. Because ultrasound power is diminished as it traverses tissue, the intensity of the returning echo, when related to the original echo, is expressed in negative terms.

3. How does the frequency of the ultrasound beam influence the depth of beam penetration and image resolution?

For maximal resolution of ultrasound, the transmitted waves should be parallel. If the target of interest is too close or too far from the transducer, divergence of the wavelength will cause distortion of the image. Hence, proper positioning of the ultrasound (US) transducer and use of the appropriate frequency are essential to provide maximum resolution.

US Frequencies	Penetration	Axial Resolution
5 MHz	8 cm	0.8 mm
10 MHz	4 cm	0.4 mm
20 MHz	2 cm	0.2 mm

4. What are the ultrasonographic properties of the common structures of the body?

Water/blood	Echo poor (black)
Collagen	Echo rich (white)
Air	Reflection (reverberation echoes)
Bone	Reflection (reverberation echoes)
Muscle	Echo poor (black)

5. Describe the key differences in the intraluminal GI ultrasound equipment currently available.

The number and variety of instruments used for intraluminal GI ultrasound have exploded in the last decade. Instruments were initially rigid and nonoptical, with fixed resolution and fixed depth of tissue penetration. Now, ultrasound scanning can be performed with optical, flexible endoscopes.

The two currently available **echoendoscopes** are manufactured by Olympus and Pentax. The Olympus upper echoendoscope offers 360° radial sector scanning. The Pentax echoendoscope offers in-line longitudinal sector scanning, which permits accurate direction of devices used to obtain submucosal biopsy or aspiration cytology.

The **miniaturized ultrasound probes** (various models by Olympus, Diasonics, and Microvasive) offer several advantages over the echoendoscopes: their small diameter enables passage though a forward-viewing endoscope; the cost is $500 for a disposable probe versus $40,000–50,000 for the reusable echoendoscopes; near-obstructing lesions may be traversed with a probe, whereas the echoendoscope cannot; they may be passed over a wire; and they may be passed without endoscopic assistance. Their disadvantages include a poorer quality of image and a lack of flexibility and maneuverability within the endoscope.

NORMAL ANATOMY

6. What determines the thickness of the echosonographic layer visualized? What is the normal endosonographic anatomy of the intestinal wall?

The thickness of the intraluminal ultrasound image of the intestinal wall does not equal the total thickness of a histologic section. Kimmey et al. have hypothesized that the overall appearance of the ultrasound image is determined by a combination of echoes from two sources: those created at interfaces between tissue layers with different acoustic impedances and those created within the internal structures of the tissue layer. Using 5-12 MHz scanning frequencies, the intestinal wall has five sonographic layers (see Figure 1).

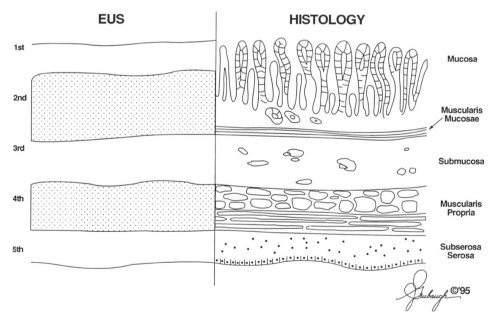

Figure 1. Correlation of endoscopic ultrasound image to the histologic composition of the bowel wall.

7. What are the imaging characteristics of a normal lymph node seen on endoscopic ultrasound (EUS)?

The high resolution of EUS imaging allows even normal lymph nodes to be visualized. A normal lymph node is characterized by the presence of internal echoes, its bean shape, and size < 1 cm. Malignant lymph nodes tend to be > 1 cm, loose their normal bean shape (becoming plump or spherical), and are hypoechoic or assume the same internal echo characteristics as the primary tumor.

8. How are blood vessels distinguished from lymph nodes on EUS?
Blood vessels generally appear as anechoic, curvilinear structures that often branch. Branching and the presence of posterior wall enhancement (hyperechoic) are helpful in distinguishing paraluminal vessels from hypoechoic lymph nodes.

9. Describe the normal EUS anatomy of the retroperitoneum. What are its major landmarks?
The pancreas and retroperitoneum are the most challenging and difficult areas to examine with intraluminal ultrasound. Familiarity with the gross and ultrasound anatomy is essential.

The examination begins with the echoendoscope at the level of the duodenal ampulla. Antimotility agents, such as glucagon, are frequently necessary. The ultrasound examination is usually conducted with a 7.5-MHz scanning frequency. The normal paraduodenal anatomy is shown in Figure 2. The normal pancreas has a homogeneous echo pattern, usually slightly more hyperechoic than the liver. There is considerable interobserver variation in measurement of the head of the pancreas, probably due to variations in the angle of view. The remainder of the pancreas is examined from a paragastric position. In the stomach, the water-filled lumen method is used.

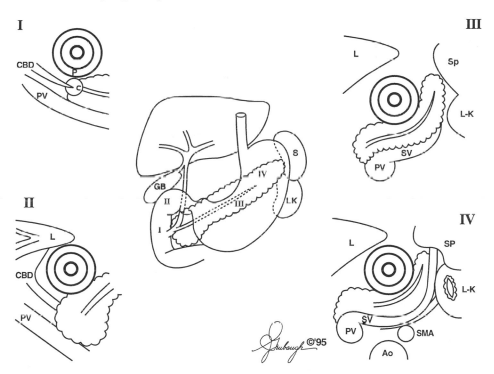

Figure 2. Four commonly used positions to examine the pancreas by EUS. **I**—transverse section at the level of the ampulla; **II**—sagittal section near the duodenal bulb; **III**—transverse section of the pancreatic body through the posterior wall of the stomach; **IV**—transverse section of the body and tail of the pancreas from the proximal stomach. (A = ampulla; CBD = common bile duct; L-K = left kidney; PV = portal vein; SV = splenic vein; L = liver; Sp = spleen; SA = superior mesenteric artery; and Ao = aorta.)

10. What are the indications for EUS examination?
Staging of GI tumors

Esophageal carcinoma	Ampullary tumors
Gastric carcinoma	Biliary tract carcinoma
Gastric lymphoma (non-	
Hodgkin's lymphoma)	Colorectal carcinoma

Pancreatic lymphoma   Colorectal adenoma
Pancreatic endocrine tumors   Submucosal tumors
Evaluation of nonneoplastic disease
  Reflux esophagitis   Portal hypertension
  Achalasia   Chronic pancreatitis
  Gastric ulcer   Common bile duct stones
  Giant gastric folds   Inflammatory bowel disease

11. How is EUS used in the clinical evaluation of esophageal cancer?
Currently, EUS has no role in the *diagnosis* of esophageal cancer. Findings from EUS provide
morphologic staging but do not supplant the need for histologic diagnosis of malignancy. EUS
has not been shown to be helpful in differentiating malignant from inflammatory strictures. It is
not sufficiently sensitive to use as a screening test for cancer (i.e., in Barrett's esophagus with dysplasia). Combined EUS and computed tomographic (CT) scanning provide the most accurate
method of TNM staging for esophageal cancer. CT should be performed first to exclude distant
metastasis (M stage), followed by EUS for precise T and N staging.

TNM Staging for Esophageal Carcinoma

Primary tumor (T)
Tx	Primary tumor cannot be assessed
T0	No evidence of primary tumor
Tis	Carcinoma in situ
T1	Tumor invades lamina propria or submucosa
T2	Tumor invades muscularis propria
T3	Tumor invades the adventitia
T4	Tumor invades adjacent structures

Regional lymph nodes (N)
Nx	Regional lymph nodes cannot be assessed
N0	No regional lymph node metastasis
N1	Regional lymph node metastasis

Distant metastasis (M)
Mx	Presence of distant metastasis
M0	No distant metastasis
M1	Distant metastasis

**12. In what ways can EUS findings impact on clinical management of patients with
esophageal carcinoma?**
- Direct stage-dependent treatment decisions
- Perform preoperative assessment of tumor resectability
- Permits a more accurate pretreatment prognosis

13. Compare the staging accuracies of EUS and CT for esophageal malignancy.

Comparison of EUS and CT in the Preoperative Staging of Esophageal Cancer

STAGE	NO.	ACCURACY	
		EUS	CT
T1	12	92%	—
T2	15	73%	11%
T3	42	93%	69%
T4	46	91%	59%
N0	42	64%	67%
N1	80	84%	36%

Data from Tio TL, et al: Gastroenterology 96:1478–1486, 1989; Ziegler K, et al: Gastroenterology 94:A267,
1988.

14. What are the problematic areas for EUS in the staging of esophageal cancer?

- At presentation, 25–50% of esophageal cancers are so advanced that passage of the echoendoscope beyond the cancer is prohibited. Because up to 85% of obstructing lesions are already stage T3 or T4, aggressive attempts to dilatate the tumor and force the passage of the echoendoscope are foolhardy, as esophageal perforation may occur. The ultrasound miniprobes may prove helpful in this situation.
- Esophageal dilatation to permit endosonography is not recommended.
- Accurate T1 staging is difficult, and overstaging of this T stage is common.
- On lymph node (L) staging, the finding of spherical, > 1-cm, hypoechoic nodes with loss of tapered or bean shape suggests malignancy. It may be impossible to distinguish inflammatory lymphadenitis from malignancy. Node size > 1 cm is probably the best discriminator of malignancy.
- Restaging after chemotherapy and/or radiation is problematic because it is frequently difficult to differentiate residual malignancy from fibrosis. Data are conflicting on the value of EUS to predict recurrence.

15. Does EUS have a role in the evaluation of gastric cancer?

EUS has no role in the initial diagnosis of gastric cancer and should not be used as a screening tool in patients at risk for this disease. However, in patients where the suspicion of **linitis plastica** is not confirmed by biopsy, identification of the typical EUS pattern of this cancer contributes significantly to the correct diagnosis (see Figure 3). Radial sector scanning in the region of the pylorus and proximal fundus can be technically difficult. If stage-dependent treatment protocols are employed, then EUS is indicated when CT shows no metastasis (M0). EUS appears to be reliable in predicting **R0 resectability** (stages T1–T3 versus T4).

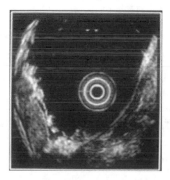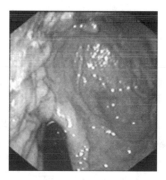

Figure 3. Endoscopic view of a gastric adenocarcinoma (*left*) compared with EUS findings (*right*) of a thickened hypoechoic tumor involving the first three echo layers, from 7–9 o'clock. The echoendoscope is located in the center of the water-filled stomach.]

16. What are the problematic areas for EUS staging of gastric malignancy?

- Overstaging of 20–30%, mainly in T2 lesions, is partly due to the peculiar histopathologic definition of stage T2 (infiltration into the submucosa) versus T3 (invasion of the serosa), a differentiation that cannot be made by EUS. Also, portions of the stomach are not covered by serosa.
- Differentiation of gastric cancer confined to the mucosa (and therefore amenable to endoscopic treatment) from cancer involving the submucosa (with an attendant increase in the incidence of lymph node metastasis) is relatively inaccurate—60–70%. Small lesions that are flat, slightly depressed, or elevated at endoscopy and cancerous on biopsy can be assumed to be confined to the mucosa if EUS does not show any abnormality of the gastric wall in relation to the tumor. Overstaging occurs predominantly with ulcerating, early carcinomas, because EUS cannot differentiate malignancy from perifocal fibrosis and inflammation.
- Differentiating benign inflammatory change in associated lymph nodes is problematic, similar to the difficulty encountered elsewhere in the GI tract.

17. What is the TNM staging classification for gastric malignancy?

TNM Staging for Primary Gastric Lymphoma

Primary tumor (T)		
	Tx	Primary tumor cannot be assessed
	T0	No evidence of primary tumor
	T1	Tumor confined to mucosa or submucosa
	T2	Tumor invades muscularis propria or subserosa
	T3	Tumor invades serosa without invasion into adjacent structures
	T4	Tumor invades adjacent structures
Regional lymph nodes		
	Nx	Regional lymph nodes cannot be assessed
	N0	No regional lymph node metastasis
	N1	Positive perigastric lymph nodes < 3 cm from the edge of tumor
	N2	Positive perigastric lymph nodes > 3 cm from the tumor edge or positive lymph nodes along the gastric, common hepatic, splenic, or celiac arteries
Distant metastasis		
	Mx	Presence of distant metastasis
	M0	No distant metastasis
	M1	Distant metastasis

Resectable stage (R0) = Stage T1–T3 or T4 chemotherapy.

18. Is EUS helpful in the evaluation of gastric lymphoma?

Yes. EUS is very accurate in determining the T stage for gastric lymphoma. However, the clinical relevance of this staging in managing these patient with surgical and/or chemotherapeutic options is uncertain. EUS trials to evaluate the depth of lymphoma tissue infiltration are needed and may determine if the echosonographic findings correlate with the risk for chemotherapy-induced perforation. EUS should also be include in surgical trials to determine its role in assessing resectability (R0). EUS staging is preferred over surgical staging in the marginal surgical candidate.

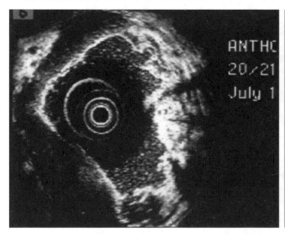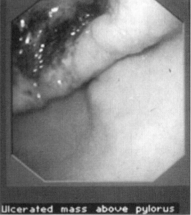

Figure 4. Endoscopic view of a gastric lymphoma (*left*) compared with EUS findings of a thickened hypoechoic tumor with foot-like (pseudopodia) extensions into the fourth echogenic layer at the 9 o'clock position. The echoendoscope is located in the center of the water-filled stomach.

19. How effective is EUS in evaluating pancreatic neoplasms?

EUS is very reliable in differentiating focal abnormalities from normal pancreatic tissue, but it is not reliable in differentiating between malignant and inflammatory tumor masses. EUS is complementary to ERCP when ultrasonography and CT findings are negative or inconclusive. Histologic proof is still mandatory, and the use of EUS-guided fine-needle aspiration awaits evaluation with suitable instruments and aspiration needles. EUS has no role in screening for pancreatic cancer.

The role of EUS to evaluate patients with vague abdominal pain (i.e., to detect pancreatobiliary abnormalities) has yet to be assessed by appropriately designed prospective studies. EUS may provide additional tumor-staging information for the patients with M0 staging by CT and ultrasound (see figure 5). In experienced hands, EUS is superior to angiography in the detection of portal vein involvement.

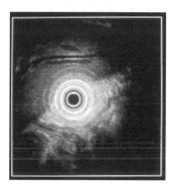

Figure 5. EUS findings of a mass in the pancreas at 6 o'clock and dilatated intrahepatic ducts at 10–12 o'clock.

20. Compare the accuracy of EUS and CT in staging pancreatic malignancy.
In a study by Rosch et al. of pancreatic cancer staging, 132 patients with suspected pancreatic tumor were evaluated by EUS, CT, ultrasound, and endoscopic retrograde cholangiography (ERCP). The final diagnosis was confirmed at surgery in 47 cases, puncture in 36, and autopsy in 3.

Pancreatic Cancer Staging

	EUS	US	CT	ERCP
Sensitivity				
All (*n* = 102)	99	66	77	90
Tumors < 3	100	50	55	90
Specificity	100	40	53	73
Positive-predictive value	100	79	85	92
Negative-predictive value	97	36	50	82

21. What are the problematic areas of EUS evaluation of pancreatic cancer?
- EUS depth of penetration may be insufficient to visualize the entire margin of large tumors.
- EUS may not reveal infiltration of arteries.
- Tumors that infiltrate the uncinate process are difficult to define by EUS.
- EUS may not reveal infiltration in the region of the confluence when the splenic vein is not involved.

22. Neuroendocrine tumors of the pancreas and peripancreas are often difficult to localize by conventional CT, ultrasound, and angiography. Does EUS examination offer any value in localizing these tumors?
Yes. EUS is the most accurate imaging method available for the localization of pancreatic endocrine tumors. When CT and ultrasound findings are negative, EUS remains 80% accurate.

When neuroendocrine tumors are extrapancreatic, the accuracy of EUS drops substantially. One needs a considerable amount of experience with EUS of the pancreas to achieve this accuracy rate.

Localization of Pancreatic Endocrine Tumors by EUS

* 37 patients from 8 centers; average age, 48 yrs
* Negative findings on CT/US; angiography positive in 27%
* 39 tumors found at surgery
* 32/39 (82%) found by EUS (mean size, 1.4 cm; range, 0.5–2.5 cm)
* 20 head of pancreas
* 9 body of pancreas
* 10 tail of pancreas

Data from Rosch T, et al: N Engl J Med 326:1721–1726, 1992.

23. Can EUS assist in the evaluation of ampullary tumors?

EUS does not contribute to the differential diagnosis of ampullary adenoma versus confined ampullary carcinoma. EUS's role in evaluating ampullary stenosis is unknown. EUS is very accurate in the staging of ampullary tumors, especially in determining intrapancreatic spread. Until the role of local tumor resection for ampullary adenomas and T1 carcinoma of the ampulla is defined and accepted as a treatment option versus Whipple's procedure for more advanced cancers (T2–T4), the clinical utility of EUS remains uncertain.

24. Is EUS helpful in evaluating biliary malignancies?

The role of EUS to define cholesterol polyps or small neoplasms of the gallbladder remains to be determined. EUS has been shown to be more accurate in the staging of gallbladder tumors than CT or ultrasound, but whether this staging will have any clinical importance has yet to be determined.

The use of EUS evaluation of indeterminate bile duct strictures has not yet been determined. EUS's value in staging proximal bile duct tumors (Klatskin tumors) is unclear. The role of the miniprobe to stage bile duct tumors is under evaluation.

25. Describe the use of EUS in the evaluation of colorectal malignancy.

EUS is very accurate in determining the T and N stage and superior to CT scanning. The combination of EUS and CT provides the most practical and accurate approach to staging rectal cancers, and the results of both tests should be considered in the planning of treatment. The choice of surgical option is largely determined by the tumor stage, with T1 appropriate for local resection and T2–T4 needing radical extirpation with or without adjuvant radiation/chemotherapy.

26. Can submucosal tumors be evaluated by EUS?

Endoscopic ultrasound is 95% accurate in distinguishing true submucosal tumors from extraluminal compression by normal or pathologic structures. Once the submucosal nature of the tumor is established, then treatment is guided by signs and symptoms as well as size of the lesion, rather than the EUS appearance. Submucosal lesions that cause obstruction and/or bleeding require treatment irrespective of the EUS findings. EUS may provide clues to the pathologic nature of the submucosal tumors but does not differentiate conclusively between benign and malignant nature, especially in myogenic tumors. Some have recommended removal of myogenic wall tumors > 3 cm, permitting prospective follow-up of myogenic tumors < 3 cm. This recommendation awaits confirmation in further studies.

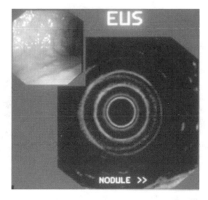

Figure 6. EUS finding of a mucosal hypoechoic carcinoid tumor and endoscopic findings.

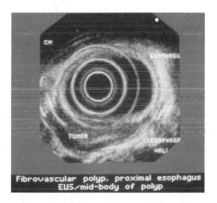

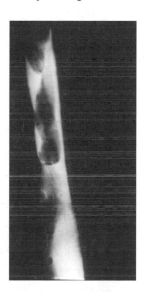

Figure 7. Esophageal fibrovascular polyp seen on barium swallow radiograph (*left*) and EUS findings (*right*).

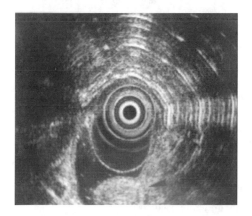

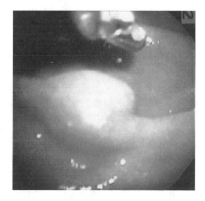

Figure 8. Endoscopic finding of a soft submucosal tumor (*left*) and EUS findings of a hyperechoic lipoma (*right*).

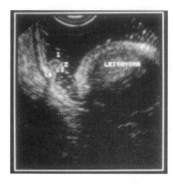 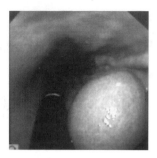

Figure 9. Endoscopic view of a submucosal tumor (*left*), confirmed to be a leiomyoma, arising from the fourth hypoechic layer (*right*).

EUS Characteristics of Submucosal Tumors

Aberrant pancreas	Submucosal; similar in echogenicity to the pancreas; hypoechoic ductular structure may be present
Bronchogenic carcinoma	Hypoechoic; disrupts submucosa and muscularis propria; usually irregular outer margin
Breast cancer	Metastatic; same as bronchogenic cancer
Carcinoid	Mucosal; hypoechoic (see figure 6)
Fibrovascular polyp	Submucosal; mixed echogenicity (see figure 7)
Gastric cyst	Anechoic; smooth border; submucosal
Granular cell tumors	Hypoechoic; submucosal; smooth margin
Lipoma	Hyperechoic; submucosal (see figure 8)
Leiomyoma	Hypoechoic; contiguous with muscularis propria; smooth outer margin (see figure 9)
Leiomyosarcoma	Hypoechoic; contiguous with muscularis propria; large lesions may have irregular outer margin; adenopathy; small lesions identical to leiomyoma
Lymphoma	Hypoechoic; may disrupt submucosa; muscularis propria and adenopathy
Pancreatic pseudocyst	Anechoic; smooth margin; compress N1 wall
Varices	Anechoic; submucosal serpentine
Vessels	Anechoic; curvilinear branching; often with through-penetration enhancement of the posterior wall

27. Is EUS useful in the evaluation of nonneoplastic disease?

- Preliminary studies of EUS in the evaluation of reflux esophagitis, achalasia, and gastric ulcer have not shown EUS to be clinically important.
- EUS evaluation of enlarged gastric folds can determine the safety of large-particle biopsy devices and exclude the presence of large intramural vascular structures. EUS findings contribute to the characterization of the etiology of the process. Thickening of the first two layers is characteristic of inflammation, Menetrier's disease, and lymphoma. Here, large particle biopsies should be safe and diagnostic. Thickening of all layers suggests lymphoma or linitis plastica. If biopsy findings are still equivocal, then exploratory laparotomy is indicated.

28. How is EUS used in the evaluation of patients with portal hypertension?

EUS can demonstrate fundal varices when endoscopic results are equivocal and define the vascular patency of the splenic vein. Some have suggested that intramural vessel enlargement can be detected in patients with portal hypertensive gastropathy. Whether EUS detection of extra-, intra-, or paramural varices after endoscopic variceal banding of injection therapy will be of value in guiding therapy or predicting relapse awaits appropriate study and evaluation.

29. Can EUS be helpful in the evaluation of chronic pancreatitis?

EUS is very accurate in detecting moderate to advanced degrees of **chronic pancreatitis.** Studies are underway to determine if it is sensitive in the diagnosis of earlier stages of the disease.

Comparative studies evaluating the accuracy of ERCP and EUS have not been conducted for the evaluation of **pancreatobiliary tract disease.** The resolution of the ductular systems offered by ERCP is generally considered to be superior, but EUS offers the advantage of no associated post-ERCP pancreatitis and more complete examination of the parenchyma and peri-hepatic/pancreatic anatomy.

EUS's role in the endoscopic management of **pancreatic pseudocyst** is still in evolution. EUS appears to be helpful in determining the site of transmural cyst puncture and provides additional safety of excluding risk of intervening vascular structures.

30. Is there any use for EUS in evaluating patients with common bile duct stones?

EUS has excellent sensitivity and specificity as shown in retrospective series. No clinical role is currently defined for EUS with respect to cholelithiasis. Studies need to be conducted to determine if EUS has a role in patients with unsuccessful endoscopic retrograde cholangiography, prior to percutaneous transhepatic cholangiography. Perhaps, EUS will be a helpful adjunctive test in the evaluation of patients with suspected cholelithiasis but who are too obese to permit diagnostic extracorporeal ultrasound.

BIBLIOGRAPHY

1. Armengol Miro JR, Benjamin S, Binmoeller K, et al: Clinical applications of endoscopic ultrasound in gastroenterology—State of the art 1993 (consensus conference). Endoscopy 25:358–366, 1993.
2. Botet JF, Lightdale CJ, Zauber AG, et al: Preoperative staging of esophageal cancer: Comparison of endoscopic US and dynamic CT. Radiology 181:419–425, 1991.
3. Boyce GA, Sivak MV, Lavery IC, et al: Endoscopic ultrasound in pre-operative staging of rectal carcinoma. Gastrointest Endosc 38:468–471, 1992.
4. Boyce GA, Sivak MV, Rosch T, et al: Evaluation of submucosal upper gastrointestinal tract lesions by endoscopic ultrasound. Gastrointest Endosc 37:449–454, 1991.
5. Caletti GC, Brocchi E, Barbara L: Role of endoscopic ultrasonography in the treatment of esophageal varices. Endoscopy 23:284–285, 1991.
6. Caletti GC, Ferrari A, Brocchi E, Barbara L: Accuracy of endoscopic ultrasonography in the diagnosis and staging of gastric cancer and lymphoma. Surgery 113:14–27, 1993.
7. Caletti GC, Zani L, Bolondi L, et al: Endoscopic ultrasonography in the diagnosis of gastric submucosal tumor. Gastrointest Endosc 35:413–418, 1989.
8. Deviere J, Dunham F, Rickaert F, et al: Endoscopic ultrasonography in achalasia. Gastroenterology 96:1210–1213, 1989.
9. Dittler HJ, Siewert JR: Role of endoscopic ultrasonography in esophageal carcinoma. Endoscopy 25:156–161, 1993.
10. Dittler HJ, Siewert JR: Role of endoscopic ultrasonography in gastric carcinoma. Endoscopy 25:162–166, 1993.
11. Frucht H, Norton JA, London JF, et al: Detection of duodenal gastrinomas by operative endoscopic transillumination. Gastroenterology 99:162–1627, 1990.
12. Lightdale C: Endoscopic ultrasonograpy. Gastrointest Endosc Clin North Am 2:557–749, 1992.
13. Lightdale CJ, Botet JF, Kelsen DP, et al: Diagnosis of recurrent upper gastrointestinal cancer at the surgical anastomosis by endoscopic ultrasound. Gastrointest Endosc 35:407–412, 1989.
14. Palazzo L, Roseau G, Salmeron M: Endoscopic ultrasonography in the preoperative localization of pancreatic endocrine tumors. Endoscopy 24:350–353, 1992.
15. Rosch T, Lightdale CJ, Botet JF, et al: Endosonographic localization of pancreatic endocrine tumors. N Engl J Med 326:1721–1726, 1992.
16. Rosch T, Lorenz R, Braig C, et al: Endoscopic ultrasound in pancreatic tumor diagnosis. Gastrointest Endosc 37:347–352, 1991.
17. Sandy H, Cooperman A, Siegel JH: Endoscopic ultrasonography compared with computed tomography with ERCP in patients with obstructive jaundice or small peripancreatic mass. Gastrointest Endosc 38:27–34, 1992.
18. Tio TL, Cohen P, Coene PP, et al: Endosonography and computed tomography of esophageal carcinoma. Gastroenterology 96:1478–1486, 1989.
19. Wierseman MJ, Hawes RH, Tao LC, et al: Endoscopic ultrasonography as an adjunct to fine needle aspiration cytology of the upper and lower gastrointestinal tract. Gastrointest Endosc 38:35–39, 1992.
20. Yasuda K, Mukai H, Nakajima M, et al: Diagnosis and staging of pancreatic cancer by endoscopic ultrasonography. Endoscopy 1993;25.

77. ENDOSCOPIC RETROGRADE CHOLANGIOPANCREATOGRAPHY (ERCP)

Gregory Zuccaro, Jr., M.D.

1. What is the distinction between diagnostic and therapeutic ERCP?

Diagnostic endoscopic retrograde cholangiopancreatography (ERCP) involves the opacification of the biliary tree and pancreatic duct via the main duodenal papilla (or on occasion, via the minor papilla). Adjunctive maneuvers of diagnostic ERCP include endoscopic biopsy of an abnormal papilla and brush cytology or biopsy of ductal strictures. Skills necessary to perform diagnostic ERCP include those of all diagnostic endoscopy, i.e., knowledge of sedation and analgesia and the ability to maneuver the endoscope.

Therapeutic ERCP involves all of the requisite elements of the diagnostic procedure, as well as additional maneuvers necessary to provide definitive therapy and/or palliation. These maneuvers include (among others) endoscopic papillotomy, stone extraction, and placement of plastic or metal stents.

2. What training is required for each form of ERCP?

Recently, there has been considerable debate among GI endoscopists regarding the need for all endoscopists performing ERCP to possess therapeutic skills. The American Society for Gastrointestinal Endoscopy has assigned threshold numbers of procedures for assessing competence for standard and advanced endoscopic procedures, 75 for diagnostic ERCP and an additional 25 for therapeutic ERCP, implying that training in diagnostic ERCP alone is an acceptable goal. Many training programs do graduate trainees with only diagnostic ERCP skills, assuming these individuals gain experience and training in therapeutic skills via proctoring or other relationships developed in their professional practice. A strong case can be made that ERCP should only be performed by individuals able to provide therapeutic interventions. With continued improvements in noninvasive imaging such as CT scanning, the necessity of ERCP to diagnose benign or malignant pancreatic disorders has decreased. Indications for therapeutic retrograde cholangiography have increased, particularly as a complement to laparoscopic cholecystectomy. Diagnosis of choledocholithiasis by an endoscopist untrained in papillotomy and stone extraction necessitates another ERCP for therapy, exposing the patient to additional sedation risk, radiation, and cost. Injection of contrast material above a biliary stricture by an endoscopist unable to provide prompt drainage increases the risk of cholangitis.

3. Are there special considerations for sedation and analgesia during ERCP?

Yes. For most standard endoscopy, a single **GI assistant** is sufficient to monitor the patient and assist with minor ancillary tasks. For ERCP, the attention of the first assistant (at the head of the bed) is often completely occupied with the preparation and movement of catheters, guidewires, and other accessories necessary for procedure completion. Therefore, a second assistant is needed whose primary task is the monitoring of the patient.

Whereas a diagnostic upper endoscopy is typically brief, ERCP takes considerably longer. The length and complexity of the procedure often require administration of higher cumulative doses of **sedative/analgesics,** which may become problematic in the elderly patient with choledocholithiasis or biliary stricture or in the patient with chronic pancreatitis who is taking daily narcotics for pain relief. In most cases, endoscopic tasks can be accomplished safely with the standard sedative/analgesic agents prudently administered by the endoscopist. **Careful monitoring,** including the use of pulse oximetry in all cases and cardiac monitoring in patients with recent history of significant cardiac disease, is essential. Supplemental oxygen is not a must at the beginning of each case but should be present in cases where relative hypoxemia occurs. Reversal agents for narcotics and benzodiazepenes should be present, as should all equipment necessary to maintain a patent airway and provide basic life support. Emergency life support measures should be immediately available. For special cases, including extremes in age and patients with conditions such as severe cardiopulmonary disease, chronic narcotic use, morbid obesity, or inability to cooperate, consultation with an anesthesiologist may be advisable.

4. What are some common indications for retrograde cholangiography?

A common indication is the investigation of obstructive jaundice or abdominal pain in which a mechanical cause, such as stone, tumor, or biliary stricture, is suspected. In virtually all of these cases, identification of these abnormalities leads to a therapeutic intervention (stone extraction, stent placement, etc.).

The advent of laparoscopic cholecystectomy has led to increased use of retrograde cholangiography. During the cholecystectomy, a cholangiogram can usually be obtained via the cystic duct. However, techniques for laparoscopic-guided extraction of common bile duct stones or common duct exploration are still under development and not widely available. Therefore, the GI surgeon will often request retrograde cholangiography for stone extraction prior to laparoscopic cholecystectomy in patients in whom choledocholithiasis is strongly suspected or after laparoscopic cholecystectomy when the operative cholangiogram reveals unexpected choledocholithiasis. Complications of laparoscopic cholecystectomy appear higher than open cholecystectomy, particularly early in the individual surgeons' experience.

Endoscopic papillotomy with or without stent placement hastens closure of the postoperative cystic duct leak. Retrograde cholangiography can identify the rare bile duct transection. Postoperative strictures can be identified and dilated and/or stented. Other indications for retrograde cholangiography include investigation of patients with recurrent acute pancreatitis, identification of sclerosing cholangitis in patients with predisposing factors (such as inflammatory bowel disease or AIDS), obtaining bile for crystal or other analyses, and performance of ancillary tasks such as biliary manometry.

5. How successful is retrograde cholangiography? What techniques might increase this rate?

In experienced hands, the rate of successful retrograde cholangiography appears to be 85–95%.

In most cases, successful opacification and/or cannulation can be achieved using standard catheters, but other catheters and devices may be helpful in difficult cases. The standard catheters accept specially coated wires that may "slip" up the bile duct and facilitate cannulation. Injection of contrast over these wires is possible but often suboptimal. Catheters with individual channels for the wire and instillation of contrast are available and do work, but potential drawbacks include increased catheter diameter or stiffness and difficulty for the assistant working with channels of decreased diameter. One useful technique is to use the guidewire with a single-lumen catheter to achieve free cannulation, then advance the catheter freely up the biliary tree. The guidewire can then be removed and contrast injected. The assistant may use the attached syringe containing contrast to aspirate air from the catheter prior to contrast injection; this may decrease the likelihood of introducing air bubbles.

Some commercially available tapered catheters have decreased diameters and stiffness compared to standard catheters, and these often allow better bowing or lifting, facilitating a bile duct approach. Many of these catheters do not accept the standard 0.035-in guidewires. A potential drawback of these catheters in the past, therefore, was that if a free cannulation was achieved and endoscopic papillotomy found to be necessary, a catheter exchange to a wire-guided papillotome had to be done over a 0.018-in wire, which can be technically difficult. Recently, intermediate 0.021- and 0.025-in wires have become available which are stiff enough for catheter exchanges or stent placements but are compatible with tapered catheters. Some endoscopists use a papillotome to achieve difficult bile duct cannulation, using variable tension on the cutting wire to bow the catheter sufficiently to achieve cannulation. The newer papillotome can be used with the specially coated guidewires, but simultaneous productive manipulation of endoscope tip, catheter, papillotome wire, and guidewire is a challenge for even the best endoscopist-assistant teams. In cases in which cholangiography is clearly indicated and the above measures fail, the interventional radiologist can often obtain a transhepatic cholangiogram. If choledocholithiasis is identified, the radiologist may pass a wire into the duodenum; this can be used by the endoscopist to guide papillotomy and stone extraction. Malignant obstructions can be brushed and stented radiographically or endoscopically via this combined technique.

6. What is a pre-cut papillotomy? Should it be employed in diagnostic cholangiography?

A pre-cut papillotomy involves creation of an incision with special catheters in the papillary area under circumstances in which a free, selective cannulation of the bile duct cannot be achieved. It may be performed using a bare wire "needle knife" papillotome or a more conventional papillotome whose cutting wire extends to the catheter tip. One reported technique involves placing these catheters into the meatus and cutting up in the direction of the bile duct, hoping to locate the duct and cannulate it after a small incision is made.

Although this technique does appear to increase the rate of successful retrograde cholangiography, the complication rate in experienced hands is two to three times that of conventional papillotomy. Stenting the pancreatic duct prior to pre-cut appears to decrease the rate of post-papillotomy pancreatitis. Pre-cutting should only be performed by experienced endoscopists in patients with strong indications for cholangiography and/or endoscopic papillotomy. One relatively strong indication for a pre-cut is the calculus impacted at the level of the papilla, where free cannulation of the biliary tree is precluded. However, even in these circumstances, a concerted attempt to achieve a free biliary cannulation using special guidewires and other techniques should precede pre-cut papillotomy.

7. Discuss the common indications for diagnostic endoscopic retrograde pancreatography.

A common indication for retrograde pancreatography is to clarify findings on noninvasive radiologic imaging of the pancreas. When a mass lesion suspicious for cancer is identified on transabdominal ultrasound or CT, a tissue diagnosis is desirable. This tissue specimen can be obtained at laparotomy, and this may be the intervention of choice if associated mechanical problems such as gastric outlet obstruction are present. A mass lesion in the pancreatic head may lead to stricture or obstruction of both the pancreatic duct and distal common bile duct, the so-called **double-duct sign** (see figure below). ERCP may afford a cytologic diagnosis and palliation of the biliary obstruction. With improvement in techniques of radiologically guided aspiration and biopsy, use of retrograde pancreatography simply to characterize or obtain brushings from cancers in the pancreatic body or tail is less frequently necessary.

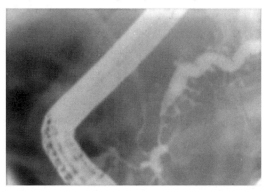

Stricture of the main pancreatic duct in the head with proximal dilatation in a patient with alcoholic chronic pancreatitis. Note the relative smooth tapering of the distal common bile duct. When a mass in the pancreatic head (neoplastic or inflammatory) leads to stricture or obstruction of the main pancreatic duct in the head, as well as narrowing or obstruction of the intrapancreatic portion of the common bile duct, this is characterized as a "double-duct sign."

Another common indication for retrograde pancreatography is to provide anatomic detail prior to surgery for chronic pancreatitis. The presence or absence of ductal dilation, obstruction due to strictures and/or calculi, and the communication of pseudocysts with the main pancreatic duct are all relevant to the likelihood of successful surgical intervention. Patients with acute, recurrent pancreatitis often undergo retrograde pancreatography to exclude anatomic abnormalities, such as pancreas divisum, neoplastic obstruction, or chronic pancreatitis (as well as cholangiography to exclude choledocholithiasis).

Retrograde pancreatography has an extremely limited role in the evaluation of abdominal pain of unknown etiology, where noninvasive pancreatic imaging is normal.

8. List five guidelines to obtaining a successful, uncomplicated biliary papillotomy for the beginner endoscopist.

1. Realize that even the best endoscopists are not always successful. The new endoscopist wants to demonstrate a high skill level and earn a reputation. However, this desire should not lead to continuing unsuccessful procedures for inordinate amounts of time (increasing the risk of complications of sedation/analgesia), repeated filling of the pancreatic duct in attempts at bile duct cannulation, or an imprudent attempt at pre cut papillotomy. Alternative interventions (a more experienced colleague and radiologic or surgical intervention) are far preferable.

2. Perform bile duct papillotomy only after a free, selective cannulation. Experienced endoscopists often begin their therapeutic cases with a papillotome rather than a standard diagnostic catheter. The less-experienced individual may find it more difficult to achieve a free cannulation with the papillotome. A standard or even tapered catheter can be used to achieve cannulation, then exchanged for a wire-guided papillotome performed over a wire.

3. Use one model of papillotome, and know its every mark. Most experienced endoscopists prefer the cutting wire to be one-half to one-third the way out of the papilla to ensure controlled cutting. They can achieve this by sight and feel. An alternative is to memorize each mark on the papillotome, particularly those coincident with the proximal and distal ends of the cutting wire, and the point half-way between. This allows the endoscopist to maneuver the catheter by following the marks and increases confidence that the cutting wire is properly situated.

4. Use a guidewire that can be left in place during papillotomy. Many guidewires must be removed before the papillotomy is performed. However, special "protected" wires that can be left safely in place are now commercially available. These provide an extra measure of confidence in withdrawal of the papillotome to its proper position, as the endoscopist need not fear the loss of selective cannulation.

5. Accept only optimal cutting wire orientation. The bile duct papillotomy is carried out along the maximal impression of the intraduodenal segment of the common bile duct. This is referred to as the "10 o'clock to 1 o'clock position." Sometimes, the cutting wire does not orient in

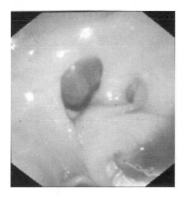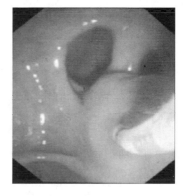

Free cannulation of the common bile duct is achieved with a papillotome. **A,** In some cases, the orientation of the cutting wire is suboptimal (in the 2 o'clock position). **B,** The cutting wire has been repositioned and is now in approximately the 12 o'clock position.

this fashion (see figure on p. 577). The endoscopist should remove the catheter from the endo-scope and try to reorient the catheter with the cutting wire to the left as the catheter bends with gradual tightening of the wire. The papillotome can then be replaced. However, if the attempt at reorientation does not result in proper placement of the cutting wire, do not accept it. Request an-other papillotome. If this happens with two papillotomes, particularly if the cutting wires are rel-atively short, request a papillotome with a long cutting wire. These sometimes orient more fa-vorably in a variety of circumstances.

9. What are some of the common complications of ERCP?

The most frequent complications of diagnostic and therapeutic ERCP include pancreatitis and cholangitis. Bleeding and duodenal perforation rarely complicate diagnostic ERCP but cer-tainly can occur with therapeutic procedures.

Pancreatitis may occur in 1–5% of patients undergoing ERCP. The cause of post-ERCP pan-creatitis is likely multifactorial. The amount of contrast infused into the main pancreatic duct may be one precipitating factor. The contrast typically used for ERCP is iodinated and of high osmo-lality (~1500 mosm/kg), although studies using lower osmolality or nonionic contrast media have not clearly established the benefit of these more costly alternatives.

Cholangitis usually occurs after instillation of contrast proximal to an obstruction in the bil-iary tree. It is more likely when adequate drainage and relief of the obstruction are not provided in a timely fashion. Patients with proximal malignant strictures are more likely than those with distal ones to develop postprocedural cholangitis. Those undergoing reopacification, i.e., multi-ple procedures to establish a diagnosis or endoscopic drainage, appear to be at increased risk. Giv-ing broad-spectrum antibiotics is prudent prior to retrograde cholangiography performed for obstructive jaundice, but it is not a substitute for definitive drainage. Proper disinfection and han-dling of endoscopes and accessories are also essential. Biliary sepsis related to *Pseudomonas* has been traced to contaminated water bottles.

Post-papillotomy **bleeding** is a recognized complication of therapeutic ERCP, occurring in 1.5–5% of cases. Bleeding may be recognized at the time of papillotomy, but can occur several days or longer after an apparently unremarkable procedure. Using blended current and a slow, controlled cut with scrupulous attention to position and orientation of the cutting wire should de-crease the likelihood of bleeding.

Perforation occurs in ~1% of patients and is often recognized during the procedure. Man-agement must be individualized, but not all perforations require immediate surgical exploration. Placement of a **nasobiliary tube** should always be strongly considered in suspected or confirmed perforation. Presumably, the papillotomy was done to remedy a structural abnormality, but the endoscopist may not be comfortable carrying out stone extraction or stent placement after perfo-ration is recognized. However, drainage of infected biliary contents occurs directly out of the tube and may limit retroperitoneal infection. Often, perforation readily seals with nasobiliary drainage and parenteral antibiotic therapy. Drainage is continued until the patient is ready to undergo de-finitive therapy for the underlying obstruction.

Oversedation is a potential complication of ERCP, as it is in all GI endoscopy in which se-dation/analgesia is administered.

Aspiration of gastric contents is rare but may occur. The patient is prone for long periods, and the attention of the assistant may be focused on the procedural tasks. If significant gastric con-tents are noted during initial endoscope passage, the risks of continuing the procedure must be weighed against the potential benefits. In extreme cases, lavage of the stomach contents and in-creased vigilance of the assistant may be beneficial.

10. How can the likelihood of post-ERCP be decreased?

Patients with a nondilated bile duct undergoing endoscopic papillotomy are more likely to experience procedure-related pancreatitis than those with a dilated duct. However, it is generally extremely difficult to predict immediately post-ERCP which patients will develop pancreatitis. Given this and the incomplete understanding of the pathophysiology, it is impossible to offer rec-ommendations to eliminate the problem, but these measures might help:

a. *Have the procedure indication in mind before beginning.* There is no reason to obtain a pancreatogram at all in a patient undergoing ERCP for choledocholithiasis. Attempt a selective cannulation of the bile duct. If the main pancreatic duct is inadvertently opacified, cease the injection immediately. Try in subsequent cannulation attempts to orient the catheter toward the bile duct.

b. *Opacify the main pancreatic duct with the minimum contrast volume* necessary to establish the diagnosis.

c. When focusing fluoroscopic attention on the main pancreatic duct in the tail during contrast injection, *do not ignore the head of the gland.* Overfilling of side branches or acinarization can occur in the head during attempts at complete filling of the duct in the tail.

d. *Listen to your assistant.* If the injection can only be made forcefully, take the time to readjust catheter position for a smoother, controlled injection.

11. Are basket catheters or balloon catheters preferable for extraction of bile duct calculi after papillotomy?

Both are effective and may complement one another. After creation of an adequate papillotomy, a **balloon catheter** can be placed above the most proximal calculus and then inflated. Balloons of varied diameters are available and can be selected as appropriate to the size of the papillotomy, degree of ductal dilation, and number or size of calculi. The inflated balloon catheter is then gradually pulled into the duodenum; an occlusion cholangiogram can be simultaneously obtained. Gentle insertion and clockwise rotation of the endoscope, along with movement of the tip away from the medial wall (using the large wheel) may facilitate delivery of the balloon through the papilla. Disadvantages of the balloon include an inability to visualize directly the clearance of calculi from the duct and a relative increased stiffness of these catheters. This increased stiffness may make the balloon catheter more challenging to insert into small papillotomies or deliver to the proximal biliary tree (particularly to the left hepatic duct). Use of a guidewire can facilitate balloon placement.

Basket catheters are used to grasp and extract individual stones (see figure below). Advantages include direct tactile and visual confirmation of stone extraction and a relative increased flexibility compared to balloon catheters. The basket itself can be manipulated by the assistant and guide the catheter into desired areas in the proximal biliary tree. Disadvantages include an inability to perform confirmatory occlusion cholangiography during or after calculus extraction. Some endoscopists are concerned about impaction of the basket around a stone that cannot be delivered through the papilla, but ancillary techniques, such as mechanical lithotripsy, can often remedy this infrequent occurrence.

One useful approach is to begin with directed stone extraction using basket catheters, followed by an occlusion balloon cholangiogram to sweep away any residual debris and confirm completion of the task.

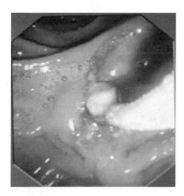 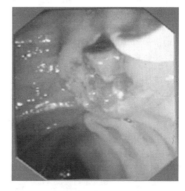

A, After successful papillotomy, a stone trapped in a retrieval basket is pulled into the duodenum. **B,** Another stone falls into the duodenum as the retrieval balloon is pulled distally through the common bile duct.

12. Should patients with cholelithiasis and acute pancreatitis undergo emergent ERCP?

Many patients with acute gallstone pancreatitis show signs of improvement very early in their hospital stay. Emergent ERCP is not generally necessary. However, as these patients do have cholelithiasis and some persistent choledocholithiasis, this should be addressed surgically or endoscopically in a timely fashion, so as to prevent further episodes of pancreatitis.

Patients with more severe gallstone pancreatitis or those in whom clear progressive improvement is not obvious are more likely candidates for emergent or urgent ERCP during the episode of pancreatitis. In many patients with severe or unresolving gallstone pancreatitis, choledocholithiasis will be identified. A stone impacted at the level of the papilla is a not infrequent discovery. Early endoscopic intervention can also decrease the incidence of cholangitis in patients with choledocholithiasis and pancreatitis and perhaps lower the overall mortality rate. This is a circumstance where an experienced endoscopist is essential. Many of these patients are quite ill. The endoscopic intervention should be carried out with all deliberate speed. Selective free cannulation of the biliary tree is important; opacification of the main pancreatic duct could theoretically worsen the pancreatitis. Pre-cut papillotomy may be necessary for extraction of a stone impacted at the level of the papilla. Placement of a nasobiliary tube may be necessary to augment biliary drainage in some cases. Occasionally, patients may require intensive care monitoring; if such a patient is transported to the endoscopy suite, all necessary monitoring should accompany them. Presence of an anesthesiologist to administer sedation/analgesia may be appropriate for the most acutely ill.

13. Should the endoscopic management of malignant biliary obstruction always involve metal stents?

Endoscopic palliation of malignant biliary obstruction with polyethylene stents is a well-established standard of care. These stents provide adequate drainage and are easily placed in most cases; some hilar strictures where both right and left systems require drainage can be a challenge to even the best endoscopist. They are subject to periodic clogging, and many endoscopists recommend regular stent change to prevent cholangitis.

Recently, metal stents have become commercially available. These are easily placed by the endoscopist or radiologist. Clogging and obstruction are less frequent. The initial cost of metal stent placement exceeds that of the polyethylene stent, but the long-term costs may be lower. Both the need for subsequent endoscopy for polyethylene stent change and total hospital days for cholangitis due to stent obstruction are less with metal stents. Another difference between polyethylene and metal stents is that although the plastic stents are easily removed, the metal ones are not. Therefore, palliation for a patient in whom surgical resection is still possible might be better managed with a plastic stent. If subsequently surgery is ruled out, a metal stent can still be placed at the time of the first scheduled stent change. Metal stents may not be cost-effective in patients with an extremely short life expectancy.

14. Is there a role for therapeutic endoscopic retrograde pancreatography?

One such circumstance is endoscopic therapy for acute, recurrent pancreatitis attributed to pancreas divisum. There does appear to be an association between divisum, which is failure of fusion of the dorsal and ventral pancreatic ducts, and pancreatitis. It is theorized that the volume of pancreatic drainage via the dorsal duct and accessory papilla in pancreas divisum exceeds their capacity, leading to episodic pancreatitis. Surgical sphincteroplasty of the accessory papilla appears to decrease or eliminate further attacks. Endoscopic therapy can also be provided. The accessory papilla may be cannulated and opacified using special tapered or fine-tipped catheters. Small-diameter stents may be placed endoscopically for a clinical trial to assess response or as a guide to endoscopic papillotomy. Both dorsal duct stent placement and stent placement with papillotomy of the accessory papilla have provided benefit to patients with acute recurrent pancreatitis in controlled clinical trials with short-term follow-up. Experience with endoscopic pancreatic duct sphincterotomy, stent placement, stone extraction, and pseudocyst drainage as therapy for sequelae of chronic pancreatitis is growing. Long-term studies are needed to determine the circumstances under which these interventions are most beneficial and to determine their efficacy compared to standard surgical and radiologic interventions.

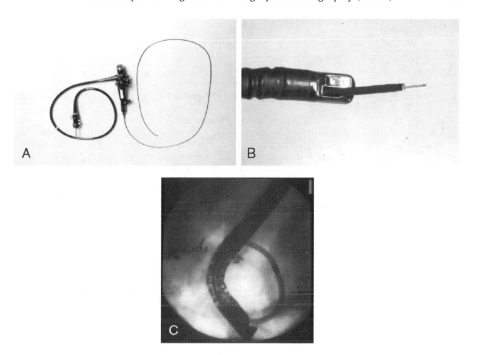

A, The Olympus CHF B20 choledochofiberscope. **B,** The choledochofiberscope passed through the operating channel of the Olympus TJF M20 duodenomotherfiberscope. The choledochoscope has a small operating channel. **C,** Radiographic image of the choledochoscope inserted into the common bile duct.

15. Does cholangioscopy have a role in the diagnosis and management of biliary tract disorders?

Rarely. Direct visualization of the bile duct or main pancreatic duct can be accomplished with special small-caliber endoscopes passed through a duodenoscope with a large operating channel (see figure above) or with special small optical fibers. The information gained during routine ERCP is sufficient to establish the diagnosis and management for most patients. In rare circumstances, cholangioscopy or pancreatoscopy might add relevant information. Occasionally, it may be difficult to distinguish a mass lesion in the biliary tree from an adherent calculus. Direct visualization of a bile duct stricture might add to the information available from cytology or noninvasive imaging, directed cytology or biopsy may be possible with some cholangioscopes. Laser or other ablative therapy for tumors or large stones will likely be performed via cholangioscopy with increasing frequency in the future.

16. What is the role of the radiologist in ERCP?

The radiologist's role varies with the institution. In many practices, ERCP is performed in the radiology suite rather than in the endoscopy unit. Often, a member of the radiology staff, either attending physician, resident physician, or technician, is in attendance. When the attending radiologist is present, interpretation of hard copy films is straightforward, as the radiologist knows the relevant history, results of correlative imaging, and sequence of procedural events. When the radiologist is not present, the endoscopist must take responsibility to identify the relevant findings fluoroscopically but also to document them on hard copy film for later reference. The endoscopist therefore must be aware of his/her role as an *archivist,* being sure to obtain the control flat plate prior to retrograde pancreatography for chronic pancreatitis. Significant actions routinely are taken by the endoscopist on the basis of fluoroscopic images, and it is prudent to document these findings carefully on hard copy film kept in the patient's permanent file.

BIBLIOGRAPHY

1. Principles of Training in Gastrointestinal Endoscopy. Manchester, MA, American Society for Gastrointestinal Endoscopy, May 1991.
2. Classen DC, Jacobson JA, Burke JP, et al: Serious pseudomonas infections associated with endoscopic retrograde cholangiopancreatography. Am J Med 84:590–596, 1988.
3. Cotton PB: Precut papillotomy—A risky technique for experts only. Gastrointest Endosc 35:578–579, 1989.
4. Cotton PB, Lehman G, Vennes J, et al: Endoscopic sphincterotomy complications and their management: An attempt at consensus. Gastrointest Endosc 37:383–393, 1991.
5. Cotton PB, William CB: Endoscopic retrograde cholangio-pancreatography (ERCP). Practical Gastrointestinal Endoscopy, 3rd ed. Boston, Blackwell Scientific, 1990, pp 85–117.
6. Deviere J, Motte S, Dumonceau JM, et al: Septicemia after endoscopic retrograde cholangiopancreatography. Endoscopy 22:72–75, 1990.
7. Fan ST, Lai EC, Mok FP, et al: Early treatment of acute biliary pancreatitis by endoscopic papillotomy. N Engl J Med 328:228–232, 1993.
8. Geenen JE, Vennes JA, Silvis SE: Resume of a seminar on endoscopic retrograde sphincterotomy (ERS). Gastrointest Endosc 7:31–38, 1981.
9. Huibregtse K, Smits ME: Endoscopic management of diseases of the pancreas. Am J Gastroenterol 88(suppl):S66–S77, 1994.
10. Knyrim K, Wagner HJ, Pausch J, et al: A prospective, randomized, controlled trial of metal stents for malignant obstruction of the common bile duct. Endoscopy 25:207–212, 1993.
11. Lans JI, Geenen JE, Johanson JF, Hogan WJ: Endoscopic therapy in patients with pancreas divisum and acute pancreatitis: A prospective, randomized, controlled clinical trial. Gastrointest Endosc 38:430–434, 1992.
12. Lehman GA, Sherman S, Hisi R, Hawes RH: Pancreas divisum: Results of minor papilla sphincterotomy. Gastrointest Endosc 39:1–8, 1993.
13. Motte S, Deviere J, Dumonceau JM, et al: Risk factors for septicemia following endoscopic biliary stenting. Gastroenterology 101:1374–1381, 1991.
14. Richter JM, Schapiro RH, Mulley AG, Warshaw AL: Association of pancreas divisum and pancreatitis, and its treatment by sphincteroplasty of the accessory ampulla. Gastroenterology 81:1104–1110, 1981.
15. Roszler MH, Campbell WL: Post-ERCP pancreatitis: Association with urographic visualization during ERCP. Radiology 157:595–598, 1985.
16. Sherman S, Lehman GA: ERCP—and endoscopic sphincterotomy-induced pancreatitis. Pancreas 6:350–367, 1991.
17. Sherman S, Ruffolo TA, Hawes R, Lehman G: Complications of endoscopic sphincterotomy: A prospective series with emphasis on the increased risk associated with sphincter of Oddi dysfunction and nondilated bile ducts. Gastroenterology 101:1068–1075, 1991.
18. Tweedle DEF, Martin DF: Needle knife papillotomy for endoscopic sphincterotomy and cholangiography. Gastrointest Endosc 37:518–521, 1991.

X. Surgery and the GI Tract

78. ESOPHAGEAL SURGERY

Robert C. McIntyre, Jr., M.D., and Greg Van Stiegmann, M.D.

GASTROESOPHAGEAL REFLUX DISEASE

1. Outline the four phases of management of gastroesophageal reflux disease. What are the indications for antireflux surgery?

Phase I: Nonmedical therapy includes changing the diet (avoid caffeine, alcohol, and chocolate), weight loss, quitting tobacco use, elevating the head of the bed, avoiding meals before bed, avoiding tight-fitting clothes and antacids.

Phase II: The diagnosis should be confirmed by endoscopic examination to evaluate the esophagus, stomach, and duodenum. If esophagitis is present, it should be documented with biopsy. More intensive medical therapy is indicated using H_2 receptor blockade or alternatives, prokinetic agents (bethanechol, metoclopramide, cisapride) and cytoprotective agents (sucralfate)

Phase III: Patients who remain symptomatic after the preceding therapy should be treated with omeprazole.

Phase IV: Patients who fail medical therapy are considered for antireflux surgery. Strong indications for antireflux surgery include refractoriness to medical therapy, erosive esophagitis unresponsive to omeprazole, strictures unresponsive to dilatation, development of Barrett's esophagus while on adequate medical therapy, and advancement of Barrett's epithelium while on adequate medical therapy. Young, good risk patients who are symptom-free on omeprazole but have recurrence of symptoms off medication should be considered for early, elective antireflux surgery.

2. Which diagnostic studies are useful in the preoperative evaluation of patients with GERD?

Upper gastrointestinal (UGI) tract barium studies: The most important role of an UGI barium study is to demonstrate and classify a hiatal hernia. Barium studies may also be used to document reflux, although the sensitivity and specificity of this study are poor. An UGI study should also confirm that the gastroesophageal junction is reducible to near or below the diaphragmatic hiatus in patients with hiatal hernia under consideration for surgery.

Esophagogastroduodenoscopy (EGD): During an EGD exam, it is possible to visualize inflammatory changes in the distal esophagus and obtain biopsy specimens for histologic confirmation of esophagitis or Barrett's epithelium. Assessment of the stomach for retained contents or outlet obstruction is also done.

24-hour pH probe: Long-term (24-hour) pH assessment is indicated in patients whose symptoms are suggestive of GERD but who do not have esophagitis on EGD and biopsy. This test is the most specific study for the diagnosis of GERD in patients without unequivocal endoscopic or histologic evidence of disease.

Esophageal manometry: Manometry alone cannot be used to diagnose GERD. It may be indicated in patients whose symptoms are not promptly relieved by medical therapy or if surgery is contemplated. Manometry is able to determine the presence and adequacy of esophageal peristalsis. Absence of esophageal peristalsis is a contraindication to antireflux surgery.

3. What are the physiologic principles of an antireflux procedure?

Operations for GERD attempt to restore the distal esophageal sphincter pressure to a level at least twice the resting gastric pressure. The main principles of antireflux procedures are restoring the anterior position of the esophagogastric junction and increasing the length of the esophagus exposed to the increased pressure of the abdominal cavity. The operation should not increase the resistance of the distal esophageal sphincter to such a level that it exceeds the ability of esophageal peristalsis to overcome it.

4. What procedures are available to prevent reflux?

Antireflux procedures may be done using either laparoscopic or open surgical techniques. The principal laparoscopic procedures include the Nissen fundoplication (360° wrap), Toupet fundoplication (posterior 270° wrap), and the round ligament cardiopexy. The most common procedure done is the Nissen fundoplication. It is most commonly performed using the technique described by DeMeester for open fundoplication, which is a 360° wrap, 2 cm in length, done over a large dilator (50–60F). Open procedures include the Nissen fundoplication, the Belsy Mark IV operation (270° wrap), Hill fundoplication (median arcuate ligament repair), and Angelchik prosthesis.

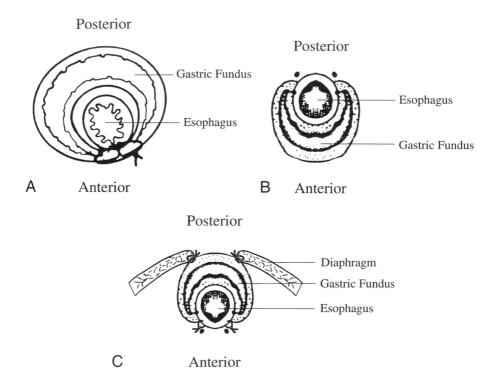

Cross-sectional view of antireflux procedures: **A,** Nissen fundoplication; **B,** Belsy Mark IV; and **C,** Toupet fundoplication. In each view, the esophagus and gastric fundus are identified. The Nissen fundoplication entails a posterior 360° wrap, the Belsy Mark IV operation is an anterior 270° wrap, and the Toupet is a posterior 270° wrap. The Toupet also involves securing the gastric fundus to the crus of the diaphragm.

5. What are the success rates of these procedures and their expected complications?

Operation controls reflux in 85–95% of cases. Side effects of operation include dysphagia (2–10%), gas bloat (0–8%), inability to vomit (5%), and gastric fistula ($< 1\%$). Late complications include reflux recurrence (0–10%) and the slipped Nissen (1–2%).

BARRETT'S ESOPHAGITIS

6. What is Barrett's esophagus?

Barrett's esophagus is an acquired condition in which damaged squamous esophageal epithelium undergoes metaplasia to columnar cells which proliferate to form an abnormal epithelium. There are two variations of Barrett's esophagus classified according to their similarity to intestinal or gastric epithelium. In nearly 15,000 patients undergoing EGD for various reasons, Barrett's epithelium was found in 7.4/1000 patients. In patients with symptoms of GERD, Barrett's was found in 80.1/1000 patients. From a functional standpoint, patients with Barrett'esophagus appear to have an increase in exposure of the distal esophagus to both acid and alkaline secretions, loss of lower esophageal sphincter pressure, delayed esophageal clearance of refluxed material, increased gastric acid production, and increased duodenogastric reflux.

7. Why is Barrett's esophagus significant?

Most esophageal adenocarcinoma appears to arise in Barrett's epithelium. The prevalence of adenocarcinoma in a Barrett's esophagus in reported series is as high as 13%. However, the risk of developing adenocarcinoma in a Barrett's esophagus is much lower. In a series of patients from the Mayo Clinic, only 2 of 104 patients with Barrett's esophagus developed cancer.

8. How should Barrett's esophagus be managed?

Despite the evidence that reflux of duodenal secretions may be an important causative factor, the current medical therapy for patients with Barrett's esophagus is acid suppression. However, acid suppression has not been demonstrated to cause regression of Barrett's epithelium. In fact, some patients may have Barrett's epithelium advance while on acid suppression (lending further support to the evidence that duodenogastric reflux is important in the pathophysiology). These patients should be considered for antireflux procedures.

Annual surveillance of patients with Barrett's esophagus is recommended. Screening for carcinoma should be done by four-quadrant biopsies every 1–2 cm. Further management of a patient depends on the results of biopsy, of which there are five options: no dysplasia, indefinite for dysplasia, low-grade dysplasia, high-grade dysplasia or carcinoma in situ, and invasive carcinoma.

ESOPHAGEAL CARCINOMA

9. What are the risk factors for esophageal carcinoma?

Esophageal carcinoma is most common in Iran, China, and South Africa. In the United States, elderly black males in the southeast have a higher risk than age-matched whites. Squamous cell carcinoma is more common in black men, whereas adenocarcinoma shows a predilection for white men. Tobacco and ethanol use lead to increased risk. Premalignant conditions include Barrett's esophagus, achalasia, Plummer-Vinson syndrome, caustic injuries, and scleroderma.

10. How is esophageal carcinoma classified according to histology and distribution?

Nearly 50% of esophageal carcinoma is adenocarcinoma occurring at the gastroesophageal junction. The remaining 50% is squamous cell carcinoma, which is in the middle third of the esophagus in 50%, lower third in 35%, and upper third in 15%. A small percentage of patients have cancer of the cervical esophagus. Carcinoma of the gastric cardia is treated in the same fashion as distal esophageal carcinoma and has a similar outcome. The incidence of adenocarcinoma of the esophagus appears to be increasing.

11. Which preoperative investigations are useful in evaluating a patient with esophageal carcinoma? What findings mitigate against a curative resection?

- Upper GI barium studies are useful and noninvasive. They allow accurate localization of the tumor and planning of the correct surgical approach.

- Esophagogastroduodenoscopy (EGD) is essential and allows biopsy confirmation of the diagnosis.
- Endoscopic ultrasound has been used for assessing the lateral spread and presence of enlarged lymph nodes (as well as for surveillance following treatment).
- Computed tomography (CT) excludes lung and liver metastasis and accurately localizes the tumor.
- Magnetic resonance (MR) imaging is no more useful than CT.

Findings that mitigate against a curative resection include a completely obstructed lesion, angulation of the esophageal lumen on UGI barium studies, an esophageal-tracheal fistula, a lesion longer than 5 cm, or recurrent laryngeal nerve or phrenic nerve paralysis.

12. Describe the options for nonoperative palliation for esophageal carcinoma.

- **Radiotherapy** used alone provides temporary relief of dysphagia in an appreciable number of patients: unfortunately the benefits are brief. The 5-year survival in patients receiving radiotherapy alone varies from 1–8%.
- **Chemotherapy** used alone has a limited role because the response rate is low (15–20%) and brief in duration. In multidrug therapy, cisplatin is usually used in combination with vindesine, bleomycin, 5-fluorouracil, or mitomycin.
- **Chemoradiotherapy** provides better relief than either radiotherapy or chemotherapy alone, with effective palliation of dysphagia in 70–80% of patients.
- **Dilatation** may provide some relief of dysphagia but is seldom long-lasting.
- **Nd:YAG** (neodymium:yttrium-aluminum-garnet) **laser** therapy may provide relief of dysphagia in up to 85% of patients.
- **Photoirradiation** is done using a hematoporphyrin derivative before treatment with an argon-pulsed dye laser. Its ultimate role is yet undetermined.
- Stents allow for rapid palliation of esophageal obstruction. The available prostheses include the conventional plastic prosthesis and the newer metal Wallstent. Complications include bleeding, obstruction of the tube, perforation, tube migration, and intractable gastroesophageal reflux.

13. What surgical options are used for resection and palliation in esophageal carcinoma?

The term *curative resection* should be reserved for a resection in which the surgeon believes there is no macroscopic residual tumor left behind. A *palliative resection* implies that the surgeon left visible tumor behind. Incurable tumors are usually left in place, and palliation is performed by nonoperative means or surgical bypass procedures.

Multiple surgical options can be used for resection of esophageal carcinoma. The traditional surgical esophageal resection is the **two-stage Ivor Lewis esophagogastrectomy.** The first stage is a laparotomy for mobilization of the stomach, and the second, a right thoracotomy for removal of the tumor and an esophagogastric anastomosis in the chest. An alternative to the two-stage resection is a three-stage resection (McKeown), which includes mobilization of the cervical esophagus for anastomosis of the esophagus to a gastric tube in the neck. The rationale for this procedure is that it allows a longer proximal resection, an anastomosis in the neck with its reduced morbidity and mortality, and a more extensive lymph node dissection. Patients with cancer of the distal esophagus or of the gastric cardia can have their tumors removed through a left thoracoabdominal exposure with an intrathoracic anastomosis.

The transhiatal **"blunt" esophagectomy** avoids the thoracotomy of the above two approaches. The esophagus is mobilized from the abdomen through an enlarged hiatus and from above through a cervical incision along the anterior border of the left sternocleidomastoid. The standard technique is to perform the mediastinal mobilization in a blind fashion; however, laparoscopic assistance allows the dissection to be done under direct vision. This technique has gained considerable popularity in North America.

The most common replacement for the esophagus is the stomach, which can be mobilized to reach the cervical esophagus. Other options include the colon and small intestine. The most common path for the replacement is in the normal posterior mediastinal position, but the replacement may be brought posterior to the sternum or, rarely, in the subcutaneous plane.

Options available to the surgeon for **palliation** include surgically placed stents, bypass of the tumor (usually done with a gastric tube placed behind the sternum), or a gastrostomy or jejunostomy for feedings.

14. What is the prognosis of esophageal carcinoma?
The goals of esophageal resection should be <5% operative mortality, 50–75% 1-year survival, and 15–20% 5-year survival. Patients should be capable of relatively normal deglutition.

15. What is the role of adjuvant therapy?
Radiotherapy is usually reserved for patients with nonresectable tumors or for patients with recurrence after a surgical resection. Radiotherapy used in conjunction with chemotherapy before surgery may have benefit in selected patients.

ACHALASIA

16. How is the patient with achalasia evaluated?
Achalasia affects both sexes equally, with a typical age range of 25–60 years. Patients have solid-food dysphagia and frequently have dysphagia for liquid. They also report fullness in the chest, regurgitation, and weight loss. Some patients report that postural maneuvers frequently are necessary to assist with passage of food. Stress may worsen the dysphagia. Chest pain and heartburn are occasional complaints, and a few patients may have episodes of aspiration pneumonia.

Plain chest radiographs may reveal a wide posterior mediastinum, an air-fluid level within the chest, an absent gastric air bubble, and evidence of chronic aspiration. Barium studies reveal ineffective peristalsis. The esophageal body is often dilatated; although early in the disease, it may not be dilatated. The lower esophageal sphincter (LES) at barium esophagography is usually visualized as a taper of the barium (often called a "bird's beak"). The LES may open partially and intermittently and is not coordinated with swallowing. Endoscopy is necessary to evaluate for the presence of a malignant tumor. Even though the LES does not open with insufflation, it will allow easy passage of the endoscope. Manometry is indicated and findings are usually absence of peristalsis, elevated esophageal pressures, abnormal LES relaxation and pressure. Patients should also be evaluated for the possibility of Chagas' disease (caused by *Trypanosoma cruzi*).

17. List the alternatives for treatment.
1. Pharmacotherapy with smooth muscle relaxants (isosorbide dinitrate, nifedipine)
2. Pneumatic dilatation (250–300 mm Hg pressure)
3. Esophagomyotomy
4. Esophagectomy

18. What are the important components of esophagomyotomy?
The **length** of the esophagomyotomy has varied from 5–15 cm proximally starting from the esophagogastric junction. Most feel that 5–6 cm is an adequate length. Preoperative manometry may be used to identify the level and length of the sphincter and to guide the myotomy. The extent of the myotomy on the stomach has ranged from 0–4 cm distally, but most agree that 0.5–1 cm is recommended. Excessive length of the gastric myotomy leads to increased incidence of postoperative reflux.

The most controversial aspect of surgery for achalasia is the inclusion of an **antireflux procedure.** Postoperative reflux depends on many factors, such as the surgical procedure, approach to the esophagus (i.e., thoracic or abdominal), length of myotomy, duration of follow-up, and method of evaluation. In collected series, the mean incidence of reflux following surgery is 8.6%. Reflux increases in patients treated for achalasia via laparotomy more than thoracotomy, with extensive dissection around the gastroesophageal junction, longer extension of the myotomy onto the stomach, and duration of follow-up. Clinical symptoms underestimate the incidence of reflux; endoscopy and 24-hour pH probe studies are more sensitive. The addition of an antireflux procedure remains controversial but probably results in an improved symptomatic outcome. It must be remembered that an antireflux procedure should not constrict the esophagogastric junction and cause dysphagia in an aperistaltic esophagus.

ESOPHAGEAL PERFORATION

19. What are the most common causes of esophageal perforation?
Cervical esophageal perforations (25%) are commonly due to penetrating trauma, instrument perforation, or foreign bodies. Patients present with pain, fever, dysphagia, and neck crepitus. **Thoracic** perforations occur secondary to endoscopy, esophageal dilatation, or trauma, or spontaneously (Boerhaave's syndrome). Patients present with fever and pain but infrequently have dysphagia. **Abdominal** esophageal perforations may occur spontaneously or during surgery. Sixty percent of perforations are iatrogenic due to instrumentation, 25% are due to trauma, and 15% are spontaneous.

20. How is perforation diagnosed?
The key to diagnosis is strong **clinical suspicion.** Cervical esophageal perforations frequently have subcutaneous tissue emphysema on plain radiographs. Chest radiographs may reveal pleural effusion with or without a pneumothorax. Infrequently, a pneumopericardium is seen. Perforation of the abdominal esophagus may cause free air under the diaphragm. An upper GI contrast study using water-soluble contrast material (Gastrografin, meglumine diatrizoate), under fluoroscopy can accurately diagnose an esophageal perforation. This initial study should be followed by a small amount of thin barium in the event that a perforation is not localized with Gastrografin.

21. Name some surgical options for treatment of esophageal perforation.
  1. Primary closure with or without tissue reinforcement (pleura, pericardium, omentum, diaphragm, intercostal muscle, stomach) is best suited for early perforations (< 24 hours).
  2. Drainage alone is most appropriate for perforations with extensive contamination >24 hours old.
  3. Insertion of a large T-tube creates a controlled external fistula. The area around the perforation should also be widely drained.
  4. Resection may be necessary for patients with a malignancy or distal esophageal stricture. Immediate reconstruction is possible when the patient is stable and there is minimal soilage; however, a cervical esophagostomy and gastrostomy followed by delayed reconstruction may be necessary when patients are unstable or there is massive soilage.
  5. Exclusion and diversion of the esophagus with a decompressive gastrostomy is advocated by some for unstable patients with extensive soilage.
  6. Nonoperative means may be used to manage selected patients. Criteria for nonoperative management include a contained mediastinal leak with drainage back into the esophagus, no signs of systemic sepsis, recent perforation, and absence of distal obstruction. Treatment is broad-spectrum antibiotics, parenteral nutrition, and careful observation.

DIVERTICULA

22. Where do diverticula occur in the esophagus? What is the etiology?
Esophageal diverticula are classified based on location:
  • **Pharyngoesophageal** (Zenker's) diverticula are mucosal outpouchings that occur in the triangular bare area between the cricopharyngeus muscle and the inferior pharyngeal constrictor. Most occur on the left side, and approximately 50% of patients have improper upper esophageal sphincter relaxation.
  • **Midesophageal** diverticula are usually traction diverticula secondary to a mediastinal inflammatory process (such as tuberculosis).
  • **Epiphrenic** diverticula occur secondary to propulsion and typically occur in elderly patients. An underlying mechanical obstruction is usually found on evaluation.

23. What are the important components of surgical therapy for esophageal diverticula?

Treatment of pharyngoesophageal diverticula should always include a cricopharyngeal myotomy. Most large and smaller diverticula may be resected flush with the esophageal wall while a 50-French dilator is in the esophagus to prevent stenosis.

Surgery for midesophageal diverticula is rarely indicated. Treatment of the underlying disorder is the mainstay of therapy. In rare cases, resection of the diverticula through a thoracotomy may be indicated for refractory symptoms.

The surgical approach to epiphrenic diverticula is through a low, left posterolateral thoracotomy. The diverticula are resected in the presence of a 50-dilator. Complete treatment requires a myotomy.

PARAESOPHAGEAL HIATAL HERNIA

24. Outline the classification of hiatal hernias.

Type I	Sliding hiatal hernia	Esophagus moves freely through the hiatus, with the gastroesophageal junction (GEJ) in the thorax or abdomen at various times.
Type II	Paraesophageal hiatal hernia	GEJ is in the normal position within the abdominal cavity, but the gastric fundus or greater curvature herniates alongside the esophagus.
Type III	Combination	GEJ is displaced into the thorax as in a type I hernia, but the gastric fundus is herniated as in a type II hernia (see figure below).

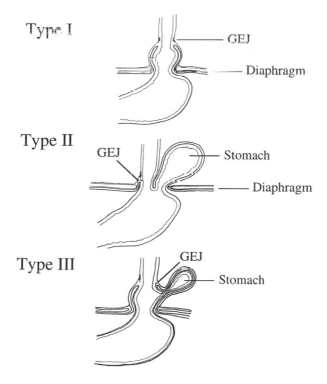

Schematic representation of type I, type II, and type III hiatal hernias.

25. When is surgery indicated in patients with hiatal hernia?
Immediate surgical correction is indicated for the patient with a paraesophageal hernia that is complicated, i.e., resulting in gastric volvulus with obstruction, hemorrhage, infarction, or perforation. On the other hand, some patients present with minimal symptoms. There is disagreement as to whether a patient who is asymptomatic or has minimal symptoms requires surgical repair, but most agree that patients with symptoms should have elective repair.

26. List the important components of surgical therapy for hiatal hernias.
The principles of repair of a paraesophageal hiatal hernia include:
  1. Reduction of the contents of the hernia into the peritoneal cavity;
  2. Maintenance of the hernia contents in the peritoneal cavity so that they cannot rotate or herniate back through the hiatus; and
  3. Closure of the hiatus.
The need for an antireflux procedure is controversial. Those who advocate the routine addition to an antireflux procedure claim that patients frequently have symptoms of gastroesophageal reflux in addition to the hernia. Additionally, a fundoplication may reduce the risk of hernia recurrence. Others do not advocate fundoplication, stating that the incidence of recurrence without it is low. Some authors advocate a gastropexy or gastrostomy to fix the stomach and prevent recurrent herniation.

CAUSTIC INJURY

27. How should the patient with a caustic ingestion be evaluated?
The severity of the injury should be assessed by thorough questioning of the patient, witnesses, and/or family about the agent and the amount ingested. Plain radiographs of the chest and abdomen should be done to assess for aspiration, pneumothorax, pneumomediastinum, or pneumoperitoneum. Endoscopy should be done to assess the severity and extent of the injury.

28. Explain the early management of patients with caustic injury to the esophagus?
Initial treatment of a caustic ingestion includes an assessment of the patient's airway and intubation for airway compromise. Respiratory therapy may be necessary to help the patient clear pulmonary secretions. Oropharyngeal suctioning is done for patients who are unable to control their saliva and secretions. Patients should be kept well-hydrated, because extensive caustic injury may cause a large amount of fluid to accumulate in the tissues resulting in hypovolemia. Total parenteral nutrition should be instituted early for patients with severe injury. Antibiotics are indicated for the treatment of a specific infection. In patients with mild injury who can eat normally, an upper GI contrast study should be done 2–4 weeks after the ingestion.

29. What are the complications of caustic injury?
  Early complications: esophageal or gastric necrosis, stricture
  Late complications: reflux esophagitis, carcinoma

30. How should the early complications of caustic ingestion be managed?
Esophageal or gastric necrosis is a devastating complication. In children, mild esophageal injury occurs in most cases, whereas adults more commonly have moderate and severe gastric injuries. Septic shock, pneumomediastinum, or pneumoperitoneum are ominous signs. Management of this condition should consist of a midline laparotomy with esophagectomy, gastrectomy, or both. A transhiatal esophagectomy can be done to avoid a thoracotomy. Immediate reconstruction may be possible in select cases; however, an esophagostomy and gastrostomy with delayed reconstruction may be necessary.
Esophageal stricture occurs in only 5% of patients following a caustic ingestion. In patients with moderate esophageal injuries (limited necrosis or ulcers), dilatation should be started approximately 10 days after the ingestion using fluoroscopic and guidewire control (Savary). On the

other hand, if the amount of necrosis is extensive, the patient should be supported with gastrostomy or jejunostomy tube feeds for 4–6 weeks. Stenotic lesions may then be dilatated with a number of different bougies. Antegrade dilatation is easiest and safest using guidewire (Savary) dilators with fluoroscopic control. Alternatively, retrograde dilation (Tucker) can be done by passing a string perorally through the stenosis and out the gastrostomy. The string is attached to the dilator, which is then drawn up through the stenosis. Patients with resistant strictures may ultimately require esophageal replacement.

31. Describe the management of the late sequelae of caustic ingestion.

Symptoms of esophageal **reflux** may occur following caustic ingestion. Patients may be treated by prokinetic agents, H_2 receptor blockade, or omeprazole. The value of fundoplication is doubtful. Ingestions occurring in childhood may result in a foreshortened esophagus, requiring esophageal replacement. The most feared late complication of a caustic ingestion is the development of squamous cell carcinoma or, less commonly, adenocarcinoma in cases of stenosis and reflux esophagitis.

FOREIGN BODY

32. How should patients with suspected esophageal foreign bodies be evaluated?

Most (80%) patients with foreign bodies entering the upper GI tract are children. Over 90% of these foreign bodies enter the GI tract, and approximately 8% enter the tracheobronchial tree. Most (80–90%) pass spontaneously, 10–20% require endoscopic removal, and a few necessitate surgery

The patient, witnesses, and family members should be questioned about the nature of the object. A history of odynophagia should be elicited. Patients should be observed for problems in handling their saliva and secretions; these findings suggest complete esophageal obstruction. Pain, swelling, tenderness, and crepitus in the neck suggest perforation.

The initial evaluation should include plain radiographs, both anteroposterior and lateral, to evaluate for radiopaque bodies. If the plain films are negative, thin barium may be used. Asymptomatic patients with negative studies need no further evaluation. Patients who ingest coins should have weekly films unless symptoms develop during observation. Endoscopy is indicated if symptoms persist for more than a few hours.

33. When is surgery indicated for removal of foreign bodies?

Children should have general anesthesia in order to undergo endoscopic removal of foreign bodies. To remove impacted objects at the cricopharyngeus in children, airway control should be done first. Adults can be given sedatives for endoscopy.

Surgery is indicated for patients with large or long objects that remain in the stomach for 5 days, perforation, bleeding, or obstruction.

ESOPHAGEAL MOTILITY DISORDER

34. What are the major esophageal motility disorders?

1. **Oropharyngeal and upper esophageal sphincter dysfunction** may result from neurologic and neuromuscular diseases or be idiopathic. Oropharyngeal dysphagia may also occur following surgery (such as tracheostomy, laryngectomy, or cervical dissection).

2. **Primary idiopathic motor disorders** include achalasia, diffuse esophageal spasm, nutcracker esophagus, hypertensive lower esophageal sphincter (LES), or nonspecific esophageal motility disorders.

3. **Reflux disease** is associated with a hypotensive LES but normal esophageal body contractile amplitude and peristalsis. Long-standing reflux disease may result in decreased contractile amplitude. Alternatively, reflux with a weak or absent LES in conjunction with absent peristalsis may be due to scleroderma.

35. What are the treatment options for esophageal dysmotility?

- Patients with cricopharyngeal dysphagia and a hypertensive upper esophageal sphincter should undergo cricopharyngeal myotomy.
- Achalasia may be treated with pharmacotherapy (isosorbide dinitrate, nifedipine), pneumatic dilatation (250–300 mm Hg pressure), or myotomy with or without an antireflux procedure.
- Diffuse esophageal spasm is amenable to treatment with smooth muscle relaxants or a long myotomy with or without an antireflux procedure.
- Nonspecific esophageal motility disorders should be evaluated for significant gastroesophageal reflux and treated for GERD if indicated.

BIBLIOGRAPHY

1. Cameron AJ, Ott BJ, Payne WS: The incidence of adenocarcinoma in a columnar-lined (Barrett's) esophagus. N Engl J Med 313:857, 1985.
2. Cameron JL, Kieffer RJ, Hendrix TR, et al: Selective nonoperative management of contained intrathoracic esophageal perforations. Ann Thorac Surg 27:404, 1979.
3. Chakkaphak S, Chakkaphak K, Ferguson MK, et al: Disorders of esophageal motility. Surg Gynecol Obstet 172:325, 1991.
4. Csendes A, Braghetto I, Henrique A, et al: Late results of a prospective randomized trial comparing forceful dilatation or esophagomyotomy in patients with achalasia of the esophagus. Gut 30:299, 1989.
5. DeMeester T, Bonavina L, Albertucci M: Nissen fundoplication for gastroesophageal reflux in patients with reflux oesophagitis. Ann Surg 204:9, 1986.
6. Earlam R, Cunha-Melo JR: Oesophageal carcinoma: II. A critical review of radiotherapy. Br J Surg 67:457, 1980.
7. Ellis FH, Croziewr RE, Shea JA: Paraesophageal hiatus hernia. Arch Surg 121:416, 1986.
8. Hinder RA, Filipi CJ, Wetscher G, et al: Laparoscopic Nissen fundoplication is an effective treatment for gastroesophageal reflux disease. Ann Surg 220:472, 1994.
9. Jamieson GG, Watson DI, Britten-Jones R, et al: Laparoscopic Nissen fundoplication. Ann Surg 220:137, 1994.
10. Kirsh MA, Peterson A, Brown JW, et al:. Treatment of caustic injuries of the esophagus: A ten year experience. Ann Surg 188:675, 1978.
11. Knyrim K, Wagner HJ, Bethge N, et al: A controlled trial of an expansile metal stent for palliation of esophageal obstruction due to inoperable cancer. N Engl J Med. 329:1302, 1993.
12. Launois B, Delarue D, Champion JP, et al: Preoperative radiotherapy for carcinoma of the esophagus. Surg Gynecol Obstet 153:609, 1981.
13. Nesbitt JC, Sawyers JL: Surgical management of esophageal perforation. Ann Surg 53:183, 1987.
14. Roussel A, Paillot B, Gillet M, et al: The value of preoperative radiotherapy in esophageal carcinoma. World J Surg 11:426, 1987.
15. Spechler S: Barrett's esophagus. Curr Opin Gastroenterol 8:573, 1992.
16. Steitz JM, Glick ME, Ellis FH: Selective use of myotomy for treatment of epiphrenic diverticula: Manometric and clinical analysis. Arch Surg 127:585, 1992.
17. Strietz JM, Williamson WA, Ellis FH: Current concepts regarding the nature and treatment of Barrett's esophagus and its complications. Ann Thorac Surg 54:586, 1992.
18. Vantrappen G, Hellemans J: Treatment of achalasia and related disorders. Gastroenterology 79:144, 1980.
19. Webb WA: Management of foreign bodies of the upper gastrointestinal tract. Gastroenterology 94:204, 1988.

79. SURGERY FOR PEPTIC ULCER DISEASE

Anne M. Flynn, M.D.

DUODENAL ULCER

1. What are the classic indications for peptic ulcer surgery?
Operative intervention is generally reserved for complications of peptic ulcer disease (PUD). The most common complications are intractability, hemorrhage, perforation and obstruction.

2. List the major goals in the surgical treatment of peptic ulcer disease.
1. Eliminate the pathology causing the ulcer
2. Treat the complications (i.e. perforation, obstruction, etc.)
3. Choose the treatment with the least amount of side effects

3. What is the role of *Helicobacter pylori* in the pathogenesis of gastric and duodenal ulceration?
There appears to be an association between *H. pylori* infection and peptic ulceration. *H. pylori* has been isolated from the gastric antral mucosa in a large percentage of cases of duodenal ulceration. However, 20% of healthy volunteers harbor *H. pylori* and are asymptomatic. This finding further supports the hypothesis that the pathogenesis of PUD is most likely multifactorial. However, if *Helicobacter* infection is identified in a patient with an active or remote history of duodenal ulcer, it should be treated.

4. Name the three surgical procedures that have been most widely employed for PUD.
Truncal vagotomy and drainage
Truncal vagotomy and antrectomy
Proximal gastric vagotomy

5. Why is a "drainage procedure" always added to a truncal vagotomy?
Truncal vagotomy involves the division of both vagal trunks at the esophageal hiatus. This denervates the mucosa in the fundus that produces acid as well as other vagally supplied viscera. However, it also significantly impairs gastric emptying. Therefore, a procedure to eliminate the pyloric sphincter function is done, usually a pyloroplasty.

6. What is the difference between a Billroth I and a Billroth II reconstruction?
The **Billroth I** procedure consists of gastroduodenostomy with anastomosis of the remaining stomach (following partial gastric resection) to the duodenum. It is considered to be more physiologic than a Billroth II.

The **Billroth II** operation consists of gastrojejunostomy with anastomosis of the gastric remnant to a loop of jejunum (side-to-side, usually posterior). A potential complication specific to the Billroth II anastomosis is afferent (Aff) loop syndrome.

7. Who was Billroth?
Christian Albert Theodor Billroth (1829–1894) was an outstanding European surgical innovator. German born and Berlin educated, he was the first surgeon to perform extensive operations on the pharynx, larynx, and stomach. He published honest reports of his results, both good and bad, and encouraged others to do the same.

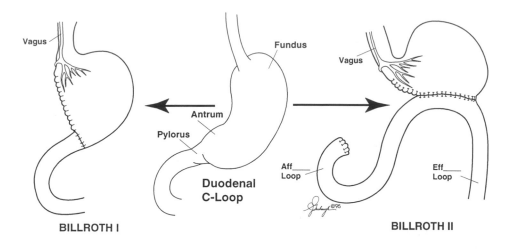

BILLROTH I

BILLROTH II

8. Define truncal vagotomy, selective vagotomy, and highly selective vagotomy.

Truncal vagotomy involves complete division of the anterior and posterior vagal trunk at the esophageal hiatus (see Figure 2).

Selective vagotomy preserves the hepatic and celiac branches of the vagi (which, when interrupted, as in truncal vagotomy, predisposes to gallstones and diarrhea). Clinical experience has *not* shown it to be superior to truncal vagotomy in the treatment of duodenal ulcer disease.

Highly selective vagotomy, also known as proximal gastric vagotomy or parietal cell vagotomy, involves dissection of the anterior and posterior vagal trunks off the esophagus (approxi-

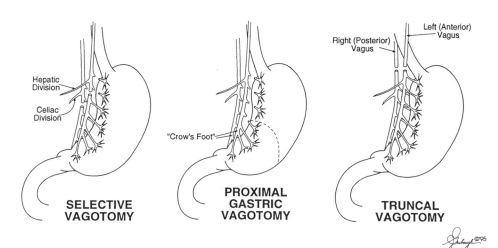

SELECTIVE VAGOTOMY

PROXIMAL GASTRIC VAGOTOMY

TRUNCAL VAGOTOMY

Figure 2. Three standard forms of vagotomy.

mately 6 cm), and then ligation and cutting of each small branch along the lesser curve (anterior and posterior), leaving intact the two terminal branches of the anterior and posterior nerves of Latarjet. This preserves the antral and pyloric innervation, thereby retaining normal antral pump function and pyloric emptying.

9. Compare the physiologic consequences of truncal vagotomy and proximal gastric vagotomy.

	TRUNCAL VAGOTOMY	PROXIMAL GASTRIC VAGOTOMY
Basal acid secretion	↓	↓
Pentagastrin-stimulated MAO	↓	↓
Postoperative gastrin level	↑	↑
Solid emptying rate	↑	No change
Liquid emptying rate	↑	↑
Pancreatic exocrine secretion	↓	No change
Post-cibal biliary secretion	↓	No change
Fecal fat excretion	↑	No change

MAO—maximum acid output.

10. How do you define intractability? What is the operation of choice?
Intractability is failure of mucosal healing with maximal medical treatment. Specific criteria for refractory ulcers include:
    (1) Persistence of ulceration at 3 months despite medical treatment;
    (2) Recurrence of ulcers within 1 year while on maintenance therapy;
    (3) Cycles of prolonged active ulcers with brief or absent remissions.
    These three criteria are indications for surgical therapy, but what operation? Most surgeons agree that proximal gastric vagotomy affords the lowest operative mortality rate (0.5%), the lowest incidence of postoperative complications (<5%), and an acceptable risk of recurrent ulcer (5–10%).

11. The advent of H_2 receptor antagonists has not changed the incidence of hemorrhagic complications associated with PUD. When, then, is operative intervention indicated?
    Upper GI endoscopy is effective in diagnosis and, on occasion, therapy for bleeding duodenal ulcers. However, 70% of bleeding duodenal ulcers will stop spontaneously (sometimes temporarily) without intervention. Some basic guidelines for indications for surgery for bleeding duodenal ulcers include:
    (1) Massive hemorrhage causing shock or cardiovascular instability (after appropriate hemodynamic stabilization)
    (2) Continued blood loss requiring multiple transfusions
    (3) Recurrent bleeding during medical therapy or after endoscopic therapy

12. What operation should be done?
Duodenotomy with direct ligation of the bleeding vessel, followed by an acid-reduction procedure, either truncal vagotomy with pyloroplasty (my first choice) or truncal vagotomy with antrectomy (less appealing since it has higher morbidity and mortality with the antrectomy, i.e., anastomotic leak, blown duodenal stump, pancreatic injury).

13. A 43-year old male smoker presents with complaints of sudden and severe epigastric pain. Physical exam reveals a temperature of 100.8°F, tachycardia, and a rigid abdomen. Upright abdominal x-ray shows free air. After resuscitation, this patient should undergo exploratory laparotomy with closure of the perforation. What operation should be done to treat the underlying PUD?
    Approximately two-thirds of all patients who present with perforation have chronic symptoms and are therefore at risk for recurrent disease. These patients should have a definitive antiulcer op-

eration. Basic criteria to assist in making the decision include (1) history or anatomic evidence of chronic ulceration (i.e., scarring); (2) no preoperative shock; (3) no life-threatening medical problems; and (4) perforation of <48 hours' duration. If above criteria are not met, then simple omental patching is probably the safest approach.

In this case, the options include (1) truncal vagotomy and pyloroplasty; (2) proximal gastric vagotomy and patch closure of the perforation; or (3) truncal vagotomy and antrectomy.

14. What is the role of endoscopy in the patient with gastric outlet obstruction?
Gastric outlet obstruction is a complication of PUD characterized by inflammation and scarring of the pylorus, preventing adequate emptying of the stomach. Upper endoscopy is employed to confirm the obstruction and to exclude neoplasm. Also, endoscopic hydrostatic balloon dilatation of the pyloric stenosis may be attempted. Occasionally, this procedure is palliative, but usually operative intervention is necessary.

15. What is the operative procedure of choice in gastric outlet obstruction?
The goals are to relieve the obstruction and to treat the underlying ulcer disease.
    1. Truncal vagotomy and antrectomy (antrectomy may be technically prohibitive in the face of marked pyloric scarring)
    2. Truncal vagotomy and drainage (either via pyloroplasty or gastroenterostomy)
    3. Proximal gastric vagotomy with pyloroplasty or posterior gastroenterostomy (controversial)

16. What are the immediate and long-term complications associated with the surgeries for PUD?

Complications Associated with Surgery for PUD

	TRUNCAL VAGOTOMY AND DRAINAGE (%)	TRUNCAL VAGOTOMY AND ANTRECTOMY (%)	PROXIMAL GASTRIC VAGOTOMY (%)
Mortality	0.5–1	1–2	0.5
Dumping			
Mild	10	10–15	<5
Disabling	1	1–2	0
Diarrhea			
Mild	25	20	<5
Disabling	2	1–2	0

17. What is the rate of recurrent ulcers associated with these procedures?

Ulcer Recurrence

Truncal vagotomy and drainage	12%
Truncal vagotomy and antrectomy	1–2%
Proximal gastric vagotomy	10–15%

18. What is alkaline reflux gastritis? How is it treated?
Alkaline reflux gastritis is usually seen following truncal vagotomy and drainage or resection. It occurs transiently in 10–20% and persists in approximately 1–2% of patients. It is defined by a triad of findings:
    a. Postprandial epigastric pain often associated with nausea and vomiting
    b. Documented reflux of bile into the stomach
    c. Histologic evidence of gastritis
After establishing the diagnosis with endoscopy and possibly a radionuclide scan, attempted management includes antacids, H_2 receptors, antagonists, bile acid chelators, and diet manipulations. However, none of these have proved to be universally beneficial. The only proven treatment has been operative diversion usually via conversion to a Roux-en-Y gastrojejunostomy with a 50–60-cm limb.

GASTRIC ULCER

19. Can benign and malignant gastric ulcers be differentiated without biopsy?

Clinically, it is usually impossible to differentiate benign from malignant gastric ulcers based on symptoms alone. On **upper GI films,** benign ulcers tend to have a smooth outline and a flat ulcer base, with radiation of the mucosal folds to the edge of the ulcer crater. Malignant gastric ulcers tend to have a mass in the vicinity of the ulcer, with a nodular or irregular ulcer base and abnormal mucosal folds. On esophagoduodenoscopy, biopsies are performed (usually 9–10) to confirm the benign or malignant status. However, there is an approximate 5% incidence of false-negatives.

20. Name the five types of gastric ulcer.

Type I   Located on body of the stomach, usually on the lesser curve (*see* Figure 3)
              Associated with low to normal acid output
              Comprise 50–60% of gastric ulcers

Type II   Located on body of the stomach, *in combination* with a duodenal ulcer
              Usually associated with high acid output
              Comprise 20% of gastric ulcers

Type III   Prepyloric ulcer
              Associated with high acid output
              Comprise 20% of gastric ulcers

Type IV   Located high on lesser curve, near gastroesophageal junction
              Incidence = <10%

Type V   Recently described ulcer
              Develops secondary to long-term use of nonsteroidal
                anti-inflammatory drugs (NSAIDs)
              Carry significant risk for perforation and hemorrhage, with patients
                remaining asymptomatic until presentation
              Misoprostol (a synthetic prostaglandin) effectively decreases the risk of
                gastric ulcers in patients taking NSAID

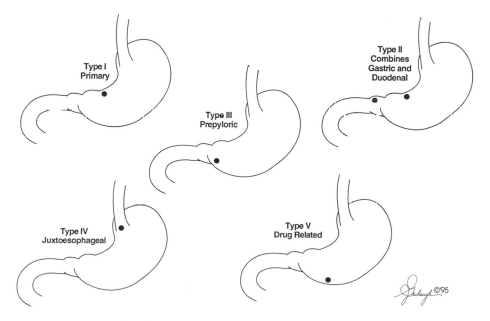

Figure 3. Anatomic sites of the five types of gastric ulcers.

21 What is the natural history of a gastric ulcer? What percentage of gastric ulcers require surgical intervention?

The natural history of gastric ulcers is characterized by episodes of quiescence and relapse, which correspond to healing and recurrence. Rates of relapse are as high as 70% in 1 year, and ulcers usually recur at the same site.

Complications requiring surgical intervention occur in 8–20% of patients. Perforation is the most frequent complication, followed by hemorrhage (35–40%) and, rarely, obstruction.

22. What are the indications for *elective* surgical treatment of a gastric ulcer? What are the key surgical goals?

The complications of gastric ulcer are similar to those of duodenal ulcer—hemorrhage, perforation, and (rarely) obstruction. These complications require surgical intervention. Indications for **elective surgical therapy** include persistent bleeding, failure to heal, recurrence, and suspicion for malignancy. Key principles in surgical therapy include total excision of the ulcer and reduction in gastric secretion.

23. What operation is indicated for the patient with a Type I gastric ulcer who presents with persistent bleeding (has required 4 units) but is still hemodynamically stable?

A Type I gastric ulcer is located on the body of the stomach, usually the lesser curve. The elective operation of choice for a Type I gastric ulcer is a distal gastrectomy (with the ulcer included) with a gastroduodenal (Billroth I) or gastrojejunal (Billroth II) anastomosis.

Operative mortality is approximately 2–3%; the recurrence rate is 3%. An alternative procedure would be proximal gastric vagotomy with excision of the ulcer.

24. How does surgical treatment differ for a Type II gastric ulcer?

Surgical therapy for a Type II gastric ulcer is based on excising the ulcer *and* reducing acid secretion. Operative options include antrectomy (which includes the ulcer) with truncal vagotomy and either a Billroth I or Billroth II reconstruction (preferably Billroth I). An acceptable alternative would be truncal vagotomy and drainage with excision of the ulcer.

25. In a 55-year-old man with a large prepyloric ulcer that has failed to heal with omeprazole, what is the procedure of choice? Why not do a proximal gastric vagotomy?

Surgical therapy for a Type III gastric ulcer is usually a vagotomy and antrectomy (to include the ulcer). Proximal gastric vagotomy has not been found to be successful in the management of pyloric channel or prepyloric ulcers, because recurrence rates have been reported to be >30%.

26. What are the surgical options for Type IV gastric ulcers?

The surgical treatment of a Type IV (or high-lying) gastric ulcer can be technically challenging. Factors to be considered include size of the ulcer, distance from the gastroesophageal junction, and degree of surrounding inflammation. One acceptable technique would be distal gastrectomy with vertical extension of the resection, to include the lesser curvature (including the ulcer), followed by gastroduodenostomy. Another approach is excision of the ulcer via an anterior gastrostomy with transverse closure of the defect.

27. What is a giant gastric ulcer? How is it treated?

A giant gastric ulcer is an ulcer whose diameter is ≥3 cm. These are most commonly located on the lesser curve. The incidence of malignancy increases with their size. They are associated with a high rate of complications, and therefore early resection is recommended.

BIBLIOGRAPHY

1. Beahrs OH, Beart RW, Pemberton JH (eds): Surgical Consultations. St. Louis, C.V. Mosby, 1993.
2. Csendes A, Maluenda F, Braghetto I, et al: Prospective randomized study comparing three surgical techniques for the treatment of gastric outlet obstruction secondary to duodenal ulcer. Am J Surg 166:45–49, 1993.

3. Donahue PE, Richter HM, Liu KJ, et al: Experimental basis and clinical application of extended highly selective vagotomy for duodenal ulcer. Surg Gynecol Obstet 176:39–48, 1993.
4. Emas S, Grupcer G, Eriksson B: Ten-year follow-up of a prospective randomized trial of selective proximal vagotomy with ulcer excision and partial gastrectomy with gastroduodenostomy for treating corporeal gastric ulcer. Am J Surg 167:596–600, 1994.
5. Feliciano DV: Do perforated duodenal ulcers need an acid-decreasing surgical procedure now that omeprazole is available? Surg Clin North Am 72:369–380, 1992.
6. Greenfield LJ, et al (eds): Surgery: Scientific Principles and Practice. New York, McGraw-Hill, 1994.
7. Jordan PH: Operations for duodenal ulcer disease. Annu Rev Med 40:1–15, 1989.
8. Miedema BW, Torres PR, Farnell MB, et al: Proximal gastric vagotomy in the emergency treatment of bleeding duodenal ulcer. Am J Surg 161:64–68, 1991.
9. Rizoli SB, Neto AC, Diorio AC, et al: Risk of complication in perforated duodenal ulcer operations according to the surgical technique employed. Am Surg 59:312–314, 1993.
10. Sabiston DC: Atlas of General Surgery. Philadelphia, W.B. Saunders, 1994.
11. Schwartz SI, Shires GT, Spencer FC (eds): Principles of Surgery, 6th ed. New York, McGraw Hill, 1994.
12. Stabile BE: Current surgical management of duodenal ulcers. Surg Clin North Am 72:335–356, 1992.
13. Zfass AM, McHenry L Jr, Sanyal AJ: Nonsteroidal anti- inflammatory drug-induced gastroduodenal lesions: Prophylaxis and treatment. Gastroenterologist 1(2):165–169, 1993.

80. SURGICAL APPROACH TO THE ACUTE ABDOMEN

Ben Eiseman, M.D.

1. What causes of abdominal pain characteristically start with an acute onset of severe pain?

Ruptured ectopic pregnancy
Renal passage of a biliary tract stone
Pancreatitis
Vascular occlusion
Twisted ovarian cyst
Small bowel obstruction caused by adhesions (sometimes)

2. What about ruptured abdominal aortic aneurysm and ruptured peptic ulcer?

Patients with a rupturing abdominal aortic aneurysm usually have initial sharp but not very severe pain radiating to the back before it develops into major discomfort. This signals that a small daughter aneurysm starts to leak into the retroperitoneal space.

Patients with a perforated duodenal or gastric ulcer usually notice some discomfort of the rupturing ulcer before perforation.

3. What are the common causes of duodenal and high small bowel obstruction in neonates and infants?

Duodenal webs and atresia (commonly accompanied by other congenital abnormalities, including Down's syndrome)
Hypertrophic pyloric stenosis
Annular pancreas
Intestinal malrotation
Small bowel atresia

4. What are the more common causes of abdominal pain in the elderly?

Small bowel ischemia caused by mesenteric artery occlusion
Cancers of various types causing obstruction
Diverticular disease
Gallstones and cholecystitis
Sigmoid volvulus
Deceptively mild course of appendicitis

5. Following penetrating injury of the torso by multiple fragments, such as produced by a bomb explosion, what is the proper management of a patient found to have multiple fragment holes, some of which have a wound of entrance in the back?

A first and most important step is to look for such holes, even though this requires rolling the patient during examination to examine the back. An experienced trauma surgeon immediately becomes suspicious of injury of the retroperitoneal duodenum, pancreas, or colon. Penetrating injuries of these viscera may not be accompanied by immediate signs of peritonitis. Other things being equal, such injuries require exploratory laparotomy with careful inspection of the retroperitoneal space and opening of the posterior peritoneum if there is any sign of injury or bleeding. Such injuries are far easier to repair in the immediate postinjury period than 2–3 days later after an abscess has formed.

6. Following severe, blunt abdominal trauma, a patient has acute abdominal pain. An ultrasound shows a crack in the liver. Is there any place for watchful waiting?

Yes. BUT, the patient must be young and healthy, he or she must remain hemodynamically stable, and there must be no evidence of other intra-abdominal injuries.

Contrary to previous teachings, a little blood and bile in the peritoneal cavity will not necessarily result in disaster. The surgical team must be ready to perform laparotomy. Occasional cases are being reported in which such liver lacerations are treated laparoscopically. If they can be so treated, they probably need no treatment, and if they are significant, they should be treated by open operation.

7. Are these warnings equally true of a cracked spleen? Is it ever prudent to watch such blunt injuries?

In general, small lacerations of the spleen and liver following blunt injury can be managed similarly. Injuries to the liver leak bile into the peritoneal cavity, and indications for laparotomy should be more liberal than for splenic injuries.

Long-term follow-up of splenic injuries shows that even separated fragments may grow back together after some months. If laparotomy is indicated, partial splenectomy sometimes is easy, but if the spleen is crushed, no heroic attempts should be made to preserve splenic tissue because of fear of subsequent overwhelming gram-positive infections in the splenectomized patient. In infants and young children (no restraining seatbelts), added efforts can justifiably be made to preserve splenic tissue, but not at the risk of prolonging laparotomy time in a youngster who usually has many other intra-abdominal injuries.

8. How long should one persist in the medical management of an obstructing duodenal ulcer?

Factors affecting this decision include:

1. **Chronicity of the ulcer:** Acute ulcers, particularly those in the pyloric channel, may resolve rapidly and not produce prolonged obstruction. Old scarred ulcers with extensive narrowing are unlikely to remain open for long, even if they open spontaneously or with balloon dilation.

2. **Recurrent obstruction:** If obstruction has occurred previously, it is likely to happen again, and early operation is advisable.

3. **Response to medical management:** If the obstruction is not relieved by medical treatment in 5–7 days, it seems logical to provide the benefit of operation. Surgery offers an early return to ability to eat and an excellent chance for relief from subsequent ulcer symptoms. The immediate need for operation has been removed for this duodenal ulcer, and now surgeons can balance factors such as cost and convenience.

4. Discovery of the role of *H. pylori* infection in prolonging symptoms of ulcer makes its vigorous antibiotic treatment a valid option instead of immediate operative intervention.

9. "One should not allow the sun to rise or set on small bowel obstruction." Is the old maxim still valid?

Yes, the principle of early operative relief of small bowel obstruction is still valid. It should be modulated by evidence of impending perforation or vascular compromise, or by evidence of relief of total obstruction. If after 12 hours, there is no improvement despite nasogastric suction and fluid and electrolyte correction, there has to be some other good reason *not* to operate if the obstruction appears to be due to mechanical causes. Delay is riskier than laparotomy.

10. If early operation is advised for small bowel obstruction, why is delay possible in large bowel obstruction?

The small bowel is more likely to perforate. The colon has much greater capacity to dilate. Its mesentery, in contrast to the small bowels, is relatively fixed and less prone to vascular impairment.

11. What are the common causes of acute abdominal pain associated with a mass in the cecal area?

- Appendiceal abscess
- Carcinoma of the cecum
- Rarely, tuberculoma, ameboma, fungal infection, or retained foreign body (sponge) following a previous laparotomy

Occasionally at the time of laparotomy, the surgeon cannot determine the cause of the mass, even with extensive biopsies. Treatment is then right colectomy with ileotransverse colon anastomosis.

12. How is right colon obstruction due to Ogilvie's syndrome treated?

Resection of the distended and adynamic portion of the colon. In my experience, cecostomy is only an acceptable option in a desperately ill patient, when the surgeons believe that more extensive procedures might be fatal. Such a procedure leaves the adynamic colon in place and, in my experience, does not relieve subsequent obstruction.

13. In a patient requiring laparotomy for Crohn's disease, how do you decide how much bowel to resect?

If the operation is for obstruction, resect only the obstructed portion. You should resist temptation to excise all involved bowel, even if this involves performing an anastomosis through a slightly diseased portion of bowel. Unfortunately, you will probably be back at a later date, and in the meantime, the patient will be grateful for all the remaining small bowel that can be saved.

14. Is balloon dilation of a Crohn's stricture worth trying?

Yes, why not? Its ultimate benefit is still not proven, but the procedure has limited morbidity, if limited to short segments of obstruction. If it does not work, laparotomy is always possible thereafter.

15. What is the surgeon's role in the management of peptic ulcer disease?

Surgery has been and still is of value in the care of complications of ulcer disease. Improved medical treatment has changed the need for operation, but the classic indications for operation remain, although their frequency has changed.

1. **Perforation:** Few will deny that operation is indicated for early perforation of a peptic ulcer, but opinions differ as to whether perforations should be closed via laparoscopy or open laparotomy. The role of definitive operation at the time of closure remains, but these are details.

2. **Obstruction:** Currently there is enthusiasm for balloon dilatation to relieve obstruction from a scarred duodenal ulcer, but its long-term usefulness remains to be proven. With adequate intravenous support, such nonoperative treatment should be tried. In marginally obstructed ulcers, such dilation may prove helpful, although more extensive fibrotic masses will be more difficult to treat via this technique. It is possible that elimination of *Helicobacter pylori,* which may play a role in causing such obstruction to persist, may have some value, but operation provides a relatively simple, quick, and immediate relief of symptoms.

3. **Intractability:** The frequency of intractable ulcers has been reduced dramatically thanks to H_2 and proton pump blockers, recognition of the role of *Helicobacter pylori,* and widespread use of surveillance by endoscopy. About the only ulcer intractable to medical management seen these days is in an intractable patient.

4. **Bleeding:** A continued meeting ground between the surgeon and clinician is at the bedside of a patient with massive bleeding caused by a peptic ulcer. Formula and guidelines have been espoused for the timing of surgery, but a simple way to look at this is to decide at what point does the risk of continued nonoperative management begin to exceed the benefit promised by surgery.

16. How has the role of *Helicobacter pylori* altered the surgical management of peptic ulcer disease?

I have already referred to how eliminating *H. pylori* apparently diminishes the number of ulcer recurrences. Since the surgeon operates for complications of ulcer disease, the index of suspicion for *H. pylori* infection should be high and patients should be examined for such by duodenal biopsy. Following operation, such infestation should be sought and, if found, treated. This presumably will improve the combined medical and surgical treatment outcome.

17. Should highly selective vagotomy (HSV) be performed at the time of closure of a perforation?
Certainly not routinely. However, there are cases in which highly selected vagotomy is justified. These are patients who have earned a definitive operation by previous history, where the perforation is recent and peritoneal soiling not too severe, and where the surgeon is skilled in performing the operation without undue waste of operating time. Popularity of HSV is waning owing to the high incidence of late ulcer recurrence.

18. Is a perforated gastric ulcer, at the time of operation, treated any differently than a perforated duodenal ulcer?
No, except that several biopsies of gastric ulcer should be performed to exclude cancer.

19. What is the proper management of a patient with a demonstrated post-traumatic hiatal hernia with stomach in the thorax, who has persistent vomiting and is deteriorating, but whose abdomen is soft?
Such patients are clinically puzzling, because the physical findings do not match their deteriorating condition. The explanation is that the stomach is incarcerated and often strangulated in the thorax—hence, the lack of abdominal signs. Gastroscopy is often impossible since the stomach takes a sharp 180° reversal at the gastroesophageal junction. Proper management is prompt laparotomy and reduction of the incarcerated hiatal hernia. The serosa of the stomach may be frighteningly dark and gangrenous looking. However, after replacement into the abdomen, the stomach is apt to turn pink. The mucosa, being so well vascularized, often is intact.

20. What is the advised treatment of acute abdominal pain in a patient with a proven duodenal ulcer and proven hypergastrinemia?
Causes of hypergastrinemia, other than those due to a pancreatic tumor (Zollinger-Ellison syndrome), must first be excluded. These include those secondary to omeprazole therapy. Associated adenopathies should then be evaluated. The final step is trying to identify the lesion(s) presumably releasing gastrin by computed tomography (CT) or magnetic resonance (MR) angiography, operative ultrasound, or, occasionally, if all else has failed, by venous sampling from suspected sites. The latter approach is decreasingly less necessary. At exploration, evidence of metastases should be sought, and if these are not found, the identified tumor should be locally excised, if possible. Total gastrectomy may be necessary.

21. What is the advised management of acute pancreatitis caused by a biliary tract stone?
Watchful waiting and close observation while the stone passes is warranted for a few hours. If the stone does not pass and the pain persists, endoscopic retrograde cholangiopancreatographic (ERCP) removal should be aggressively attempted. The endoscopist must persist, and the obstruction either bypassed or removed. The major sin is to instrument the pancreatic and biliary ducts and fail to relieve the obstruction. If this cannot be done, a surgeon should immediately perform a laparotomy and manually remove the stone. Following this, recovery is prompt. If not, an aggressive and even fatal pancreatitis can develop.

22. When is laparotomy indicated in a patient with proven acute pancreatitis not associated with a biliary tract stone?
If after 24–28 hours of maximum supportive treatment, the patient is deteriorating as judged by Ranson's criteria, a diagnosis of progressive hemorrhagic or necrotizing pancreatitis can be assumed and laparotomy may be advisable, when all other measures are proved worthless.

What is done, once severe pancreatitis is found at laparotomy, is a matter of continued debate. Such patients have a mortality of perhaps 40%, regardless of treatment. I personally advocate necrosectomy, i.e., removing all dead liquified pancreas and saving the gastroduodenal artery and a rim of pancreas surrounding it, along the lesser curve of the duodenum. Others now believe packing the pancreatic bed and leaving the abdomen widely drained is worth a trial. Many other procedures have been tried, but none obviously is totally beneficial.

23. What is the treatment of a patient with severe abdominal pain from proven pancreatic pseudocysts?

If the patient is not septic and there is no question of a pancreatic abscess, this condition is seldom an emergency requiring immediate laparotomy. However, cysts which on a CT scan are > 2 cm in diameter are unlikely to disappear spontaneously. If they enlarge and cause pain or discomfort, they should be drained by a cystogastrostomy. A preliminary trial with percutaneous drainage is worth trying and, if successful, will avoid laparotomy. These cysts contain thick grumous material as well as fluid, and the floating pancreatic debris does not easily drain through a small percutaneously placed catheter. ERCP drainage through the pancreatic duct, using a stent to keep the duct open, occasionally is feasible.

24. What if this pseudocyst or pancreatic mass becomes septic? What do you do?

Ubi pus, ibi evacua. This maxim pertains to pus in the pancreas just as it does to pus anywhere else. Drain it one way or another—the sooner and the more complete, the better. An abscess in the pancreas is a timebomb sitting on the splenic artery and vein, boring away at its base. No time should be lost. Needle drainage may be tried given 18–24 hours to obtain complete drainage and improvement in signs of infection, but if this fails, prompt wide operative drainage should be performed. If there are multiple abscesses or infected cysts, each should be drained individually. Do not try to poke an exploring finger from one cavity to another through the friable vascular pancreatic bed; disaster will follow.

25. How can you make an early diagnosis of small bowel ischemia due to vascular obstruction?

I wish I knew. A high index of suspicion is necessary in an elderly person with more than usual complaints of abdominal pain, mild leukocytosis, and a vaguely tender abdomen that does not improve.

26. Is base deficit in electrolyte studies useful to the diagnosis of small bowel ischemia?

The test is nonspecific. Arteriography, of course, is more specific, but by the time it is considered, it is better to perform either laparotomy, laparoscopy, or even a diagnostic peritoneal lavage.

27. What are the common causes of ischemic small bowel due to vasculitis, and how should such patients be managed?

For some reason, this problem seems to be increasing in frequency, whether due to increased use of drugs that cause such pathology or simply better recognition. Common causes include the autoimmune diseases, such as polyarteritis nodosum, scleroderma, or systemic lupus erythematosus.

The clinical picture is one of diffuse abdominal discomfort and, sometimes, perforation or generalized peritonitis. By the time surgery is considered, the patient is generally in serious condition. At laparotomy, there usually are multiple areas of ischemia along the small bowel. If any is frankly gangrenous, it must be resected. The anastomosis may be through questionably involved adjacent bowel. Some pass an endoscope both above and below the enterotomy to help evaluate adjacent small bowel involvement. The surgeon should be conservative in resecting small bowel, settling instead for removing the obviously dead gut and hoping that anti-inflammatory medications will stop the inflammatory process. These patients may require a second look in a day or so. In other situations where the viability of the adjacent gut is dangerously compromised, the two ends of the involved small bowel should be exteriorized. They can be re-anastomosed when the process has been brought under control.

28. Following resection and primary anastomosis for small bowel ischemia, do you routinely advise a "second-look" laparotomy 24 hours later to detect unsuspected ischemic bowel segments?

No. I believe this depends upon the primary cause of the ischemia. Obviously this is not sensible if the ischemia is caused by torsion around an adhesion. Similarly, I am hesitant to re-operate lacking other signs if mesenteric artery obstruction is due to an embolus, such as might result from a fibrillating left auricle. If caused by "trash from an atherosclerotic plaque in the mesenteric artery," I would be suspicious of extension. This leaves the difficult problem of mesenteric artery ischemia caused by various types of vasculitis. Unfortunately in such cases, the area of frank bowel gangrene is often accompanied by suspiciously dusky patches of small bowel scattered elsewhere. It is here that a second look might occasionally be indicated. However, in my experience in such patients, even a second or third resection has no better than approximately a one-in-three chance of ultimate success. The problem in such patients is that we have not eradicated the underlying cause of the disease.

29. In a patient with small bowel infarction, where essentially the entire small intestine except a few inches of proximal jejunum and a similar short segment of terminal ileum remains viable, is there a place for performing a very high ileostomy just proximal to the duodenum and a terminal ileostomy of the ileal stump?

This is a difficult call because it depends on one's philosophy. Theoretically, it sounds appealing in lieu of doing nothing and allowing the patient to expire in dignity in a few days. In infants and newborns, perhaps it has more logic. If there are 25 cm of viable small bowel remaining, it certainly is logical. If not, I am plagued by memories of many unhappy patients who for months were maintained in a sorry existence on parenteral nutrition, and fruitless operations to make better use of remaining gut. Currently a procedure using a stapler to make a small-gauge, double-barrel shotgun out of a large bore rifle is being evaluated. I am skeptical, since no new small bowel mucosa is being added. I hope I am proved to be wrong. It wouldn't be the first time.

30. How do you manage a patient with right lower quadrant discomfort, mild tenderness, and diarrhea?

The suspicion is appendicitis versus infectious colitis. Appendicitis is seldom accompanied by diarrhea: one, or rarely, two stools, but no more. If diarrhea exists, operative restraint is justified while stools are examined and cultured. Sigmoidoscopy may be used to try to establish the diagnosis of such infections as *Clostridium difficile*.

31. Is caecum mobilis a cause of acute abdominal pain, and is it an indication for emergency laparotomy?

Rarely. Other causes of such discomfort should be investigated. About the only time that this anatomic variant warrants operation is when there is frank and obvious cecal volvulus—and that is usually obvious by x-ray examination of the abdomen or colonoscopy.

32. Accepted wisdom is to excise the perforated diverticulum of the sigmoid at the time of initial laparotomy. Do you always resect such diverticular abscesses?

The principle is correct, since there will be serious morbidity in about 40% of patients in whom the abscessed sigmoid is left. However, some of these old folks are hemodynamically unstable, and I think it perfectly appropriate to violate the rule on occasion, merely draining the abscess and performing a proximal diverting colostomy. Such a decision accepts the possible morbidity to minimize the chance of a mortality. When the patient is stable and the perforated sigmoid more mobile, the involved defunctionalized distal segment of bowel can be excised more safely.

33. What is the role of nonoperative treatment of sigmoid volvulus in an elderly patient?

Diagnosis usually can be made on the basis of history, physical examination, and an abdominal x-ray. Rarely is a contrast study of the large bowel necessary. When a barium enema is indicated, the radiologist might as well try reduction.

When the twist in the sigmoid cannot be relieved, however, I advocate placing the patient in the jackknife position on the operating table, which in itself often reduces the volvulus. If it does not, then a flexible proctosigmoidoscope can be inserted, which reduces the volvulus in about 90% of cases. This approach is safer (less chance of perforation) and cheaper than colonoscopy, which can be performed if sigmoidoscopy fails.

34. Is there any place for immediate laparotomy for reduction of such volvulus?
Yes. In the rare case in which nonoperative reduction fails. In addition, however, if the elderly patient is in good condition, immediate — or early — laparotomy with sigmoid resection is indicated because the probability of recurrent volvulus after reduction is 50–90%. After sigmoid colectomy, if the diameter of the reduced volvulus is adequately small, a primary anastomosis is possible. If the bowel proximal to the volvulus is unduly distended, then a colostomy is indicated, with later anastomosis to the severed distal rectosigmoid.

35. How do you manage the occasional case of complete large bowel obstruction due apparently to an intrinsic sigmoid mass where endoscopic biopsy cannot establish a diagnosis of cancer, but to the examining finger, the palpable mass feels certain to be neoplasm?
Assuming the obstruction cannot be relieved, laparotomy is indicated, at which time the pelvis characteristically is socked in with a solid mass. Assuming the liver and regional lymph nodes are free of tumor, then the diagnosis, despite the pelvic mass, is probably diverticular disease. A proximal, totally defunctionalizing colostomy should be performed. The mass — if indeed due to diverticular disease — will gradually resolve and a few months later the involved sigmoid can be resected and anastomosis performed.

36. In a patient with a perforated distal sigmoid diverticulum, where other diverticula are noted up to the transverse colon, do you resect all large bowel containing diverticula or merely the area of inflammation?
Only the inflamed and perforated area. For reasons unclear, the proximal diverticula seldom cause subsequent trouble.

37. Any special preoperative treatment of a patient requiring colectomy for an obstructing or acutely inflamed diverticular mass in the rectosigmoid area?
I advocate preoperative placement of a left ureteral catheter to facilitate intraoperative identification of the left ureter, which invariably is encased in the inflammatory mass. Such a palpable catheter minimizes chances of damaging the ureter.

38. How do you manage toxic megacolon in a patient with chronic ulcerative colitis?
These patients usually require intense supportive management in the ICU with massive fluid replacement, blood transfusions, intravenous corticosteroids, and antibiotics. If they fail to improve within 48 hours, a total abdominal colectomy and Brooke ileostomy should be performed.

39. How do you manage a patient with perforated large bowel due to chronic ulcerative colitis?
As soon as the patient is hemodynamically stable, laparotomy should be performed. If the perforated segment can be exteriorized as a loop colostomy, that should be performed. If not, then the site of perforation should be exteriorized by a Turnbull "blow hole" to provide temporary diversion of the fecal stream. In these patients with generalized peritonitis, it is seldom wise to perform a total abdominal colectomy removing all diseased colon. Seldom is this the place for one-stage heroics.

40. Is routine operative cholangiogram advised at the time of cholecystectomy?
Assuming that an ERCP has not been performed preoperatively, and no evidence at exploration suggests the need for common duct exploration, I believe that such an intraoperative dye study is indicated at the time of open laparotomy. The rationale is that in about 5% of patients, an unsuspected stone will be found. This classic teaching must now be modified, however, since a retained common duct stone can be removed more easily via an endoscope. It does not require operation.

The answer is not yet certain concerning cholangiography during laparoscopic cholecystectomy. Those with a good deal of experience can perform such a study in a short time. If a stone is found, then the options are (1) explore the duct via the laparoscope, (2) convert the procedure to laparotomy and explore the duct, or (3) leave the stone and have it removed by ERCP following the laparoscopic cholecystectomy. The best answer is evolving.

41. How long can you treat a patient with suspected appendicitis nonoperatively?
In general, laparotomy is advisable after 18–24 hours if the patient is not improving or another diagnosis is not established. In some cases, laparoscopy is helpful, and of course, laparoscopic appendectomy can be performed.

If such a patient has been observed overnight—and somehow this seems to be the usual case—make the decision to operate before 7 AM, when the next day's operating schedule starts. A decision after about 5 AM usually means that an elective case can be bumped, or the operation for appendicitis delayed until the next afternoon.

42. How do you differentiate between right-sided pelvic inflammatory disease (PID) and appendicitis in a young woman?
Ask about the obvious risk factors of gonorrhea or chlamydia, as well as the recent insertion of an intrauterine device. Discomfort and tenderness are characteristically greater in the pelvis than in the lower abdomen in PID, but this can be confusing. Cervical smear or culture is positive in about 30% of cases for chlamydia or gonococcus. Sometimes, a pelvic ultrasound, culdoscopy, or laparoscopy is advisable.

43. If you performed laparotomy in such a patient and found PID, what should you do?
Assuming there is not an established abscess, simply remove the appendix and get out. The gynecologist can treat the infected fallopian tube with antibiotics. If there is an established abscess, it should be drained widely. There is no longer any indication for performing a total abdominal hysterectomy and bilateral tubo-ovarian resection, as was formerly advocated. These days, the threat of generalized infection is minimized.

44. What is the management of a twisted ovarian cyst causing acute abdominal pain?
In addition to history and physical examination, ultrasound should be diagnostic. If the twisted cyst is ischemic, its base should be clamped (not untwisted) before its excision. Release of the ischemic cyst by untwisting can flood the patient with cytokines caused by the ischemic mass and produce profound shock.

45. During surgery to explore abdominal pain, you discover a solid mass in the ovary > 5 cm in diameter. What should you do?
If a gynecologist is not available for consultation, such a solid mass should be assumed to be an ovarian cancer in a woman over 40. The other ovary should be palpated. A bilateral mass increases the likelihood of malignancy. The solid mass should be removed, but first, the tumor should be staged by obtaining peritoneal washings for tumor cells and excising regional and periaortic nodes.

If the ovary and the mass is < 5 cm in diameter, and particularly in a younger woman, then the mass may be left and followed carefully after the operation.

46. What is the current treatment of hypertrophic pyloric stenosis in a child?
About the same as it has been for 50 years: early operation through a small RUQ incision and a pyloromyotomy. Ultrasound may confirm a pyloric "olive" caused by the hypertrophied muscle encircling the pylorus.

47. How do you manage a patient with persistent upper abdominal and back pain following an ERCP?
This problem was more common a decade ago, when surgeons and gastroenterologists were learning the techniques and were unfamiliar with the mild discomfort that often follows ERCP. Now, the mystique has disappeared from endoscopy, and generalists and nonphysician technicians are becoming skilled in surveillance endoscopy.

Abnormal pain raises suspicion of a bile leak from a perforation in the bile or pancreatic duct. Films taken during the procedure should be reviewed for evidence of leak, and the patient observed closely if none is found. If an obvious bile leak is found, it may be treated by repeating endoscopy and placing a catheter above the leak, bypassing the tear. If there is any question, however, the time for operative repair is immediately. If it is done while the tissue is still firm, it is relatively easy. Two or more days later, the area is inflamed, and little more than T-tube placement and drainage of the area are feasible. Lacking evidence of bile duct perforation, the patient is treated for pancreatitis primarily by watchful waiting and support.

48. Following esophagogastroscopy for achalasia, a patient complains of left chest and abdominal pain. You suspect esophageal perforation. What should be done?
Posteroanterior and lateral films of the chest and abdominal x-rays may show free air beneath the diaphragm, or pneumothorax. Contrast studies of the esophagus seldom are necessary or demonstrate the small perforation. In such a patient, early thoracotomy should be performed, and the perforation in the distal esophagus closed. This should be followed by a definitive Heller myotomy from a point well on the stomach up to the arch of the aorta. A wrap of the fundus of the stomach around the site of perforation is advisable and helps to seal the leak.

49. What are the more common causes of acute abdominal pain in a patient with AIDS?
In addition to conditions that might cause abdominal pain in other patients, one must also consider the following:
Discomfort due to drugs commonly used in treatment of AIDS
Pancreatitis
Diverticulitis
Small bowel inflammation, ulceration, and, occasionally, perforation caused by iatrogenic
     infections, such as cytomegalovirus or sporotrichosis
Small bowel lymphoma

BIBLIOGRAPHY

1. Cope Z, Silen W: Early Diagnosis of the Acute Abdomen, 18th ed. Oxford, Universal Press, 1991.
2. Norton L, Steele G, Eiseman B: Surgical Decision Making, 3rd ed. Philadelphia, W.B. Saunders, 1993.

81. COLORECTAL SURGERY

Bradley G. Bute, M.D.

POLYPOSIS SYNDROMES AND INFLAMMATORY BOWEL DISEASE

1. What are the different types of intestinal polyps?
Neoplastic, hamartomatous, inflammatory/lymphoid, and hyperplastic.

2. What is a hamartoma?
A hamartoma is an exuberant growth of normal tissue in an abnormal amount or location. An isolated hamartomatous polyp has no malignant potential.

3. Which intestinal polyposis syndromes are associated with hamartomatous polyps?
Peutz-Jeghers syndrome
Juvenile polyposis (familial or generalized)
Cronkhite-Canada syndrome (hamartomatous polyps with alopecia, cutaneous pigmentation, and toenail and fingernail atrophy)
Intestinal ganglioneuromatosis (isolated or with von Recklinghausen's disease or multiple endocrine neoplasia type 2)
Ruvalcaba-Myrhe-Smith syndrome (polyps of colon and tongue, macrocephaly, retardation, unique facies, pigmented penile macules)
Cowden's disease (GI polyps with oral and cutaneous verrucous papules [tricholemmomas], associated with breast cancer, thyroid neoplasia, and ovarian cysts)

4. How is Peutz-Jeghers syndrome manifest?
This autosomal dominant trait is often heralded by the presence of melanin spots on the lips and buccal mucosa. Hamartomas are almost always present on the small intestine and occasionally hamartomas on the stomach and colon.

5. Do the hamartomatous polyposis diseases have malignant potential?
In the past, the malignant potential for hamartomatous polyps was considered nil. Recent reviews have suggested an increased incidence of GI cancers in patients with multiple hamartomatous polyposis syndromes. A hamartoma-adenoma-carcinoma sequence has been postulated for Peutz-Jeghers syndrome, and these patients also seem to be at increased risk for extraintestinal cancers, including sex cord tumors and pancreatic and breast cancer. Generalized juvenile polyposis is now considered to be a premalignant state as well, with associated malignant degeneration of the polyps.

6. Describe familial adenomatous polyposis (FAP).
FAP is a mendelian-dominant, non–sex-linked disease in which >100 adenomatous polyps affect the colon and rectum. One-third of patients present as the propositus case (presumed mutation) with no prior family history. The disease invariably leads to invasive colon cancer if not treated. The average age at diagnosis of colon cancer is 39 years, as compared with 65 years for routine colon cancer.

7. What extracolonic abnormalities are associated with FAP?

BENIGN	MALIGNANT
Congenital hypertrophy of retinal pigment epithelium (CHRPE)	Gastric cancer
	Periampullary carcinoma
Gastric fundic gland polyps	Duodenal adenocarcinoma
Antral adenomas	Pancreatic adenocarcinoma
Duodenal adenomas	Cholangiocarcinoma
Jejunoileal adenomas	Small intestinal carcinoma
Desmoid tumors	Ileal carcinoids
Adrenal adenomas	Adrenal adenocarcinoma
Pituitary adenomas	Medulloblastoma
	Turcot's syndrome or glioblastoma
	Thyroid carcinoma
	Osteogenic sarcoma
	Hepatoblastoma

8. What is Gardner's syndrome?

FAP plus fibromas of the skin, osteomas (typically of the mandible, maxilla, and skull), epidermoid cysts, desmoid tumors, and extra dentition.

9. How does one screen for FAP?

Historically, rigid proctosigmoidoscopy beginning at about puberty was used to look for rectosigmoid polyps. This method has been replaced by flexible sigmoidoscopy. Screening is recommended every 6–12 months until age 40, after which age the development of FAP is rare (although occasionally it develops between ages 40–60.)

State-of-the-art presymptomatic detection utilizes molecular genetic screening. FAP is caused by mutation in the adenomatous polyposis coli (APC) gene on the long arm of chromosome 5 at the 5q21–q22 locus. Restrictive fragment length polymorphism linkage analysis can determine if an individual is affected with >95–99% certainty if genetic material is available from affected and unaffected individuals in the kindred. Direct determination of somatic mutations in the APC gene may be detectable in spontaneous cases of FAP.

Ophthalmoscopic examination for congenital hypertrophy of the retinal pigment epithelium (CHRPE) can detect involved individuals as early as 3 months of age with a 97% positive predictive value for developing FAP. CHRPE is present in 55–100% of FAP patients and is documented with wide-angle fundus photography.

10. What is Crohn's disease?

A nonspecific inflammatory disease that may involve any portion of the GI tract; regional enteritis commonly causes abdominal pain and diarrhea. The distribution of disease in the GI tract may be discontinuous. Presenting patterns are ileocolic in about 40%, colonic Crohn's alone in 30%, small bowel involvement alone in 25%, and anorectal disease alone in 5%.

11. What is ulcerative colitis?

It is also a nonspecific inflammatory bowel disease that involves the colon and rectum. Bloody diarrhea is the classic presenting symptom. Disease may be limited to the rectum (proctitis), left colon (proctosigmoiditis), or entire colon (pancolitis). The rectum is *always* involved; the disease process is one of continuous inflammation (no skip areas).

12. How does one differentiate Crohn's disease from ulcerative colitis?

Comparison of Ulcerative Colitis and Crohn's Colitis

	ULCERATIVE COLITIS	CROHN'S COLITIS
Clinical manifestations		
Bleeding per rectum	3+	1+
Diarrhea	3+	3+
Abdominal pain	1+	3+ (esp with ileal involvement)
Fever	R	2+
Palpable abdominal mass	R	2+
Internal fistula	R	4+
Intestinal obstruction (stricture or infection)	0	4+
Rectal involvement	4+	1+
Small bowel involvement	0	4+
Anal and perianal involvement	R	4+
Thumbprinting sign on barium enema	R	1+
Risk of cancer	2+	1+
Clinical course	Relapses/ remissions	Slowly progressive
Gross appearance		
Thickened bowel wall	0	4+
Shortening of bowel	2+	R
Fat creeping onto serosa	0	4+
Segmental involvement	0	4+
Aphthous ulcer	0	4+
Linear ulcer	0	4+
Microscopic picture		
Depth of involvement	Mucosa and submucosa	Full thickness
Lymphoid aggregation	0	4+
Sarcoid-type granuloma	0	4+
Fissuring	0	2+
Surgical treatment		
Total proctocolectomy	"Gold standard"	Indicated in total large bowel involvement
Segmental resection	Infrequent	Frequent
Ileal pouch procedure	Excellent option in selected patients	Contraindicated
Recurrence after surgery	0	3+

Symbols: R = rare; 0 = not found; 1+ = may be present; 2+ = common; 3+ = usual finding; 4+ = characteristic (not necessarily common).
From Nivatvongs S: The colon, rectum and anal canal. In James EC, Corry RJ, Perry JF Jr (eds): Basic Surgical Practice. Philadelphia, Hanley & Belfus, 1987, p 325.

13. What are the surgical indications for ulcerative colitis?

Intractability or failure of medical management
Fulminant colitis
Toxic megacolon
Massive bleeding
Prophylaxis of carcinoma (presence of high-grade dysplasia)
Treatment of carcinoma
Palliation of cutaneous and systemic (extracolonic) manifestations.

14. Identify the extracolonic manifestations of ulcerative colitis.

Skin—pyoderma gangrenosum, erythema nodosum
Liver—fatty infiltration of the liver, pericholangitis, cirrhosis
Biliary—Primary sclerosing cholangitis, bile duct carcinoma

Eye—uveitis, episcleritis, conjunctivitis, retrobulbar neuritis
Joints—monoarticular arthritis, ankylosing spondylitis, sacroiliitis
Mouth—aphthous ulcers, stomatitis
Renal—pyelonephritis, nephrolithiasis
Systemic—amyloidosis, thromboembolic disease, hypercoaguability, vasculitis, pericarditis

15. What are the elective surgical options for FAP and chronic ulcerative colitis?
- Total proctocolectomy with end (Brooke) ileostomy
- Total proctocolectomy with continent ileostomy reservoir (Kock pouch) (see figure below)
- Abdominal colectomy with ileorectal anastomosis
- Near-total proctocolectomy ± rectal mucosectomy, and ileal pouch–anal anastomosis (IPAA) with J, S, W, or H pouch) (see figures below)

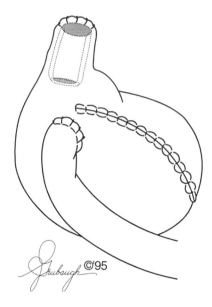

Kock pouch.

16. Why should one *not* perform ileal pouch–anal anastomosis for colonic Crohn's disease?
The high rate of recurrence of disease in the pouch, with resultant inflammation and fistulae, requires eventual excision of the pouch in 24–30% of cases. Fifty percent or more of patients suffer postoperative complications.

17. Can one always tell the difference between Crohn's disease and ulcerative colitis?
No. Colitis that cannot be categorized as definitely Crohn's or ulcerative colitis is called indeterminate colitis and may account for 5–10% of cases referred for surgical consideration. The postoperative result when IPAA is performed for indeterminate colitis has generally been held to be the same as that obtained with definite ulcerative colitis. However, a recent Mayo Clinic review notes pouch failure in indeterminate colitis to be twice that of ulcerative colitis, 18% and 9%, respectively.

18. What is pouchitis?
Pouchitis is one of the most frequent long-term complications of IPAA, a nonspecific acute and/or chronic inflammation of the reservoir. Pouchitis is found in 7–44% of patients with IPAA; it presents with watery, bloody stools, urgency, frequency, abdominal pain, fever, malaise and possible exacerbation of extraintestinal manifestations of inflammatory bowel disease. The cause of

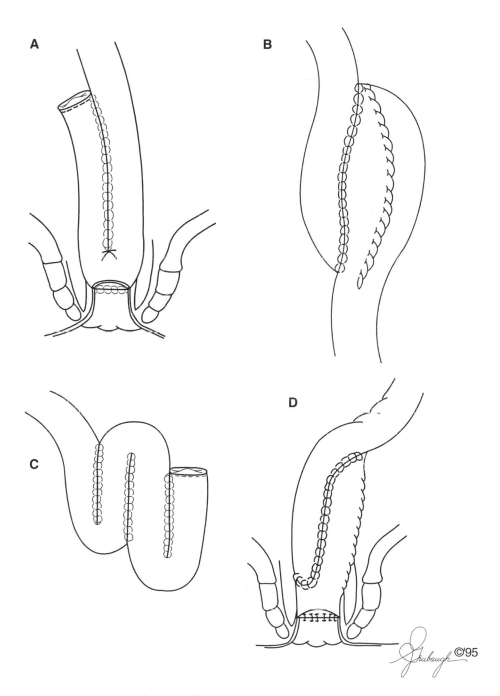

A, J pouch; **B,** S pouch; **C,** W pouch; **D,** H pouch.

pouchitis is uncertain, with a greater risk of development in chronic ulcerative colitis as opposed to familial polyposis. Pouch stasis, bacterial overgrowth, colonification of ileal mucosa, ischemia, pelvic sepsis, oxygen-derived free radicals, altered immune status, and lack of mucosal trophic factors have been proposed as etiologies.

Successful treatment regimens have included metronidazole and other antianaerobic antibiotics, as well as steroid or 5- aminosalicylate enemas. Topical volatile fatty acids and glutamine have been used with variable success. Although half of patients with pouchitis will at some time suffer a recurrence, very few develop intractable involvement requiring pouch excision.

19. Does a defunctionalized colon develop colitis?

Yes. Perhaps 30% of patients with a portion or all of the colon out of the fecal stream develop an inflammation difficult to distinguish from ulcerative colitis on biopsy. The diagnosis of **diversion colitis** is suggested when bloody mucopus is passed from the separate colorectal segment. The colon may be isolated by diverting ileostomy, end or loop colostomy, mucous fistula, or Hartmann's procedure. It is believed that short-chain fatty acids normally produced by anaerobic bacteria serve as a trophic factor for the colonocytes. The diversion colitis quickly resolves on restoration of intestinal continuity; in cases in which this is not possible, the administration of short-chain fatty acid enemas is beneficial.

CONTROVERSY

20. What are some current controversies in the surgical technique of ileal pouch–anal anastomosis (IPAA)?

- Should the anorectum be everted to allow a more complete or longer rectal mucosal stripping?
  Eversion of the anorectum to ensure complete removal of the mucosa was commonly used in the past. However, the pudendal nerves may be damaged by stretching during eversion, leading to continence problems. Shorter rectal muscle cuffs are now used to avoid abscesses between the pouch and cuff; adequate stripped cuff length can be obtained without eversion with several rectal retractors now available.
- Should the rectal mucosectomy be done trans-anally or abdominally?
  The dissection can be done from either direction. The shorter rectal cuffs now in vogue are easily performed from the perineal (trans-anal) approach.
- Should a mucosectomy be done at all?
  Mucosectomy removes part or all of the anal transition zone, a highly sensitive area that may be important for critical discrimination of pouch content and continence. Studies can be found favoring either leaving or removing this mucosa. Mucosa left in place is at risk for persistent inflammation, dysplasia, or development of carcinoma in ulcerative colitis or FAP. No mucosectomy may be preferable in the elderly (with less time at risk to develop a carcinoma, and a relatively greater need for all maneuvers to preserve continence).
- Should the IPAA be stapled or hand-sewn?
  If a mucosectomy is performed, a hand-sewn anastomosis of the pouch to the dentate line is created. If the anal transition zone mucosa is preserved, a stapled anastomosis may be performed at the top of the anorectal ring.
- Should IPAA be a one- or two-stage operation?
  The procedure has classically been two-staged, with construction of a temporary ileostomy followed at an interval by ileostomy takedown. Recent experience has shown that the morbidity of a one-stage IPAA may be less *if* the patient is on no or low-dose steroids and the operation is performed without complication. This is an operation at which there is really only "one shot" at getting it right; intraoperative judgment is at a premium in such cases.
- What type of pouch should be used?
  Higher volume pouches are being advocated. W (quadruplicated) pouches have a greater capacity than do S (triplicated) pouches and J (two-limbed) pouches. The functional re-

sults may not be all that different. Shorter efferent limbs (for S pouches) are also being used to avoid outlet obstruction.

The author prefers a noneverted trans-anal mucosal stripping with a hand-sewn anastomosis of a 15-cm long J pouch in a one-stage approach, when feasible. A stapled anastomosis preserving the anal transition zone is used in older patients with ulcerative colitis.

ANORECTAL DISEASE

21. Where are anal fissures usually located?
In the posterior (90%) or anterior (10%) midlines of the anal canal.

22. What should laterally situated anal fissures prompt one to consider?
Crohn's disease, ulcerative colitis, syphilis, tuberculosis, leukemia, carcinoma, and AIDS.

23. What would anorectal manometry demonstrate in a patient with an anal fissure?
After transient relaxation, the internal sphincter would show a prolonged elevation in pressure above the normal baseline, the "overshoot" phenomena associated with the pain/spasm cycle of fissure disease.

24. How does one manage an acute fissure?
Conservative treatment consists of stool softeners and bulk agents to avoid hard bowel movements, sitz baths to help decrease sphincter spasm, and topical anesthetics for pain relief. Suppositories should generally be avoided as they may induce anal spasm.

25. What are the signs of a chronic anal fissure? What do these signs imply?
A chronic anal fissure can be identified by the presence of a sentinel pile (skin tag or hemorrhoid), anal ulcer (with fibropurulent material or visible internal sphincter muscle in the base), and a hypertrophied anal papilla arising from the dentate line (see figure below). A chronic anal fissure will not usually respond to conservative treatment, and surgical intervention is in order.

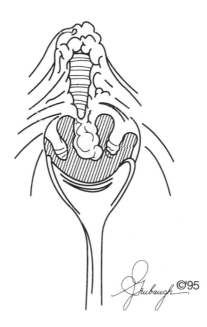

Chronic anal fissure.

26. Which surgical procedures are available for treatment of a chronic anal fissure?
Open or closed lateral internal sphincterotomy, excision (ulcerectomy), excision and Y-V or other anoplasty, or anal dilation.

27. Why has posterior anal sphincterotomy fallen out of favor?
It can result in a posterior anal canal "keyhole" defect with resultant anal seepage.

28. What are hemorrhoids?
Hemorrhoids can be very difficult to define precisely. Everyone has vascular cushions in the anal canal that contain veins (and arteries), elastic and connective tissue, and smooth muscle. They are not "varicose veins of the anus"; hemorrhoids may play a role in fine control of anal continence. It has been suggested that the term "hemorrhoid" be reserved for symptomatic involvement of these structures.

29. How are hemorrhoids classified?
   External hemorrhoids originate distal to the dentate line of the anus and are covered by squamous epithelium. External hemorrhoids may thrombose or become filled with clotted blood.
   Internal hemorrhoids arise above (proximal to) the dentate line and are covered with transitional and columnar epithelium. *First-degree* hemorrhoids swell and bleed. *Second-degree* hemorrhoids prolapse and spontaneously reduce. *Third-degree* hemorrhoids prolapse and can be manually reduced, whereas *fourth-degree* hemorrhoids are irreducible.

30. Where in the anal canal are hemorrhoids classically found?
Left lateral, right anterior, and right posterior locations for hemorrhoids are typical. The use of clockface times as descriptions of hemorrhoids (e.g., "large bundle at 9 o'clock") is confusing and should be avoided, as patients may be examined in lithotomy, jackknife, or decubitus positions by different examiners with resulting confusion.

31 How does a popular proprietary ointment containing the active ingredients shark liver oil and skin respiratory factor work to treat hemorrhoids?
I have no idea.

32. List several minimally invasive outpatient treatments of internal hemorrhoids.
   Rubber band ligation
   Bipolar cautery
   Direct current electrical therapy
   Infrared coagulation
   Sclerotherapy
   Cryotherapy

33. How is an acute thrombosed external hemorrhoid best treated?
Excision of the clot and involved hemorrhoidal complex (as opposed to incision alone) will better prevent future recurrence at the same site.

34. Explain the cause of anorectal abscesses and fistulae.
   They seem best explained by a cryptoglandular origin. Four to ten anal glands enter the anal canal at the level of the crypts in the dentate line. The glands extend back into the internal sphincter two-thirds of the time and into the intersphincteric space half the time. A blockage of the gland leads to an overgrowth of bacteria with resultant pressure necrosis and abscess formation.

An abscess or infection that causes an abnormal communication between two surfaces (such as between the anal canal and perianal skin) has created a fistula. These infections can extend in fairly standard fashion along anatomic planes to produce clinical abscesses and their potential related fistulae.

35. What are the various types of anorectal abscesses.
Submucosal, intersphincteric, perianal (anal verge), ischiorectal (perirectal), and supralevator.

36. What is a horseshoe abscess?
A perirectal abscess that connects the ischiorectal fossae bilaterally through the deep postanal space posteriorly.

37. How does one best treat an anorectal abscess?
With prompt **incision and drainage!** There is little or no role for antibiotics (exceptions being the immunocompromised and those with prosthetic heart valves or severe cellulitis) and equally no reason to wait for the abscess to "point" or become fluctuant before surgical treatment.

38. What is Goodsall's rule?
This rule helps predict the location of the internal opening of an anal fistula based on the site of its external opening (see figure below). Accurately determining the "criminal crypt" of fistula origin on the dentate line is important at the time of surgical treatment, generally fistulotomy. If the anus is divided into imaginary anterior and posterior halves in the coronal plane, posterior fistulae tend to curve into the posterior midline. Anterior fistulae shorter than 3 cm tend to proceed radially to the dentate line, while anterior fistulae longer than 3 cm *may* track back to the posterior midline.

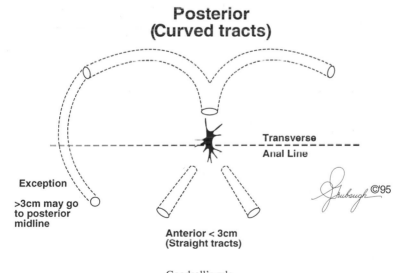

Goodsall's rule.

39. How does one differentiate true rectal prolapse from a circumferential hemorrhoidal mucosal prolapse enlargement?
The folds of tissue are concentric rings in rectal prolapse, whereas they are radially oriented in hemorrhoidal disease.

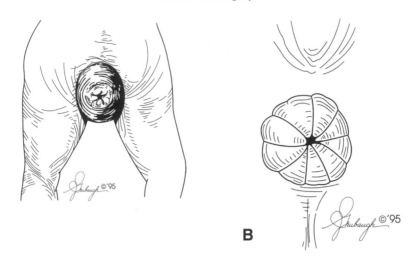

A, Rectal prolapse shows concentric rings of tissue. **B,** Tissue folds in hemorrhoids are radially oriented.

40. What patient characteristics are associated with rectal prolapse?
According to Dr. Marvin Corman:

Chronic constipation	Deep pouch of Douglas
Neurologic disease	Patulous anus
Female sex	Diastasis of the levator ani muscles
Nulliparity	Lack of fixation of the rectum to the sacrum
Redundant rectosigmoid colon	Previous anorectal surgery

41. How can a patient demonstrate a rectal prolapse during physical exam?
It is possible for some patients to prolapse the rectum voluntarily with Valsalva maneuvers and straining as if to defecate. However, this may be impossible in the commonly used jackknife or decubitus examination positions. A useful technique is to examine after the patient has strained while sitting on a toilet or, better yet, observe through a transparent elevated toilet.

42. What radiologic procedure may document a prolapse that one cannot reproduce in the office?
(Cine)defecography may reveal an internal intussusception beginning on the anterior rectal wall several centimeters above the anal verge, which can possibly progress to complete prolapse.

43. What is the relationship between rectal prolapse and anal continence?
Some degree of incontinence almost always accompanies rectal prolapse. Surgical repair may not correct incontinence problems. Abdominal approaches tend to have higher success rates for continence than do perineal operations, but the results vary widely.

44. What surgical options are available for rectal prolapse?
In general, procedures can narrow the anal orifice (Thiersch operations), obliterate the pouch of Douglas (Moschcowitz procedure), restore the condition of the pelvic floor (levator plication), excise (abdominally or perineally) the excess rectosigmoid colon, and/or fixate or suspend the rectum. Combinations of these options are often used.

45. How is rectal prolapse handled in pediatric patients?
Most prolapse in children is a mucosal prolapse alone. It is usually successfully handled with a bowel management program to reduce constipation and straining. Surgical or invasive methods, such as sclerosis, encirclement, or excision, are rarely necessary.

BENIGN COLON AND SMALL BOWEL DISEASE

46. Which type of colonic volvulus is most common?
Sigmoid volvulus (see figure below) accounts for 75% of cases seen in the United States. It is far more common than **cecal** volvulus.

47. Is volvulus a "constant" disease worldwide?
No. In the United States, volvulus causes only 10% of colonic obstruction cases. In the past, more than 50% of colonic obstructions in Iran, Ethiopia, and Russia have been attributed to volvulus. The disease process tends to present at an older age in the United States than in more rural countries.

48. What are characteristics of a typical American patient with colonic volvulus?
Male, black, elderly, and possibly from a nursing home or mental institution.

49. What does one see on plain abdominal film and contrast enema study of sigmoid volvulus?
The plain film demonstrates a "bent inner tube" or "coffee bean" sign of massively dilated, air-filled sigmoid colon arising out of the pelvis. The contrast enema would show a "bird's beak" appearance as the colon narrows at the twist at the rectosigmoid junction.

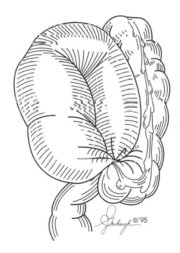

Sigmoid volvulus.

50. How does one treat a nonstrangulated sigmoid volvulus?
Rigid or flexible sigmoidoscopic or colonoscopic decompression, followed by elective sigmoid resection.

51. Why should elective surgery be performed after a successful endoscopic detorsion and decompression of a sigmoid volvulus?
Recurrence is the rule with sigmoid volvulus. Elective sigmoid resection of prepped and decompressed bowel generally can be accomplished with mortality well less than 10%. Emergency operation for a sigmoid volvulus involves a mortality of 35–80%.

52. Name the two types of large bowel obstruction.
There are **dynamic** (mechanical) and **adynamic** causes for obstruction.

53. What is the most common cause of mechanical obstruction in western society?
Carcinoma far outnumbers diverticular causes and volvulus.

54. What does plain x-ray study of the abdomen reveal in large bowel obstruction?
Differential air-fluid levels (stair steps) of the small intestine or a massively dilated colon. The colon is identified by the presence of haustral folds, as compared to the valvulae conniventes of the small intestine. The rectum is usually gasless, although gas distal to a colonic obstruction may not have completely cleared the distal colon. A picture resembling a small bowel obstruction alone may appear in a very proximal colon obstruction. Colonic pseudo-obstruction may also give a similar roentgenographic picture to a true obstruction.

55. How can one safely differentiate true from false colonic obstruction?
A water-soluble enema contrast study would reveal the presence or absence of an organic obstructing lesion. It is best to avoid barium, as a perforation during the study or a leak of colonic contents and barium at the time of surgery could lead to a severe barium peritonitis.

56. List the classes of prokinetic agents.

Cholinergic agonists	Bethanechol
Benzamides	Metoclopramide, cisapride
Dopamine antagonists	Domperidone
Macrolide antibiotics	Erythromycin
Opiate antagonists	Naloxone
Somatostatin analogs	Octreotide

57. Which lower intestinal motility disorders might respond to the use of prokinetic agents?
Irritable bowel syndrome, acute colonic psuedo-obstruction, chronic intestinal pseudo-obstruction, idiopathic constipation, chronic constipation associated with neurologic etiologies, idiopathic megacolon/megarectum.

58. What is a bezoar?
It is a concretion formed in the alimentary tract that may produce an obstruction. It can be caused by vegetable matter (phytobezoar), hair (trichobezoar), or a combination of hair and food (trichophytobezoar).

59. Which food is most commonly associated with the development of phytobezoars?
Persimmons.

60. What antecedent surgical history accompanies most cases of small intestinal bezoars?
A recent review found 76% of cases to have had previous peptic ulcer disease surgery. A vagotomy and pyloroplasty or antrectomy is believed to allow a large bolus of relatively undigested food to pass into the small intestine, where obstruction is possible.

61. What does endometriosis have to do with the alimentary system?
Endometriosis is the presence of functioning endometrial tissue outside the uterus. When this hormonally active tissue implants on intestinal surfaces, it can cause pain, cyclical bleeding, and obstructive symptoms.

62. What common symptoms are seen in women requiring surgery for endometriosis?

Pelvic pain	85%
Dyspareunia	64%
Rectal pain	52%

63. Which area of the GI tract is most often involved with endometriosis?
The rectum/cul de sac is involved in over 90% of cases requiring surgery.

64. How is a postoperative ileus differentiated from a postoperative small bowel obstruction (SBO)?

This distinction can be extremely difficult. A postoperative ileus is generally believed to occur up to 1 week after operation, whereas a postoperative SBO may last 7–30 days or longer. A SBO has nausea, vomiting, distention and abdominal pain, but an ileus may be a painless failure to pass bowel movements. The radiographic picture may or may not include differential air-fluid levels in each.

65. Is the treatment of a postoperative SBO different than treatment of an SBO remote from surgery?

Yes. Generally, one will wait out a postop obstruction for an indefinite period of time, as long as there is no evidence of strangulation or impending perforation. Approximately 80% resolve without surgery. Nasogastric suction is the mainstay of treatment for postoperative SBO, whereas "the sun never sets" upon a suspected mechanical SBO remote from surgery; one generally operates as soon as the diagnosis of complete obstruction is made with non-postop SBO.

66. What are the pathologic findings of late radiation enteritis?

It is an obliterative arteritis. There is severe fibrosis commonly accompanied by telangiectasia formation. The pelvis may be "frozen" due to incredibly dense adhesions and fibrosis.

67. What are general principles of managing radiation enteritis?

Medical management options are generally exhausted before surgery is contemplated or attempted. Cholestyramine, elemental diets, and total parenteral nutrition are commonly used. Although surgery is not withheld for urgent indications (complete obstruction, perforation, abscess not amenable to percutaneous drainage, bleeding, or unresponsive fistulae), operation carries a significant morbidity (to 65%) and mortality (to 45%). Enterolysis, or separating of adhesions, in radiated bowel is associated with a high rate of fistula formation. Anastomosis can be safely performed if at least one end of bowel to be connected has not been radiated. Intestinal bypass pro cedures without resection may be necessary.

BIBLIOGRAPHY

1. Bailey HR, Ott MT, Hartendorp P: Aggressive surgical management for advanced colorectal endometriosis. Dis Colon Rectum 37:747, 1994.
2. Bapat BP, Parker JA, Berk T, et al: Combined use of molecular and biomarkers for presymptomatic carrier risk assessment in familial adenomatous polyposis: Implications for screening guidelines. Dis Colon Rectum 37:165, 1994.
3. Bubrick MP: Volvulus of the colon. In Gordon PH, Nivatvongs S (eds): Principles and Practice of Surgery for the Colon, Rectum and Anus. St. Louis, Quality Medical Publishing, 1992.
4. Corman ML: Colon and Rectal Surgery. Philadelphia, J.B. Lippincott, 1993.
5. Escamilla C, Robles-Campos R, Parrilla-Paricio P, et al: Intestinal obstruction and bezoars. J Am Coll Surg 179:285, 1994.
6. Gordon PH, Nivatvongs S: Principles and Practice of Surgery for the Colon, Rectum and Anus. St. Louis, Quality Medical Publishing, 1992.
7. Hizawa K, Iida M, Matsumoto T, et al: Neoplastic transformation arising in Peutz-Jeghers polyposis. Dis Colon Rectum 36:953, 1993.
8. Jagelman DG: Familial polyposis coli. In Fazio VW (ed): Current Therapy in Colon and Rectal Surgery. Philadelphia, B.C. Decker, 1990.
9. Keighley MR, Williams NS: Surgery of the Anus, Rectum and Colon. London, W.B. Saunders, 1993.
10. Longo WE, Vernava AM III: Prokinetic agents for lower gastrointestinal motility disorders. Dis Colon Rectum 36:696, 1993.
11. McIntyre PB, Pemberton JH, Wolff BG, et al: Indeterminate colitis: Long term outcome in patients after ileal pouch-anal anastomosis. Dis Colon Rectum 38:51, 1995.
12. Mignon M, Stettler C, Phillips SF: Pouchitis—a poorly understood entity. Dis Colon Rectum 38:100, 1995.
13. Pickleman J, Lee RM: The management of patients with suspected early postoperative small bowel obstruction. Ann Surg 210:216, 1989.
14. Sudduth RH, Bute BG, Schoelkopf L, et al: Small bowel obstruction in a patient with Peutz-Jeghers syndrome: The role of intra-operative endoscopy. Gastrointest Endosc 38:69, 1992.

82. PANCREATIC SURGERY

Jeffrey Clark, M.D.

A surgeon's reflection on the pancreas

A certain mystique surrounds the pancreas because of circumstances unique to this organ.

1. The pancreas is responsible for one of mankind's most common afflictions—diabetes mellitus.
2. The etiology of many pancreatic diseases defies logical explanation (pancreatitis).
3. Considerable controversy exists regarding what is appropriate therapy for all pancreatic diseases. [Interpretation: Controversy is a polite way of saying we don't know what we are doing.]
4. Surgical intervention is frequently associated with high mortality and morbidity because the pancreas:
   a. has a retroperitoneal location and close proximity to vital structures (aorta, vena cava, superior mesenteric vein and artery, hilum of kidneys).
   b. shares a common blood supply with duodenum, necessitating removal of both when resecting either.
   c. contains potent indiscriminate digestive enzymes that will just as readily digest the host if uncontained.
   d. has parenchyma that is very fragile and difficult to suture, resulting in anastomotic leaks, fistulas, and bleeding.
5. Questions on the pancreas are the resident's worst nightmare. Numerous exotic endocrine tumors give rise to a disproportionate number of questions far in excess of the prevalence of the diseases these tumors produce.
6. The pancreas is unjust and unpredictable. Operations in close proximity and carefully performed may occasionally elicit its wrath (splenectomy) and even remote operations (open heart) may elicit pancreatitis.

In conclusion, it is easy to understand why the experienced surgeon approaches the pancreas with a great deal of respect and humility and will give all considerations for surgery on this organ a great deal of deliberation. [Interpretation: When you don't know what you are doing, be very, very careful.]

ACUTE PANCREATITIS

1. What is acute pancreatitis?

Inflammation of the pancreas with variable involvement of regional tissues and remote organ systems. Mild acute pancreatitis is accompanied by minimal organ dysfunction and has an uncomplicated recovery. Severe acute pancreatitis is associated with distant organ failure and defined as follows:

Pulmonary	PO_2 <60 mm Hg
Renal	Creatinine > 2 mg/dl
Cardiac	Blood pressure <90 mm Hg
Hematopoietic	Disseminated intravascular coagulation
Metabolic	Hypocalcemia and hyperglycemia
Gastrointestinal	Bleeding >500 ml/24 h
Complications	Pancreatic necrosis, abscess, pseudocyst, others

2. How common is acute pancreatitis?

Common. There are >100,000 hospital admissions and >2000 deaths a year in the United States.

3. What are the etiologies of acute pancreatitis?

Alcohol	40%
Gallstones	40%
Miscellaneous	10%
(drugs, toxins, trauma, hyperlipidemia, hypercalcemia, etc.)	
Idiopathic	10%

4. What is the pathogenesis?

The pathogenesis of acute pancreatitis remains unclear, but current hypotheses suggest pancreatic enzymes (trypsin) are activated intracellularly by lysosomal enzymes secondary to the direct action of toxins (alcohol) and/or pancreatic ductal obstruction (gallstones). This causes ductal hypertension, which overwhelms the natural trypsin inhibitors. The process is enhanced by the presence of bile, bile salts, and duodenal contents refluxing into the pancreatic duct. Trypsin activates the other potent digestive enzymes (phospholipase A, elastase, lipase), and the gland is autodigested. The damage is immediate, necrosis occurs quickly, and inflammatory mediators (cytokines and acute phase reactants) are activated and released systemically.

5. How is the diagnosis of acute pancreatitis established?

A. **History:** Sudden onset of constant and unrelenting epigastric pain ranging from mild to catastrophic, radiating straight through to the back, relieved by sitting position and leaning forward.

B. **Physical findings:** Upper abdominal pain and tenderness up to and including rigidity and rebound. (The presence of acute surgical abdomen with acute pancreatitis does not indicate emergency surgical exploration.)

C. **Laboratory findings:** Elevations of serum amylase (half-life, hours) and lipase (half-life, days) remain the gold standards. Diagnostic accuracy increases with rising levels so that amylase levels >1000 IU/l are virtually diagnostic of acute pancreatitis.

D. **Surgical findings:** Diagnosis of acute pancreatitis may be made during operation unexpectedly, when the abdomen is explored for another reason (i.e., appendicitis, cholecystitis).

6. List the differential diagnosis of acute pancreatitis.

1. **Small bowel obstruction**—especially closed loop; rule out with Gastrografin upper GI series.
2. **Perforated viscus**—especially duodenal ulcer; rule out with upright chest x-ray for free air.
3. **Bowel infarction**—rule out with arteriogram.

7. Are there tests that can determine severity and predict outcome?

Yes. The following tests are most commonly used.

Ranson's criteria. Ranson's original description of these prognostic indicators was published in 1974, but significant improvements in ICU care, operative management techniques, and antibiotics have lowered the high mortality originally reported. Nevertheless, the criteria continue to reflect accurately the severity of acute pancreatitis.

APACHE II (acute physiology and chronic health evaluation). Patients are assigned points for advancing age, abnormal physiology, and presence of severe organ dysfunction. Scores >10 are associated with increased morbidity and mortality in acute pancreatitis.

Pancreatic necrosis. Presence of 30% necrosis on dynamic CT scan (performed on patients with >3 Ranson's criteria or APACHE II scores >10).

Ranson's Prognostic Indicators for Severity of Acute Pancreatitis

---

Initial findings
 Age >55 yrs
 WBC >16,000/mm^3
 Glucose >200 mg/dl
 Lactate dehydrogenase >350 IU/d
 Aspartate aminotransferase >250 IU/dl
Develop during first 48 hrs
 Hematocrit fall >10%
 Blood urea nitrogen >8 mg/dl
 Ca^{2++} <8 mg/dl
 PO_2 <60 mm Hg
 Base deficit >6 meq/l
 Fluid sequestration >6 l
Mortality rates
 <3 = 10%
 3–4 = 15%
 5–6 = 40%
 >7 = 100%

APACHE II Scoring System for Severity of Acute Pancreatitis

Age: >45 years of age assigned ascending points to age 75 (6 point maximum)
Acute physiology score: Points are assigned for abnormal values (50 points maximum).
 Vital signs
 Arterial blood gases
 Electrolytes
 Glasgow coma scale (actual number)
Chronic health points: (2 points each)
 Liver—cirrhosis
 Lung—severe chronic obstructive pulmonary disease
 Renal—on dialysis
 Heart—congestive heart failure or angina at rest
 Immunocompromise—on chemotherapy, radiation therapy, or diagnosis of AIDS

---

8. What are some physical and radiologic signs associated with pancreatitis?

1. Gray Turner sign: Hemoglobin dissecting through tissue causes a bruise to the flank 3–5 days after acute necrotizing pancreatitis with hemorrhage.

2. Cullen's sign: Same as Gray Turner sign except bruise appears around the umbilicus.

3. Colon cut-off sign: Distended transverse colon overlying inflammatory process in pancreas seen on upright abdominal x-ray.

4. Sentinel loop: same as colon cut-off sign except paralytic loop of air-filled jejunum.

9. In managing acute pancreatitis, which steps are appropriate?

1. Admission to the hospital for all initial attacks. Recurrent mild attacks of pancreatitis may be managed as outpatients.

2. Admission to ICU for all severe acute pancreatitis.

3. Gallbladder ultrasound rule out gallstones as the etiology.

4. Dynamic CT scan is indicated when >3 Ranson's criteria or APACHE II scores >10 are present. CT scan should be performed to determine the extent of necrosis.

5. Laboratory studies include complete blood count, blood urea nitrogen, creatinine, calcium, LDH, lactate dehydrogenase, aspartate aminotransferase, bilirubin, glucose, arterial blood gases (all used to determine Ranson's prognostic criteria).

6. Narcotics are given as necessary. (Use meperidine, not morphine, which causes sphincter of Oddi contraction.)

10. Which steps are not necessary initially?

1. Nasogastric tube is needed only for severe cases, not for routine cases.

2. The prophylactic use of antibiotics has inconclusive benefits. Therapeutic use is indicated only when superinfection is definitely established.

3. Somatostatin analog has no proven benefit.

11. When should a surgeon be consulted about a case of acute pancreatitis?

When **gallstones** are discovered, when significant pancreatic **necrosis** is present, when **infection** is suspected, or when the patient is so ill as to require **admission to ICU.**

12. What are the complications of pancreatitis?

Superinfection
Pseudocyst
Pancreatic ascites and pancreatic pleural effusion
Endocrine malfunction (diabetes)
Exocrine malfunction (steatorrhea and malabsorption)

13. Is there any way to predict who will get superinfected pancreatitis?

Infection is unusual unless necrosis is present. The more extensive the necrosis, the higher the chances of infection (up to 80%).

14. How is super infection diagnosed?

CT-guided fine-needle aspiration with Gram stain and culture (and sensitivity screening).

15. Are there different types of infection?

Yes. Three distinct types of infection are found, each with different treatments and prognoses.

1. **Infected pancreatic pseudocyst:** Treatment is external drainage via exploratory laparotomy (open) or percutaneous drainage (closed).

2. **Pancreatic abscess** (well-defined loculated cavity): Treatment is external drainage, open or closed.

3. **Infected pancreatic necrosis:** Treatment is open operation only, with removal of the necrotic pancreas. The abdomen is either left open and reexplored to remove additional necrotic pancreas via multiple "second-look" procedures or large-bore sump catheters are left in place through which large-volume peritoneal lavage is performed. (Total pancreatectomy is no longer indicated for this condition, as the morbidity and mortality are too high.)

16. What are the indications for surgery in acute severe pancreatitis with necrosis?

• When superinfection has been diagnosed.
• When the patient is nonresponsive to intensive care management techniques and is dying despite all efforts (see algorithm on next page).

17. What is the prognosis when aggressive surgical techniques are applied for pancreatic necrosis and superinfection?

Mortality is decreased from >80% to <25%.

18. What are the types of fluid accumulation that occur with acute severe pancreatitis?

Acute fluid collections are located in or near the pancreas, occur early in the disease course, lack a defined wall, and usually resolve spontaneously. **Pancreatic pseudocysts** are collections of pancreatic juice confined by a discrete wall of fibrous tissue and occur later in the course of the disease (average, 4–6 weeks). **Pancreatic abscess** is a well-defined pus-filled cavity in proximity to the pancreas, usually without pancreatic juice and without necrosis. **Pancreatic necrosis** is nonviable pancreatic tissue caused by enzymatic autodigestion.

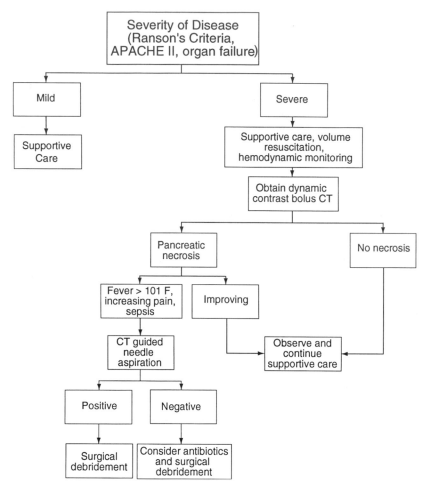

Treatment algorithm for acute pancreatitis.

19. How often do pseudocysts form?
Fluid collections associated with acute pancreatitis are common and usually resolve spontaneously. Only 1–2% of all cases of pancreatitis develop pseudocysts that persist beyond 6 weeks.

20. What symptoms are associated with pseudocysts?
Chronic pain and persistently elevated amylase level.

21. How is the diagnosis made?
CT scan.

22. What are the indications of pseudocyst therapy?
Presence of a pseudocyst >5 cm for 6 weeks.

23. What are the procedures available for treatment of chronic pseudocysts?
    1. *Percutaneous external catheter drainage:* Length of treatment is prolonged; secondary infection rate is high.
    2. *Excision:* For pseudocyst in the tail of the pancreas.

3. *Internal drainage:* Into stomach, duodenum or roux-en-Y limb of jejunum.

4. *Endoscopic cystogastrostomy*

24. What complications do neglected pseudocysts cause, and what is the therapy for each?

- **Superinfection:** External drainage, open or closed, with or without somatostatin analog.
- **Erosion into adjacent blood vessels:** Arteriographic embolization.
- **Free rupture into abdominal cavity:** Emergency laparotomy with external drainage and/or pancreatic resection.
- **Obstruction** via compression of bile ducts, stomach, or intestinal tract: Internal drainage into duodenum or stomach or roux-en-Y limb of jejunum.

25. What factors are considered in determining the correct timing of surgery for gallstone pancreatitis?

1. The gallstone usually only transiently obstructs the pancreatic duct and then passes into duodenum. Amylase levels return to normal quickly, and the patient rapidly recovers (usual case, 90%).

2. Pancreatic necrosis is unusual in gallstone pancreatitis.

3. Early operations (within 48 hours) do not improve survival or enhance recovery.

4. Operations delayed beyond 6 weeks result in 50% recurrence of gallstone pancreatitis.

Therefore, most surgeons prefer to remove the gallbladder laparoscopically during the initial hospitalization (3–8 days), after the amylase has returned to normal. If necrotizing pancreatitis is present, most surgeons would delay cholecystectomy until pancreatitis is totally resolved (see algorithm below).

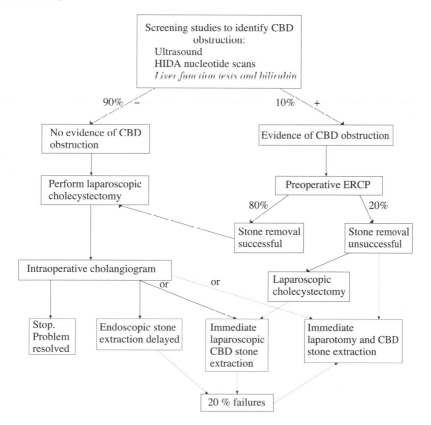

Treatment algorithm for gallstone pancreatitis.

26. What is pancreas divisum? How is it implicated in pancreatitis?
Failure of fusion of the dorsal pancreatic duct of Santorini with the ventral pancreatic duct of Wirsung occurs in approximately 5% of the population. Obstruction of the minor pancreatic ampulla (Santorini duct) may result in recurrent episodes of pancreatitis. Sphincterotomy of this minor ampulla may cure this congenital condition.

CHRONIC PANCREATITIS

27. What are the characteristic features of chronic pancreatitis?
1. Recurrent attacks
2. Mild elevation of amylase
3. Destruction and fibrous replacement of parenchyma
4. Loss of exocrine and endocrine function
5. Disabling pain.

28. How does chronic pancreatitis differ from acute pancreatitis?

Comparison Between Acute and Chronic Pancreatitis

	ACUTE	CHRONIC
Recurrent "attacks"	Rare	Classic
Reversible parenchymal changes	Yes	No
Fibrosis	No	Yes
Ductal dilations and obstructions	Rare	Common
Pancreatic calcifications	Never	Common
Peripancreatic digestion	Yes	No
Diabetes	Rare	Common
Exocrine dysfunction	Rare	Common
Etiology	Gallstones	Alcohol
Pseudocysts	1+	4+
Secondary infection	Common	Almost never
Amylase elevation	Higher	Lower
Surgical procedure	Debride and drain	Resect/drain duct

29. How is diagnosis of chronic pancreatitis established?
A history of recurrent episodes of disabling pain with mild elevations of amylase; confirmed by abdominal films showing calcifications and endoscopic retrograde pancreatography revealing duct dilations and obstructions (chain of lakes). Not all cases of chronic pancreatitis, however, have calcifications and ductal abnormalities, but when these are present, they are diagnostic of the disease.

30. What is the medical therapy for chronic pancreatitis?
Symptomatic treatment only is the rule, with pain control, alcohol abstinence, and insulin and pancreatic enzyme replacement as necessary. Antibiotics, nasogastric tubes, and somatostatin analogs are of no value. This disease is not as life-threatening as acute pancreatitis, and management is frustrating, palliative, and noncurative.

31. Who is a candidate for surgical therapy?
Patients with recurrent attacks who require repeated hospitalizations and have disabling pain causing employment disruption and narcotic addition are legitimate surgical candidates.

32. What is role of ERCP in chronic pancreatitis?
• It is used to establish diagnosis, visualizing the dilated duct with obstructions (chain of lakes).
• Preoperatively to define pancreatic duct anatomy and help plan surgery, ERCP is done within 12–24 hours of the planned surgery with antibiotic coverage.

33. What are the surgical options in chronic pancreatitis?

1. Anastomoses of the pancreatic duct side-to-side with roux-en-Y limb of jejunum (**Puestow procedure**) is used when the pancreatic duct is a "chain of lakes" (see figure below).

2. **Distal resection** and drainage to roux-en-Y limb of jejunum is used when the pancreatic duct is dilatated with proximal obstruction.

3. **Total pancreatectomy** should be performed only rarely in a patient who has previously failed other procedures and is already exocrine- and endocrine-deficient.

4. **Nerve ablation** procedures, such as celiac ganglionectomy, are infrequently combined with the other approaches to alleviate pain.

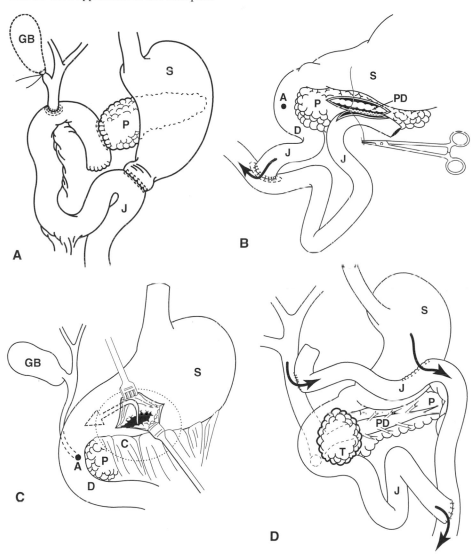

Surgical procedures for chronic pancreatitis **A,** Pylorus-preserving pancreaticoduodenectomy (Whipple procedure). **B,** Roux-en-Y side-to-side pancreaticojejunostomy. **C,** Pancreatic pseudocystogatrostomy. **D,** Roux-en-Y choledochogastrojejunostomy (palliative biliary gastric bypass) for a tumor of the head of the pancreas. (S = stomach; D = duodenum; J = jejunum; P = pancreas; C = pseudocyst of the pancreas; T = tumor of the head of the pancreas; GB = gallbladder; A = ampulla; and PD = pancreatic duct.)

34. What is pancreatic ascites?
When pancreatic ductal disruption occurs in chronic pancreatitis secondary to alcoholism and rarely trauma, the pancreatic juice leaks into the free peritoneal cavity. This ascites differs from ascites secondary to cirrhosis in two ways: (1) its amylase content is very high, in the thousands, and (2) the protein concentration is >2.5 gm/dl. Even more rarely, a pleural effusion with the same characteristics may result when the pancreatic ductal disruption communicates with the pleural space. The digestive enzymes in pancreatic ascites are not activated, so digestion of surrounding tissues does not occur.

35. How is the diagnosis of pancreatic ascites or pancreatic pleural effusion made?
Tap fluid and measure amylase and protein.

36. How is pancreatic ascites treated?
Conservative therapy resolves the ascites in 50% of the cases within 4–6 weeks and consists of NPO and somatostatin to decrease pancreatic secretion; total parenteral nutrition, to correct the malnutrition; and peritoneal or pleural taps, to relieve the pressure (as necessary).

If conservative therapy fails, a preoperative endoscopic pancreatography is performed to localize the leak, and a pancreatic resection and/or anastomosis of the leaking duct to a roux-en-Y limb of jejunum is performed. The mortality for these conditions remains high (20%) secondary to underlying cirrhosis, alcoholism, and cachexia frequently found in these patients.

CANCER OF PANCREAS AND PERIAMPULLARY REGION

37. What are the cancers of the periampullary region? Why are they lumped together?
Cancers of the pancreas (70%), ampulla of Vater (10%), duodenum (10%), and distal common bile duct (10%) all present with similar features:

Signs and symptoms	Obstructive jaundice
	Weight loss
	Abdominal pain
	Palpable gallbladder (30%)
Laboratory data	Elevated obstructive enzymes (alkaline phosphatase and gamma-glutamyl transpeptidase)
	Direct bilirubin
Diagnostic evaluations	Ultrasound
	CT scan
	ERCP (in that order)
Treatment	Whipple procedure (pancreaticoduodenectomy)

38. What are the 5-year survival rates of periampullary cancers resected with Whipple procedure for cure?
Pancreas—<10% if nodes positive, as high as 50% if nodes are negative.
Ampulla—30–40%
Duodenum—15–30%
Distal common bile duct—30–40%

39. Describe the typical patient with pancreatic cancer.
The patient typically is a middle-aged black man, a smoker and diabetic, with a history of alcoholism and pancreatitis. He presents with a dull aching pain, weight loss, and palpable gallbladder. Obstructive enzymes are elevated, and hepatocellular enzymes are normal; direct bilirubin is elevated.

40. What is the best serum marker for cancer of the pancreas?
CA 19-9, with sensitivity and specificity of about 90% each.

41. What is the "double duct" sign?
On ERCP, when both the distal common bile duct and proximal pancreatic duct are obstructed and dilatated, there is a very high probability of pancreatic cancer.

42. What is Courvoisier's sign?
Palpable gallbladder in a jaundiced patient secondary to malignant obstruction of the common bile duct. It is present in 25–40% of periampullary cancers.

43. What percentage of patients with pancreatic cancer present with localized disease that can be potentially cured by surgery?
Of 30,000 cases diagnosed annually in the United States, only about 1500 Whipple procedures are performed (5%). Eighty percent of cases have positive nodes, 50% have distant disease, and 40% have locally advanced disease. Almost all patients eventually die of their disease, 95% within a few months. Over 90% of patients who have surgical exploration are unresectable for cure.

44. Should all patients with pancreatic cancer be referred for surgical exploration to determine resectability or to bypass the GI tract and biliary tree when unresectable?
No. CT scan, endoscopic ultrasound, or arteriography may reveal unresectability (liver metastases, malignant ascites, invasion of the portal vein or inferior vena cava, or bulky lymphadenopathy). In these cases, fine-needle aspiration to confirm the diagnosis precedes endoscopic or transhepatic percutaneous stent decompression of the common duct obstruction.

45. Is there a role for laparoscopy in periampullary cancer?
Yes. Not for resection but for determination of resectability short of formal open surgical exploration.

46. When cancer arises in the body and tail of the pancreas, what is the prognosis?
Incurable. Virtually never resectable.

47. What is the standard operative approach to periampullary cancer?
Exploratory laparotomy is used initially. If there is no evidence of distant positive lymph nodes or metastases, and there is no invasion into inferior vena cava, portal vein, or adjacent organs, then a Whipple procedure is performed to remove the distal stomach, duodenum, head of the pancreas, and distal common bile duct.

48. What is a pylorus-preserving Whipple procedure? When should it be performed?
When the cancer does not involve the stomach and the first 2.0 cm of the duodenum, these structures can be preserved. Thus, the complications of partial gastrectomy are avoided, and yet, long-term survival is preserved.

49. When should preoperative biliary decompression be performed?
Very rarely. When ascending cholangitis is present or delay for nutritional support is deemed important, decompression is indicated. Most often, surgery can be performed in the presence of obstructive jaundice without increasing mortality and morbidity.

50. At the time of surgery, should the pancreas be biopsied to verify cancer?
This is a question that will probably never be settled! Surgeons who **favor biopsy** argue that since the operative mortality of a Whipple procedure is 10–20% (community practice) and 5-year survival is low (<5%), one should never proceed without pathologic confirmation of cancer. Furthermore, biopsy is harmless, with a low complication rate (especially with fine-needle aspiration), and roux-en-Y choledochojejunostomy and gastrojejunostomy provide respectable long-term palliation.

Surgeons who will proceed with a **"blind" Whipple** procedure argue that the clinical accuracy of the detection of pancreatic cancer by the experienced surgeon is >95%, and thus delay for pathologic confirmation is avoided. Mortality at large centers performing many Whipple procedures is <5%, and palliation is best when resection of the cancer is performed.

However, a word of caution is appropriate here. Just because the mortality of a pancreaticoduodenectomy at several centers of excellence has been lowered to 1%, this does not mean necessarily that the same mortality can be duplicated across the spectrum of community hospitals. Interpret these data within the context and results of your own hospital and staff. Certainly, attempts to duplicate these results are most appropriate when feasible, but the safe surgeon will acknowledge the limits of his or her ability and hospital and will refer complex cases to a center of excellence.

51. Because pancreatic cancer is multicentric and many complications are related to the pancreatic anastomosis, why not remove the entire pancreas?
Survival is not improved, and the diabetes that results is very difficult to control. The combination of loss of insulin and glucagon and the presence of malabsorption requiring pancreatic enzymes entails erratic glucose metabolism.

52. Is there anything that can be done to prevent pancreatic anastomotic complications?
Yes. Somatostatin analog, 100 μg subcutaneously every 8 hours, will decrease these complications.

53. Is advanced age considered a contraindication to Whipple resection?
No. This view is controversial, but most recent experience in larger centers indicates age is no contraindication. Common sense would indicate that the elderly should be in excellent health without comorbid conditions and the individual surgeon's results should be superlative to escape criticism of such a position.

54. Should the Whipple procedure be performed if regional lymph nodes are positive?
Probably not. Prognosis is dismal in this situation, and palliation only is the most logical approach.

54. Is there a role for arteriography in periampullary cancer?
Yes. Arteriography is routinely performed by some surgeons to identify anomalous anatomy and determine if encasement of blood vessels by cancer has occurred (evidence of unresectability).

56. When resection for cure is not possible, should biliary and stomach bypass procedures always be performed?
Always bypass the biliary tree, and if intestinal obstruction appears imminent, bypass the stomach also because up to 30% will eventually obstruct the GI tract.

57. Is adjuvant therapy helpful in pancreatic cancer?
Yes. The application of chemotherapy and radiation therapy when all gross cancer is removed (adjuvant therapy) doubles the 2-year survival in patients with pancreatic cancer (43% versus 18%).

ENDOCRINE TUMORS OF THE PANCREAS

58. What is an insulinoma?
A very rare tumor of pancreatic islet B cells that produces excess insulin, causing either symptoms relating to CNS hypoglycemia (confusion, erratic behavior, seizures, and coma) or symptoms relating to excess compensary catecholamine release (sweating, tachycardia, and palpitations).

59. What is Whipple's triad?
1. Symptoms precipitated by fasting.
2. Blood sugar < 50 mg/dl.
3. Symptoms reversed by glucose.

60. How is the diagnosis established?
An in-hospital, observed 72-hour fast with simultaneous blood glucose and insulin measurements will diagnose all patients with insulinoma, usually within the first 24 hours. An insulin/glucose ratio of >0.3 is diagnostic (μU/ml:mg/dl).

61. What is the rule of 10's?
As applied to insulinoma, roughly 10% are malignant, 10% are multiple, 10% are associated with multiple endocrine neoplasia type I, and most are about 10 mm in size.

62. How are insulinomas located in the pancreas?
　　CT
　　Angiograms (vascular blush seen 90% of the time)
　　Intraoperative ultrasound (finds the remaining lesions)

63. Who should be offered surgical exploration?
Everyone, because surgery is highly curative (90%) and even patients with metastatic disease are palliated with debulking of these endocrine tumors.

64. What surgical procedures are offered?
1. Simple enucleation for benign tumors.
2. Resection of pancreas, nodes, and liver for metastatic lesions.

65. Can the pathologist diagnose endocrine malignancy by cellular appearance alone?
Usually not, because all endocrine tumors can manifest bizarre nuclear atypia and still behave in a benign fashion. The only proof of endocrine malignancy is metastasis.

66. What is the most common benign tumor of the pancreas?
Cystadenoma of the pancreas. This tumor occurs most frequently in younger females, presents as a painless mass in the body or tail, and has columnar epithelium lining the cyst spaces. It is prone to malignant degeneration (cystadenocarcinoma) and therefore is treated by surgical resection.

67. What are the other pancreatic endocrine tumors?

Rare Pancreatic Endocrine Tumors

	CELL ORIGIN	HORMONE	MULTICENTRIC	MALIGNANT	MEN	SIGNS AND SYMPTOMS
Glucagonoma	A	Glucagon	No	70%	Rare	Hyperglycemia, anemia, necrolytic migratory erythema, cachexia
VIPoma Verner-Morrison syndrome Pancreatic cholera WDHA	II	Vasoactive intestinal peptide	No	60%	Rare	Cachexia, watery diarrhea, hypokalemia, achlorhydria (WDHA)
Somatostatinoma	D	Somatostatin	No	90%	No	Hyperglycemia, cachexia, gallstones, diarrhea, steatorrhea, achlorhydria

MEN = multiple endocrine neoplasia, WDHA = watery diarrhea, hypokalemia, achlorhydria syndrome.

BIBLIOGRAPHY

1. Bradley EL: Classification for acute pancreatitis. Arch Surg 128:586–90, 1993.
2. Bradley EL: Experience with open drainage for infected pancreatic necroses. Surg Gynecol Obstet 177:215–222, 1993.
3. Buchler M: Role of octreotide in the prevention of postoperative complications following pancreatic resections. Am J Surg 163:125, 1992.
4. Cameron JL: Factors influencing survival after pancreaticoduodenectomy for pancreatic cancer. Am J Surg 161: 120–125, 1991.
5. Cameron JL, et al: One hundred and forty-five consecutive pancreaticoduodenectomies without mortality. Am Surg 217:430–435, 1993.
6. Grace PA: Pylorus preserving pancreaticoduodenectomy: An overview. Br J Surg 77:968–974, 1990.
7. Gumaste VV: Diagnostic tests for acute pancreatitis. Gastroenterologist 2:119–130, 1994.
8. Imrie CW, et al: Predictions of outcome in acute pancreatitis. Br J Surg 77:1260–1264, 1990.
9. Marshall JB: Acute pancreatitis: A review. Arch Intern Med 153:1185–1198, 1993.
10. Pellegrini CA: Surgery for gallstone pancreatitis. Am J Surg 165:515–518, 1993.
11. Posner MR, et al: The use of serologic markers in gastrointestinal malignancies. Hematol/Oncol Clin North Am 8:533–553, 1994.
12. Ranson JHC: Prognostic signs and the role of surgery in acute pancreatitis. Surg Gynecol Obstet 139: 69–81, 1974.
13. Ranson JHC: The role of surgery in acute pancreatitis. Am Surg 211:382–393, 1990.
14. Warshaw AL, et al:Early debridement of pancreatic necroses is beneficial. Am J Surg 163:105–110, 1992.
15. Whittington R, et al: Adjuvant therapy for cancer of pancreas. Int J Radiat Oncol Biol Phys 21(5):1137–1143, 1991.

83. HEPATOBILIARY SURGERY

Phillip L. Mallory, II, M.D.

BILIARY DISORDERS

1. What is the most common cause of benign biliary strictures?

The most common etiology is operative injury to the bile ducts, particularly during cholecystectomy. Even with the advent of laparoscopic cholecystectomy, bile duct injury is conservatively estimated to occur in 1 per 200–300 operations.

2. What factors contribute to operative injury?

A myriad of factors have been suggested as predisposing to operative injury. These include congenital anatomic variations, the difficult cholecystectomy, and bile duct ischemia induced by excessive dissection around the bile ducts.

3. Bile duct strictures are identified or suspected in what postoperative time frame?

In only 10% of cases are bile duct strictures suspected in the first week after cholecystectomy; 70% are identified within the first 6 months of operative injury; and at 1 year, 80% of bile duct strictures have been identified. Biliary drainage is the predominant feature of the early presenters. Painless jaundice is the major feature of patients who present in months to years after operative injury.

4. What is the preferred diagnostic modality for postoperative bile duct strictures?

Cholangiography remains the *sine qua non* of diagnosing postoperative bile duct strictures. Percutaneous transhepatic cholangiography (PTC) or endoscopic retrograde cholangiopancreatography (ERCP) are both equally acceptable modalities. A temporizing stent can be passed with either technique. However, when there is duct discontinuity, PTC is preferable because the proximal biliary anatomy is better visualized.

5. Which surgical options are possible in repairing a postoperative bile duct stricture?

Immediate end-to-end repair has been associated with a high re-stricture rate. The preferable option is a hepaticojejunostomy over a stent with a roux-en-Y jejunal loop.

6. What is a choledochal cyst? Is it related to Caroli's disease?

A choledochal cyst is a cystic dilatation of the extrahepatic bile duct, occurring in approximately 1 in 2 million live births. Caroli's disease refers to intrahepatic cystic dilatation of the bile ducts. See chapter 32.

Todani Classification of Biliary Cysts

Type I	Cystic dilatation of the common bile duct (most common, 80–90%)
Type II	Diverticulum of the common bile duct (2%)
Type III	Terminal cystic dilatation of the bile duct (1–5%)
Type IVA	Multiple cysts of intra/extrahepatic bile ducts (19%)
Type IVB	Multiple cysts of extrahepatic bile ducts only (rare)
Type V	Caroli's disease

7. What is the classic triad of a choledochal cysts?

Abdominal pain, jaundice, and abdominal mass comprise the classic triad, but it is present in only 3% of patients. Forty to sixty percent of patients present before age 10. Other presenting symptoms include bile peritonitis (if rupture occurs), pancreatitis, or ascending cholangitis. Liver function tests are frequently abnormal but are not diagnostic. Imaging may be accomplished with ultrasound, HIDA scan, or computed tomography (CT), but cholangiography is definitive.

8. Describe the operative management of choledochal cysts.
Formerly, internal drainage of the choledochal cyst was the preferred management, but because of various complications and a reoperation rate of 50%, this approach has been abandoned. Total excision of the cyst with Roux-en-Y hepaticojejunostomy reconstruction is now the preferred surgical management.

9. Outline the epidemiology, distribution, histology, and morphology of bile duct cancers?
Bile duct cancers account for approximately 3% of all cancers. There is no sex predilection. Cholelithiasis is not an associated risk factor, but the risk is clearly increased in patients with choledochal cysts. Two-thirds of all bile duct cancers occur at or above the junction of the cystic duct with the hepatic duct. The overwhelming majority are adenocarcinomas, which tend to be mucin-producing, slow-growing, and locally invasive. Morphologically, bile duct cancers tend to be sclerosing, nodular, or papillary. Sclerosing is the most common morphology, but papillary portends the best prognosis.

10. What is a Klatskin's tumor?
This has been a favorite question of surgical staff for decades and simply refers to a bile duct cancer strategically located at the bifurcation of the left and right hepatic ducts. This bifurcation tends to be extrahepatic.

11. What are the clinical features of bile duct cancer?
Clearly, jaundice is the predominant symptom in most patients. Less common symptoms, in order of frequency, include weight loss, abdominal pain, fever, and a palpable abdominal mass. Serum alkaline phosphatase and gamma-glutamyl transpeptidase levels are the most useful markers of biliary obstruction.

12. Which diagnostic modality is the most sensitive in establishing a tissue diagnosis of bile duct cancer?
This is an area fraught with difficulty, controversy, and a plethora of choices. Cytologic samples may be recovered through duodenal aspiration, ERCP, PTC, CT-guided percutaneous fine-needle aspiration, and intraoperative fine-needle aspirations. Although biliary aspiration in the setting of PTC or ERCP will detect 33% of pancreaticobiliary malignancies, biliary brush cytology has emerged as a more sensitive technique. With a mass lesion, percutaneous CT-guided and intraoperative fine-needle aspiration have a diagnostic yield of 50% and 80%, respectively. Despite the improvement in cytologic collection techniques, further refinements must be made in histologic evaluation of samples to better differentiate inflammatory from neoplastic changes.

13. What constitutes an adequate preoperative evaluation for resectability? What are the criteria for nonresectability (inoperable)?
The ultimate discriminator for resectability remains surgical exploration, but useful preoperative studies include cholangiography, hepatic arteriography, portal venography, CT, and ultrasound. Duplex sonography may be of value in assessing hepatic veins and hilar vessels. None of these modalities is very sensitive for lymph node metastasis. Criteria of unresectability include extensive bilateral intrahepatic bile duct involvement, main portal vein invasion, and bilateral hepatic artery or portal vein invasion.

14. Discuss the surgical options in the management of bile duct cancer.
Distal bile duct tumors, if resectable, are managed with a Whipple procedure (radical pancreaticoduodenectomy). For more proximal bile duct cancers, resection of the bile duct tumor

with adequate margins and a hepaticojejunostomy is the acceptable surgical management. For more proximal hilar bile duct tumors, a concomitant hepatic lobectomy may also be required. Improved techniques of hepatic resection have allowed this aggressive approach. Intrahepaticojejunostomy would be required for reconstruction.

In a recent Mayo Clinic study of 171 patients who underwent operative exploration, only 49 patients (29%) were resectable. The 5-year survival of these patients who underwent a curative resection was 44%, compared with 16% for all patients who underwent a noncurative resection or palliative stenting. The operative mortality was 5%.

15. Which is better, operative or nonoperative palliative stenting?

In patients in whom the overall medical condition is surgically prohibitive or in whom preoperative studies clearly indicate unresectability, then nonoperative palliative stenting is preferable. However, in those patients who undergo exploration but are deemed unrespectable, then operative stenting offers comparable palliation. Regardless of modality, median survival is 12 months.

HEPATIC DISEASES

16. What is the major antecedent cause of pyogenic liver abscesses?

Hepatic abscesses are either of pyogenic or amebic origin. The major causes of pyogenic abscess include ascending biliary infection, portal vein hematogenous spread, hematogenous spread via the hepatic artery, and intraperitoneal direct extension. Ascending biliary infection from calculi or biliary carcinoma is now the major antecedent cause of pyogenic hepatic abscesses. These abscesses usually have mixed isolates, including *Escherichia coli, Staphylococcus, Streptococcus, Proteus, Klebsiella,* and *Bacteroides.*

17. List the common clinical manifestations of pyogenic liver abscesses.

Fever, chills, nausea, vomiting, pain, jaundice, and hepatomegaly. Fever is the most common symptom and is usually of the "picket-fence" configuration. Leukocytosis, anemia, abnormal alkaline phosphatase, positive blood cultures, right hemidiaphragm elevation, and air-fluid levels on ultrasound, liver-spleen scan, or CT all may suggest the diagnosis.

18. How are pyogenic hepatic abscesses best managed?

The mainstay of management is CT- or ultrasound-guided percutaneous catheter drainage in conjunction with intravenous antibiotics. This treatment regiment is effective in 80% of cases. Surgery is reserved for treatment failures, and on rare occasion, when multiple abscesses are confirmed to a lobe, hepatic resection may be indicated.

19. What is the most common complication of amebic abscesses?

Entamoeba histolytica is ubiquitous, and the amebas reach the liver from intestines via the portal venous system. The ensuing **hepatic abscess** is usually single, located in the right lobe, and shows the characteristic anchovy paste on aspiration. Fever and liver pain are the predominant symptoms. The indirect hemagglutination test is almost always positive. The most common complication is **secondary infection.** Less commonly, the abscess may rupture freely into the peritoneal cavity, thoracic cavity, pericardial sac, or adjacent viscus. Metronidazole is the mainstay of therapy, as it attacks both hepatic and intestinal phases of parasite. This may be combined with closed aspiration. Open surgical drainage is reserved for treatment failures or secondary infection.

20. Name the major common benign tumors of the liver.

Cavernous hemangioma, hepatic adenoma, focal nodular hyperplasia, and bile duct adenoma (hamartoma). With the advent of more diagnostic imaging techniques (i.e., CT), there is an increasing awareness of benign liver tumors, the so-called incidentalomas of the liver.

21. When is surgical resection of a cavernous hemangioma indicated?

Cavernous hemangiomas are benign, congenital, vascular hamartomas. They may reach enormous size but generally are <3 cm. Spontaneous rupture, regardless of size, is rare. When cavernous hemangiomas exceed 10 cm, they may produce nonspecific abdominal complaints, such as fullness, early satiety, vague abdominal pain, nausea, and vomiting. Platelet sequestration may occur with the larger hemangioma. Rare presentations include jaundice and gastric outlet obstruction. Contrast CT is the mainstay for diagnosis. Angiography is preferable when considering resection. Thus, surgical resection is only undertaken for **large symptomatic (.10 cm) cavernous hemangiomas.** A preoperative biopsy is usually not required. Surgical intervention may require a formal lobectomy.

22. Which entity is more associated with oral contraceptive use, hepatic adenoma or focal nodular hyperplasia?

Hepatic adenomas are more commonly associated with oral contraceptives. Other associated risk factors for this tumor include pregnancy, diabetes, and adenomatosis syndromes. The major risk of these benign tumors is hemorrhage, and there is a substantially lesser risk of hepatocellular malignant transformation. CT or ultrasound can accurably demonstrate these lesions. In good-risk patients, resection is favored.

Focal nodular hyperplasia occurs in females of reproductive age, but there is no demonstrable correlation with oral contraceptive use. These benign tumors appear to be a reactive injury to an existing spiderlike vascular malformation. Angiography demonstrates a typical sunburst hypervascular pattern. These lesions do not require resection, as hemorrhage or malignant transformation is rare.

23. Spillage or rupture intra-abdominally of this hepatic cyst can result in an anaphylactic reaction. What type of cyst?

Cystic disease of the liver can arise from a wide variety of etiologies, but in clinical practice, one encounters simple cysts, cysts in conjunction with polycystic disease of the liver (usually in females), and **hydatid disease.** Hydatid disease occurs worldwide and is usually caused by the parasite *Echinococcus granulosus.* It has a predilection for the right lobe of the liver in 85% of patients and may cause multiple cysts in as many as 25–33% of patients. Intra-abdominal rupture is heralded by abdominal pain and signs of anaphylactic shock. These cysts may also rupture into the biliary tract, suppurate, or extend into the thoracic cavity.

CT and the indirect agglutination test are the mainstays of diagnosis. Treatment is surgical and consists of sterilization with a scolicidal agent, followed by careful evacuation along the cleavage planes. The residual cavity is managed with omentum. For multiple or larger cysts, hepatic resection may be indicated.

24. What are the major etiologic factors of hepatocellular carcinoma (HCC)?

Of the primary malignant tumors of the liver, hepatocellular carcinoma or its immature variant, hepatoblastoma, is the most common. Implicated etiologic factors include *Aspergillus flavus* aflatoxin, cirrhosis, hemochromatosis, and hepatitis B and C.

25. What are the clinical manifestations of HCC?

Weight loss, weakness, and abdominal pain are the major presenting symptoms of HCC. Because cirrhosis is a frequent companion of HCC, the stigmata of portal hypertension are occasionally seen. Splenic enlargement, ascites, and jaundice are also frequent findings.

26. Which diagnostic laboratory tests are useful in HCC?

Of the liver function tests, alkaline phosphatase is most frequently abnormal. 5-Nucleotidase is usually elevated. Alpha-fetoprotein is a useful tumor marker, but is positive in only 30% of cases of HCC in the United States.

27. What is the major determinant of recurrence after hepatic resection for HCC?

Because cirrhosis underlies most cases of HCC, the state of the hepatic remnant defines postoperative recovery. Intraoperative ultrasound allows the performance of precise, limited, nonanatomic resection. Even in favorable curative resections, the long-term prognosis is bleak. Slightly better survival has been achieved with hepatic transplantation.

28. For which malignancies metastatic to the liver does surgical resection confer a survival benefit?

With the exception of colorectal carcinoid and Wilm's tumor, few patients significantly benefit from the resection of hepatic metastases. There has been widespread enthusiasm for the resection of **colorectal hepatic metastases** in properly selected patients. Prognostic factors include stage of the primary tumor, number of metastases, disease-free interval prior to hepatic resection, size and location of metastases, and age. Fifteen percent of patients with metastatic liver masses will have disease confined to the liver. Of these patients, only 30% will be amenable to hepatic resection. Synchronous lesions (i.e., those present at the time of colon resection) should be managed on a staged basis after appropriate workup. An exception to this would be a small peripheral synchronous lesion amenable to a nonanatomic or segmental resection.

The surgical margin of hepatic resection significantly impacts survival. Patients with a >1-cm surgical margin had a 47% 5-year survival compared with 23% when the margin is <1 cm. A patient over age 70, with stage C disease, and who later develops three or more hepatic metastases is unlikely to benefit from hepatic resection.

Intraoperative ultrasound is a valuable tool in the management of colorectal hepatic metastases. In the author's experience, intraoperative ultrasound influenced the decision to perform a trisegmentectomy as opposed to a right hepatectomy by disclosing a previously unrecognized lesion in the medial segment of the left hepatic lobe. This patient survived an additional 3 years before succumbing to metastatic disease. Secondary resection for colorectal hepatic metastases has been shown to be technically feasible and does confer a survival advantage.

BIBLIOGRAPHY

1. Blumgart, et al: Improvement in survival by aggressive resections of hilar cholangiocarcinoma. Ann Surg 27:20–27, 1993.
2. Cameron JL, et al: Unrespectable hilar cholangiocarcinoma: Percutaneous versus operative palliation. Surgery 115:597–603, 1994.
3. Forteh PG: Diagnosis of cancer by cytologic methods performed during ERCP. Gastrointest Endosc 40:249–252, 1994.
4. Goodnight JE, et al: Hepatic resection of metastases. Surg Gynecol Obstet 170:454–460, 1991.
5. Lilly JR, et al: Congenital biliary tract disease. Surg Clin North Am 70:1403–1418, 1990.
6. Melleham KW, et al: The current role of U tubes for benign and malignant biliary obstruction. Ann Surg 218:621–629, 1993.
7. Nagorney DM, et al: Outcomes after curative resections of cholangiocarcinoma. Arch Surg 128:871–879, 1993.
8. Schwartz S, et al (eds): Principles of Surgery. New York, McGraw Hill, 1994, pp 1326–1340.
9. Siegel JH, Cohen SA: Endoscopic treatment of laparoscopic bile duct injuries. Gastroenterologist 2:5–13, 1994.
10. Vauthey J-N, Blumgart LH: Recent advances in the management of cholangiocarcinomas. Semin Liver Dis 14:109–114, 1994.
11. Willemore KD, Pitt HA, Cameron JL: Postoperative bile duct strictures. Surg Clin North Am 70(6):1355–1379, 1990.
12. Yeo CJ, Pitt HA, Cameron JL: Cholangiocarcinoma. Surg Clin North Am 70(6):1429–1441, 1990.

84. LAPAROSCOPIC SURGERY

Anthony J. LaPorta, MD, and Michael R. Marohn, D.O.

1. What is minimally invasive surgery?

Few developments have changed modern surgery more dramatically and rapidly than laparoscopic cholecystectomy. First performed in 1985 in France, then laparoscopic laser cholecystectomy was introduced to the United States in 1988. The subsequent explosion of efforts to perform conventional surgery through minimal-access incisions has been unprecedented in surgical history.

In addition to laparoscopic surgery, an increasing number of minimal-access surgery, video endoscopic surgery, or minimally invasive surgery procedures utilize alternative routes to the organ of interest, suggesting that the nomenclature *minimally invasive surgery* best describes this emerging group of procedures. Driven by consumer demand to minimize the impact of surgery, along with socioeconomic pressures to decrease hospital stays and return patients to the workplace sooner, surgical innovation and modern technology advances gave birth to the minimally invasive surgery era. The drive to accomplish surgical goals of diagnosis, staging, resection, and reconstruction by approaches with minimal physical, biochemical, and psychological insult has irrevocably changed modern surgery.

2. What are the advantages and disadvantages of *minimally invasive surgery?*

ADVANTAGES	DISADVANTAGES
Better visualization	2-Dimensional representation of a 3-dimensional operative field
Reduced postoperative pain, reduced postoperative stress	Loss of ability to palpate
Improved cosmetic result	Longer operating times; increased operating room costs
Reduced hospital stay, overall reduced hospital costs	Unique problems with specimen handling
Earlier return to normal activity; socioeconomic savings	High-tech, labor intensive, intimidating video-game environment
Minimal disruption of immune system	Need for unique video-endoscopic hand–eye surgery skills

3. How many laparoscopic cholecystectomies are performed annually in the United States?

About 600,000 cholecystectomies are performed annually in the United States.

4. Has demand for cholecystectomy increased with the introduction of the laparoscopic approach?

A retrospective study using insurance company data compared the frequency of cholecystectomy before and after the introduction of laparoscopic cholecystectomy. The frequency of cholecystectomy was 1.35/1000 in 1988, compared with 2.15/1000 in 1992 (59% increase). Savings from decreased hospital costs for laparoscopic cholecystectomies were offset by an increase in demand with an overall net increase in total costs of gallbladder surgery of 11.4%. A statewide review of all acute care hospitals in Maryland found a similar increase in the incidence of cholecystectomy from 1.65/1000 in 1985 to 2.17/1000 in 1992 (32% increase). The introduction of laparoscopic cholecystectomy may have shortened hospital stays and costs, but it has increased demand, overwhelming the cost savings originally envisioned.

5. List the advantages and disadvantages related to the use of carbon dioxide as an insufflation gas over other gases.

CO_2 as an Insufflation Gas

ADVANTAGES	DISADVANTAGES
CO_2 suppresses combustion and therefore is felt to be ideal for operative laparoscopy.	CO_2 is rapidly absorbed and thus can raise arterial PCO_2 and lower pH, with adverse potential metabolic and hemodynamic consequences in susceptible patients.
CO_2 has a high diffusion coefficient, reducing the risk of a serious gas embolism. Up to 100 ml/min of CO_2 can be injected directly into the bloodstream of animals without adverse outcome.	Insufflation of cold CO_2 ($0.3°$ C), especially in high-flow systems or long procedures, can result in a drop in core temperature with resultant hypothermia.
CO_2 is safely absorbed and can be effectively eliminated by the lungs with moderate hyperventilation.	Tension CO_2 pneumothorax, either from occult defects in the diaphragm or in the absence of diaphragmatic injury (typically in subhiatal laparoscopic surgery), has been reported.
CO_2 is inexpensive and readily available.	CO_2 gas embolism can occur, even without direct venous insufflation into mesenteric veins.

6. Are there alternative gases that can be used for laparoscopy?

Room air, oxygen, nitrous oxide, helium, and carbon dioxide have all been used for pneumoperitoneum for laparoscopy, but CO_2 is the most commonly used. Research is ongoing to identify alternative gases for pneumoperitoneum. Helium shows promise; in an experimental animal model of chronic obstructive pulmonary disease, helium insufflation was compared with CO_2, and showed far less arterial CO_2 retention than from an equivalent pneumoperitoneum using CO_2.

7. What are the respiratory and cardiovascular consequences of pneumoperitoneum (planned intra-abdominal hypertension)?

Respiratory effects: Pneumoperitoneum alters respiratory mechanics. Intra-abdominal hypertension results in elevation of the diaphragm, functional residual capacity falls, total lung volume decreases, and ventilation-perfusion inequalities and atelectasis result. Some patients may require increased peak inspiratory pressure to compensate for decreased respiratory compliance. No significant change occurs in arterial oxygenation in healthy patients under pneumoperitoneum, but in patients with cardiopulmonary compromise, arterial oxygen desaturation has been reported, presumably secondary to mechanical pulmonary dysfunction.

Hemodynamic effects: Mean arterial blood pressure (MAP) and systemic peripheral resistance are increased (up to 35% and 160%, respectively) at operative levels of pneumoperitoneum (12–15 mm Hg), considered secondary to sympathetic vasoconstriction from hypercarbia. Cardiac index may decrease 20%. As intra-abdominal pressure increases more than 20 mm Hg, cardiac output falls and abdominal venous compliance decreases, reaching a point at which effective inferior vena cava resistance increases, venous return decreases, and hypotension occurs. Trendelenberg position and higher pneumoperitoneum can combine in the patient with preexisting cardiopulmonary disease to produce potential hemodynamic compromise. Portal venous blood flow is reduced by 70% when intra-abdominal pressure reaches 25 mm Hg. Many workers similarly believe that, though not well documented, there is a decrease in renal blood flow, and therefore glomerular filtration rate, with pneumoperitoneum > 12–15 mm Hg.

In summary, intra-abdominal hypertension > 15 mm Hg can result in significant changes in central hemodynamics and even more pronounced changes in splanchnic circulation.

8. What is recommended as the maximum safe insufflator pressure setting for a CO_2 insufflator?

Based upon the potential adverse cardiopulmonary effects of intra-abdominal hypertension, the maximum recommended insufflation pressure setting is 15 mm Hg.

9. What are current *contraindications* to laparoscopic surgery?

Patient selection criteria for laparoscopy have changed over the past 5–8 years. Fundamental to safe patient selection is the surgeon's skill level at the time of the proposed procedure. More difficult surgeries require advanced skills and may require higher conversion rates. The decision to convert a "closed" procedure to an "open" surgery should never be viewed as surgeon failure but as good judgment for patient safety.

The list of contraindications to laparoscopy is decreasing. Currently, only an uncorrectable coagulopathy is an absolute contraindication. Other conditions requiring special attention include:

Generalized peritonitis

Carcinoma

Inability to tolerate general anesthesia

Morbid obesity

Porcelain gallbladder

Prior abdominal surgery

Intestinal obstruction

Acute and chronic inflammation

Cirrhosis

Minor bleeding disorders

Pacemaker

Pregnancy

Ventriculoperitoneal shunt

Comorbid conditions warrant identification and evaluation in all patients, regardless of surgical approach. The risk of a given procedure is not automatically reduced because it is performed via a minimally invasive route.

10. A thin, 68-year old woman with chronic obstructive pulmonary disease (COPD) from 52 years of smoking undergoes laparoscopic cholecystectomy for acute cholecystitis. Because she has had a previous lower midline abdominal incision, you choose the "open," Hasson technique for initial trocar placement and have no difficulties with access to the peritoneal cavity. You immediately insufflate with a flow rate of 10 l/min to a pneumoperitoneum of 12 mm Hg and then proceed with laparoscopic cholecystectomy. Fifteen minutes into the procedure, the anesthesiologist observes that the patient's end tidal CO_2 ($ETCO_2$) is elevated and he plans to draw an arterial blood gas (ABG). Before he can obtain the ABG, the patient experiences several episodes of ventricular tachycardia and arrests. What is the pathophysiology behind these events?

Insufflated carbon dioxide is directly absorbed through the peritoneum into the capillary bed and bloodstream. Typically, the patient's PCO_2 and $ETCO_2$ increase only slightly, but there are circumstances when the patient's PCO_2 can rise dramatically, causing a significant drop in pH, with the resulting acidemia aggravating any preexisting cardiac condition. Most patients adapt to the absorbed CO_2 by maximizing plasma and intracellular buffering systems, accelerating CO_2 transport and elimination with mild hyperventilation, but some patients have impaired CO_2 clearance mechanisms. Patients who cannot handle an acute change in PCO_2 are those with high metabolic and cellular respiratory rates (e.g., septic patients), those with large ventilatory deadspace (e.g., COPD patients), and those with poor cardiac output (e.g., cardiac failure patients).

During laparoscopy, special care and monitoring should be provided to prevent significant hypercarbia and acidemia. Rapid shifts in intra-abdominal pressure (with attendant pCO_2 absorption gradients) should be avoided, as would follow an initial insufflation at a high flow rate with a resultant sudden large gradient between intra-abdominal CO_2 pressure and PCO_2. Equilibrium between CO_2 pressure in blood and tissues occurs at about 20 minutes. After initial insufflation, arterial PCO_2 steadily rises for about 20 minutes, then plateaus.

This septic patient with preexisting COPD was subjected to rapid CO_2 insufflation which resulted in hypercarbia, peaking 15–20 minutes after rapid insufflation, with consequent acidemia, triggering ventricular irritability and arrest.

11. Is the risk of deep venous thrombosis, and therefore the risk of pulmonary embolus, increased with upper abdominal laparoscopic surgery? Should we use routine thromboembolic prophylaxis?

Intuitively, several factors inherent in laparoscopic upper abdominal surgery would predict that there should be an increased incidence of deep venous thrombosis (DVT), and therefore an increased risk for pulmonary embolus. Use of reverse Trendelenberg and modified lithotomy positions, long operative times, and elevated intra-abdominal pressure all favor decreased venous return with pooling of blood in the lower extremities. Data to date have not demonstrated an increased incidence of pulmonary embolus in large series of laparoscopic cholecystectomies. However, Beebe performed duplex scanning and direct right femoral venous pressure measurements before and after abdominal insufflation and found increased venous pressure and slowed peak blood velocity without change in cross-sectional area after insufflation. Insufflation also eliminated venous pulsatility in 75% of patients. All parameters normalized after desufflation.

Although no studies have documented DVT formation, these findings support the prediction that DVT risk is increased with upper abdominal laparoscopic surgery. Wilson's group subsequently demonstrated that pneumoperitoneum creates resistance to venous return that is effectively counteracted by compression stockings. Routine use of thromboembolic prophylaxis is recommended, either with pneumatic sequential compression stockings or subcutaneous heparin, for laparoscopic general surgery patients.

12. Who introduced electrocautery to the medical community? Why is the alternating cycle (AC) frequency typically used?

The "Bovie" nickname for electrosurgical units in most operating rooms acknowledges the introduction in 1929 of electrocautery by **William Bovie** and **Harvey Cushing.** In most American homes, the alternating current (AC) that powers our appliances and lights alternates at 60 cycles/sec. However, in the operating room or endoscopy suite, the electrosurgical unit alternates between 400,000 and 2,000,000 cycles/sec. This high-frequency electrical current is essential to avoid neuromuscular stimulation. Lower-frequency currents, as the standard 60 cycle AC current, can cause tetany and electrocution.

Electrosurgery units work by producing heat at the cellular level. When the electrosurgical unit is on **cut,** the current is "on" nearly 100% of the time, but at a lower voltage (e.g., 100 V) than during **coagulation** (e.g., 600 V), when the current is "on" in bursts typically 5–10% of the time and "off" 90% of the time. The various blends of cut and coagulation modes combine lower voltages than used with coagulation (but higher than with cut) with varying percentages of time that the current is "on" for optimal effect.

Though the precise mechanisms are not known, the cut mode of electrosurgery generates an uninterrupted current with movement of ions within the cell, vaporizing the cell. The release of vaporized (boiled) cell content from the disrupted cell dissipates the heat, accounting for the lack of damage to surrounding tissue. In the coagulation mode, the higher-voltage but short-duration energy bursts lead to a cellular insult but not vaporization. The drying effect on the cells during the "off" part of the cycle (i.e., cellular desiccation) leaves an area of increased resistance to electron flow, and thus more heat dissipation and progressive insult to deeper tissue layers. This can be explained partially by the formula $p = I^2 R$, where power (p, or relative heat per unit time) is equal to a given current (I) through a certain resistance (R). This subject is more complex than this simple formula, as various body tissues have different levels of conductivity and resistance. This explains why some structures may be affected by electrosurgical energy while other structures are spared injury.

13. Is the incidence of silent gastroesophageal reflux (GER), and therefore possible risk of aspiration pneumonia, increased during laparoscopic surgery?

The combination of Trendelenburg position and pneumoperitoneum was initially presumed to predispose to "silent" GER during laparoscopic surgery. However, continuous esophageal pH monitoring performed during laparoscopic cholecystectomy has demonstrated no increased GER. Halevy studied 14 patients with distal esophageal pH monitoring during laparoscopic cholecystectomy. Only 2 patients suffered a single short episode of reflux (0.1-minute durations with pH 3.3 in one and pH 3.7 in the other). Lind first noted that increased intra-abdominal pressure resulted in an increase in lower esophageal sphincter pressure and a net overall increase in barrier pressure. In addition, Jones et al. found this response to be present during laparoscopy. These studies argue that there is *no* increased danger of GER due to the intra-abdominal hypertension attendant with laparoscopic surgery. Nonetheless, empiric studies on the incidence of clinically significant gastric reflux range from 0.002% to 2.0 for elective laparoscopic surgery cases and up to 20% for emergency laparoscopic surgery cases.

Risk factors for GER during laparoscopy include obesity, pregnancy, diabetes mellitus, gastroparesis, aerophagia, Trendelenberg position, and hiatal hernia. Prophylactic measures to reduce the likelihood of GER during laparoscopy should include administration of a promotility agent (e.g., metoclopramide, 10 mg orally or intravenously), administration of an H_2 blocker (e.g., cimetidine or ranitidine), and decompression of the stomach with an orogastric tube.

14. Morbid obesity, defined as > 100 lbs above ideal body weight, is no longer a contraindication to laparoscopic cholecystectomy, but successful outcomes require special considerations. Describe the technical changes necessary for successful laparoscopic cholecystectomy for the morbidly obese patient.

Safe access and adequate visualization of the porta hepatis structures are the major concerns for safe laparoscopic cholecystectomy in the morbidly obese patient. One important technical consideration addresses selection of the optimal site for the telescope trocar, typically at the umbilicus for the normal-weight patient. For obese patients, particularly with taller patients, shifting the umbilical trocar site 1–5 inches cephalad from the umbilicus allows optimal visualization of the portal structures with a 0° telescope. Visualization from an umbilical port is often obscured by the bowel horizon in the upper abdomen or by the heavy pannus which the insufflation cannot sufficiently elevate.

Some physicians prefer to gain access to the peritoneum in the obese patient using the "closed" Verress needle approach through the umbilicus, and then pass an extra long trocar from the skin level at a previously determined supraumbilical position following insufflation. Preperitoneal insufflation is a common problem in obese patients because, even with mechanical elevation of the interior abdominal wall, the posterior fascia often does *not* become elevated. We favor an "open" Hasson approach at a supraumbilical location.

Another technique to improve visualization of the porta hepatis in morbidly obese patients involves use of a 30° angled telescope; this may obviate the need for a supraumbilical trocar site selection. Care must be taken with placement of lateral trocars to avoid skiving to a preperitoneal position.

Placement of a fifth 5-mm subcostal trocar either medially or laterally may be necessary to facilitate adequate retraction and exposure. Some surgeons employ a 5-mm fan-type retractor to press down the duodenum or transverse colon. Care should be employed, however, with these retractors, particularly if they are positioned "off" camera, to avoid injury from the retractors.

Operative times for laparoscopic cholecystectomy among morbidly obese patients are longer than those for normal-weight patients. No increased conversion rates nor increased complication rates have been reported. Laparoscopic cholecystectomy has become the treatment of choice for the morbidly obese patient with symptomatic cholelithiasis, but special skills and techniques are required.

15. Describe the pathophysiologic features of acute cholecystitis that increase the likelihood of technical difficulties. What techniques are necessary to overcome these features?

The rate of conversion to open cholecystectomy from laparoscopic cholecystectomy for acute cholecystitis is two to four times higher than for chronic cholecystitis (typically reported at 3–5%) among experienced laparoscopic surgeons, even when special techniques are employed. When approaching the patient with acute cholecystitis, the distended, inflamed, thick-walled gallbladder presents the first challenge. Decompression of the distended gallbladder with a special trocar, or even percutaneously (under direct visualization) with a central venous pressure catheter, makes it easier to grasp the gallbladder with laparoscopic grasping forceps. It may be necessary to use traumatic/toothed, grasping forceps, but because these graspers tend to puncture the gallbladder wall, once applied they should be left in place to minimize bile spillage. When there is an area of bile leakage, either from the percutaneous drainage site or a tear from a traumatic grasper in the gallbladder wall, a suture or loop ligature can be used to close a small rent in the gallbladder wall. There remain some acutely inflamed gallbladders that cannot be grasped with conventional graspers, and for these, one solution is use of commercial "screw-like" devices, such as the Reddick screw, that can facilitate retraction of the gallbladder.

Despite the best efforts by experienced surgeons, bile spill is seen in 30–50% of laparoscopic cholecystectomies. Sterile laparoscopic specimen bags are indicated to retrieve lost gallstones, to remove a friable, disrupted gallbladder, or to remove detached, necrotic tissue. Use of closed suction drains should follow the same guidelines employed at open surgery.

Another difficulty performing laparoscopic cholecystectomy for acute cholecystitis relates to securing the cystic duct and cystic artery; the degree of inflammation may make utilization of laparoscopic clip devices inadequate. In these cases, pre-tied loop ligatures can be employed to control the cystic duct or cystic artery.

16. What are the *key principles for safe porta hepatis dissection?*

Keys Strategies for Safe Laparoscopic Cholecystectomy:

1. Dissection from the infundibulum down toward the cystic duct
2. Dissection from lateral to medial
3. Adequate lateral traction to open the triangle of Calot
4. Dissection to develop continuity both laterally and medially from the neck of the gallbladder onto the cystic duct
5. Divide no structure without certainty as to its identity

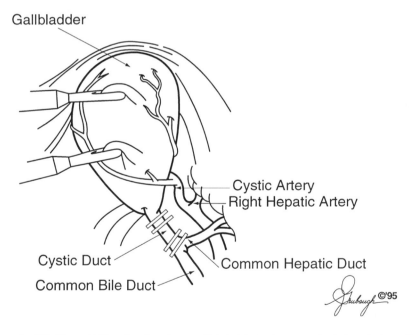

Gallbladder

Cystic Artery
Right Hepatic Artery

Cystic Duct

Common Bile Duct

Common Hepatic Duct

©'95

Diagram of gallbladder and biliary ductal anatomy as distorted during laparoscopic cholecystectomy. (From Zucker KA, Bailey RW, Reddick EJ (eds): Surgical Laparoscopy. St. Louis, MO, Quality Medical Publishing, 1991, p 157; with permission.)

A key potential danger of laparoscopic cholecystectomy is bile duct injury. With acute inflammation, there may be a shortened cystic duct, distorted anatomy, or simply loss of distinctive features in the porta hepatis, making identification of key structures difficult at laparoscopic dissection (see figure below). Accordingly, consideration of routine intraoperative cholangiography is essential to delineate often difficult or distorted anatomy. If biliary ductal anatomy cannot be determined with 100% certainty by either laparoscopic dissection and/or intraoperative cholangiogram, conversion to open, traditional cholecystectomy should be considered for *safety*. Laparoscopic cholecystectomy can be performed safely for acute cholecystitis with an acceptable conversion rate (as low as 8%), shortened hospital stay, and speedy return to work.

17. What is the incidence of bile duct injury during open cholecystectomy versus laparoscopic cholecystectomy? When do most injuries occur?

Major bile duct injuries have been a focus of attention with laparoscopic cholecystectomy because they often represent a devastating surgical injury and because early experience suggested that the incidence is higher with laparoscopic cholecystectomy than with open cholecystectomy. Data from large, contemporary, open cholecystectomy series cite bile duct injury rates ranging from 0.1–0.4%. Bile duct injury rates during laparoscopic cholecystectomy vary widely, but when 90% of published data are pooled, the incidence is about 0.1–0.6%.

Of note, every major study of laparoscopic cholecystectomy has found that **surgeon experience** matters. The U.S. Military review of 99.4% of all laparoscopic cholecystectomies performed worldwide, beginning with case 1 at the introduction of this procedure, found an acceptable rate of bile duct injury of 0.57%, which also included several injuries that occurred *after* conversion to open surgery (this would correct the value to 0.48%). Of interest, 92.5% of the bile duct injuries occurred on or before the 10th case in the surgeon's laparoscopic experience, echoing the finding from the Southern Surgeons Club that *inexperience* is a major variable in bile duct injury rates. In the U.S. Military data, for example, excluding the first 10 cases of a surgeon's experience would reduce the bile duct injury rate from 0.57% to 0.1%. Even though most of the data for laparoscopic cholecystectomy are from the early 1990s, when most surgeons' experience remained limited, data examining bile duct injury rates for open versus laparoscopic cholecystectomy appear comparable.

18. How are bile duct injuries classified?

Reports describing bile duct injuries have often used the Bismuth classification system to describe the type and level of bile duct injury, but this system was originally designed to classify postoperative biliary strictures from open surgery and may not be applicable for laparoscopic bile duct injuries. Wherry and colleagues proposed an alternate classification system that is simple, has prognostic implications, and allows comparison between groups of patients. By their BDICS system, a Class I injury can result from a lateral injury to the common bile duct (CBD) by a surgeon preparing to perform and intraoperative cholangiogram but mistaking the CBD for the cystic duct. Prompt recognition of this Class I bile duct injury (prior to converting it to a Class II with transection) could be managed with simple lateral repair over a T-tube. In contrast, *all* Class III injuries with transection and resection of a portion of the bile duct system, even if discovered at the time of injury, require an enterobiliary anastomosis, with a more morbid long-term outcome than for a Class I injury simple repair.

Bile Duct Injury Classification System (BDICS)

CLASS I	CLASS II	CLASS III
Simple lateral or partial injury to a bile duct	Transection of a bile duct	Both transection and resection of a portion of the bile duct system

From Wherry DC, Rob CG, Marohn MR, et al: An external audit of laparoscopic cholecystectomy performed in medical treatment facilities of the Department of Defense. Ann Surg 220:626–634, 1994; with permission.

19. Should routine or selective intraoperative cholangiography (IOC) be performed during laparoscopic cholecystectomy?

A fundamental principle of safe biliary tract surgery is careful identification of biliary anatomy before any structure is ligated or divided. This objective is best accomplished by careful dissection of the triangle of Calot. But early laparoscopic surgeons, fearing injury to major biliary structures during this dissection, shifted from the traditional focus of open cholecystectomy dissection—identification of the junction of the common hepatic duct with the cystic duct to form the CBD—to an approach employing routine use of IOC to verify the necessary anatomic landmarks. Laparoscopic cholecystectomy dissection strategy has evolved to focus on the gallbladder neck, identifying continuity, laterally *and* medially, with the proximal cystic duct. Controversy regarding the necessity of performing routine IOC continues partly due to the extra time, cost, expertise, and equipment required to accomplish this task; partly due to early lack of focus as to the best dissection strategy at laparoscopic cholecystectomy; and partly due to the fact that this argument was never settled for open cholecystectomy.

Advantages of Routine IOC during Laparoscopic Cholecystectomy

- Verifies identification of ductal anatomy
- Allows recognition of abnormal anatomy (seen in 10% of patients)
- Allows identification of cystic duct and CBD stones (unsuspected choledocholithiasis in 7–12%)
- Allows identification of unintended bile duct injuries, can allow earlier identification of bile duct injuries, and can reduce the severity of bile duct injuries (e.g., prevent conversion from a BDICS Class I to Class II or III bile duct injury)
- Ensures and maintains necessary surgeon proficiency when IOC is essential

Point: Routine IOC is essential for safety during laparoscopic cholecystectomy and provides useful information. Advocates of routine IOC during laparoscopic cholecystectomy argue that it prevents bile duct injury by illuminating difficult or abnormal anatomy, detects CBD stones, ensures a surgeon's cholangiography skills when cholangiogram is absolutely indicated, and helps the surgeon develop skills required for laparoscopic bile duct exploration. **Some 31–47% of surgeons perform routine IOC.**

Review of CBD injury cases finds that cholangiography is *rarely* performed in these cases, favoring that routine IOC could reduce either the frequency or severity of bile duct injuries. Tertiary referral center experience does not suggest that small, lateral duct injuries (BDICS Class I) would be reduced by routine IOC, because duct misidentification occurs before the cholangiogram, but does suggest that IOC can reduce the severity of the injury by allowing identification of confusing or misidentified anatomy *before* bile duct transection (BDICS Class II) or, worse, bile duct transection and resection (BDICS Class III).

Advocates of routine IOC acknowledge the shortcomings of static IOC and recommend **fluoroscopic cholangiography.** Routine IOC identifies unsuspected CBD stones in 7–12% of cases. Most of these stones will pass without clinical sequelae, but some overlooked stones result in ascending cholangitis, gallstone pancreatitis, or biliary obstruction, and it is difficult to predict which stones will pass uneventfully. Accordingly, many surgeons favor efforts to identify all CBD stones at the time of cholecystectomy and leave only small stones (90% of retained stones < 6 mm pass spontaneously) in normal CBDs.

Disadvantages of Routine IOC During Lapararoscopic Cholecystectomy

- Adds time and expense (operating room time, equipment costs, radiologist fees)
- Results in low yield of useful information, either in detecting common bile duct stones (< 2–5% are clinically signficant), abnormal anatomy (< 10%), or unrecognized biliary duct injuries (< 1%)
- Many common bile duct stones are of no clinical significance; those which are can usually (> 90%) be managed without surgery by postop endoscopic retrograde cholangiopancreatography (ERCP)
- May result in ductal injury (improper entry site, catheter or clip trauma, etc.)
- Does not reduce bile duct injuries
- False-positives (as high as 20%) may result in unnecessary and potentially morbid common bile duct exploration (CBDE) or ERCP

Counterpoint: Selective IOC saves resources. In patients without specific indications for cholangiography, laparoscopic cholecystectomy is safe without IOC, with little risk of bile duct injury or retained calculi. A strong case for selective use of IOC during laparoscopic cholecystectomy can be made. **About 52% of surgeons selectively perform IOC.** Experienced surgeons argue that careful dissection is the key to safe laparoscopic cholecystectomy and that routine cholangiography has not been proved to enhance safety. Further, advocates of selective cholangiography note the limitations of technique and technology with cholangiography, its cost, its low yield, and the potential for harm when abnormal findings that may not require intervention induce pursuit. Overlooked CBD stones or biliary misadventures have been reported at < 1% of cases when selective cholangiography is used; other reviewers have placed the incidence of significant *missed* important information with selective cholangiography at closer to 3–5%. The yield from IOC of clinically significant pathology is < 3% in patients in whom there is no history of pancreatitis, normal liver-associated enzyme tests, and a CBD < 5 mm diameter. Because this group represents up to 50% of elective laparoscopic cholecystectomy patients, the argument for selective cholangiogram in this group is strong if the surgeon has clearly identified intraoperative anatomy.

Summary: The Consensus Statement on Gallstones and Laparoscopic Cholecystectomy from the National Institutes of Health emphasized the necessity of clear identification of ductal anatomy prior to excision of the gallbladder, emphasizing that high-quality cholangiography should be available and that cannulation of the cystic duct should be part of the training of all surgeons performing laparoscopic cholecystectomy. This group did not, however, conclude that *routine* IOC was necessary.

20. Are there alternatives to intraoperative cholangiography (IOC)?

1. **Translaparoscopic transcystic choledochoscopy:** Translaparoscopic transcystic choledochoscopy through the cystic duct could replace cholangiography, but this is unlikely. The technology for introducing a choledochoscope the size of a cholangiocatheter through a cystic ductotomy is currently available, and choledochoscopy previously has been shown to be more accurate in avoiding retained stones. Potential difficulties relate to the requirements for additional equipment, cost, and expertise; to the same requirement as cholangiography for dissecting the biliary anatomy before it is defined; and to the problem that even at open surgery, transcystic choledochoscopy can only articulate to examine the proximal common hepatic and intrahepatic radicals 50% of the time. Still, with development of further technology and endoscopic skills, the choledochoscope could supplant the cholangiogram, with its added benefit of therapeutic as well as diagnostic capability.

2. **Translaparoscopic intraoperative ultrasound:** This technique used to detect bile duct stones and delineate biliary anatomy can be performed with greater sensitivity that cholangiography, yet without risking bile duct injury, misidentification of anatomy, contrast reaction, or radiation exposure. As translaparoscopic ultrasound probes evolve, the limiting factor will be less the technology than surgeon inexperience with ultrasound principles. The potential, however, of delineating biliary anatomy before performing potentially damaging dissection, particularly with acute cholecystitis, is enticing.

21. What are the costs related to IOC, retained stones, and bile duct injuries?

Physician fees for laparoscopic cholecystectomy run about $1400 per case, with total costs averaging $5420. IOC adds $500–700. Conversion to open cholecystectomy with cholangiography results in total costs averaging $6680, or an additional cost of about $1260. ERCP with stone extraction and/or sphincterotomy costs $1170 in physician fees, $145 in radiology fees, and $1000 in facility fees, for an average total of $2315. A crude cost analysis finds that costs for laparoscopic cholecystectomy with IOC and conversion to open surgery if needed are less than costs for laparoscopic cholecystectomy with postoperative ERCP. Further, postop ERCP fails in 10% of cases and carries a 10% morbidity and 1% mortality.

Management of a BDICS type II or III bile duct injury costs about $30,000 (not including medicolegal fees). Phillips has argued that avoiding one major complication for every 1000 laparoscopic cholecystectomy cases would pay for all of the unnecessary cholangiograms.

22. What to do with spilled bile and gallstones?

Point: Spilled gallstones are not significant and can be ignored. The spillage of gallstones during laparoscopic cholecystectomy has been reported at rates up to 30–50%, but postsurgical intra-abdominal abscess rates are reported at only 0.1–0.3%. Soper reported a gallbladder perforation (bile spills) rate of 32% among 250 patients undergoing laparoscopic cholecystectomy.

There were no differences in outcomes, specifically, in postoperative infection rates, between the group with bile spills and the group without bile spills. Recognition of the statistical disconnection in outcome data between bile and gallstone spillage and subsequent intra-abdominal abscess formation has prompted many surgeons to conclude that there is no reason to be significantly concerned by the intraoperative spillage of bile and/or gallstones at laparoscopic cholecystectomy.

Counterpoint: Spilled gallstones are a potential source for abscess or fistulization and should be recovered at the initial laparoscopic cholecystectomy. Despite the incongruity between the incidence of gallstones spilled and the number of associated complications, the magnitude, type, and time delay for these complications warrant concern. Experimental work with an animal model found that gallstones left in the peritoneal cavity, in combination with sterile or infected bile, had an increased rate of abscess and adhesion formation, supporting recommendations to attempt recovery of spilled stones in laparoscopic cholecystectomy patients. Major intra-abdominal abscesses, fistulization, and even "cholelithoptysis" are of such significance as to warrant focused effort at recovery for larger or multiple spilled gallstones. Sterile laparoscopic specimen bags and special spoon instruments can facilitate stone retrieval.

23. Should we routinely use prophylactic antibiotics for laparoscopic cholecystectomy?
Because the rate of bile spills during laparoscopic cholecystectomy in most reports runs 30–50%, because basic science data suggest that normal bile is colonized in 30–40%, and because positive bacterial cultures are obtained in acute cholecystitis 60% of the time, most surgeons provide patients with routine rather than selective antibiotic prophylaxis. For routine laparoscopic cholecystectomies, a first-generation cephalosporin should provide adequate prophylaxis for most common organisms, though many surgeons employ a second-generation cephalosporin. A prospective, randomized study to answer this question for laparoscopic cholecystectomy remains to be performed.

24. At 24 hours postoperatively, patients having undergone open upper abdominal surgery utilizing subcostal incisions show a decrease in FVC, FEV-1, and FEV 25%-75% of nearly 50% of normal function. Following laparoscopic cholecystectomy, what decreases would one expect in these pulmonary functions at 24 hours?

Postoperative Pulmonary Function Tests (PFTs): Open versus Laparoscopic Surgery

| | PERCENTAGE OF PREOPERATIVE VALUE | |
MEASURED PFTS AT 24 HRS AFTER SURGERY	OPEN SURGERY	LAPAROSCOPIC SURGERY
Forced vital capacity (FVC)	54%	73%
Forced expiratory volume at 1 sec (FEV-1)	52%	72%
Forced expiratory flow at 25%–75% (FEF 25%–75%)	53%	81%

Pulmonary function measured at 24 hours after laparoscopic cholecystectomy found a decrease in pulmonary function of approximately half of that seen at open surgery. In a related study, age-, gender-, and size-matched patients were prospectively randomized to open versus laparoscopic cholecystectomy, and then pulmonary function tests were measured pre- and postoperatively. FVC and FEV-1 were similarly decreased, but less with laparoscopic than with open surgery. FRC was significantly higher at 72 hours after laparoscopic than after open surgery. After laparoscopic surgery, respiratory function is less impaired and recovery improved compared with open surgery.

25. An 18-year-old woman with a hemoglobinopathy is admitted for elective laparoscopic cholecystectomy. The procedure was performed uneventfully, but following surgery, her umbilical dressing is persistently wet. Collection of this fluid for chemistries demonstrates a creatinine value of 20 mg/dl. A Foley urinary catheter was placed during the procedure, making the surgeon confident that no urinary bladder injury had occurred. What is the diagnosis? What key historical fact could have prevented this complication?
The patient has a persistent congenital anomaly, a vesicoumbilical fistula or persistent urachal sinus/diverticulum, that was injured during trocar placement. The easily obtainable history of chronic or episodic drainage from her umbilicus would have prompted an investigation into the

possibility of a urachal remnant, allowing repair of this problem in conjunction with her laparoscopic cholecystectomy, rather than as a complication repair postoperatively. In general, it is not uncommon for patients to have some trocar site leakage of irrigation fluid for up to 8–12 hours postoperatively, but persistence of fluid drainage beyond 24 hours warrants further evaluation to rule out an occult intra-abdominal injury.

26. What central principle should guide decision-making in minimally invasive surgery?

The surgeon should strive to perform video endoscopic surgery procedures in keeping with established principles and techniques of conventional, open surgery. Minimally invasive surgery is *not* a *new* surgical discipline, but a new way of approaching *old* surgical objectives of diagnosis, staging, resection, or repair. The principles of surgery have *not* changed. The burden for today's surgeon is not only to learn new video endoscopic skills but also to apply them according to established principles of surgery for optimal patient safety and outcome.

BIBLIOGRAPHY

1. Beebe DS, McNevin MP, et al: Evidence of venous stasis after abdominal insufflation for laparoscopic cholecystectomy. Surg Gynecol Obstet 176:443–447, 1993.
2. Brooks DC: Techniques in laparoscopy: Training, credentialing, and socioeconomic considerations. In Brooks DC (ed): Current Techniques in Laparoscopy. Philadelphia, Current Medicine, 1994, pp 1–2.
3. Cho JM, LaPorta AJ, Clark JR, et al: Response of serum cytokines in patients undergoing laparoscopic cholecystectomy. Surg Endosc 8:1380–1384, 1994.
4. Crist DW, Gadacz TR: Complications of laparoscopic surgery. Surg Clin North Am 73(2): 1993.
5. Fitzgerald SD, Andrus CH, Baudendistel DF, et al: Hypercarbia during carbon dioxide pneumoperitoneum. Am J Surg 163:186–190, 1992.
6. Flowers JL, Zucker KA, Bailey RW: Complications. In Ballantyne GH, Leahy PF, Modlin IM (eds): Laparoscopic Surgery. Philadelphia, W.B. Saunders, 1994, p 81.
7. Frazee RC, Roberts JW, Okeson GC, et al: 'Open' versus laparoscopic cholecystectomy: A comparison of postoperative pulmonary functions. Ann Surg 213:651–653, 1991.
8. Jones MJ, Mitchell RW, Hindocha N: Effect of increased intra abdominal pressure during laparoscopy on the lower esophageal sphincter. Anesth Analg 68:63 65, 1989.
9. Joris JL, Noirot DP, Legrand MJ, et al: Hemodynamic changes during laparoscopic cholecystectomy. Anesth Analg 76:1067–1071, 1992.
10. Legorreta AP, Silber JH, et al: Increased cholecystectomy rate after introduction of laparoscopic cholecystectomy. JAMA 270:1429 1432, 1993.
11. McLucas B, March C: Urachal sinus perforation during laparoscopy: A case report. J Reprod Med 35:573–574, 1990.
12. Moosa AR, Easter DW, Van Sonnenberg E, et al: Laparoscopic injuries to the bile duct: A cause for concern. Ann Surg 215:203–208, 1992.
13. Phillips EH: Routine vs. selective cholangiography. Am J Surg 165:505–507, 1993.
14. Rattner DW, Ferguson C, et al: Factors associated with successful laparoscopic cholecystectomy for acute cholecystitis. Ann Surg 217:233–236, 1993.
15. Reddick EJ, Olsen DO, Daniell JF, et al: Laparoscopic laser cholecystectomy. Laser Med Surg News Adv 7:38–40, 1989. [1st US report]
16. Roberts DJ, Goodman NW: Gastro-esophageal reflux during elective laparoscopy. Anesthesia 45:1009–1011, 1990.
17. Schirmer BD, Dix J, Edge SB, et al: Laparoscopic cholecystectomy in the obese patient. Ann Surg 216:146–152, 1992.
18. Stiegmann GV, McIntrye R: Principles of endoscopic and laparoscopic ultrasound. Surg Endosc 7:350–361, 1993.
19. Steiner CA, Bass EB, et al: Surgical rates and operative mortality for 'open' and laparoscopic cholecystectomy in Maryland. N Engl J Med 330:403–408, 1994.
20. Talamini MA, Gadacz TR: Equipment and instrumentation. In Zucker KA, Bailey RW, Reddick EJ (eds): Surgical Laparoscopy Update. St. Louis, Quality Medical Publishing, 1993, p 14.
21. Trokel MJ, Bessler M, Treat MR, et al: Preservation of immune response after laparoscopy. Surg Endosc 8:1385–1388, 1994.
22. Wherry DC, Rob CG, Marohn MR, et al: An external audit of laparoscopic cholecystectomy performed in medical treatment facilities of the Department of Defense. Ann Surg 220:626–634, 1994.
23. Voyles CR, Tucker RD: Education and engineering solutions for potential problems with monopolar electrosurgery at laparoscopy. Am J Surg 164:57–62, 1992.

INDEX

Page numbers in **boldface type** indicate complete chapters.